W0227972

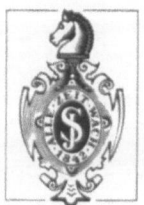

Bone Scanning in Clinical Practice

Edited by Ignac Fogelman

With 217 Figures

Springer-Verlag
London Berlin Heidelberg New York
Paris Tokyo

Ignac Fogelman BSc, MD, MRCP
Consultant Physician,
Department of Nuclear Medicine,
Guy's Hospital,
St. Thomas Street,
London SE1 9RT.

ISBN-13: 978-1-4471-1409-3   e-ISBN-13: 978-1-4471-1407-9
DOI: 10.1007/978-1-4471-1407-9

Library of Congress Cataloging-in-Publication Data
Bone scanning in clinical practice.
Includes bibliographies and index.
1. Bones—Diseases—Diagnosis.   2. Radioisotope scanning.   I. Fogelman, Ignac, 1948–   .   [DNLM: 1. Bone and
Bones—radionuclide imaging.   2. Tomography, Emission Computed. WE 225 B7128] RC930.5.B65   1986
616.7'107575 86–13824

BAS Printers Limited, Over Wallop, Hampshire

2128/3916/543210

This book is dedicated to
Coral, Gayle and Richard

Preface

The most frequently requested investigation in any nuclear medicine department remains the technetium-99m (^{99m}Tc)-labelled diphosphonate bone scan. Despite rapid advances in all imaging modalities, there has been no serious challenge to the role of bone scanning in the evaluation of the skeleton. The main reason for this is the exquisite sensitivity of the bone scan for lesion detection, combined with clear visualisation of the whole skeleton. In recent years several new diphosphonate agents have become available with claims for superior imaging of the skeleton. Essentially, they all have higher affinity for bone, thus allowing the normal skeleton to be visualised all the more clearly. However, as will be discussed, this may occur at some cost to the principal role of bone scanning, lesion detection.

The major strength of nuclear medicine is its ability to provide functional and physiological information. With bone scanning this leads to high sensitivity for focal disease if there has been any disturbance of skeletal metabolism. However, in many other clinical situations, and particularly in metabolic bone disease, more generalised alteration in skeletal turnover may occur, and quantitation of diphosphonate uptake by the skeleton can provide valuable clinical information.

The use of single photon emission tomography (SPECT) for imaging the skeleton is increasingly being shown to be of value in problematic cases where results from planar images may be equivocal. Measurement of bone mineral content by single and dual photon absorptiometry is currently of considerable interest as physicians and the public alike become more aware of the major health issues relating to osteoporosis. These are some of the newer aspects of the use of radioisotopes in the investigation of bone disease which have been included in the present text.

In *Bone Scanning in Clinical Practice* a group of experts from the UK and North America have joined forces to bring together their experience with "bone scanning". Topics covered, in addition to the aforementioned, include the history of bone scanning, mechanisms of uptake of diphosphonate in bone, the normal bone scan, and the role of bone scanning in clinical practice. The aim of this book is to provide a source of reference relating to bone scan imaging for all those who are interested in the skeleton. While I believe the information presented will be of value to those in nuclear medicine, I hope that others in fields such as endocrinology, rheumatology, orthopaedics and oncology will find much of relevance to their clinical practice.

London, 1986   Ignac Fogelman

Contents

7   The Bone Scan in Metabolic Bone Disease

8   The Bone Scan in Paget's Disease

9   The Role of Bone Scanning, Gallium and Indium Imaging in Infection

10   The Bone Scan in Traumatic and Sports Injuries

11   The Bone Scan in Arthritis

12   The Bone Scan in Avascular Necrosis

Contributors

B. D. Collier MD
Director, Nuclear Medicine, Medical College of Wisconsin, Milwaukee, Wisconsin, USA.

I. Fogelman BSc, MD, MRCP
Consultant Physician, Department of Nuclear Medicine, Guy's Hospital, London, England.

M. D. Francis BA, MA, PhD
Senior Scientist, Norwich Eaton Pharmaceuticals, A Procter and Gamble Company, Norwich, New York, USA.

I. Gordon FRCR
Senior Lecturer in Diagnostic Radiology, Institute of Child Health, and Consultant Radiologist, Department of Paediatric Radiology, Hospital for Sick Children, London, England.

H. W. Gray MD, FRCP
Consultant Physician, University Department of Medicine, Royal Infirmary, Glasgow, Scotland.

P. Matin MD, FACNP
Associate Clinical Professor, University of California, Davis, and Chairman, Department of Nuclear Medicine, Roseville Community Hospital, Roseville, California, USA.

I. R. McDougall MB, ChB, PhD, FRCP, FACP
Professor of Radiology and Medicine, Division of Nuclear Medicine, Stanford University School of Medicine, Stanford, California, USA.

J. H. McKillop MB ChB, PhD, MRCP
Senior Lecturer and Consultant Physician, University Department of Medicine, Royal Infirmary, Glasgow, Scotland.

M. V. Merrick MSc, MRCP, FRCR
Consultant in Nuclear Medicine and Senior Lecturer in Medicine and Radiology, Western
General Hospital, Edinburgh, Scotland.

K. Mido MD
Resident in Nuclear Medicine, Division of Nuclear Medicine, Stanford University School of
Medicine, Stanford, California, USA.

D. A. Navarro MD
Resident in Nuclear Medicine, Division of Nuclear Medicine, Stanford University School of
Medicine, Stanford, California, USA.

A. M. Peters BSc, MD, MRCPath
Honorary Consultant Radiologist, Department of Paediatric Radiology, Hospital for Sick
Children, and Department of Diagnostic Radiology, Royal Postgraduate Medical School,
London, England.

L. Rosenthall MD
Professor of Radiology, McGill University, and Director, Division of Nuclear Medicine, The
Montreal General Hospital, Montreal, Quebec, Canada.

G. M. Segall MD
Resident in Nuclear Medicine, Division of Nuclear Medicine, Stanford University School of
Medicine, Stanford, California, USA.

M. L. Smith BSc, MB ChB, MRCP
Senior Registrar in Nuclear Medicine, Department of Nuclear Medicine, Addenbrooke's
Hospital, Cambridge, England.

H. W. Wahner MD, MS
Professor of Laboratory Medicine, Mayo Medical School, and Consultant in Nuclear
Medicine, Mayo Clinic, Rochester, Minnesota, USA.

Introduction

I. Fogelman

It is generally accepted that the bone scan is more sensitive than radiography in detecting skeletal disease; however, it is important to be aware that each of these investigations assesses different parameters in relation to bone. X-ray absorption reflects bone mineral content and shows the net result of bone destruction and repair. The bone scan, however, is a study of function depending upon osteoblastic activity and, to a lesser extent, skeletal vascularity for uptake of tracer (Davis and Jones 1976). In the context of disease the scan indicates the dynamic response of bone to whatever insult is present, be it traumatic, inflammatory or neoplastic.

If involvement of the skeleton by malignancy is chosen as a specific example of disease, then when tumour cells invade bone they produce two basic effects: bone destruction, usually mediated via osteoclasts, and an osteoblastic reaction, which represents attempts by the surrounding bone to repair the destructive effects (Milch and Changus 1956). Radiographs demonstrate both processes; bone destruction is seen as radiolucencies (osteolytic areas) and bone repair as radiodensities (osteosclerotic areas). Bone destruction, however, must be advanced before an abnormality is seen on the radiograph, and it has been suggested that a lesion in trabecular bone must be greater than 1–1.5 cm in diameter, with loss of approximately 50% of bone mineral before radiolucencies will be apparent on a conventional radiograph (Edelstyn et al. 1967). Early in bone repair, insufficient mineral has been laid down to be visualised radiographically as radiodensities. For these reasons the radiograph is normal during the early phase of tumour involvement, and several studies have confirmed that histologically proven metastases may not be detected by radiography (Borak 1942; Shackman and Harrison 1948). The bone scan is based on an entirely different principle. Tracer uptake is not directly dependent on bone destruction, but reflects the functional reaction of the bone to tumour invasion. There is an increase in new bone formation with increased skeletal blood flow following tumour invasion and this is demonstrated by high uptake of a bone-seeking radiopharmaceutical. It is important to note that the increased concentration of tracer is not due to or directly dependent on the metabolism of the tumour cells themselves, but is directly related to the local changes in bone metabolism consequent upon tumour invasion.

Thus, early in bone invasion by tumour, a positive bone scan may be associated with normal radiography. As the tumour progresses, the bone destruction it causes will become visible on the radiograph as an osteolytic lesion. In these circumstances bone reaction is considerable, and the bone scan result is also strongly positive. If the tumour does not progress, calcium will be laid down during the healing process in such quantities that sclerotic areas will be visible on the radiograph. At this stage the results of both investigations are positive. Eventually, if the lesion heals completely, there will be extensive calcification producing a dense appearance on the radiograph. At this stage the bone scan may appear normal.

As the bone scan depends on the metabolic reaction of the bone, it is clear that if there is little or no bone reaction to tumour invasion, the scan may be normal or near normal despite radiographic evidence of bone destruction. This occurs infrequently but may be found in some cases of myeloma (Leonard et al. 1981) and, rarely, with rapidly growing anaplastic carcinoma or, conversely, in cases of indolent tumours such as thyroid cancer (Charkes 1970). If bone destruction is extensive (Goergen et al. 1974), or if bone metabolism is modified by radiotherapy (Cox 1974), a "cold" area may be seen, corresponding to the area of diminished bone activity.

Similarly, in the metabolic bone disorders considerable alteration in bone calcium may occur without detectable change on the radiograph. If there is net balance between bone formation and bone resorption, albeit if both are increased, then these changes may theoretically never be revealed by radiography (De Nardo 1966). Radioactive tracer techniques may circumvent these difficulties since they depend only upon increased bone turnover regardless of the net calcium balance. It is clear, however, that the techniques of skeletal radiography and scintigraphy are in many instances complementary, and maximum diagnostic information can often be obtained by performing both studies.

References

Borak J (1942) Relationship between the clinical and roentgenological findings in bone metastases. Surg Gynecol Obstet 75: 599–604

Charkes ND (1970) Bone scanning: principles, technique and interpretation. Radiol Clin North Am 8: 259–270

Cox PH (1974) Abnormalities in skeletal uptake of ^{99m}Tc polyphosphate complexes in areas of bone associated with tissues which have been subjected to radiation therapy. Br J Radiol 47: 851–856

Davis AG, Jones AG (1976) Comparison of ^{99m}Tc-labeled phosphate and phosphonate agents for skeletal imaging. Semin Nucl Med 6: 19–31

De Nardo GL, Volpe JA, Captain MC (1966) Detection of bone lesions with the strontium-85 scintiscan. J Nucl Med 7: 219–236

Edelstyn GA, Gillespie PJ, Grebell FS (1967) The radiological demonstration of osseous metastases: experimental observations. Clin Radiol 18: 158–162

Georgen T, Halpern S, Alazraki N, Heath V, Taketa R, Ashburn W (1974) The "photon defficient" area: a new concept in bone scanning. J Nucl Med 15: 495 (abstract)

Leonard RCF, Owen JP, Proctor SJ, Hamilton PJ (1981) Multiple myeloma: radiology or bone scanning? Clin Radiol 32: 291–295

Milch RA, Changus GW (1956) Response of bone to tumour invasion. Cancer 9: 340–351

Shackman R, Harrison CV (1948) Occult bone metastases. Br J Surg 35: 385–389

1 · The Bone Scan—Historical Aspects

I. Fogelman

Introduction

The earliest indication that radionuclides could accumulate in the skeleton originated from observations in painters of luminous watch dials who developed bone necrosis, osteomyelitis and bone tumours following chronic exposure to radium (Blum 1924; Hoffman 1924). It was initially thought that this radionuclide was taken up by reticuloendothelial cells, until autoradiography of human post-mortem material revealed that the bone itself was radioactive (Martland 1926). Nevertheless, it was widely believed that bone was metabolically inactive until Chiewitz and Hevesy (1935) demonstrated incorporation of ^{32}P phosphate into the skeleton of adult rats.

Although we now know that the skeleton is composed of living tissue and is metabolically active, many deficiencies remain in our understanding of the aetiology and pathophysiology of bone disease. However, with the development of the current bone-seeking radiopharmaceuticals—the technetium -99m (^{99m}Tc)-labelled diphosphonates—agents became available that were extremely sensitive for the detection of alterations in skeletal metabolism and the identification of disease.

While the bone scan is currently accepted as a powerful investigational tool in the evaluation of patients with both benign and malignant skeletal disease, it is worth reflecting that it is only a mattter of some 10 years since the introduction of the "new" radiopharmaceuticals which made clear visualisation of the skeleton possible. The bone scan as we recognise it today results from the development of ^{99m}Tc-labelled polyphosphate by Subramanian in 1971 (Subramanian and McAfee 1971). That report is the foundation on which the subsequent development of ^{99m}Tc-labelled bone-seeking agents is based. The excellent physical characteristics of ^{99m}Tc are well documented (Harper et al. 1965; McAfee and Subramanian 1975). The short physical half-life of 6.02 h is ideal for many studies. The monoenergetic gamma emission of 140 keV is easily collimated and the absence of biologically hazardous beta decay reduces the absorbed dose of radiation. Thus the introduction of a bone-scanning agent which could be labelled with ^{99m}Tc was clearly a major advance; indeed, ideal physical properties combined with relatively low cost and easy availability make ^{99m}Tc the radionuclide of choice in radioisotope imaging procedures for nearly every major organ system in man (Harper et al. 1965). In addition to the introduction of ^{99m}Tc-labelled bone-scanning agents there was continuing development of nuclear medicine imaging devices with improvement in their resolution (Anger 1964; Cooke and Kaplan 1972). These factors combined to allow clear visualisation of the skeleton and to produce the bone scan that we are familar with today.

Bone Scanning With Strontium-85 and Fluorine-18

The history of bone scanning commences some 10 years earlier than Subramanian's important publication, and the first report of skeletal imaging with a radionuclide was from Fleming et al. (1961) using strontium-85 ([85]Sr). They found that [85]Sr localised at areas of increased osteoblastic activity, and the scan could be used as an index of bone repair; they concluded that scanning of bone lesions was practical and informative. However, the increasing use of bone scanning in clinical practice throughout the 1960s was greatly influenced by the efforts of Drs. Sklaroff and Charkes. In many articles (Charkes and Sklaroff 1964; Charkes et al. 1964; Sklaroff and Charkes 1964; Charkes et al. 1966; Sklaroff and Charkes 1968; Charkes et al. 1968) they demonstrated that bone scan imaging had a primary role to play in the detection of skeletal metastases. Their extensive experience was supported by a series of reports from De Nardo and colleagues (De Nardo 1966; De Nardo et al. 1966; De Nardo 1968; De Nardo et al. 1972) confirming the practicality and usefulness of bone imaging. The cumulative experience with [85]Sr showed clearly that bone scanning consistently detected lesions months before radiographs of the skeleton became abnormal. Thus by 1970 the bone scan had already become a clinically acceptable procedure, but radiostrontium—initially [85]Sr and later [87m]Sr (Charkes 1969)—the most practical bone agent available, was far from ideal (Fig. 1.1). The low gamma yield, gut excretion of tracer which could interfere with lesion visualisation, limitation of use to patients with malignant disease because of high radiation dose, and prolonged delay from injection to imaging led to increasing dissatisfaction with [85]Sr. It is of interest today that a bone scan with [85]Sr could only be obtained after a delay of some 24–48 h following injection to allow excretion of non-skeletal tracer via bowel and urinary tract (Sklaroff and Charkes 1964), and a single view of pelvis could take 30–45 min to obtain (De Nardo 1966). On the other hand, [87m]Sr had a short physical half-life (2.8 h) and larger activities could be injected, making it possible to obtain scans of high count density with relatively short patient scanning times (Volpe 1971). However, the main disadvantage of [87m]Sr was the slow blood clearance of tracer. High background activities in blood and soft tissues resulted in low target background ratios and thus relatively poor visualisation of normal and pathological bone until many hours after injection (Weber et al. 1969). The

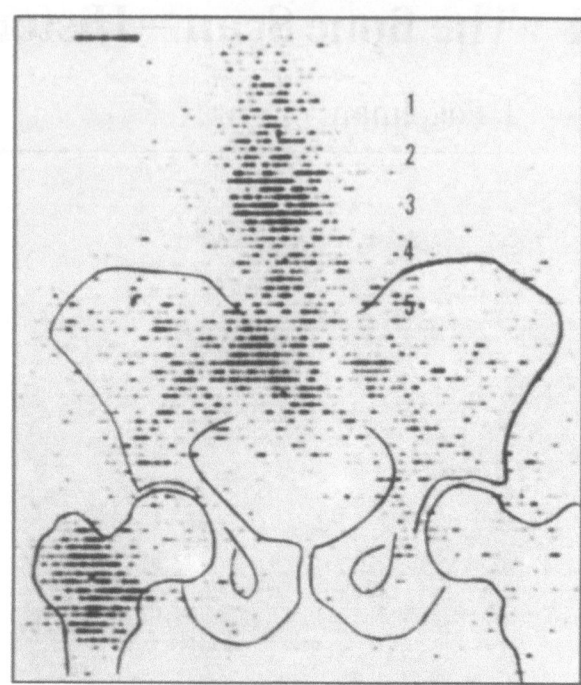

Fig. 1.1 [85]Sr scan of anterior pelvis (with overlay to define outline of pelvis) with metastases present in pelvis, spine and femora. (From Sklaroff and Charkes 1964. Reproduced by courtesy of Dr. N. D. Charkes and with permission from the *Journal of the American Medical Association*. Copyright 1964, American Medical Association)

short physical half-life of [87m]Sr, however, precluded waiting until background levels were low, when optimum target/background ratios would be obtained. It was reported that the high blood and extracellular fluid activities of [87m]Sr could lead to erroneous false-positive diagnoses (Charkes 1969).

Some of the disadvantages of imaging with the strontium isotopes had already been overcome with the introduction of fluorine-18 (^{18}F) by Blau and associates (Blau et al. 1962). With more favourable radiation dosimetry and faster blood clearance, it was possible to administer larger activities resulting in greater count density and faster scanning speeds. Visualisation of the entire skeleton thus became practical with ^{18}F; it quickly replaced the strontium isotopes as the scanning agent of choice and extensive experience was accumulated with its use (Blau et al. 1962; French and McCready 1967; Blau et al. 1972; Sharma and Quinn 1972; Fordham and Ramachandran 1974; Shirazi et al. 1974). However ^{18}F required cyclotron production and was expensive; these disadvantages, combined with its short physical half-life, (1.83 h), created insoluble problems regarding widespread distribution of this radionuclide. Thus only relatively few centres could use ^{18}F, which precluded general acceptance of this reliable and effective radionuclide.

The search for a satisfactory bone scan compound continued. Many alternative nuclides and radiopharmaceuticals were considered. These included gallium-68 (^{68}Ga; Hayes et al. 1965; Edwards et al. 1966) and ^{99m}Tc pertechnetate (Tow and Wagner 1967). Because of the chemical similarity to calcium, several nuclides of the alkaline earth element barium (Ba) were evaluated. Both ^{131}Ba and ^{135m}Ba were found to have excellent physical characteristics and rapid blood clearance (Lange et al. 1970; Spencer et al. 1970; Subramanian 1970). Another promising group of agents were chelates of the rare earth elements (the lanthanides) (O'Mara et al. 1969). Of these compunds the N-hydroxyethylene diamine triacetic acid (HEDTA) chelate of dysprosium-157 (^{157}Dy) appeared to have the most suitable properties (Subramanian et al. 1971; Yano et al. 1971).

While some initial excitement was generated by the agents described above, their roles as bone-scanning agents in clinical practice were completely supplanted by the introduction of ^{99m}Tc polyphosphate by Subramanian and McAfee (1971).

Introduction of ^{99m}Tc Phosphate

Animal studies using polyphosphate labelled with phosphorus-32 (^{32}P) were first carried out by Fels and co-workers in 1959 (Fels et al. 1959). They demonstrated that the accumulation of tracer in bone relative to soft tissue was greater for polyphosphate than orthophosphate. There were major therapeutic implications from this work regarding the possibility of delivering higher amounts of ^{32}P selectively to sites of bone metastases; indeed, subsequent studies (Kaplan et al. 1960) on human subjects with carcinoma of the prostate verified increased localisation of polyphosphate ^{32}P in bone in proportion to the severity of malignant disease. If polyphosphate with increased skeletal affinity had applications in the realm of therapy, could it not also be of use in the diagnosis of disease?

Several years earlier Neuman and Neuman (1953) had described localisation of anionic metal complexes in bone. As ^{99m}Tc readily forms anionic complexes, it was considered feasible to obtain selective osseous localisation of this radionuclide (Subramanian and McAfee 1971). The polyphosphates, also known as condensed phosphates, are compounds which possess chains of –P–O–P– units

joined together. Their ability to prevent deposition of calcium carbonate from solution is well known (Fleisch and Russell 1970), and it was predicted that polyphosphates would have strong affinity for hydroxyapatite crystals in the mineral phase of bone, in particular for sites of new bone formation. Such affinity had been previously demonstrated in autoradiographic studies using ^{32}P-labelled polyphosphate (Fels et al. 1959). Techniques were already available for reducing ^{99m}Tc pertechnetate with stannous chloride (Eckelman and Richards 1970) which made it possible to label phosphate compounds with ^{99m}Tc.

This was the background to that initial publication from Subramanian and McAfee (1971). A compound with high skeletal affinity was combined with a radionuclide with near-perfect physical properties, thus introducing ^{99m}Tc-labelled phosphate bone-scanning agents (Fig. 1.2) to clinical practice (Subramanian et al. 1972a). While the first bone scans may have had rather high body background activity, the skeleton was nevertheless clearly discernible.

Following the initial development and introduction of ^{99m}Tc polyphosphate, attention turned to other phosphates which might be suitable bone-scanning agents. ^{99m}Tc pyrophosphate (Fig. 1.2) appeared promising. Pyrophosphate is believed to be important in regulating the calcification process in bone, although its precise role in calcium metabolism and in disorders of bones and teeth is not well defined (Fleisch and Russell 1970, 1972). When labelled with ^{99m}Tc, pyrophosphate provided improved bone to background activity ratios, and satisfactory scans were obtained in experimental animal and early patient studies (Perez et al. 1972; Fletcher et al. 1973; Hosain et al. 1973; Huberty et al. 1974). Bone scanning was now rapidly becoming established in clinical practice as scans looked like bone surveys—an advantage Sklaroff and Charkes did not have with ^{85}Sr and ^{87m}Sr.

Shortly after the introduction of ^{99m}Tc polyphosphate and ^{99m}Tc pyrophosphate, yet another group of bone-scanning agents, the diphosphonates (Fig. 1.2), became available. The development of the diphosphonates stemmed from the search for a therapeutic agent in bone disease which combined the biological properties of pyrophosphate and polyphosphate, together with resistance to enzymatic destruction in vivo (Fleisch et al. 1969; Francis et al. 1969). While the possibility of using both polyphosphate and pyrophosphate as therapeutic agents had been considered (Russell and Smith 1973), their rapid destruction by tissue phosphatases made this impossible. During the late 1960s, however, a diphosphonate (hydroxy-

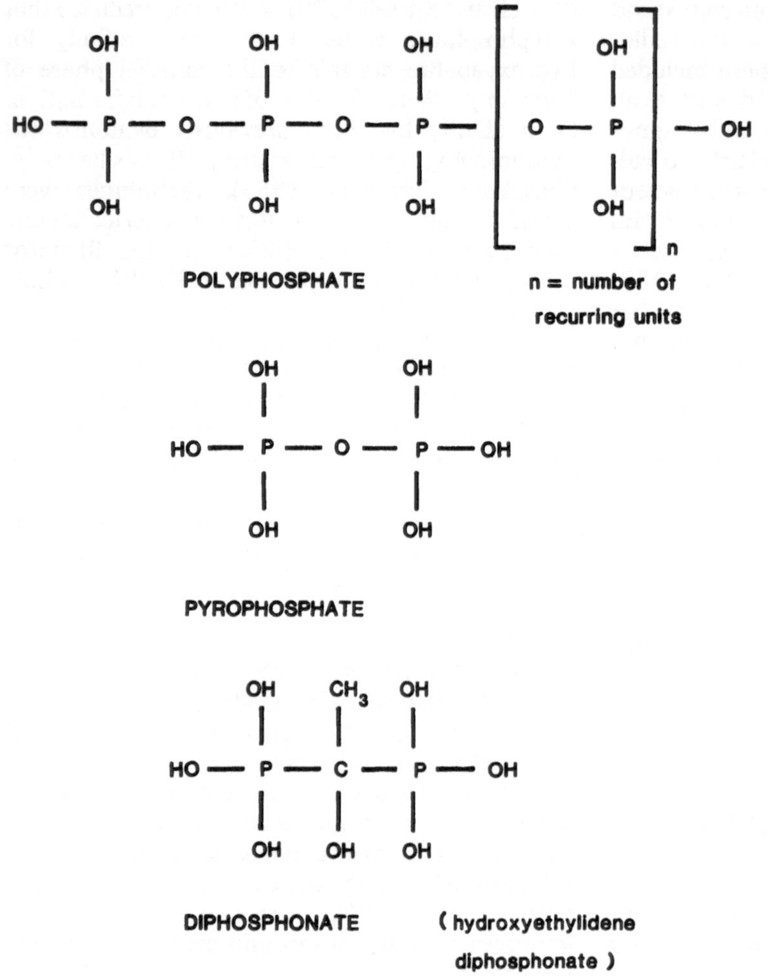

POLYPHOSPHATE

n = number of
recurring units

PYROPHOSPHATE

DIPHOSPHONATE   (hydroxyethylidene

diphosphonate)

Fig. 1.2 Chemical structure of
polyphosphate, pyrophosphate and
diphosphonate.

ethylidene diphosphonate) was shown to be of value in the treatment of myositis ossificans (Bassett et al. 1969) and was soon after evaluated in Paget's disease (Smith et al. 1971). Today, diphosphonates are a standard therapy for Paget's disease (Russell et al. 1974; Khairi et al. 1977), and many other potential clinical applications have been suggested (Russell and Smith 1973). ^{99m}Tc-labelled diphosphonate (hydroxyethylidene diphosphonate) as a bone-scanning agent was independently proposed and evaluated by several groups of workers (Castronovo and Callahan 1972; Tofe and Francis 1972; Subramanian et al. 1972b; Yano et al. 1973), and evidence was obtained that diphosphonate provided improved scans when compared with either ^{99m}Tc pyrophosphate (Citrin et al. 1975; Fogelman et al. 1977) or [18]F (Silberstein et al. 1973). Within a year a major clinical study from Pendergrass et al. (1973) using ^{99m}Tc diphos-

phonate summarised their experience with 500 bone scans. It had taken Sklaroff and Charkes almost 8 years to obtain similar numbers of patient studies using [85]Sr (Charkes et al. 1968).

Thus, within a short period of time, three new, good bone-scanning agents had become available (^{99m}Tc polyphosphate, pyrophosphate and diphosphonate). Since then, cumulative experience has shown that the diphosphonates are the bone-scanning agents of choice (Dunson et al. 1973; Krishnamurthy et al. 1974; Serafini et al. 1974) with superior detection of lesions in metastatic disease (Citrin et al. 1975; Fogelman et al. 1977; Silberstein et al. 1978). While other agents such as ^{99m}Tc monofluorophosphate (Citrin et al. 1974), ^{99m}Tc sodium trimetaphosphate (Nelson et al. 1975) and ^{99m}Tc imidodiphosphate (Subramanian et al. 1975a) have since been evaluated, none has presented a serious challenge to ^{99m}Tc hydroxyethylidene diphosphonate. However, Subramanian and colleagues in 1975 introduced a new diphosphonate, methylene diphosphonate (Subramanian et al. 1975b). This compound had more rapid blood clearance than hydroxyethylidene diphosphonate and higher skeletal affinity. It is currently the most widely used bone-scanning agent. Nevertheless, the search for a better scanning agent has by no means stopped, and at present two further diphosphonate compounds (hydroxymethylene diphosphonate and dicarboxypropane diphosphonate) are available. While these agents appear to have higher absolute bone uptake than methylene diphosphonate, they have not yet been shown to have any clinical advantage.

References

Anger HO (1964) Scintillation cameras with multichannel collimators. J Nucl Med 5: 515–531

Bassett CAL, Donath A, Macagno F, Preisig R, Fleisch H, Francis MD (1969) Diphosphonates in the treatment of myositis ossificans. Lancet II: 845 (letter)

Blau M, Nagler W, Bender MA (1962) Fluorine-18: a new isotope for bone scanning. J Nucl Med 3: 332–334

Blau M, Ganatra R, Bender MA (1972) ^{18}F-Fluoride for bone imaging. Semin Nucl Med 2: 31–37

Blum T (1924) Osteomyelitis of the mandible and maxilla. J Am Dent Assoc 11: 802–805

Castronovo FP, Callahan RJ (1972) New bone scanning agent: ^{99m}Tc-labeled 1-hydroxy-ethylidene-1, 1-disodium phosphonate. J Nucl Med 13: 823–827

Charkes ND (1969) Some differences between bone scans made with ^{87m}Sr and ^{85}Sr. J Nucl Med 10: 491–494

Charkes ND, Sklaroff DM (1964) Early diagnosis of metastatic bone cancer by photoscanning with strontium-85. J Nucl Med 5: 168–179

Charkes ND, Sklaroff DM, Bierly J (1964) Detection of metastatic cancer to bone by scintiscanning with strontium 87m. Am J Roentgenol Radium Ther Nucl Med 91: 1121–1127

Charkes ND, Sklaroff DM, Young I (1966) A critical analysis of strontium bone scanning for detection of metastatic cancer. Am J Roentgenol Radium Ther Nucl Med 96: 647–656

Charkes ND, Young I, Sklaroff DM (1968) The pathologic basis of the strontium bone scan. JAMA 206: 2482–2488

Chiewitz O, Hevesy G (1935) Radioactive indicators in the study of phosphorus metabolism in rats. Nature 136: 754–755 (letter)

Citrin DL, Bessent RG, Greig WR (1974) Clinical evaluation of ^{99m}Tc-labelled monofluoro-phosphate: a comparison with ethane-hydroxy diphosphonate. J Nucl Med 15: 1110–1112

Citrin DL, Bessent RG, Tuohy JB, Elms ST, McGinley E, Greig WR, Blumgart LH (1975) A comparison of phosphate bone-scanning agents in normal subjects and patients with malignant disease. Br J Radiol 48: 118–121

Cooke MBD, Kaplan E (1972) Whole-body imaging and count profiling with a modified Anger camera. 1. Principles and application. J Nucl Med 13: 899–907

De Nardo GL (1966) The ^{85}Sr scintiscan in bone disease. Ann Intern Med 65: 44–53

De Nardo GL (1968) Clinical application of bone scintiscans. Clin Med 75: 22–32

De Nardo GL, Volpe JA, Captain MC (1966) Detection of bone lesions with the strontium-85 scintiscan. J Nucl Med 7: 219–236

De Nardo GL, Jacobson SJ, Raventos A (1972) ^{85}Sr bone scan in neoplastic disease. Semin Nucl Med 2: 18–30

Dunson GL, Stevenson JS, Cole CM, Mellor MK, Hosain F (1973) Preparation and comparison of technitium-99m diphosphonate, polyphosphate and pyrophosphate in nuclear bone imaging radiopharmaceuticals. Drug Intell Clin Pharmacol 7: 470–474

Eckelman W, Richards P (1970) Instant ^{99m}Tc-DTPA. J Nucl Med 11: 761

Edwards CL, Hayes R, Ahumada J, Kniseley RM (1966) Gallium-68 citrate: a clinically useful skeletal scanning agent. J Nucl Med 7: 363–364

Fels IG, Kaplan E, Greco J, Veatch R (1959) Incorporation in vivo of P^{32} from condensed phosphates. Proc Soc Exp Biol Med 100: 53–55

Fleisch H, Russell RGG (1970) Pyrophosphate and polyphosphate. In: Rasmussen H (ed) International encyclopedia of pharmacology and therapeutics. Section 51, vol 1. Pergamon, Oxford, pp 61–100

Fleisch H, Russell RGG (1972) A review of the physiological and pharmacological effects of pyrophosphate and diphosphonates on bones and teeth. J Dent Res 51 (suppl): 324–332

Fleisch H, Russell RGG, Francis MD (1969) Diphosphonates inhibit hydroxyapatite dissolution in vitro and bone resorption in tissue culture and in vivo. Science 165: 1262–1264

Fleming WH, McIlraith JD, King ER (1961) Photoscanning of bone lesions utilising strontium-85. Radiology 77: 635–636

Fletcher JW, Solaric-George E, Henry RE, Donati RM (1973) Evaluation of ^{99m}Tc-pyrophosphate as a bone imaging agent. Radiology 109: 467–469

Fogelman I, McKillop JH, Citrin DL (1977) A clinical comparison of ^{99m}Tc-hydroxyethylidene diphosphonate (HEDP) and ^{99m}Tc-pyrophosphate in the detection of bone metastases. Clin Nucl Med 2: 364–367

Fordham EW, Ramachandran PC (1974) Radionuclide imaging of osseous trauma. Semin Nucl Med 4: 411–429

Francis MD, Russell RGG, Fleisch H (1969) Diphosphonates inhibit formation of calcium phosphate cyrstals in vitro and pathological calcification in vivo. Science 165: 1264–1266

French RJ, McCready VR (1967) The use of ^{18}F for bone scanning. Br J Radiol 40: 655–661

Harper PV, Lathrop KA, Jiminez F, Fink R, Gottschalk A (1965) Technetium 99m as a scanning agent. Radiology 85: 101–109

Hayes RL, Carlton JE, Byrd BL (1965) Bone scanning with gallium-68: a carrier effect. J Nucl Med 6: 605–609

Hoffman FL (1924) Radium (Mesothorium) necrosis. JAMA 85: 961–965

Hosain F, Hosain P, Wagner HN, Dunson GL, Stevenson JS (1973) Comparison of ^{18}F, ^{87m}Sr and ^{99m}Tc-labelled polyphosphonate, diphosphonate, and pyrophosphate for bone scanning. J Nucl Med 14: 410

Huberty JP, Hattner RS, Powell MR (1974) A ^{99m}Tc-pyrophosphate kit: a convenient, economical, and high quality skeletal-imaging agent. J Nucl Med 15: 124–126

Kaplan E, Fels IG, Kotlowski BR, Greco J, Walsh WS (1960) Therapy of carcinoma of the prostate metastatic to bone with P^{32} labelled condensed phosphate. J Nucl Med 1: 1–13

Khairi MRA, Altman RD, De Rosa GP, Zimmermann J, Shenk RK, Johnston CC (1977) Sodium etidronate in the treatment of Paget's disease of bone. A study of long-term results. Ann Intern Med 87: 656–663

Krishnamurthy GT, Tubis M, Endow JS, Singhi V, Walsh CF,

Blahd WH (1974) Clinical comparison of the kinetics of ^{99m}Tc-labelled polyphosphate and diphosphonate. J Nucl Med 15: 848–855

Lange RC, Treves S, Spencer RP (1970) ^{135}Ba and ^{131}Ba as bone scanning agents. J Nucl Med 11: 340–341 (abstract)

McAfee JG, Subramanian G (1975) Radioactive agents for imaging. In: Freeman LM, Johnston PM (eds) Clinical scintillation imaging. Grune and Stratton, New York, pp 55–59

Martland HS (1926) Microscopic changes of certain anemias due to radioactivity. Arch Pathol Lab Med 2: 465–472

Nelson MF, Melton RE, Van Wazer JR (1975) Sodium trimetaphosphate as a bone-imaging agent. 1. Animal studies. J Nucl Med 16: 1043–1048

Neuman WF, Neuman MW (1953) The nature of the mineral phase of bone. Chem Rev 53: 1–45

O'Mara RE, McAfee JG, Subramanian G (1969) Rare earth nuclides as potential agents for skeletal imaging. J Nucl Med 10: 49–51

Pendergrass HP, Potsaid MS, Castronovo FP (1973) The clinical use of ^{99m}Tc-diphosphonate (HEDSPA). Radiology 107: 557–562

Perez R, Cohen Y, Henry R, Panneciere C (1972) A new radiopharmaceutical for ^{99m}Tc bone scanning. J Nucl Med 13: 788–789 (abstract)

Russell RGG, Smith R (1973) Diphosphonates—experimental and clinical aspects. J Bone Joint Surg [Br] 55: 66–86

Russell RGG, Smith R, Preston C, Walton RJ, Woods CG (1974) Diphosphonates in Paget's disease. Lancet I: 894–898

Serafini AN, Watson DD, Nelson JP, Smoak WM (1974) Bone scintigraphy—comparison of ^{99m}Tc-polyphosphonate and ^{99m}Tc-diphosphonate. J Nucl Med 15: 1101–1104

Sharma SM, Quinn JL (1972) Sensitivity of ^{18}F bone scans in the search for metastases. Surg Gynecol Obstet 135: 536–540

Shirazi PH, Rayudu GVS, Fordham EW (1974) ^{18}F bone scanning: review of indications and results of 1500 scans. Radiology 112: 361–368

Silberstein EB, Saenger EL, Tofe AJ, Alexander GW, Pack H-M (1973) Imaging of bone metastases with ^{99m}Tc–Sn–EHDP (diphosphonate), ^{18}F, and skeletal radiography. A comparison of sensitivity. Radiology 107: 551–555

Silberstein EB, Maxon HR, Alexander GW, Rauf C, Bahr GK (1978) Clinical comparison of technetium-99m diphosphonate and pyrophosphate in bone scintigraphy: concise communication. J Nucl Med 19: 161–163

Sklaroff DM, Charkes ND (1964) Diagnosis of bone metastases by photoscanning with strontium 85. JAMA 188: 1–4

Sklaroff DM, Charkes ND (1968) Bone metastases from breast cancer at the time of radical mastectomy. Surg Gynecol Obstet 127: 763–768

Smith R, Russell RGG, Bishop M (1971) Diphosphonates and Paget's disease of bone. Lancet I: 945–947

Spencer RP, Lange RC, Treves S (1970) ^{131}Ba: an intermediate-lived radionuclide for bone scanning. J Nucl Med 11: 95–96

Subramanian G (1970) ^{135m}Ba: preliminary evaluation of a new radionuclide for skeletal imaging. J Nucl Med 11: 650–651

Subramanian G, McAfee JG (1971) A new complex of ^{99m}Tc for skeletal imaging. Radiology 99: 192–196

Subramanian G, McAfee JG, Blair RJ, O'Mara RE, Greene MW, Lebowitz E (1971) ^{157}Dy-HEDTA for skeletal imaging. J Nucl Med 12: 558–561

Subramanian G, McAfee JG, Bell EG, Blair RJ, O'Mara RE, Ralston PH (1972a) ^{99m}Tc-labeled polyphosphonate as a skeletal imaging agent. Radiology 102: 701–704

Subramanian G, McAfee JG, Blair RJ, Mehter A, Connor T (1972b) ^{99m}Tc-EHDP: a potential radiopharmaceutical for skeletal imaging. J Nucl Med 13: 947–950

Subramanian G, McAfee JG, Blair RJ, Rosenstreich M, Coco M, Duxbury CE (1975a) Technetium-99m-labeled stannous imidodiphosphate, a new radiodiagnostic agent for bone scanning: comparison with other ^{99m}Tc complexes. J Nucl Med 16: 1137–1143

Subramanian G, McAfee JG, Blair RJ, Kallfelz FA, Thomas FD (1975b) Technetium-99m-methylene diphosphonate—a superior agent for skeletal imaging: comparison with other technetium complexes. J Nucl Med 16: 744–755

Tofe AJ, Francis MD (1972) In vitro optimization and organ distribution studies in animals with the bone scanning agent ^{99m}Tc-Sn-EHDP. J Nucl Med 13: 472 (abstract)

Tow DE, Wagner HN (1967) Scanning for tumors of brain and bone. JAMA 199: 610–614

Volpe JA, (1971) The radioisotope skeletal survey. J Surg Oncol 3: 43–51

Weber DA, Greenberg EJ, Dimich A, Kenny PJ, Rothschild EO, Myers WPL, Laughlin JS (1969) Kinetics of radionuclides used for bone studies. J Nucl Med 10: 8–17

Yano Y, Van Dyke DC, Verdon TA, Anger HO (1971) Cyclotron-produced ^{157}Dy compared with ^{18}F for bone scanning using the whole body scanner and scintillation counter. J Nucl Med 12: 815–821

Yano Y, McRae J, Van Dyke DC, Anger HO (1973) Technetium-99m-labeled stannous ethane-1-hydroxy-1 1-diphosphonate: a new bone scanning agent. J Nucl Med 14: 73–78

2 · ^{99m}Tc Diphosphonate Uptake Mechanism on Bone

M. D. Francis and I. Fogelman

Introduction

Bone scanning or scintigraphy is directed towards identifying sites of altered skeletal metabolism and abnormal foci of calcium phosphate deposition, such as heterotopic ossification and soft tissue calcification. The requirements of an ideal bone-scanning agent are excellent imaging properties of the nuclide, high concentration of the nuclide at the abnormal site, little or no extraosseous or non-calcification site uptake, minimum tissue radiation, simple and safe preparation of the agent and ready availability of the nuclide. No scanning agent has all these ideal characteristics but the ^{99m}Tc diphosphonates come closest to satisfying the above criteria. ^{99m}Tc is easily obtained from a molybdenum-99/technetium-99m generator. The scheme, abundances, half-lives and energies are shown in Fig. 2.1.

Reduction of ^{99m}Tc O_4^-

When ^{99m}Tc(VII)O_4^- is eluted from a generator for bone scanning, it must be reduced to a lower oxidation state ^{99m}Tc(III, IV or V) for effective complexing with ligands which will direct the nuclide to bone (Russell et al. 1978; Steigman et al. 1978; Wilson and Pinkerton 1985). Diphosphonates and pyrophosphate are the most commonly used ligands for bone scanning. Stannous tin (SnII) is generally used for reducing the ^{99m}TcO$_4^-$ in commercial bone-scanning kits (Srivastava et al. 1977), but reduction and complexing can also be achieved chemically by other agents (Fritzberg et al. 1977; Deutsch et al. 1980), electrolytically by amperometric titration (Russell 1977) or by polarography (Grassi et al. 1979). The similarity in biological uptake of ^{99m}Tc reduced by three separate methods and complexed with a diphosphonate is shown in Fig. 2.2. There

Fig. 2.1. The decay scheme of molybdenum-99 into technetium-99m and finally into technetium-99. The half-life of each nuclide is shown in parenthesis in hours (h) or years (y). The abundance of the energy forms are shown in percentages, and the various gamma radiation energies of molybdenum and technetium are given in tabular form on the *right* in keV.

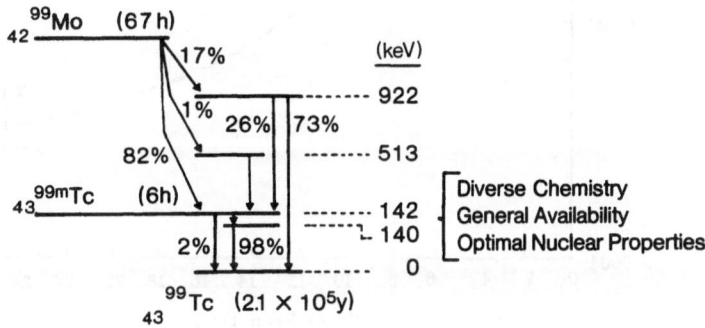

is essentially no difference in biodistribution of ^{99m}Tc in either soft or hard tissue among the three differently reduced complexes.

The difference in uptake and clearance from bone of the Sn(II) reduced ^{99m}Tc hydroxyethylidene diphosphonate (^{99m}Tc-HEDP) complex and unreduced ^{99m}TcO$_4^-$ is shown in Fig. 2.3. The unreduced ^{99m}TcO$_4^-$ has little or no retention on bone while the reduced diphosphonate complex ^{99m}Tc-HEDP has approximately 1000 times more retained dose (Francis et al. 1976).

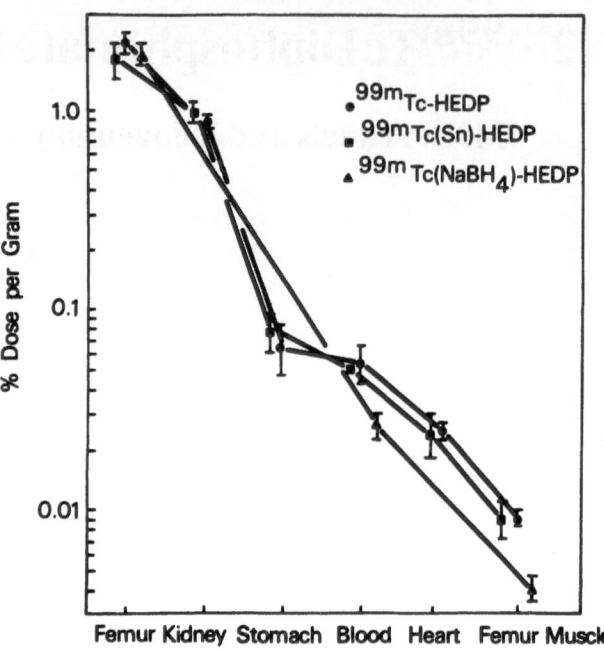

Fig. 2.2. Comparative biodistributions of ^{99m}Tc in Sprague Dawley rats. The ^{99m}TcO$_4^-$ was reduced by three different chemical methods, HBr, NaBH$_4$ or SnCl$_2$, and complexed with hydroxyethylidene diphosphonate (*HEDP*). (Deutsch et al. 1980)

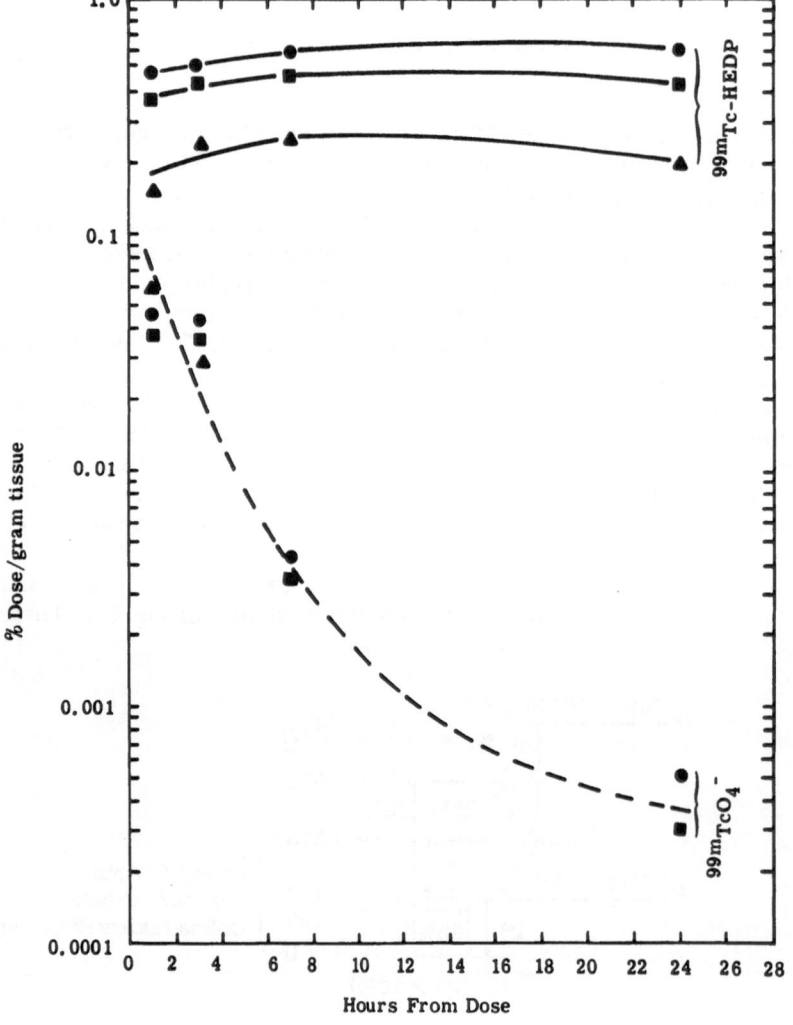

Fig. 2.3. The uptake and rate of clearance of intravenous ^{99m}Tc in the reduced complex (^{99m}Tc-HEDP) form or unreduced pertechnetate (^{99m}TcO$_4^-$) form from rabbit bones. (●, iliac crest; ■, femur metaphysics; ▲, femur diaphysis.) (Francis et al. 1976)

Calcium Content of Tissues

The uptake and retention of the reduced ^{99m}Tc diphosphonate complex in all tissues (soft and hard) seems to be, in general, a function of the calcium content of the tissue (Silberstein et al. 1975). This is shown in Fig. 2.4 where it can be seen that as the tissue calcium content rises from very low values in such soft tissues as muscle (0.005% Ca) and thyroid (0.03% Ca) to hard tissue where calcium is very high (14%–24% Ca), the percentage of ^{99m}Tc retained at 3 h after dose in rats rises from 0.005% dose/g to about 0.7% dose/g respectively (Silberstein et al. 1975). Furthermore, in hard tissue the metabolic activity of the bone and surface bone area available to the extracellular fluid and vascular flow also strongly influence the uptake and retention of ^{99m}Tc diphosphonate, as can be seen from the insert in Fig. 2.4. The metabolically active and vascular metaphysis region (14.3% Ca), which is rapidly turning over, has a retention of ^{99m}Tc of 0·77%

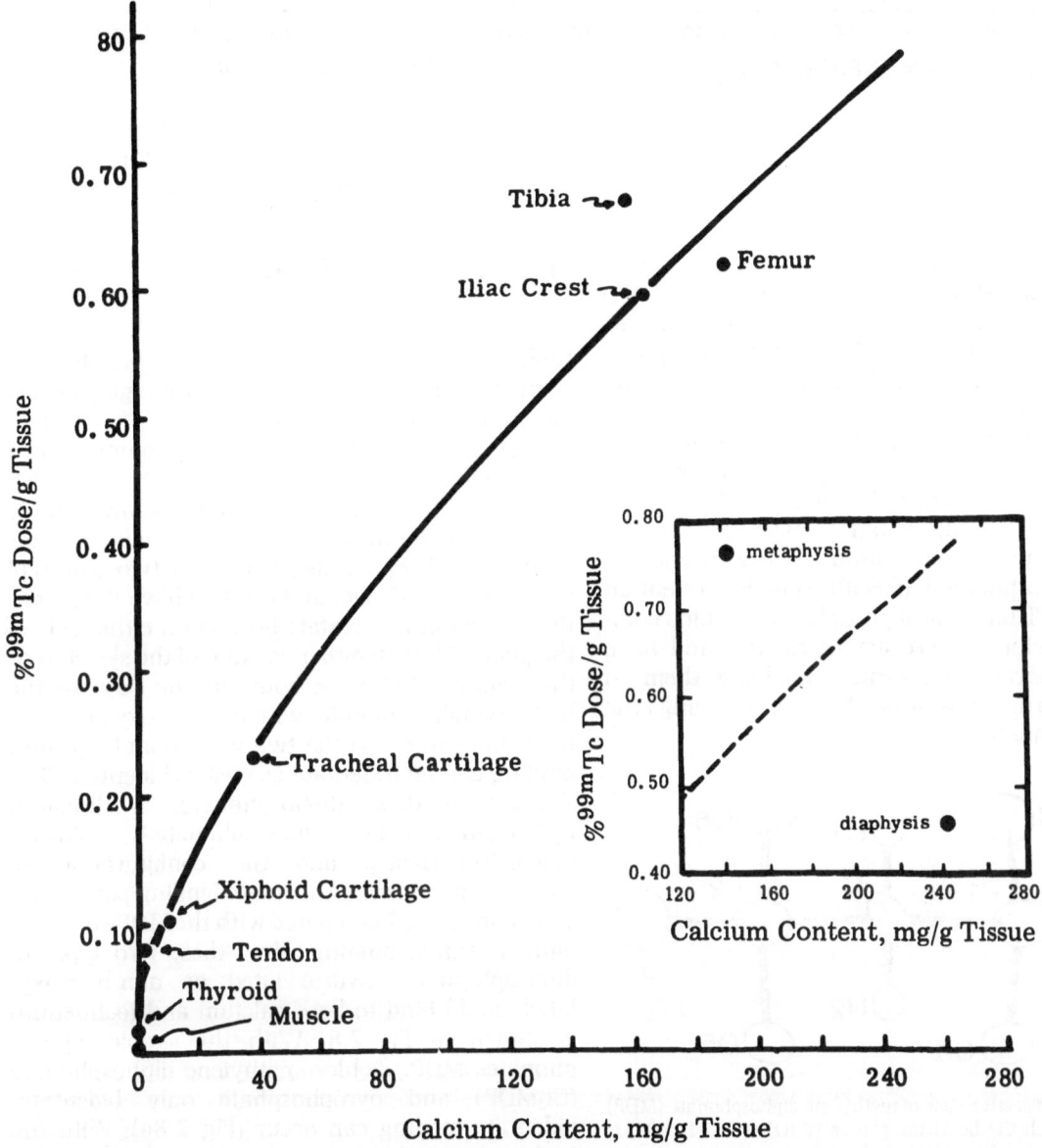

Fig. 2.4. Tissue retention of bone-scanning agent ^{99m}Tc diphosphonate at 3 h after administration in the adult rat as a function of calcium content of various tissues. The *dashed line* in the *insert* is a segment of the *solid line* in the main graph. The uptake and retention of ^{99m}Tc in the metaphysis and the diaphysis regions of the femur in the *insert* are plotted in relation to the overall tissue uptake curve. (Adapted from Silbertstein et al. 1975)

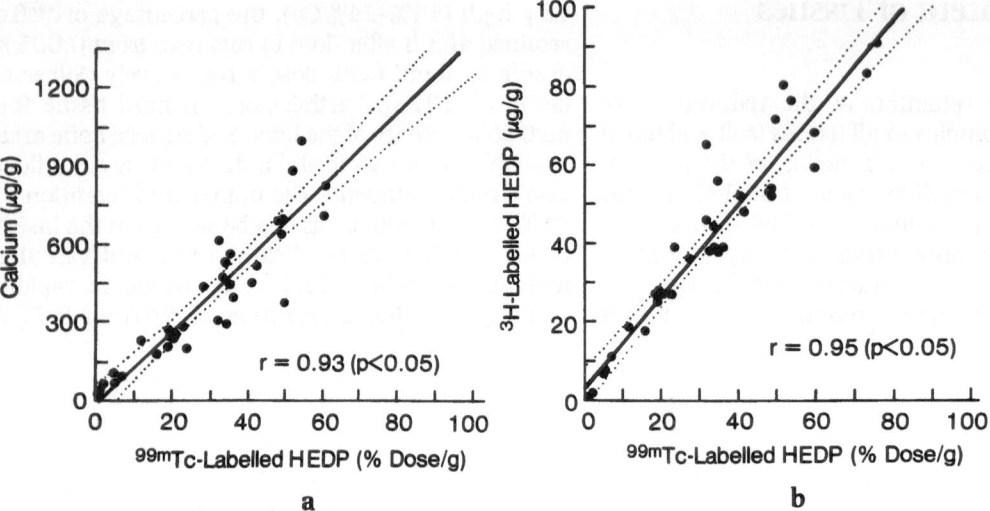

Fig. 2.5a, b. Correlation plots between calcium content of myocardial infarct tissue and 99mTc-HEDP (hydroxyethylidene diphosphonate) retention (**a**) and between retention of 3H-HEDP and 99mTc-HEDP in myocardial infarct tissue (**b**). (After Buja et al. 1977)

dose/g, while the less active and less vascular diaphysis with a higher calcium content (23.9% Ca) has a retention of only 0·46% dose/g at 3 h in rats (Silberstein et al. 1975). This metabolic phenomenon is readily seen on bone scan images of long bones from children.

The correlation ($r = 0.93$) between calcium and dose retention of 99mTc diphosphonate is also true in the infarcted heart, as shown in Fig. 2.5a. There is also a very high correlation ($r = 0.95$) between the pure diphosphonate retention (3H-HEDP) and the 99mTc diphosphonate (HEDP) complex retention (Fig. 2.5b). That is, the diphosphonates which complex the reduced 99mTc act as carriers and have residual coordination centres enabling them to adsorb onto tissue calcium while still "carrying" the nuclide technetium.

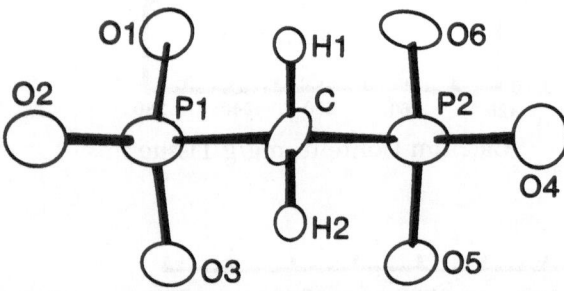

Fig. 2.6. A perspective view of methylene diphosphonate (MDP) ligand in which the backbone planar W (O2–P1–C–P2–O4) is perpendicular to the plane of the paper and the potential unprotonated coordinating oxygens O1, O6 and O3, O5 extend out on either side of the W plane. (Reprinted with permission from Deutsch and Barnett 1980. Copyright 1980 American Chemical Society).

Diphosphonate Structure

Diphosphonate ligands are the most widely used compounds to prepare 99mTc skeletal imaging agents in conjunction with reduction of the 99mTc(VII)O$_4^-$ ion. The simplest of all the diphosphonates is disodium methylene diphosphonate (MDP), $CH_2(PO_3HNa)_2$. The structure of this ligand is shown simply in Fig. 2.6 without the hydrogen and sodium atoms on the two phosphonate groups. The two groups of two oxygens (O1, O6, and O3, O5) have the potential to bind in a bidentate fashion on either side of the planar W with either calcium of the skeleton or the reduced 99mTc, or both. In the case of the hydroxydiphosphonates with the hydroxy group on the same carbon as the two phosphonate groups, binding can be tridentate as well as bidentate. The simplest of these diphosphonates is disodium hydroxymethylene diphosphonate (HMDP), $CH(OH)(PO_3HNa)_2$, and the configuration of oxygens engendering tridentate binding potential is shown in Fig. 2.7 compared with the MDP structure with bidentate binding. How these two types of diphosphonates, hydroxylated or non-hydroxylated, could bind to both calcium and technetium is shown in Fig. 2.8. With the simple diphosphonates MDP, dichloromethylene diphosphonate (Cl$_2$MDP) and pyrophosphate only bidentate-bidentate binding can occur (Fig. 2.8a). With the hydroxylated diphosphonates, however, possible modes of binding with technetium and hydroxyapatite are bidentate-tridentate and the inverse, shown also in Fig. 2.8b, c. Substituents (R$_1$, R$_2$), however, on the central carbon atom, $C(R_1)(R_2)(PO_3HNa)_2$ can markedly alter the binding to technetium and calcium as is manifest in Cl_2MDP, where R_1, and R_2 are chlorine groups. It is well recognised that Cl_2MDP makes a very poor bone-scanning agent. Even though bidentate-bidentate binding is feasible with Cl_2MDP the complex with technetium is very unstable. Hydroxylated diphosphonates like HMDP and HEDP most probably bind at the bone surface through the tridentate ligation since this configuration (Fig. 2.8b) completes the trigonal antiprismatic coordination of calcium at the OO1 face of hydroxyapatite (the most rapidly growing face of the crystal). This structural configuration is shown in Fig. 2.9.

Diphosphonate Chain Length

The effect of chain length of simple diphosphonates on the retention of ^{99m}Tc in bone-scanning complexes has been investigated by Benedict and Van Duzee (1982). The series of n-alkyl-1, 1-diphosphonates (carbon chain lengths of 1, 2, 5 and 9) and 1-hydroxy-n-alkyl-1, 1-diphosphonates (carbon chain lengths 1, 2, 4, 6 and 9) were synthesised (Benedict and Van Duzee 1982) and made into bone-scanning complexes with $^{99m}TcO_4^-$ and stannous chloride ($SnCl_2$). Rat biodistribution studies were conducted (Benedict and Van Duzee 1982)

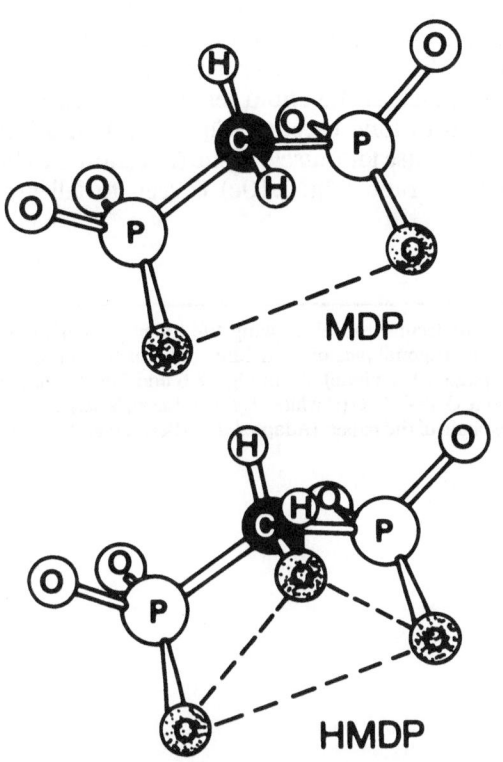

Fig. 2.7. Structures of methylene diphosphonate (*MDP*) and hydroxymethylene diphosphonate (*HMDP*) are shown with the coordinating oxygens (unprotonated) on one side of the planar W (see Fig. 2.6) *stippled* to show bidentate (*MDP*) and tridentate (*HMDP*) binding potential for calcium or reduced ^{99m}Tc (see Fig. 2.8). (After Bevan et al. 1979)

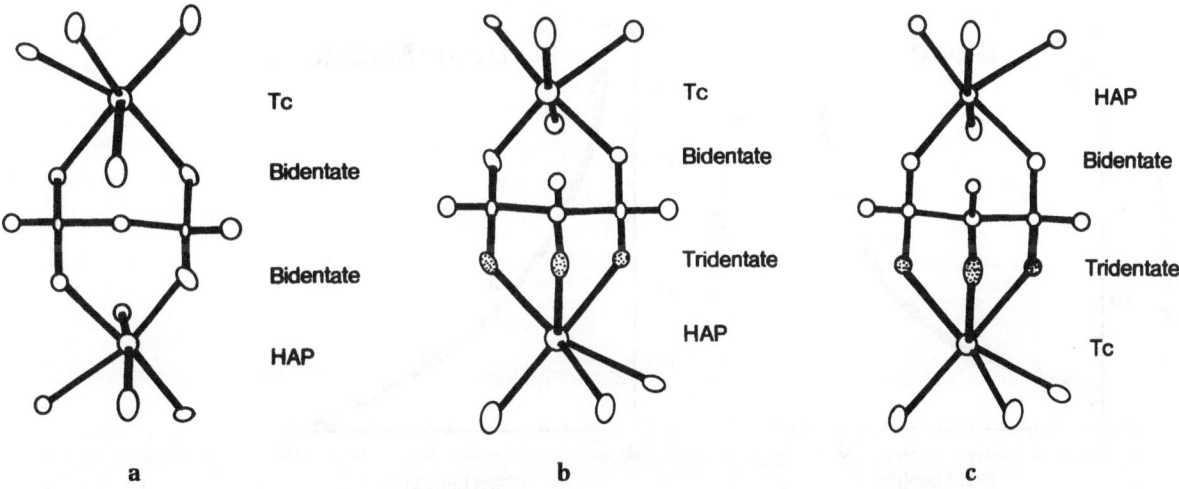

Fig. 2.8. Structures of diphosphonates are shown bonding to reduced technetium (*Tc*) and to hydroxyapatite (*HAP*) in a bidentate-bidentate bridge, as would occur in methylene diphosphonate (a). Diphosphonate is shown binding in a tridentate configuration (*stippled*) with HAP and bidentate with Tc (b). Tridentate binding with Tc and bidentate with HAP is also shown (c). In each case the planar W backbone O–P–C–P–O (see Fig. 2.6), is perpendicular to the plane of the paper with the bidentate or tridentate binding mode on either side of the W as would occur in hydroxymethylene diphosphonate. (Adapted from Deutsch and Barnett 1980)

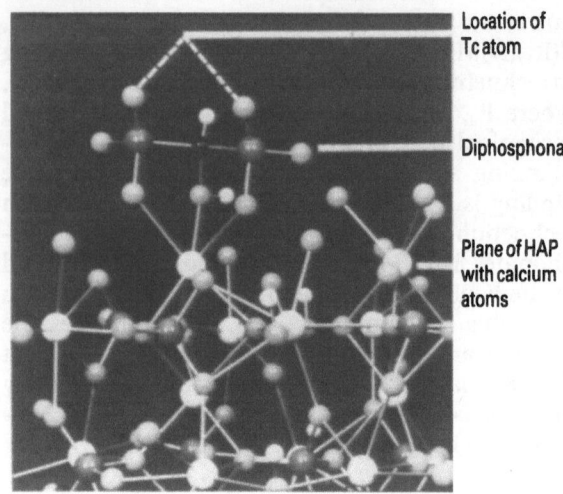

and these are shown in Fig. 2.10a–c. In bone there was very little difference in the uptake of ⁹⁹ᵐTc from the different chain lengths studied (Fig. 2.10a). The retention in blood (lack of clearance), however, rose over 100 times as the chain length changed from one carbon to nine carbons (Fig. 2.10b), and this was also the case for muscle tissue (not shown). The bone/muscle ratio (Fig. 2.10c) is seen to fall pre-

Fig. 2.9. A molecular model showing the tridentate binding of HMDP to the trigonal face of a calcium centre at the surface of hydroxyapatite (001 plane). As in Figs. 2.6 and 2.8 the planar W backbone O–P–C–P–O (O *white*, P *gray*, C *black*), is perpendicular to the plane of the paper. (Adapted from Deutsch and Barnett 1980)

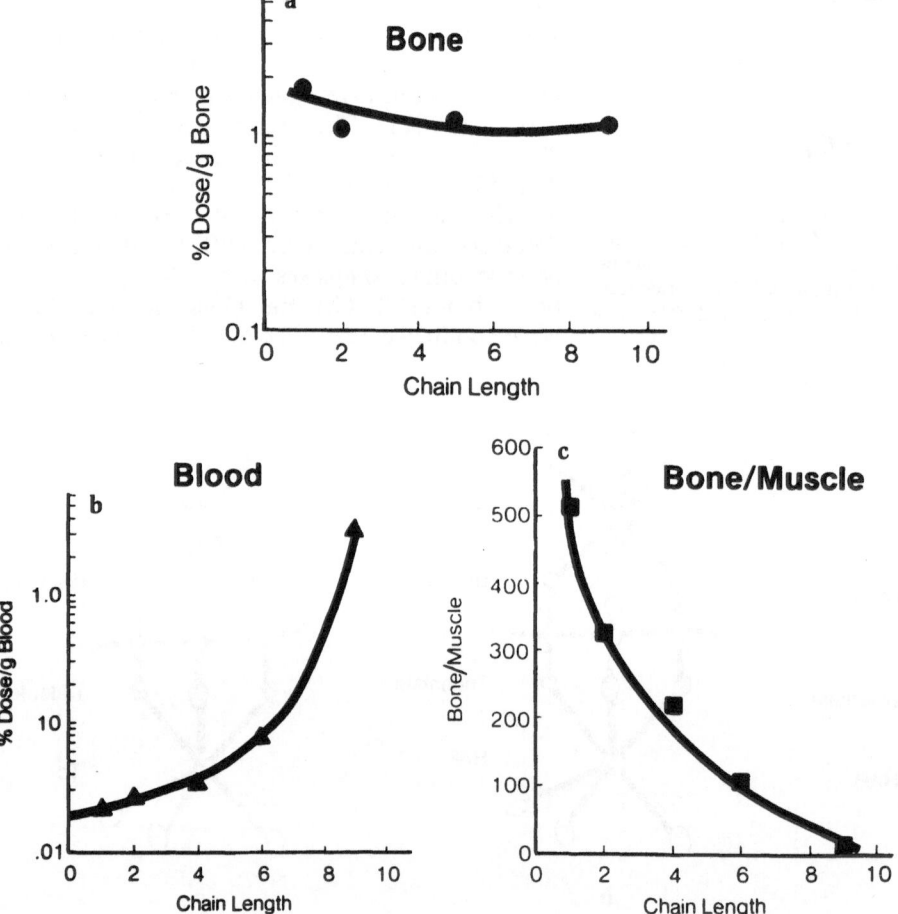

Fig. 2.10a–c. Bone, blood and muscle retention in the rat of ⁹⁹ᵐTc bone-scanning agents made from a series of *n*-alkyl-1, 1-diphosphonate and 1-hydroxy-*n*-alkyl-1, 1-diphosphonates using ⁹⁹ᵐTc pertechnetate and stannous chloride. **a** Bone retention of ⁹⁹ᵐTc dose as a function of increasing chain length of *n*-alkyl-1, 1-diphosphonates. **b** Blood retention of ⁹⁹ᵐTc as a function of increasing chain length of 1-hydroxy-*n*-alkyl-1, 1-diphosphonates. **c** Bone/muscle retention ratios of ⁹⁹ᵐTc dose as a function of increasing chain length of 1-hydroxy-*n*-alkyl-1, 1-diphosphonates.

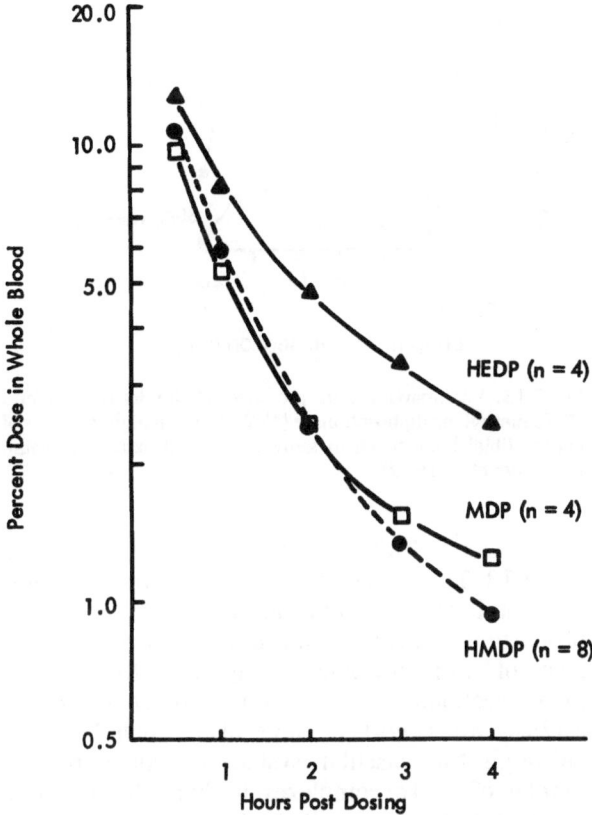

Fig. 2.11. Blood clearance of ^{99m}Tc-hydroxyethylidene diphosphonate (*HEDP*), ^{99m}Tc methylene diphosphonate (*MDP*) and ^{99m}Tc hydroxymethylene diphosphonate (*HMDP*) in dogs as a function of time. (Bevan et al. 1979)

cipitously with increasing chain length from one to nine carbons for the diphosphonates because muscle retention rose while bone retention was almost constant. This striking change in soft tissue retention is due to the greater lipophilicity with longer chain and hence a greater interaction and retention in blood and muscle, probably on cell membranes. The calcium coordinating properties of all these geminal diphosphonates changed only very marginally.

The change in blood clearance of ^{99m}Tc with three widely used diphosphonates can probably also be related to their relative lipophilicity (Fig. 2.11). HEDP is the slowest to be cleared, is structurally similar to HMDP but has one more carbon (methyl group rather than hydrogen). MDP and HMDP have the same number of carbons, but the hydroxy group in HMDP rather than hydrogen in MDP reduces the lipophilicity (increases hydrophilicity), and hence MDP is cleared slighly less effectively than HMDP at 4 h.

The whole-body retention in normal subjects of the above three ^{99m}Tc diphosphonate complexes and the percentage dose per gram of dog bone of each are shown together in Fig. 2.12. The interrelationship of the ^{99m}Tc retention in whole-body studies (Fogelman et al. 1981) and in studies directly on dog bone (Bevan et al. 1979) is remarkable. HMDP shows the highest retention, MDP shows slightly less and HEDP shows the least (Fig. 2.12). Moreover, the dog rib bones, which are highly active

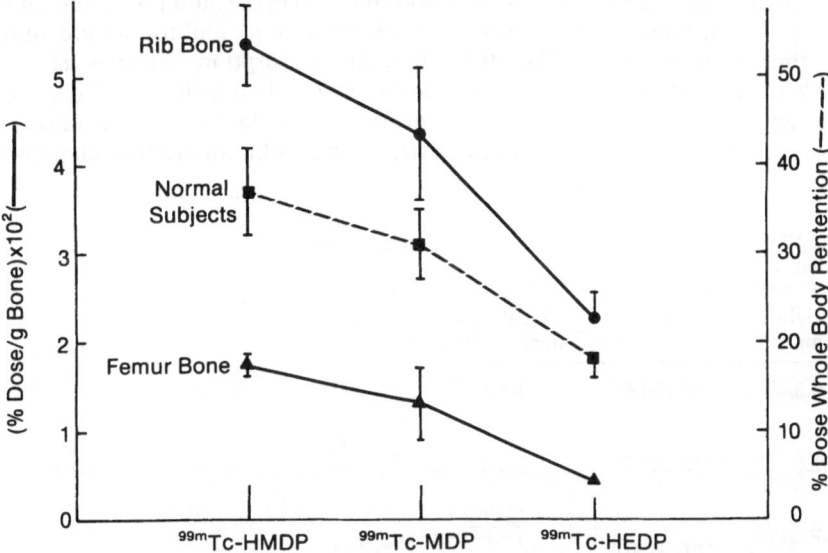

Fig. 2.12. The retention of ^{99m}Tc hydroxymethylene diphosphonate (^{99m}Tc-*HMDP*), ^{99m}Tc methylene diphosphonate (^{99m}Tc-*MDP*) and ^{99m}Tc-1-hydroxyethylidene diphosphonate (^{99m}Tc-*HEDP*) in the rib and femur bones of dogs (*solid lines, left ordinate*) and in normal human subjects using whole-body retention (*dashed lines, right ordinate*). (After Bevan et al. 1979 and Fogelman et al. 1981)

metabolically, and primarily trabecular bone with very thin cortices, show the higher retention with all three agents, while femora with high cortical bone content and relatively low metabolic activity show the lower retention. The summation uptake of all bones (whole-body retention; Fogelman et al. 1981) gives the same relationship of bone uptake to direct bone analysis in dogs with all of the three scanning agents. Thus even though some small error may be made in whole-body retention studies by the soft tissue retention of ⁹⁹ᵐTc, from a clinical standpoint whole-body retention measurements provide valid assessments of skeletal retention and the relative metabolic activity of bone. Numerous other comparisons of these agents and others have recently been presented (Schwarz and Kloss 1981; Fogelman 1982; Littlefield and Rudd 1983; Pauwels et al. 1983).

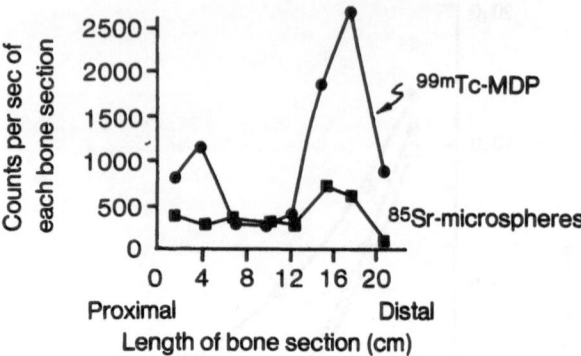

Fig. 2.13. A comparison of the presence of ⁸⁵Sr microspheres and ⁹⁹ᵐTc methylene diphosphonate (*⁹⁹ᵐTc-MDP*) in eight sections of canine tibial bone taken in sequence from proximal to distal. (Lavender et al. 1979)

Mechanism of ⁹⁹ᵐTc Diphosphonate Adsorption on Bone

There seems little doubt that skeletal uptake of a ⁹⁹ᵐTc-labelled bone-scanning agent is dependent upon the vascular supply to the bone. In numerous instances, such as in a pagetic bone lesion, increased bone uptake is associated with increased vascularity. However, another factor perhaps as important in ⁹⁹ᵐTc uptake is the nature of the calcium phosphate (Ca-P) deposited. This difference in reactivity of the Ca-P deposit is in the composition of the Ca-P, the particle size of the solid Ca-P, the surface area and state of hydration of the low-density deposit (Landis 1985). The hypothesis that other factors are involved is suggested by the lack of proportional uptake of ⁹⁹ᵐTc scanning agents with vascularity and is demonstrated by a comparison of ⁸⁵Sr micros-

pheres and ⁹⁹ᵐTc-MDP in bone sections, as seen in Fig. 2.13. This data clearly shows that the proximal and distal ends of the tibia do *not* show ⁹⁹ᵐTc uptake proportional to the vascularity, as indicated by the levels of ⁸⁵Sr microspheres compared with the ⁹⁹ᵐTc in the sections of bone examined (Lavender et al. 1979). Other workers have also concluded that although the vascular system is crucial to the uptake of ⁹⁹ᵐTc complexes in bone it does not account for the unusually high uptake of scanning agents found at sites of rapid formation such as the epiphyseal plate of long bones, metabolic bone tumours and healing fractures (Charkes et al. 1978; Sager et al. 1978).

In order to investigate this non-vascular component of skeletal uptake and retention, the role of bone matrix and the form of calcium phosphate has been studied with respect to diphosphonate and ⁹⁹ᵐTc diphosphonate adsorption (Francis et al. 1980). The earliest stage of biological Ca-P deposition, such as at a rapidly califying front, is known to be of low Ca/P molar ratio, highly hydrated and

Table 2.1. Adsorption of ¹⁴C-HEDP or ⁹⁹ᵐTc-HMDP on bone matrix and inorganic calcium phosphate. Non-competitive and competitive adsorption

System	Type	Weight (mg)	Adsorbant	¹⁴C-Adsorbed (moles × 10⁷)	Ratio
Calcium phosphate (Ca-P) alone	NC	9.3	¹⁴C-HEDP	8.82	
Bone matrix (BM) alone	NC	2.6	¹⁴C-HEDP	1.16	7.6
Ca-P + BM (combined)	C	{Ca-P: 200, BM: 56}	⁹⁹ᵐTc-HMDP	% Dose Ca-P: 89.9 BM: 2.2	41.8

Abbreviations: NC, non-competitive; C, competitive; HEDP, hydroxyethylidine diphosphonate; HMDP, hydroxymethylene diphosphonate low density (Landis 1985). To simulate this and determine the effect of this kind of Ca-P compared with the mature Ca-P found in cortical bone, both a rapidly precipitated, immature, amorphous Ca-P (Ca/P = 1.35) and crystalline mature hydroxyapatite (Ca/P = 1.66) were synthesised. The adsorption of three ^{14}C diphosphonates (HMDP, MDP or HEDP) on the above two Ca-P solids was then investigated.

With all three diphosphonates the adsorption on the immature, low Ca/P calcium phosphate was higher (1.8 times) than on the mature crystalline hydroxyapatite on a mole of diphosphonate per mole of calcium basis (Francis et al. 1980). In addition to the vascularity and state of the Ca-P in bone, it has been suggested that the matrix of bone may be a selective source of deposition of ^{99m}Tc-diphosphonate skeletal agents (Rosenthall and Kaye 1975; Francis et al. 1979). To examine the importance of bone organic matrix relative to the inorganic component of bone, the adsorption of the diphosphonate, ^{14}C-HEDP, on each component was examined separately (Francis et al. 1979). The adsorption of ^{99m}Tc-HMDP on both matrix and calcium phosphate components combined was then determined. The results are shown in Table 2.1 (Francis et al. 1981). The *non-competitive* adsorption of ^{14}C-HMDP on a per gram basis was about 2.1/1:

Ca-P/matrix or in the approximate weight ratio of each component to be found in bone it was 7.6/1 (Table 2.1). However, when the Ca/P and matrix were mixed uniformly and then reacted with ^{99m}Tc-HMDP (conditions under which each component was *competing* for the bone agent) the ratio of the ^{99m}Tc on the Ca-P inorganic fraction compared with the organic matrix fraction was 41.8/1 (Table 2.1). This pronounced selectivity of adsorption of the diphosphonate or the ^{99m}Tc diphosphonate for the inorganic or mineral component of bone is strikingly demonstrated by autoradiographic studies of rabbit bone. Whether the endosteal surface is a resorption cavity with no surface osteoid (organic matrix) or whether it is an actively forming bone surface with a significant lining of osteoid covering the inorganic bone, the silver grains resulting from deposition of ^{3}H-HEDP are on the inorganic surface (mineral layer) of bone (Fig. 2.14). This means that even though the complex has had to diffuse through the osteoid layer to reach the inorganic component, under competitive circumstances, such as in an in vivo bone scan, the deposition of diphosphonate will take place almost entirely on the inorganic Ca-P surface of bone rather than on the organic matrix. This has also been demonstrated in autoradiography studies using ^{99m}Tc-labelled bone-scanning agents (Tilden et al. 1973; Guillemart et al. 1980).

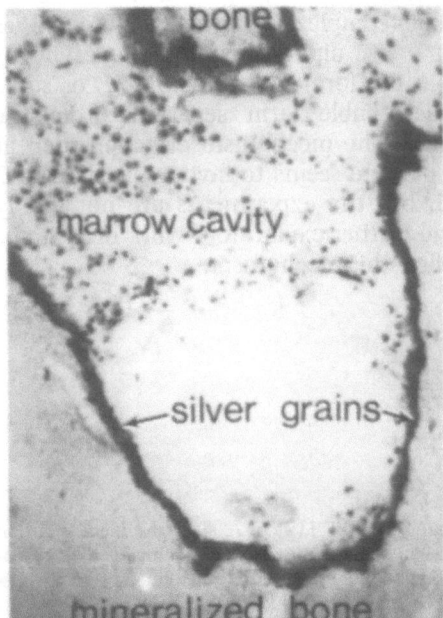 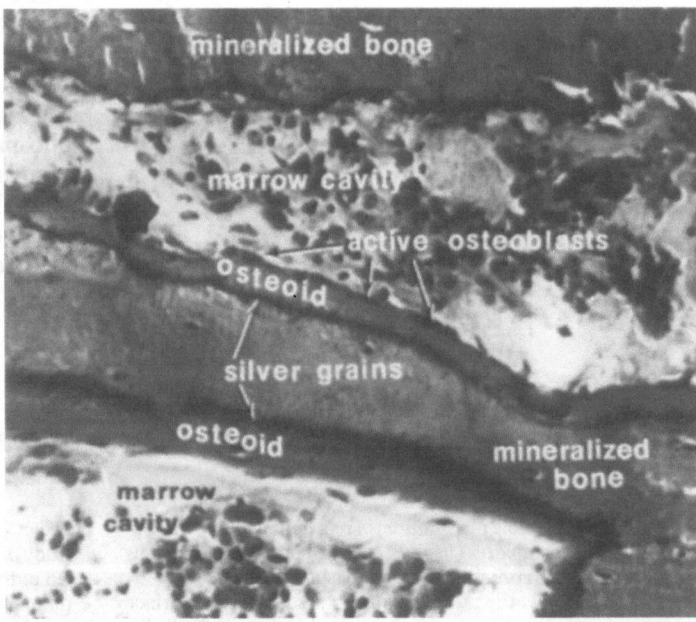

a   b

Fig. 2.14a, b. Microautoradiographs of the endosteal surface of rabbit bone in which ^{3}H-HEDP was administered intraperitoneally. The concentration of silver grains indicating the adsorption of ^{3}H-HEDP on the bone surface is seen totally lining the resorption cavity (a). The heavy concentration of silver grains (b) appear below the osteoid layers on either side of the spicule of bone and below the osteoblasts lining the surface of the osteoid.

Considerable work is being carried out to determine the nature of the ^{99m}Tc complexes that form and interact with bone tissue (Deutsch and Barnett 1980; Wilson and Pinkerton 1985). The reactivity of the apparently multiple complexes, complex charges and polymeric forms of the complexes are currently being rigorously studied. The absolute separation without alteration of each unique complex in the scanning agents is very difficult, however, and much of this work is in a state of flux.

Among the remaining mechanistic questions regarding the reaction of ^{99m}Tc skeletal agents with bone is what happens to the complex at the surface of the bone. Figure 2.15 shows two of the most likely mechanisms which would be totally consistent with the autoradiographic and quantitative distribution data just cited. To investigate which of these two mechanisms might pertain, in vitro and in vivo experiments were performed (Francis 1980, 1981, unpublished work). Solid hydroxyapatite crystals

were reacted with ^{99m}Tc-^{14}C-HEDP or ^{99m}Tc-^{14}C-HMDP. The solid was washed and then immediately flooded five times with 2% non-tagged diphosphonate to desorb the diphosphonate-^{99m}Tc-complex from the apatite (Francis et al. 1980). Only about 50% of the ^{99m}Tc could be desorbed by this technique, suggesting about half the ^{99m}Tc might be adsorbed on the Ca-P as the complete desorbable complex (mechanism 1, Fig. 2.15), but the other half of the adsorbed ^{99m}Tc seemed to be in a non-labile form (not desorbable) suggesting mechanism 2. To test the mechanism more realistically, rats were given an intravenous dose of ^{99m}Tc-^{14}C-HEDP and then 16 h later half the animals were used to determine the ratio of ^{99m}Tc to ^{14}C on bone. As expected, radioassay of bones indicated that ^{99m}Tc and ^{14}C were both adsorbed. The other half were given a very high intraperitoneal dose of non-radiolabelled HEDP (25 mg/kg) to flood and saturate the in vivo bone system. Blood samples were taken at 1, 1$\frac{1}{2}$, and 2 h later. Only ^{14}C-HEDP showed a spike in the blood over the background levels at 16 h indicating desorption of free ^{14}C-HEDP. ^{99m}Tc blood levels did not rise over background with the high dose of HEDP. This implies that the ^{99m}Tc on the bone in the rats at 16 h after dose was in a non-desorbable form (mechanism 2, Fig. 2.15), while the uncomplexed ^{14}C-HEDP on the bone was desorbable by the non-radioactive HEDP (Francis 1981, unpublished work). It appears that after some period of time, the adsorbed ^{99m}Tc part of the ^{99m}Tc-^{14}C diphosphonate complexes on bone is no longer present as a ^{99m}Tc diphosphonate complex but is most likely in the form of insoluble TcO_2 or some other non-desorbable form separated from the diphosphonate. The mechanism of action then at the surface of bone seems to favour mechanism 2 in Fig. 2.15, but the experiments are not totally definitive and further exploratory work needs to be done to confirm this mechanism.

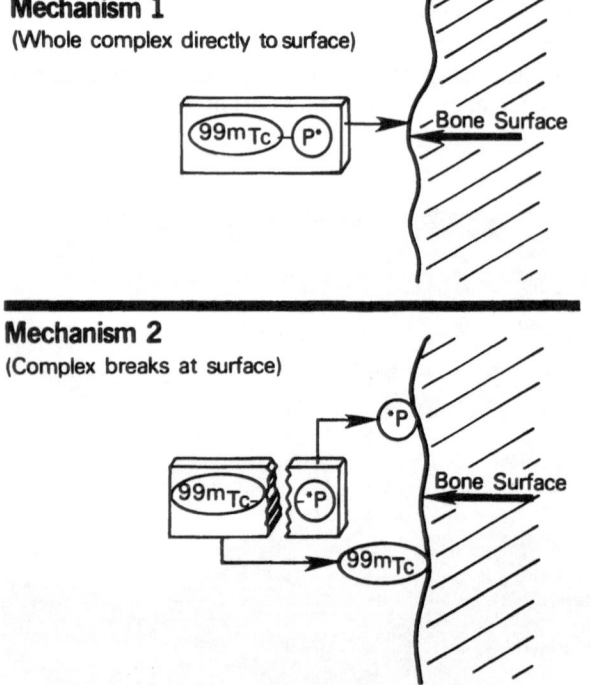

Mechanism 1
(Whole complex directly to surface)

Mechanism 2
(Complex breaks at surface)

Fig. 2.15. Two possible mechanisms of reaction of the ^{99m}Tc-^{14}C-diphosphonate complexes (^{99m}Tc-P*) with a bone surface such as seen in Fig. 2.14, (Francis 1981, unpublished work).

In **mechanism 1**, the skeletal complex adsorbs to the surface intact and remains there in the ratio of administered ^{99m}Tc-P*. In **mechanism 2** at the surface, the complex breaks and the diphosphonate adsorbs to the calcium phosphate surface separately (see Fig. 2.9) while the released ^{99m}Tc(IV) ion would hydrolyse, migrate and adsorb separately on the bone surface as highly insoluble ^{99m}TcO_2$.

References

Benedict JJ, Van Duzee BF (1982) A structure/biodistribution study of ^{99m}Tc-diphosphonate skeletal imaging agents. Presented at the international symposium on technetium in chemistry and nuclear medicine, Padua, Italy, 9 Sept 1982

Bevan JA, Tofe AJ, Francis MD, Barnett BL, Benedict JJ (1979) Tc-99m hydroxymethylene diphosphonate (HMDP): a new skeletal imaging agent. In: Sorenson JA (ed) Radiopharmaceuticals II, proceedings of the 2nd international symposium on radiopharmaceuticals. New York, Society of Nuclear Medicine, pp 646–654

Buja LM, Tofe AJ, Kulkarni PV et al. (1977) Sites and mechanisms of localization of technetium-99m phosphorus radiopharmaceuticals in acute myocardial infarcts and other tissues. J Clin Invest 60: 724–740

Charkes ND, Makler PT Jr, Phillips C (1978) Studies of skeletal tracer kinetics. 1. Digital computer solution of a five-compartment model of (^{18}F) fluoride kinetics in humans. J Nucl Med 19: 1301–1309

Deutsch E, Barnett BL (1980) Synthetic and structural aspects of technetium chemistry as related to nuclear medicine. In: Martell AE (ed) Inorganic chemistry in biology and medicine. ACS symp series No 140, pp 103–119

Deutsch E, Libson K, Becker CB et al. (1980) Preparation and biological distribution of technetium diphosphate radiotracers synthesized without stannous tin. J Nucl Med 21: 859–866

Fogelman I (1982) Diphosphonate bone scanning agents—current concepts. Eur J Nucl Med 7: 506–509

Fogelman I, Pearson DW, Bessent RG, Tofe AJ, Francis MD (1981). A comparison of skeletal uptakes of three diphosphonates by whole-body retention: concise communication. J Nucl Med 22: 880–883

Francis MD, Slough CL, Tofe AJ, Silbertstein EB (1976) Factors affecting uptake and retention of technetium-99m-diphosphonate and 99m-pertechnetate in osseous, connective and soft tissues. Calcif Tissue Res 20: 303–311

Francis MD, Tofe AJ, Benedict JJ, Bevan JA (1979) Imaging the skeletal system. In: Sorenson JA (ed) Radiopharmaceuticals II, proceedings of the 2nd international symposium on radiopharmaceuticals. New York, Society of Nuclear Medicine, pp 603–614

Francis MD, Ferguson DL, Tofe AJ, Bevan JA, Michaels SE (1980) Comparative evaluation of three diphosphonates: in vivo adsorption (C-^{14} labelled) and in vivo osteogenic uptake (Tc-99m complexed). J Nucl Med 21: 1185–1189

Francis MD, Horn PA, Tofe AJ (1981) Controversial mechanism of technetium-99m deposition on bone. J Nucl Med 22: 72 (abstract)

Fritzberg AR, Lyster DM, Dolphin DH (1977) Evaluation of formamidine sulfinic acid and other reducing agents for use in the preparation of Tc-99m labelled radiopharmaceuticals. J Nucl Med 18: 553–557

Grassi J, Devynck J, Tremillon B (1979) Electrochemical studies of technetium at a mercury electrode. Anal Chem 107: 47–58

Guillemart A, Le Pape A, Galy G, Besnard JC (1980) Bone kinetics of calcium-45 and pyrophosphate labelled with technetium-96. An autoradiographic evaluation. J Nucl Med 21: 466–470

Landis WJ (1985) Characterization of the mineral phases initially deposited in calcifying vertebrate tissues. In: Klee WE (ed) Proceedings of the conference on crystal deposition and dissolution in tissues, Evian, France, 26–28 Sept, pp La 1–18

Lavender JP, Khan RAA, Hughes SPF (1979) Blood flow and tracer uptake in normal and abnormal canine bone: comparisons with Sr-85 microspheres, Kr-81m, and Tc-99m MDP. J Nucl Med 20: 413–418

Littlefield JL, Rudd TG (1983) Tc-99m hydroxymethylene diphosphonate and Tc-99m methylene diphosphonate: biological and clinical comparison: concise communication. J Nucl Med 24: 463–466

Pauwels EKJ, Blom J, Camps JAJ, Hermans J, Rijke AM (1983) A comparison between the diagnostic efficacy of ^{99m}Tc-MDP, ^{99m}Tc-DPD and ^{99m}Tc-HDP for the detection of bone metastases. Eur J Nucl Med 8: 118–122

Rosenthall L, Kaye M (1975) Technetium-99m-pyrophosphate kinetics and imaging in metabolic bone disease. J Nucl Med 16: 33–39

Russell CD (1977) Carrier electrochemistry of pertechnetate: application to radiopharmaceutical labelling by controlled potential electrolysis at chemically inert electrodes. Int J Appl Radiat Isot 28: 241–249

Russell CD, Majerik JE, Cash AG, Lindsay RH (1978) Technetium pyrophosphate, a mixture?—Preparation and comparative biologic properties of Tc(III) and Tc(IV) pyrophosphate. Int J Nucl Med Biol 5: 190–194

Sagar V, Piccone JM, Charkes ND, Makler PT Jr (1978) Skeletal tracer uptake and bone flow in dogs. J Nucl Med 19: 705–706

Schwarz A, Kloss G (1981) Beziehungen zwischen chemischer Structure und Skelettfixierung verschiedener Tc-99m-Phosphonsäuren. Nuklearmedizin Suppl 18: 120–124

Silberstein EB, Francis MD, Tofe AJ, Slough CL (1975) Distribution of ^{99m}Tc-Sn-diphosphonate and free ^{99m}Tc pertechnetate in selected soft and hard tissues. J Nucl Med 16: 58–61

Srivastava SC, Meinken G, Smith TD, Richards P (1977) Problems associated with stannous ^{99m}Tc-radiopharmaceuticals. Int J Appl Radiat Isot 28: 83–95

Steigman J, Meinken G, Richards P (1978) The reduction of pertechnetate-99m by stannous chloride—II. The stoichiometry of the reaction in aqueous solutions of several phospherous (V) compounds. Int J Appl Radiat Isot 29: 653–660

Tilden RL, Jackson J, Enneking WF (1973) ^{99m}Tc-polyphosphate: histological localization in human femurs by autoradiography. J Nucl Med 14: 576–578

Wilson GM, Pinkerton TC (1985) Determination of charge and size of technetium diphosphonate complexes by anion-exchange liquid chromatography. Anal Chem 57: 246–253

3 · The Normal Bone Scan

M. V. Merrick

Introduction

The bone scan is the most frequently performed nuclear medicine investigation, the commonest indication being the detection of occult metastases, for which purpose the entire skeleton should be imaged. For other purposes it is often adequate to examine only part of the skeleton. The amount of isotope taken up at any site depends primarily on the local rate of bone turnover rather than on bone mass. The scintigraphic appearance therefore does not necessarily correlate with the radiographic one; however, as there is a relationship between the rate at which bone is replaced and the quantity of bone which is present at any point, the two appearances are not entirely unrelated.

Recognition of abnormality is based on a detailed knowledge of normal scintigraphic appearances, which may be affected not only by skeletal physiology and anatomy but also by a variety of technical factors which can influence image quality.

Technical Considerations

Radiopharmaceutical

The only compounds still in general use for bone scintigraphy are diphosphonate chelates of ^{99m}Tc(IV), the most popular of which is methylene diphosphonate. The relative merits of the different diphosphonates are discussed in Chapter 4.

In the normal subject the absolute amount of diphosphonate taken up by bone depends on the compound used (Fogelman et al. 1981). Variations in soft tissue uptake may also occur (Eckelman et al. 1974; Citrin et al. 1975a), but with modern-day agents, appearances are generally similar irrespective of the radiopharmaceutical employed. The kidneys are readily visualised in the majority of normal subjects (Hattner et al. 1975; Sy et al. 1975), but other soft tissues are barely seen at exposure settings correct for the axial skeleton.

Radiopharmaceutical Quality

It is relatively uncommon to encounter poor-quality bone scans resulting from radiopharmaceutical problems. However, abnormally high levels of tissue background may be due to the presence of free pertechnetate or free reduced technetium, although in many cases no definite cause can be found. On a single examination it is rarely possible to distinguish normal interpatient variation from fluctuations in radiopharmaceutical quality, unless there is evidence of free pertechnetate, which is always a radiopharmaceutical fault. Reduced free technetium can only be distinguished clinically from the normal interpatient variation if several patients have received the same preparation. Free pertechnetate may be distinguished from other causes of a high soft tissue background because it accumulates in the gastric mucosa as well as the thyroid. In the presence of free pertechnetate, activity is also seen in the stomach, often in small bowel and, if the interval before imaging is long enough, in large bowel. Uptake of pertechnetate in the thyroid gland itself is always accompanied by gastric uptake. A study with detectable free pertechnetate is unsatisfactory for diagnostic purposes and should be repeated.

Timing of Images

Timing of images may depend upon the clinical problem under investigation (see individual chapters). In some circumstances a "three-phase" examination will provide valuable additional information (Maurer et al. 1981). This involves a dynamic flow study of the area of interest with rapid sequential images taken every 2–3 s for 30 s. This is followed by a blood pool image at 1 min, when the radiopharmaceutical is still predominantly within the vascular compartment. Delayed static images are then obtained 2–4 h and, rarely, 24 h later as dictated by the clinical situation and by the workload of the department.

There is at present no general agreement as to the optimum time interval between injection and static imaging. Normal bone uptake of tracer is maximal by 2 h, but differential uptake in lesions is higher at 4 h (Citrin et al. 1975b; Fogelman et al. 1979). Image quality is affected not only by absolute bone uptake, but also by the contrast between bone and soft tissue, which is greatest at 6 h (Makler and Charkes 1980).

In general, imaging should not be performed earlier than 2 h after injection, and, where local conditions permit, a 4-h wait will improve image quality. On rare occasions 24-h images may be useful in confirming lesions that appear equivocal at 4 h (Merrick 1975; Hardoff and Front 1978).

Equipment

Technical factors are of considerable importance in bone scintigraphy. Perhaps surprisingly there is no evidence that, for the range of instruments currently available, the resolution of the imaging device has any effect on sensitivity or accuracy. High-resolution images are undoubtedly aesthetically more attractive, but a fundamental problem with all the diphosphonates currently in general use is the high uptake in normal bone, with correspondingly relatively low contrast between normal and abnormal areas.

Although scintigraphy is most commonly performed with a gamma camera, the appearance of the images obtained is influenced to only a minor extent by the type of instrumentation used. Any scanning gamma camera which produces a single image of the entire skeleton has a lower resolution than the same camera used in the static mode, when several images are required to include the whole skeleton. This is partly a consequence of the compromises which must be made when a gamma camera is adapted for scanning. However, the difficulties are considerably compounded by the requirement that the head of the camera when scanning is at some distance from the patient, whereas in the static mode it is possible to position the patient directly against the collimator face. With all gamma cameras the resolution falls rapidly as the distance from the collimator face increases. In consequence, static or "spot" views will always be sharper than those obtained with a scanning mechanism.

A further advantage of static images is that the patient can, if necessary, be repositioned for each projection, for example to allow for a kyphosis. The actual number of individual projections depends on the field of view of the particular camera and the size of the patient. When a camera with a small field of view is employed the loss of resolution may be less important than the uncertainty engendered when 20 or more views, each including only a little of the skeleton, are evaluated. Static images are undoubtedly preferable when using a camera with a large field of view.

Multi-detector scanners are probably the best instruments for skeletal whole-body imaging because their collimators are designed to minimise the effect of depth on resolution and sensitivity. However, they are less versatile than gamma cameras and can be justified only in departments with a large workload of whole-body skeletal scintigraphy.

Count Density

For maximal diagnostic accuracy the number of counts collected is more important than the resolution of the imaging device. Although a number of workers have advocated rapid images with low count densities, there is ample evidence that this is an unreliable technique and should not be employed under any circumstances. It was shown some years ago (Merrick 1973) that the minimum acceptable count density is 360 counts/cm^2 from normal areas of spine. There may well be an advantage in using a higher count density, although this is unproven.

The number of counts per view should not be preset to an identical value for all projections. The preferred technique is to take an image of an area, such as the thorax, which does not contain bladder or kidney, and to collect approximately one million counts using a camera with a large field of view. All other projections should be taken for the same time. If this is not done, views of the pelvis may obtain very few counts from bone, most of the counts coming from activity in the bladder (unless this is completely empty). The importance of an adequate count density is illustrated in Figs. 3.1 and 3.2. Figure 3.1 is a conventional whole-body image obtained with a multi-detector scanner, with an adequate count density over the spine but not over the periphery. Figure 3.2 is an image of the knees of the same patient, showing uptake in the medial tibial plateau not visible on the whole-body image, which contains too few counts from this region. Inadequate count densities are a major source of error, substantially reducing the sensitivity of the examination.

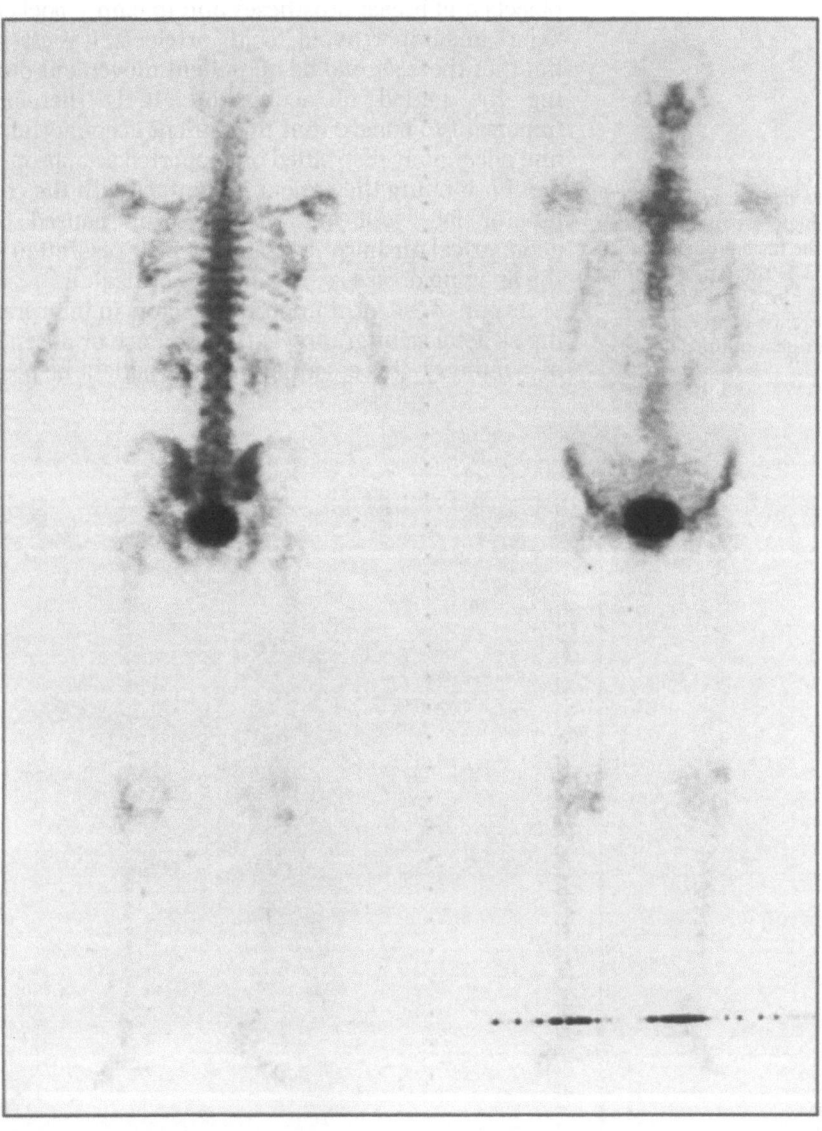

Fig. 3.1. Posterior whole-body image obtained using a multi-detector scanner. The image on the *left* is the posterior and that on the *right* the anterior projection. In the posterior projection the vertebrae, posterior ribs, scapulae and pelvis are clearly visualised. In the comparison with the higher resolution camera pictures, the disc spaces cannot be readily identified, even though the spinous processes and pedicles of the lumbar and lower thoracic vertebrae are readily identifiable. There is slight asymmetry in the rate of drainage from the two kidneys. Note the very low count rate along the shafts of the long bones.

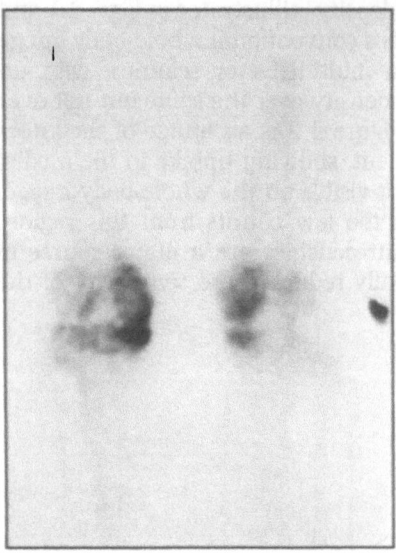

Fig. 3.2. Image of the knees of the same patient as in Fig. 3.1, acquired on the same day using a high-resolution gamma camera. Increased uptake is visible in the medial tibial plateau of the left knee. This is not evident in Fig. 3.1. This image contains 500 000 counts. The equivalent area in Fig. 3.1 contains approximately 50 000 counts. The difference between the two images is due to the difference in count rate, not the differences in resolution.

Radiographic Technique

Since diphosphonate is excreted by the kidneys, patients should be encouraged to drink fluids (at least a litre, if possible) in the interval between injection and imaging. This ensures faster clearance of non-skeletal tracer from the urinary tract, thereby decreasing soft tissue background and the absorbed radiation dose to the bladder, which is the critical organ. Complete bladder emptying just prior to scintigraphy is thus mandatory to ensure adequate views of the pelvis.

Patients must be asked to remove jewellery, metal objects and breast prostheses and to empty pockets before imaging to avoid "cold" artefacts. It is essential that there should be no patient movement during the period of acquisition. It is therefore important to ensure that the patient is comfortable and adequately restrained or supported as appropriate. Positioning the patient in contact with the collimator face will minimise blurring caused by geometrical unsharpness. The intrinsic resolution of the imaging device is probably less critical.

As one of the most important factors in interpreting skeletal scintigraphy is the presence or absence of symmetry, it is essential that the patient be posi-

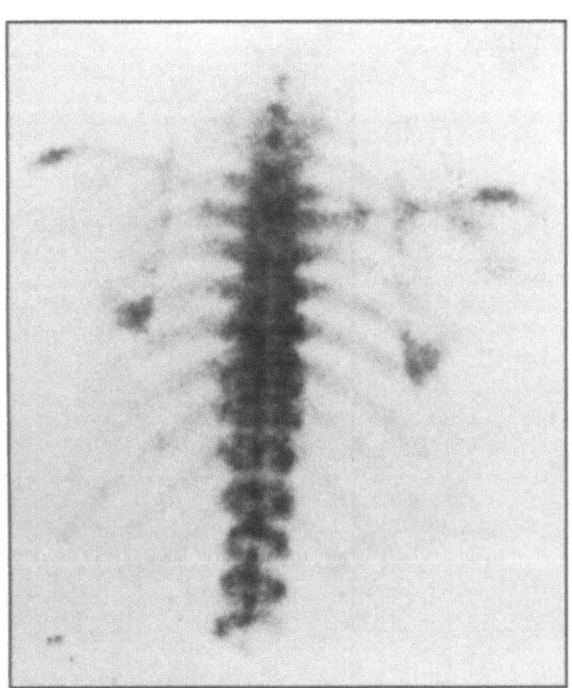

a

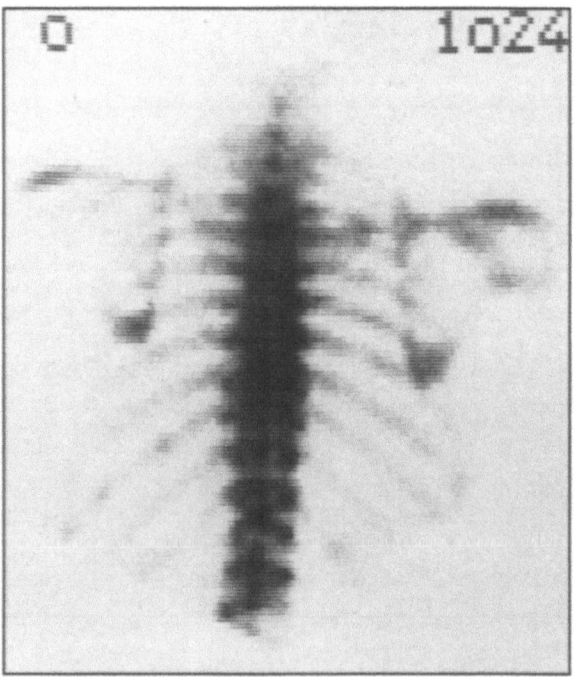

b

Fig. 3.3.a. Analogue image of the posterior thorax of an adult, obtained by collecting one million counts with a high-resolution gamma camera. b. Simultaneously acquired digital image of the same patient. Despite the coarse (128 × 128) acquisition matrix, the amount of information present in this film is identical to that present in a.

tioned straight. Where the field of view of the detector is not large enough to include both of paired structures, positioning of the two sides should be closely controlled to be as similar as possible. Supplementary oblique or lateral projections are occasionally helpful (Schutte 1980) but they cannot be accepted on their own as a substitute for straight anterior and posterior views. Vertex projections of the skull substantially increase the detection rate in this region (Smith et al. 1982).

Patient Factors

In addition to the technical considerations already discussed, image quality can also be adversely affected by various factors such as impaired renal function, gross cardiac failure, obesity and possibly old age (Wilson 1981; Adams and Shirley 1983).

Digital Imaging

Examples of analogue and digital images, obtained simultaneously, are shown in Fig. 3.3a, b. In practice, there is nothing to choose between a digital image and a correctly exposed analogue one, although digital acquisition allows subsequent skeletal numeration (see Chap. 16). The use of quantitative criteria for interpretation increases the number of faint lesions detected (Pitt and Sharp 1985), but at the cost of a clinically unacceptable rise in the false-positive rate. The only as yet proven advantage of digital imaging is that, whereas if the

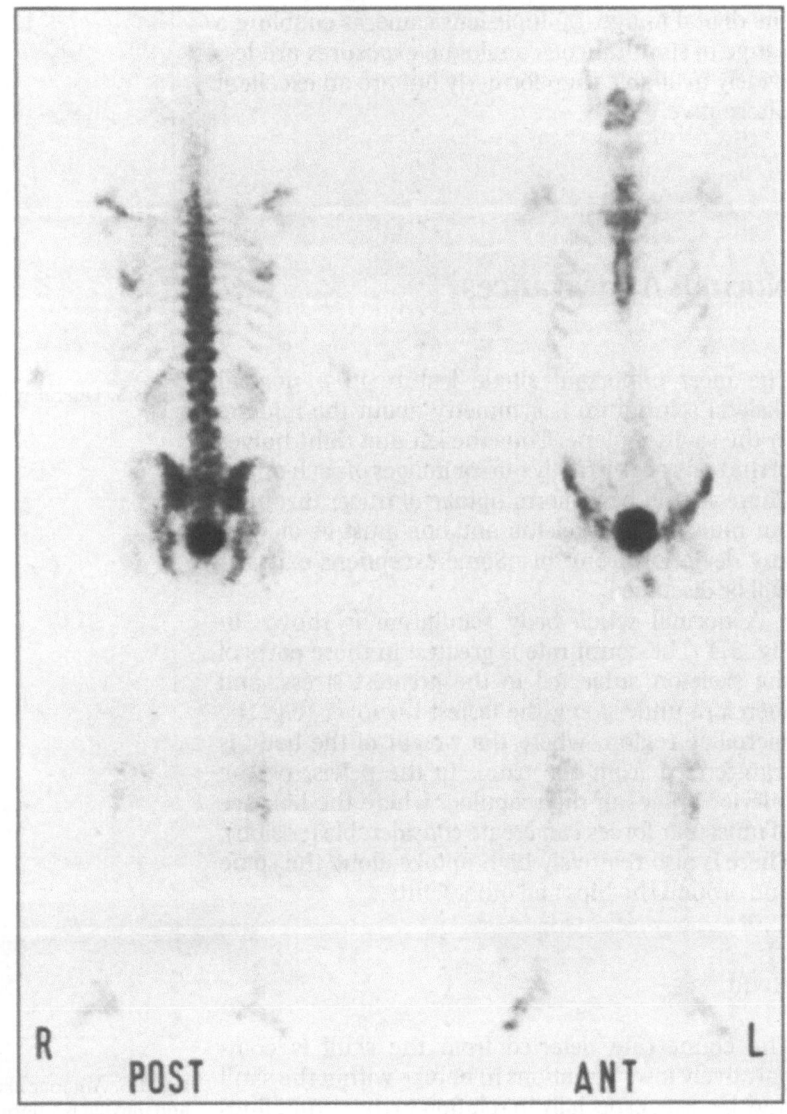

Fig. 3.4. Posterior and anterior whole-body images obtained with a multi-detector scanner.

photographic exposure is incorrect for an analogue picture the examination must be repeated, if it is incorrect for a digital image only the photographic film needs to be repeated, which does not require the presence of the patient.

There is no point in employing an excessively fine matrix. Increasing the number of points in a matrix reduces the number of counts per cell and therefore increases the statistical noise. Nothing is to be gained, and indeed information may be concealed in noise and consequently missed if a matrix finer than 256 × 256 is employed with a 40-cm diameter field. Occasionally, if there are abnormalities with very high count rates, it may not be possible to obtain a correctly exposed film showing both the very high and the very low count rate areas. This can easily be remedied, if digital images have been acquired, by taking two exposures at different intensity settings or by using a non-linear grey scale for the digital image. Multiple lens cameras enabling a range of simultaneous analogue exposures are less widely available than formerly but are an excellent alternative.

Normal Appearances

The most important single feature in a normal skeletal scintigram is symmetry about the midline in the sagittal plane. Thus the left and right halves of the body are virtually mirror images of each other. There should be uniform uptake of tracer throughout much of the skeleton and one must be alert to any deviation from this. Some exceptions exist, as will be discussed.

A normal whole-body scintigram is shown in Fig. 3.4. The count rate is greatest in those parts of the skeleton subjected to the greatest stress, and therefore undergoing the fastest turnover (e.g. the sacroiliac region, where the weight of the body is transferrred from the trunk to the pelvis, or the inferior angles of the scapulae, where the balance of muscular forces can create considerable tension). There is also relatively high uptake along the spine and around the hips and other joints.

Head

The count rate detected from the skull is comparatively low. Variations in uptake within the skull may be seen, especially in relation to the suture lines

(Fig. 3.5). A recent study has suggested that around 1% of patients may show this variant (Harbert and Desai 1985). This may cause quite intense tracer uptake and may be due to subradiographic cartilaginous rests, sutural foramina or Pacchionian granulations (arachnoid extensions into the lumen of the dural sinuses). Harbert and Desai (1985) concluded that foci of increased uptake in the line of the sutures are likely to be benign.

In the anterior projection the orbits and facial bones are clearly visualised. A higher count rate is observed from the facial bones, especially the maxilla and ethmoids (Fig. 3.6), where the stresses resulting from mastication are transmitted to the facial skeleton. In older children and adolescents dif-

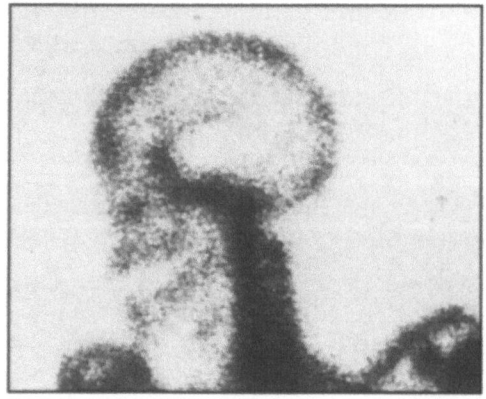

Fig. 3.5. Lateral view of adult skull showing uptake in suture lines.

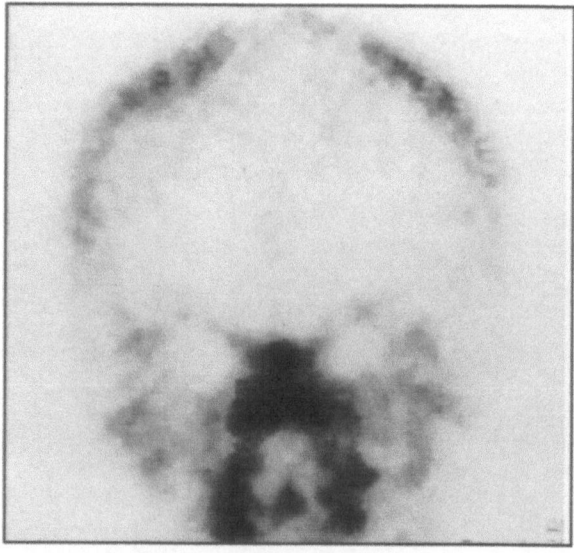

Fig. 3.6. Anterior skull projection. The uptake in the ethmoids and maxilla is a normal feature.

ficulty may arise if it is not appreciated that there is an important suture, which can be very active, between the sphenoid and the basiocciput (Fig. 3.7). This is a normal feature and should not be confused with sphenoidal sinusitis or pathology in the region of the clivus. During the eruption of dentition uptake in the maxilla and mandible may be uneven (Fig. 3.8).

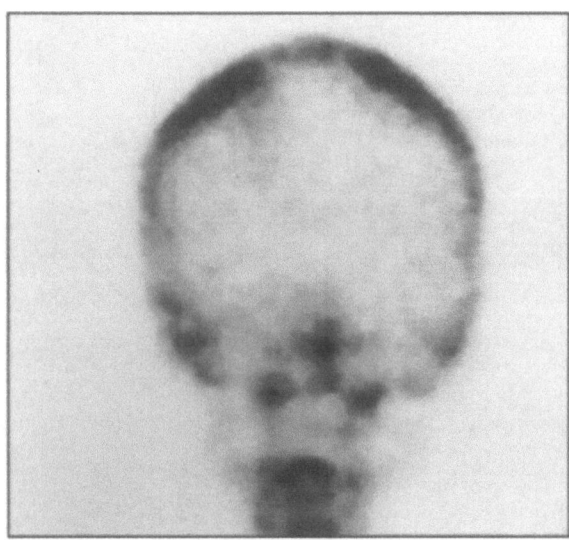

Fig. 3.9. Posterior projection of the skull of an 11-year-old girl. Individual cervical vertebrae are just resolvable, and the odontoid and atlas can be seen. There is no uptake in the skull sutures.

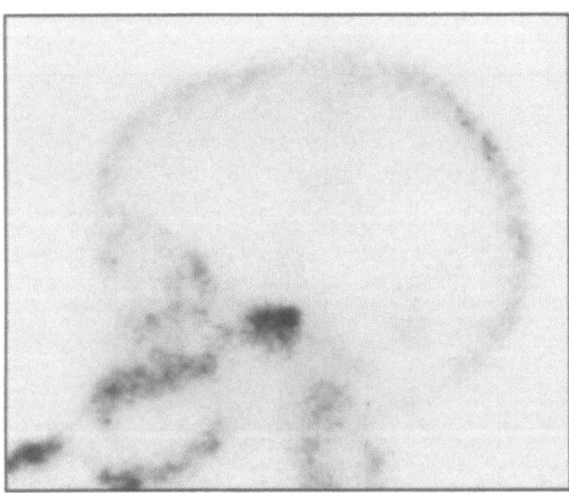

Fig. 3.7. Lateral projection of the skull of a 7-year-old child. The high uptake in the base is due to the suture between the sphenoid and the basiocciput, which was in process of fusion. Note also the relatively high uptake in the maxilla compared with the mandible. This reflects the state of dentition.

Neck

The individual bones of the cervical spine can be separately resolved only with high-resolution instruments (Fig. 3.9). The axoatlantal and atlanto-occipital joints are not easily seen except in agile subjects, and are often difficult to project clear of other structures. The spinous process of the vertebra prominens (C–7) is usually visible and distinct (See Fig. 3.3a, b) and may have a higher count rate than adjacent bones. Uptake in the neck in the absence of free pertechnetate is usually in the thyroid cartilage (which is not necessarily calcified radiologically) or hyoid (Oppenheim and Cantez 1977; Lin et al. 1981) rather than thyroid gland (Fig. 3.10).

Thorax

In the anterior projection of the thorax the sternum is clearly seen and, particularly in older subjects, the thyroid cartilage may be identified above it (Fig. 3.10). The sternomanubrial joint is often relatively active, particularly in older subjects (Fig. 3.10), and in occasional individuals there is high tracer uptake at the sternoclavicular joints. The clavicles are not well seen, but the acromio-clavicular joints often exhibit relatively high but usually symmetrical uptake. Calcified costal cartilages are often visualised in older subjects.

All of the ribs should be visible in the posterior projection of the thorax. The count rate in the ribs

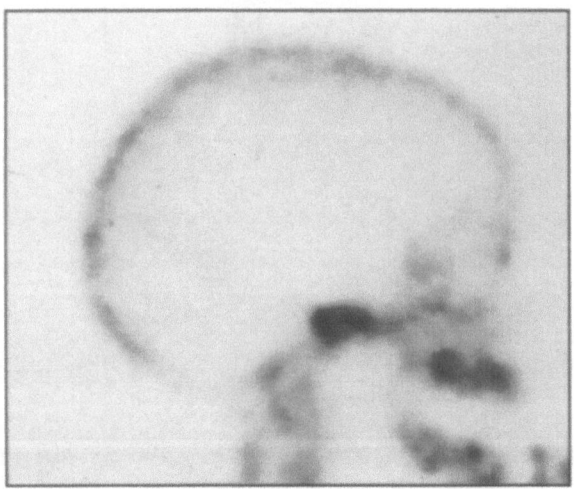

Fig. 3.8. Lateral skull of a 10-year-old child. The suture between the sphenoid and the basiocciput is much more active than in the subject shown in Fig. 3.7, and there is much more asymmetry in the maxilla because of the eruption of various teeth.

is comparatively low and is usually uniform, although "stippling" of the ribs caused by the insertions of the ileocostalis thoracis portion of the erector spinae muscles may be seen as a normal variant in about 7% of patients (Fink-Bennett and Johnson 1985). The scapulae are well seen, uptake being mainly concentrated at the angles, where muscle stresses are greatest. Where they overlie ribs, abnormalities may be difficult to distinguish, especially if the scapulae are not absolutely symmetrical. Rib deposits at this site are easily overlooked, or, if the

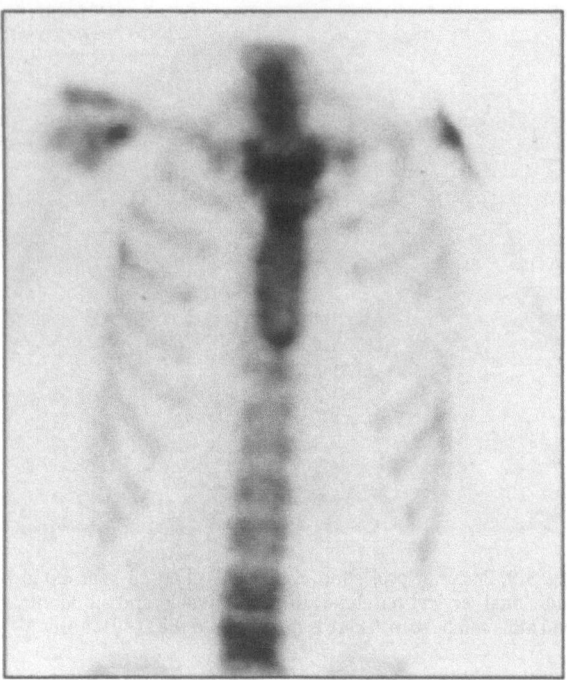

Fig. 3.10. Anterior projection. Note the high activity at the sternoclavicular joint and the sternomanubrial joint. There is uptake in the thyroid cartilage and in the acromioclavicular joints.

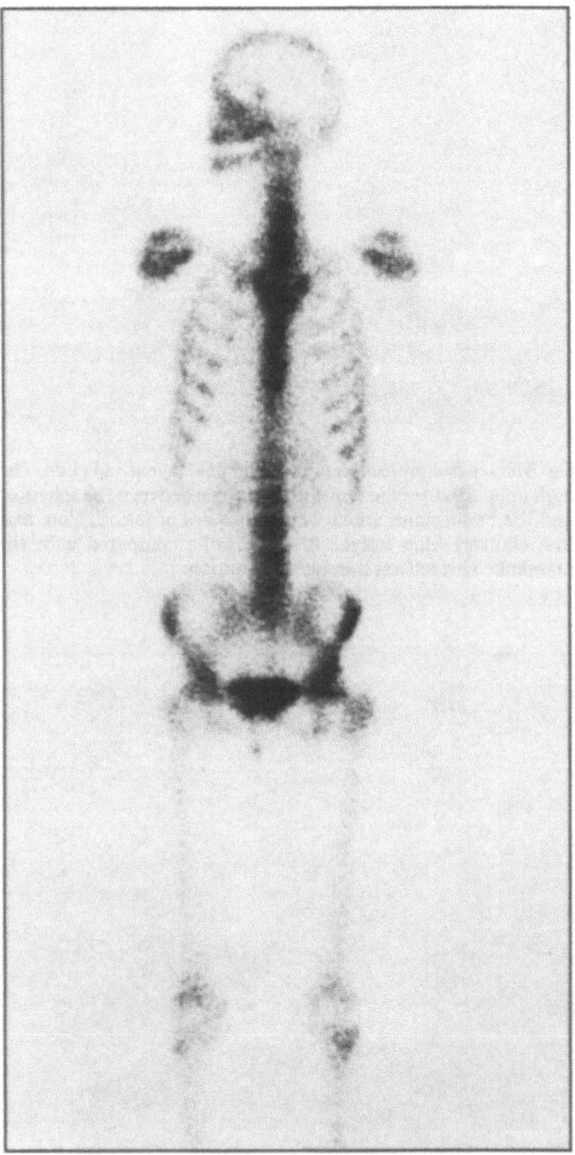

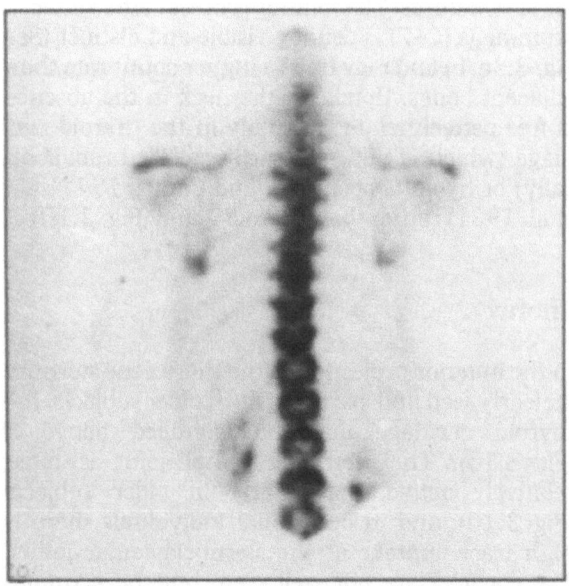

Fig. 3.11. Posterior thorax of a young adult. Using a high-resolution camera the individual vertebrae and interverterbral discs are clearly visible, as are the costotransverse joints. Note the symmetry of the scapulae and high uptake at the inferior angle and at the acromioclavicular joints.

Fig. 3.12. Anterior whole-body bone scan showing prominence of lower lumbar vertebrae caused by lumbar lordosis. Note also periarticular activity.

patient is askew, overdiagnosed. The costotransverse joints are visible in some subjects, parallel to the thoracic spine (Fig. 3.11).

Spine

The upper thoracic vertebrae cannot be individually identified, but there should be no difficulty in visualising the disc spaces between the lower ones. In the normal subject lower thoracic and lumbar pedicles and spinous processes are readily identified (see Figs. 3.1, 3.4), but it is not possible to distinguish the apophyseal joints separately from the pedicles except on oblique projections. The normal lumbar lordosis often makes the lower lumbar vertebrae appear prominent on anterior views of the spine (Fig. 3.12). The kidneys are seen in views of the lumbar spine, but the collecting system and ureters are not visualised at all unless there is urinary tract outflow obstruction.

Pelvis

There is usually perfect axial symmetry, but this may be disturbed by asymmetrical uptake in the ischiopubic synchrondosis (Cawley et al. 1983). There is often some residual activity in the bladder, the apparent position and shape of which differs in the anterior and posterior projections and may also change between supine, prone and erect. Bladder diverticulae and variations in shape are common and can be difficult to distinguish. The symphysis and adjacent parts of the pubis and ischium are consequently often obscured. A pelvic inlet projection, with the patient seated on the camera, is often helpful in this situation. Difficulty in interpretation sometimes arises in patients who have had urinary diversions, when activity is present in the bowel or a bag. Wherever possible these should be emptied prior to imaging, but in the case of a bowel diversion this may not be possible.

Limbs

There is relatively low uptake in the limbs, with the greatest concentration in the periarticular areas (Fig. 3.12). The normal femoral heads are seen only faintly in the adult, although the region of the greater trochanter and the intertrochanteric ridge can usually be identified (Fig. 3.13). In children the epiphysis for the greater trochanter as well as that for the head of the femur are readily visible. Uptake in the femoral head itself is adequate for avascular

regions to be identified as photon-deficient areas in high-resolution "pin-hole" images.

The shafts of the long bones are virtually invisible at intensity settings suitable for displaying the rest of the skeleton, but uptake can just be seen around the shoulders, elbows, knees, ankles and feet (Charkes et al. 1973; Merrick 1975, 1984; see Fig. 3.4). Muscle insertions, such as the deltoid tuberosity (Fink-Bennett and Vicuna-Rios 1980), are sometimes visible and are commonly asymmetrical as turnover is related to local stress. Other sites which may have a high enough concentration of tracer to give rise to diagnostic difficulty include the patella (Fogelman et al. 1983), the distal femur (Velchik et al. 1984) and accessory ossicles (Apple et al. 1984), although it is not clear to what extent visualisation of the latter is secondary to minor trauma. An artefact due to extravasation of tracer may be seen at the injection site, which should be documented in each patient.

In childhood, growth occurs principally in the epiphyses adjacent to the knee and away from the elbows. The activity of the epiphyses varies considerably with age (Figs. 3.14–3.17). The age at which epiphyses fuse radiographically is well documented, but there has been no systematic study of how this affects scintigraphic appearances. Most epiphyses appear to become more active shortly before fusion. While fusion is usually symmetrical, some asymmetry can occasionally be seen.

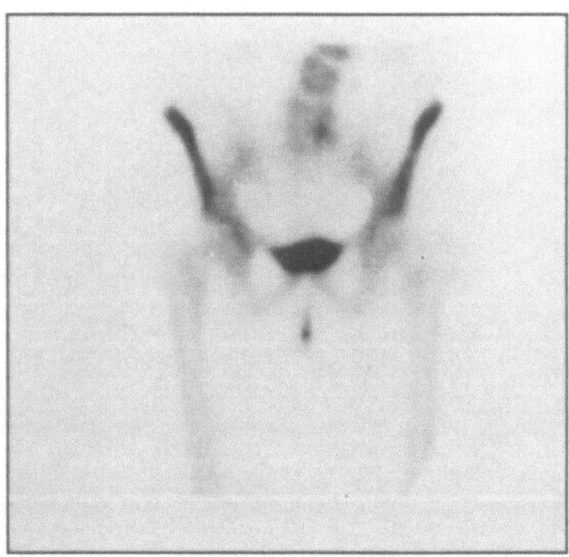

Fig. 3.13. Uptake in the neck and head of the normal femora is low and is only just discernible above background. The intertrochanteric ridge is well seen. Note that the patient has a scoliosis.

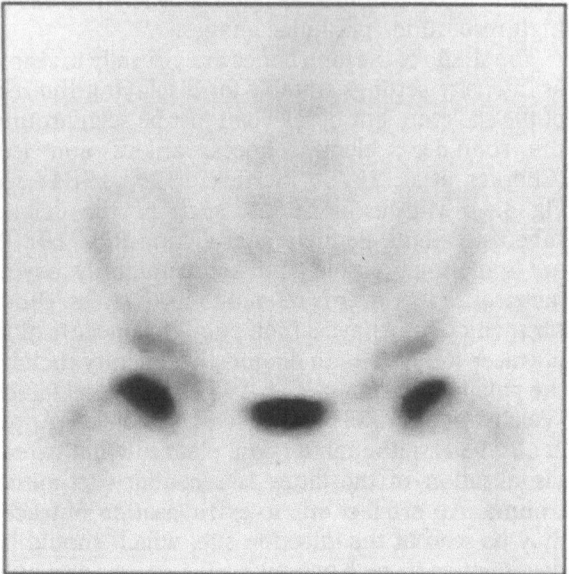

Fig. 3.14. Pelvis and hips of a 4-year-old child. There is high activity in the epiphyses of the femoral head, but the epiphyses of the greater trochanter are barely discernible.

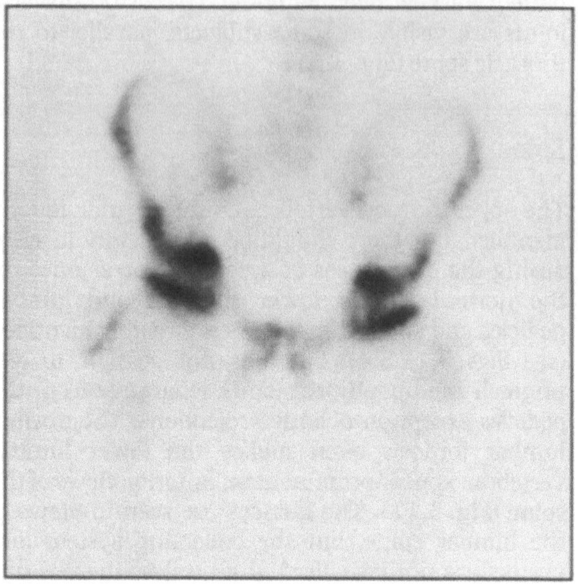

Fig. 3.16. Pelvis of an 8-year-old child. The epiphyses of the greater trochanter on the right is clearly visible but is much less active than the head epiphyses. Note that at this age there is considerable activity in the triradiate cartilages.

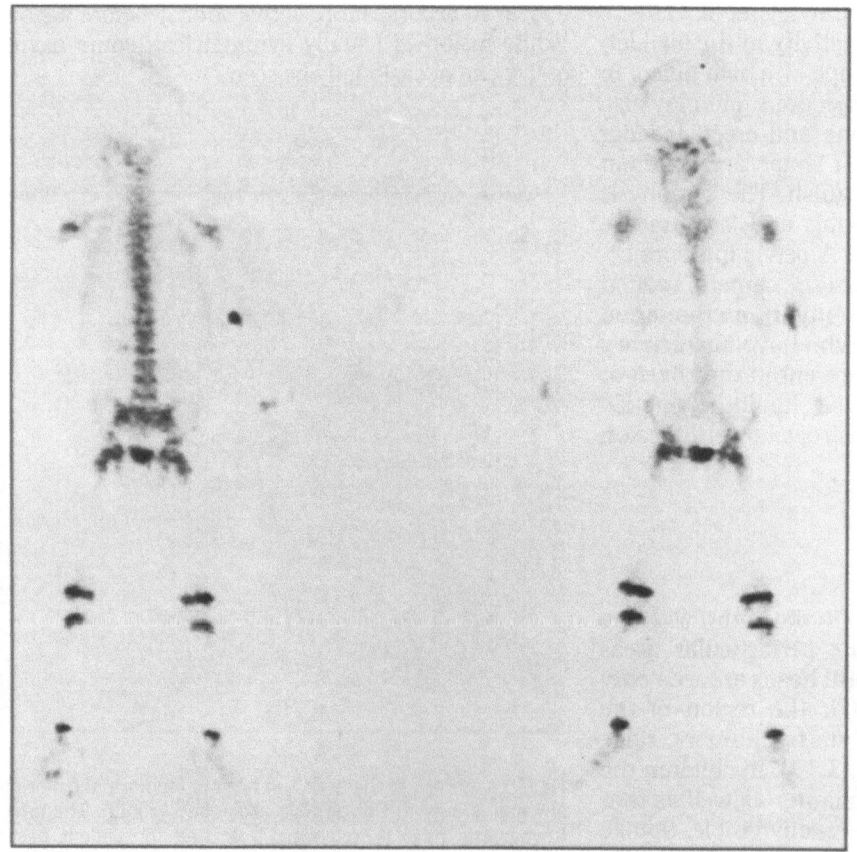

Fig. 3.15. Whole-body anterior and posterior images of a 5-year-old child. Note the substantial differential in count rate between the upper and lower limbs. Note that at this age there is high uptake in the distal tibial epiphyses.

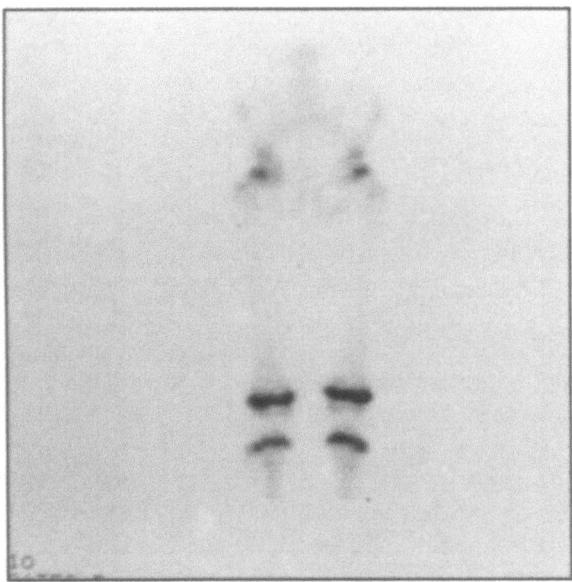

Fig. 3.17. Lower limbs of a 10-year-old child. At this age activity around the knee is much greater than at the proximal end of the femur, as this is where the greater part of growth is occurring. There is nevertheless some asymmetry.

Conclusion

Accurate bone scan diagnosis depends on high-quality images and a detailed appreciation of normal appearances. There should be an awareness of the variations that can occur as the result of technical factors and normal skeletal physiology.

References

Adams FG, Shirley AW (1983) Factors influencing bone scan quality. Eur J Nucl Med 8: 436–439

Apple JS, Martinez S, Nunley JA (1984) Painful os styloideum: bone scintigraphy in Carpe Bossu disease. AJR 142: 181–182

Cawley KA, Dvorak AD, Wilmot MD (1983) Normal anatomic variant: scintigraphy of the ischiopubic synchondrosis. J Nucl Med 24: 14–16

Charkes ND, Valentine G, Cravitz B (1973) Interpretation of the normal ^{99m}Tc polyphosphate rectilinear bone scan. Radiology 107: 563–570

Citrin DL, Bessent RG, Tuohy JB et al. (1975a) A comparison of phosphate bone-scanning agents in normal subjects and patients with malignant disease. Br J Radiol 48: 118–121

Citrin DL, Bessent RG, McGinley E, Gordon D (1975b) Dynamic studies with ^{99m}Tc-HEDP in normal subjects and in patients with bone tumours. J Nucl Med 16: 886–890

Eckelman WC, Reba RC, Kubota H, Stevenson JS (1974) ^{99m}Tc-pyrophosphate for bone imaging. J Nucl Med 15: 279–283

Fink-Bennett D, Johnson J (1985) Stippled ribs—a potential pitfall in bone scan interpretation. J Nucl Med 26: 82 (abstract)

Fink-Bennett D, Vicuna-Rios J (1980) The deltoid tuberosity—a potential pit-fall (the "delta sign") in bone scan interpretation: concise communication. J Nucl Med 21: 211–212

Fogelman I, Citrin DL, McKillop JH, Turner JG, Bessent RG, Greig WR (1979) A clinical comparison of Tc99m HEDP and Tc99m MDP in the detection of bone metastases: concise communication. J Nucl Med 20: 98–101

Fogelman I, McKillop JH, Gray HW (1983) The "hot patella" sign: is it of any clinical significance? Concise communication. J Nucl Med 24: 312–315

Fogelman I, Pearson DW, Bessent RG, Tofe AJ, Francis MD (1981) A comparison of skeletal uptakes of three diphosphonates by whole-body retention: concise communication. J Nucl Med 22: 880–883

Harbert J, Desai R (1985) Small calvarical bone scan foci—normal variations. J Nucl Med 26: 1144–1148

Hardoff R, Front D (1978) The value of delayed (24-hour) bone scintigraphy. Clin Nucl Med 3: 39–42

Hattner RS, Miller SW, Schimmel D (1975) Significance of renal asymmetry in bone scans: experience in 795 cases. J Nucl Med 16: 161–163

Lin D, Alavi A, Dalinka M (1981) Scintigraphic evaluation of the hyoid bone and the thyroid-cricoid cartilage. Int J Nucl Med Biol 8: 96–104

Makler PT Jr, Charkes ND (1980) Studies of skeletal tracer kinetics. IV. Optimum time delay for Tc-99m (Sn) methylene diphosphonate bone imaging. J Nucl Med 21: 641–645

Maurer AH, Chen DCP, Camargo EE, Wong DF, Wagner HN, Alderson PO (1981) Utility of three-phase skeletal scintigraphy in suspected osteomyelitis. J Nucl Med 22: 941–949

Merrick MV (1973) Detection of skeletal metastases: a comparison of three radioisotope techniques using ^{18}F and radiology. Br J Radiol 46: 968–971

Merrick MV (1975) Review article. Bone scanning. Br J Radiol 48: 327–351

Merrick MV (1984) Essentials of nuclear medicine. Churchill Livingstone, London

Oppenheim BE, Cantez S (1977) What causes lower neck uptake in bone scans? Radiology 124: 749–752

Pitt WR, Sharp PF (1985) Comparison of quantitative and visual detection of new focal bone lesions. J Nucl Med 26: 230–236

Schutte HE (1980) Some special views in bone scanning. Clin Nucl Med 5: 172–173

Smith HL, Beal W, Chaudhuri T (1982) Significance of skull vertex in bone scintigraphy. J Nucl Med 23: 78

Sy WM, Patel D, Faunce H (1975) Significance of absent or faint kidney sign on bone scan. J Nucl Med 16: 454–456

Velchik MG, Heyman S, Makler PT et al. (1984) Bone scintigraphy: differentiating benign cortical irregularity of the distal femur from malignancy. J Nucl Med 25: 72–74

Wilson MA (1981) The effect of age on the quality of bone scans using technetium-99m pyrophosphate. Radiology 139: 703–705

4 · ^{99m}Tc Diphosphonate Bone-scanning Agents

I. Fogelman

Introduction

The ability to image the skeleton by bone scanning, with its sensitivity for disease, is a relatively recent phenomenon and dates back to the development of ^{99m}Tc-labelled polyphosphate by Subramanian and McAfee in 1971. This important advance meant that a compound with high skeletal affinity could at last be combined with a radionuclide with near-ideal physical properties. Nevertheless, there was a continuing search for further improvement and several phosphate compounds rapidly became available (Subramanian et al. 1972a; Fletcher et al. 1973; Citrin et al. 1974). A ^{99m}Tc-labelled diphosphonate (hydroxyethylidene diphosphonate) bone-scanning agent was independently proposed and evaluated by several groups of workers (Castronovo and Callahan 1972; Subramanian et al. 1972b; Tofe and Francis 1972; Yano et al. 1973). Since their introduction, cumulative experience has shown that the diphosphonates are the bone-scanning agents of choice (Subramanian et al. 1972b; Pendergrass et al. 1973; Silberstein et al. 1973; Citrin et al. 1975; Fogelman et al. 1977).

At the present time ^{99m}Tc-labelled methylene diphosphonate (Subramanian et al. 1975) is the most widely used bone-scanning agent. However, several new diphosphonate compounds have recently become available, and there is a clear trend amongst radiopharmaceutical companies to develop agents with relatively high skeletal affinity, leading to greater absolute uptake of tracer by bone. While the resulting improved contrast between bone and background soft tissue may lead to more pleasing images being obtained in normal subjects, it is not clear that higher bone uptake will be equally valuable in the identification of disease. In this chapter the properties required of an ideal bone-scanning agent in both benign and malignant disease are discussed and, in addition, the clinical studies which have evaluated diphosphonate bone-scanning compounds are summarised.

Properties Required of a Bone-scanning Agent

The search for metastatic disease remains the most important single indication for performing a bone scan. Abnormalities in this situation are identified by the presence of focal lesions. Visualisation of a focal lesion depends upon the contrast between the lesion and the surrounding bone, that is to say the ratio of counts in the lesion to those in background bone (L/B; Fig. 4.1b). The contrast between bone and soft-tissue (B/ST) is important for visualisation of the skeleton itself; for a normal subject, a higher B/ST ratio will lead to an improved bone scan (Fig. 4.1a). However, a higher B/ST ratio does not signify that lesions will be better visualised on the bone scan, nor that disorders leading to diffuse abnormality on the bone scan, such as metabolic bone disease, will be more easily identified.

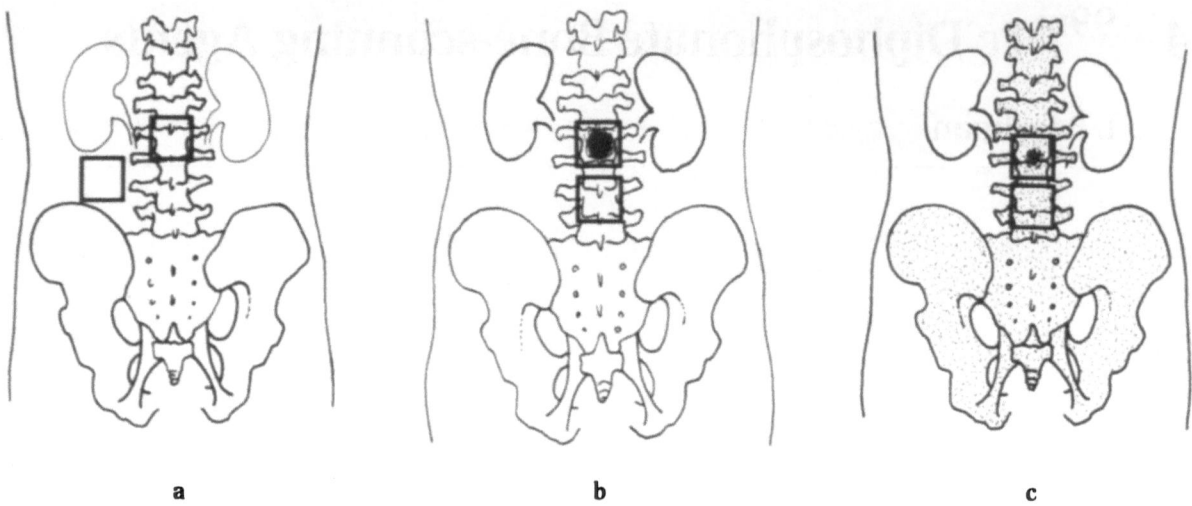

Fig. 4.1. a Regions of interest (ROI) selected over bone and soft tissue. B/ST ratio will reflect skeletal contrast. b ROI over normal bone and vertebra with lesion (L/B ratio). c As in b, but there is higher skeletal affinity for tracer, and, while B/ST ratio will be higher, lesion contrast (L/B ratio) is lower.

It is even possible that different bone-scanning agents may be preferred in various clinical situations. Where visualisation of normal skeletal anatomy is required (although the bone scan is not the technique of choice for this), high uptake of tracer throughout the skeleton is desirable. In metastatic disease the contrast between tumour and background bone is of more importance, and it may be argued that if there is high background uptake of tracer then lesions may be less clearly seen against this background (Fig. 4.1c), unless there is even higher specific uptake of tracer by bone involved with tumour. In the metabolic bone disorders recognition of generalised high uptake of tracer depends upon a subjective evaluation of the scan, and it is also likely that lesions will be more difficult to recognise against high background uptake of tracer by the skeleton.

Thus if a satisfactory bone-scanning agent is available, then on theoretical grounds it would seem that no clear advantage is to be derived from further increasing skeletal uptake of tracer by the normal skeleton. Certainly, if two bone-scanning agents are to be compared in metastatic disease then a simple subjective evaluation of scan appearances or even measuring B/ST ratios is not adequate, as it does not really matter if one scan looks nicer than the other. What is relevant is lesion visualisation and the L/B ratios. Similarly, to state that one agent has faster blood clearance than another does not imply that it is a better agent in clinical practice. If other properties are similar then the agent with higher skeletal affinity will have the faster blood clearance.

It should be apparent that it is not possible to evaluate a bone-scanning agent by randomly allocating patients with metastatic disease to one or another agent and then measuring B/ST ratios or subjectively evaluating the visual quality of these scans. Paired studies, using both agents, should be performed in individual patients. Lesion counts and L/B ratios must be obtained.

^{99m}Tc Diphosphonate Bone-scanning Agents (Fig. 4.2)

^{99m}Tc Hydroxyethylidene Diphosphonate (HEDP)

^{99m}Tc-HEDP was the first diphosphonate to be introduced into clinical practice and is undoubtedly the diphosphonate that has been most extensively evaluated. Several early studies demonstrated that HEDP had improved biological properties, with faster blood clearance, when compared with polyphosphate or pyrophosphate (Dunson et al. 1973; Ackerhalt et al. 1974; Krishnamurthy et al. 1974; Hughes et al. 1975). Not all reports, however, were favourable. In an evaluation of 140 patient studies Nelson et al. (1977) considered HEDP to be inferior to both pyrophosphate and trimetaphosphate. Also Weber et al. (1976) in 90 patient studies preferred pyrophosphate to HEDP. However, in both cases

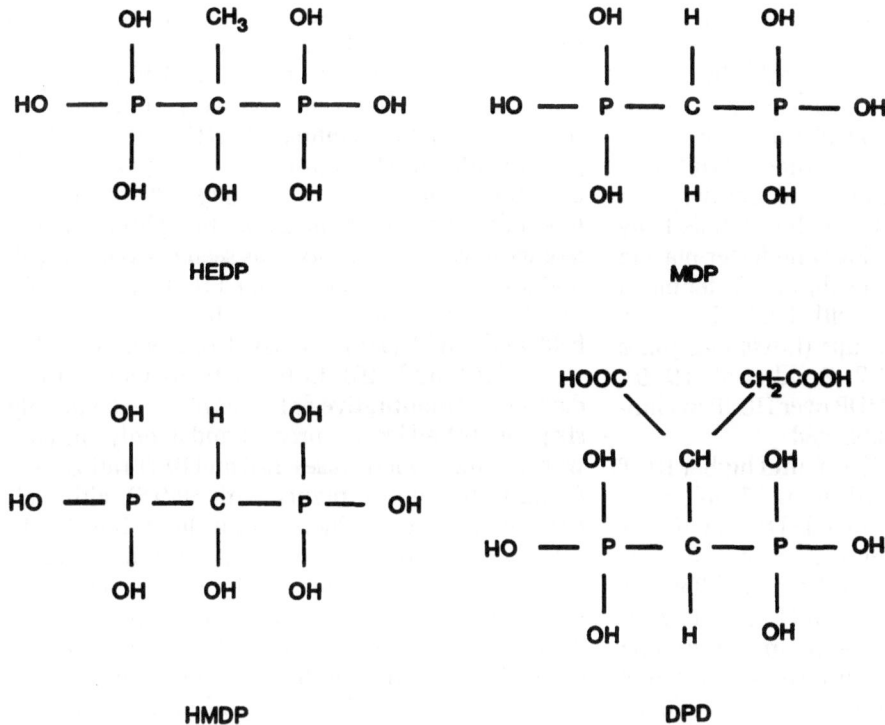

Fig. 4.2. ⁹⁹ᵐTc diphosphonate bone-scanning agents.

evaluation was essentially based on normal scans, and paired studies using both agents in individual patients were not obtained.

Silberstein et al. (1973) carried out paired studies using both HEDP and ¹⁸F in 10 patients with carcinoma and found that ¹⁸F detected only 56% of the lesions seen with HEDP. Pendergrass et al. (1973) reviewed their experience with over 500 scan studies using HEDP and concluded that HEDP was more sensitive for detection of skeletal metastases than ¹⁸F.

Serafini et al. (1974) compared HEDP and pyrophosphate in 18 paired studies: 7 normal subjects and 11 with lesions present on scan. In general it was felt that pyrophosphate gave more variable results and, while the lesion detection rate was the same with both agents, L/B ratios were higher with HEDP in approximately half the cases. In no case was the L/B ratio higher than with pyrophosphate. Silberstein et al. (1978) compared HEDP and pyrophosphate in paired studies in 30 patients with carcinoma. While it was considered that there was no difference in scan quality between agents, 10 of 30 lesions detected with HEDP were not seen with pyrophosphate. Citrin et al. (1975), in a study of 29

patients with skeletal metastases, compared HEDP, pyrophosphate and polyphosphate. All patients had studies with at least two of the three agents. Citrin concluded that HEDP was clearly superior to the other agents and showed that significantly higher L/B ratios were obtained with HEDP when compared with either pyrophosphate or polyphosphate. Fogelman et al. (1977) confirmed these findings in a smaller study of 11 patients with metastatic diseases in which the quality of scan image, lesion detection and L/B ratios were all shown to be superior with HEDP as compared with pyrophosphate.

Lundell et al. (1975) studied nine women who had radiographically proven metastases with HEDP, pyrophosphate and polyphosphate. The scans were visually evaluated, and, while no significant difference in lesion detection was found, it was concluded that HEDP provided superior images with higher lesion to bone contrast. In addition, computer quantitation of the scan images was obtained in three patients (B/ST and L/B ratios), and, although these results were not presented, the authors commented that the findings were in agreement with the visual interpretation.

^{99m}Tc Methylene Diphosphonate (MDP)

Following the introduction of ^{99m}Tc-MDP by Subramanian et al. in 1975, MDP is currently the most widely used bone-scanning agent. However Subramanian's original suggestion that MDP was superior to HEDP as a scanning agent was based on higher bone uptake in rats, higher whole-body retention of tracer in beagle dogs and faster plasma clearance in human volunteer subjects. Faster blood clearance of MDP compared with HEDP has now been confirmed by many groups (Davis and Jones 1976; Rosenthall et al. 1977; Rudd et al. 1979). However, the superiority of MDP over HEDP in clinical practice has not been established.

While Rosenthall et al. (1977) found higher B/ST ratios with MDP than with HEDP in 11 volunteer and 20 patient studies, and concluded that MDP was the preferred radiopharmaceutical, only 7 patients had skeletal metastases, and in these no difference in lesion detection was found. Rudd et al. (1979) carried out paired studies comparing MDP and HEDP in ten patients (six with carcinoma) and found higher B/ST ratios with MDP. They concluded that MDP produced superior images, although no difference in lesion detection was seen. Indeed, Rudd commented that in various clinical situations MDP and HEDP may have different binding mechanisms: In one patient with prostatic carcinoma a lesion was better visualised with HEDP, whereas in a patient with benign vertebral collapse the lesion was better visualised with MDP. Fogelman et al. (1979) compared MDP and HEDP in paired studies in 17 patients with skeletal metastases. Although no difference in the number of lesions detected was found, L/B ratios were significantly higher with HEDP.

^{99m}Tc Hydroxymethylene Diphosphonate (HMDP)

Recently a new diphosphonate, ^{99m}Tc-HMDP, has become available for clinical practice. Early studies demonstrated that it had faster blood clearance (Bevan et al. 1980) and higher skeletal uptake (Bevan et al. 1980; Francis et al. 1980; Fogelman et al. 1981) than MDP.

Domstad et al. (1980) randomly allocated 102 patients to either HMDP or MDP and found higher B/ST ratios with HMDP. However, overall image quality, bone delineation, soft-tissue uptake and L/B ratios were the same with both agents. Silberstein (1980) compared HMDP and HEDP in paired studies in 20 patients with carcinoma and found that HMDP provided superior images in about half the

cases. Quantitative data were only available in seven cases, and L/B ratios in four. Only marginal differences in L/B ratios between HMDP and HEDP (although in HMDP's favour) were found. Rosenthall et al. (1981) compared HMDP and MDP in paired studies in 10 volunteers and 20 patients with carcinoma and found scan quality, B/ST ratios and lesion detection to be the same. In addition, no difference in blood clearance was seen between HMDP and MDP, and it was concluded that there was no significant difference between these agents. Littlefield and Rudd (1983) carried out paired studies with HMDP and MDP in ten patients with various diagnoses. Quantitative data was obtained, but only six patients had lesions present and in only one case was this due to metastases. L/B and B/ST ratios were found to be slightly higher with HMDP, although not significantly so. There was a slight, but significant, observer preference for HMDP when images were evaluated together, but no significant difference was found when the images were independently evaluated; indeed, the MDP images actually scored higher. The number of lesions was found to be too low to assess the efficacy of either agent with regard to lesion detection. In this study it was also shown that HMDP had slightly more rapid blood clearance than MDP. This is somewhat different from the biological data presented by Rosenthall et al. (1981). The reason for this is not known but it is possible that it is in some way related to the method which was used to prepare the radiopharmaceutical. Littlefield injected 20 mCi (740 MBq) ^{99m}Tc into a vial for each patient dose, whereas Rosenthall injected a large dose, of several hundred millicuries, into a vial and obtained multiple patient doses.

Pauwels et al. (1983) evaluated 20 patients with bone metastases. Paired studies were carried out using MDP and either HMDP or dicarboxypropane diphosphonate (DPD). There was no difference seen in location or number of lesions between agents. Furthermore, it was considered that there was no difference in lesion intensity. B/ST ratios were significantly higher with HMDP and DPD than with MDP, but MDP had significantly higher L/B ratios than the other two agents. It was commented upon that the differences in these ratios were generally not appreciated during visual inspection of the bone scan images. It was concluded that HMDP and DPD do not possess clinical advantages over MDP for the detection of skeletal metastases. Van Duzee et al. (1984) compared bone scan images in 28 patients with skeletal metastases at 2 and 4 h after injection with MDP and with HMDP. There was no significant difference in lesion identification with either agent at 2 or 4 h. Quantitation of images was carried out;

L/B ratios were marginally higher with HMDP, although this difference was not significant. B/ST ratios, however, were significantly higher with HMDP and image quality was considered subjectively to be better than with MDP. Delaloye et al. (1985) have reported results from a multicentre investigation involving six departments in five countries in which paired studies using HMDP and MDP were performed in 33 patients with skeletal metastases at 2 and 3 h after injection. There was no difference in lesion detection between agents even when 2-h images were compared with 3-h ones. HMDP had higher B/ST ratios, but no significant difference was found for L/B ratios, although values were marginally higher for MDP. Image quality was felt to be improved with HMDP, but it was stated that the quality of 2-h HMDP scans did not reach that of 3-h MDP scans, which were clearly superior.

⁹⁹ᵐTc Dicarboxypropane Diphosphonate (DPD)

⁹⁹ᵐTc-DPD is the newest of the available diphosphonates and, as with HMDP, it is claimed that DPD has significantly higher skeletal uptake than MDP. Schwarz and Kloss (1981) found DPD to have 15% higher bone uptake when compared with MDP in rat studies. In addition, in 300 patient studies it was considered that DPD showed superior skeletal visualisation when compared with MDP. Hale et al. (1981), in 60 patient studies comparing DPD and MDP, also found improved skeletal visualisation and higher B/ST ratios with DPD.

Buell et al. (1982) evaluated a total of 839 bone scans obtained with MDP (636) and DPD (203) in patients with a variety of disorders. Bone scans were obtained at approximately 2 h after injection, and the B/ST ratios were measured at 2 sites—the femoral diaphysis, considered to be a "low-uptake" area, and the sacrum, a "high-uptake" area. Higher values for both ratios were found for DPD than for MDP. In addition, higher values were found for B/ST ratios in patients who had a history of malignant disease, even when metastases were not visualised.

Mele et al. (1983) studied 18 normal subjects, 9 each with MDP and DPD. There was no difference seen in scan quality. In this study quantitative data was generated using compartmental kinetic analysis. Results suggested that MDP had higher bone uptake and lower soft tissue retention than DPD.

Schroth et al. (1984) randomly allocated ten patients with carcinoma of the thyroid to be given bone scans with either MDP or DPD. They found that clearance of MDP from the blood was slightly faster than DPD up to 4.5 h, and no significant difference in B/ST ratios were shown. However, urinary excretion of MDP was higher throughout a 10-h period. In addition, a single paired study (using both MDP and DPD scans) was carried out in a patient with multiple skeletal metastases. No difference in L/B ratios was found, and the authors concluded that MDP was not better than DPD in detecting bone lesions. One may feel that it is difficult to justify such a conclusion on the basis of a single study in a patient with extensive skeletal disease.

As stated previously, Pauwels et al. (1983) carried out paired studies comparing MDP and DPD in ten cases with skeletal metastases. They did not find any difference in lesion detection. Studies with DPD had higher B/ST ratios, but those with MDP had the higher L/B values.

Discussion

There seems to be little doubt that the ⁹⁹ᵐTc-labelled diphosphonates deserve their virtual monopoly in the bone-scanning field. Early studies exhaustively evaluated ⁹⁹ᵐTc-HEDP and showed it to be clearly superior to the other available agents at that time— ¹⁸F, ⁹⁹ᵐTc pyrophosphate and ⁹⁹ᵐTc polyphosphate. However, the later diphosphonates with their increased uptake in bone have not been as extensively evaluated, and, as has been shown, there is no evidence that any of these diphosphonates is superior to ⁹⁹ᵐTc-HEDP as regards lesion detection in malignancy. Nevertheless, current bone scans do look much improved, and this presumably reflects the combination of advances in gamma camera technology together with higher skeletal uptake of radiopharmaceutical. However, one must not confuse the two quite separate issues of a good-looking bone scan in a normal subject and sensitivity for identification of skeletal lesions, particularly metastases. Moreover, just because the bone scan is already the most sensitive means of identifying metastases we should not become complacent and must be receptive to the possibility of further advances with regard to improved sensitivity. As discussed previously, the identification of metastases depends upon L/B ratios and not B/ST ratios. In the only study comparing L/B ratios in scans obtained with both ⁹⁹ᵐTc-MDP and ⁹⁹ᵐTc-HEDP, higher values were obtained with ⁹⁹ᵐTc-HEDP (Fogelman et al. 1979). Arnold et al. (1978), using a computerised technique for subtracting blood and soft tissue backgrounds from sequential images of bone, found that marked differences exist between the kinetic behaviour of ^{99m}Tc-MDP and ^{99m}Tc-HEDP, with each having different binding characteristics. It was suggested that while ^{99m}Tc-MDP may be the better agent for imaging the skeleton, ^{99m}Tc-HEDP may image osteoblastic lesions better. However, while this evidence perhaps marginally favours ^{99m}Tc-HEDP over ^{99m}Tc-MDP with regard to lesion detection, ^{99m}Tc-HEDP is no longer commercially available and ^{99m}Tc-MDP is currently the most popular bone-scanning agent. More recently, Pauwels et al. (1983) have shown that ^{99m}Tc-MDP has higher L/B ratios than ^{99m}Tc-HMDP and ^{99m}Tc-DPD, two newer agents which have even higher absolute skeletal uptake. Subramanian et al. (1983) used a rabbit model where lesions were drilled in bone and also found lower L/B ratios with ^{99m}Tc-DPD and ^{99m}Tc-HMDP when compared with ^{99m}Tc-MDP. These findings support the view that the higher the background bone uptake of tracer, the lower the L/B ratio is likely to be. Although one can certainly argue about the theoretical advantages of one diphosphonate as compared with another with regard to lesion detection, in multiple comparative studies of bone-scanning agents no commercially available diphosphonate has been shown to identify lesions missed by another.

Two recent reports of a "new" diphosphonate bone-scanning agent ^{99m}Tc dimethyl-amino diphosphonate (DMAD) (Fig. 4.3) have stated that several of the lesions identified were not seen on the MDP scan (Rosenthall et al. 1982; Smith et al. 1984).

However, ^{99m}Tc-DMAD is not commercially available and has been provided to investigators by Dr. Subramanian. There is extremely low uptake of ^{99m}Tc-DMAD by normal bone and the images obtained would be of unacceptable quality to most nuclear medicine physicians; however, there is high uptake of ^{99m}Tc-DMAD in lesions and this, therefore, gives rise to extremely high L/B ratios. Certainly, it is only with ^{99m}Tc-DMAD that I personally have been convinced that it is possible to see lesions that are not visualised with another diphosphonate (Fig. 4.4). In both reports of ^{99m}Tc-DMAD, studies were performed in patients with widespread metastases. Although one would anticipate that a "low-uptake" agent would have increased sensitivity in the identification of early disease, this has still to be proven. I now believe that there is a strong case to be made for the availability of a low-uptake agent such as ^{99m}Tc-DMAD. It is clear that this would not be acceptable for routine use but may have a valuable role to play in selected cases, e.g. when an equivocal lesion is noted in the spine, or if a patient with a known primary tumour is complaining of bone pain and yet no abnormality is seen on the initial scan. A potential disadvantage of ^{99m}Tc-DMAD is that because of its poor uptake in normal bone one may well miss photon-deficient lesions. However, these are relatively uncommon and would presumably be identified on the standard ^{99m}Tc-MDP scan.

In Fig. 4.5, the relative skeletal uptake of ^{99m}Tc-DPD, ^{99m}Tc-HMDP, ^{99m}Tc-MDP and ^{99m}Tc-HEDP obtained by the 24-h whole-body retention (WBR) of diphosphonate technique (Fogelman et al. 1978) is shown. This confirms that both ^{99m}Tc-DPD and ^{99m}Tc-HMDP do indeed have higher skeletal uptake than ^{99m}Tc-MDP, although there has been some suggestion that ^{99m}Tc-DPD may have slightly higher muscle uptake than other diphosphonates (Subramanian et al. 1983), and it is not clear to what extent this is reflected in the WBR result. WBR measurements have also been obtained with ^{99m}Tc-DMAD; this diphosphonate has extremely low uptake at around 12% in normal subjects at 24 h (Rosenthall et al. 1982). It is apparent that slight alterations in molecular structure can have a significant effect on affinity for skeletal surfaces. However, it would appear that each diphosphonate behaves in a characteristic way, as Fogelman et al. (1981) have shown that the pattern of uptake of three different diphosphonates (HEDP, MDP and HMDP) was the same in studies performed on 20 volunteer subjects (Fig. 4.6).

Where quantitative 24-h WBR of diphosphonate measurements have been used to identify patients with increased bone turnover, it has previously been

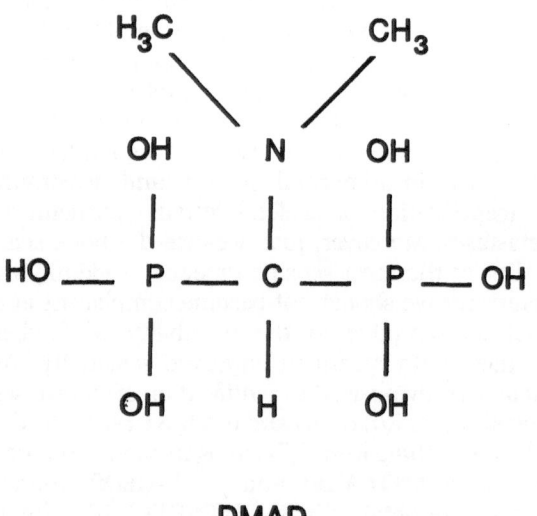

DMAD

Fig. 4.3. ^{99m}Tc dimethyl-amino diphosphonate (DMAD).

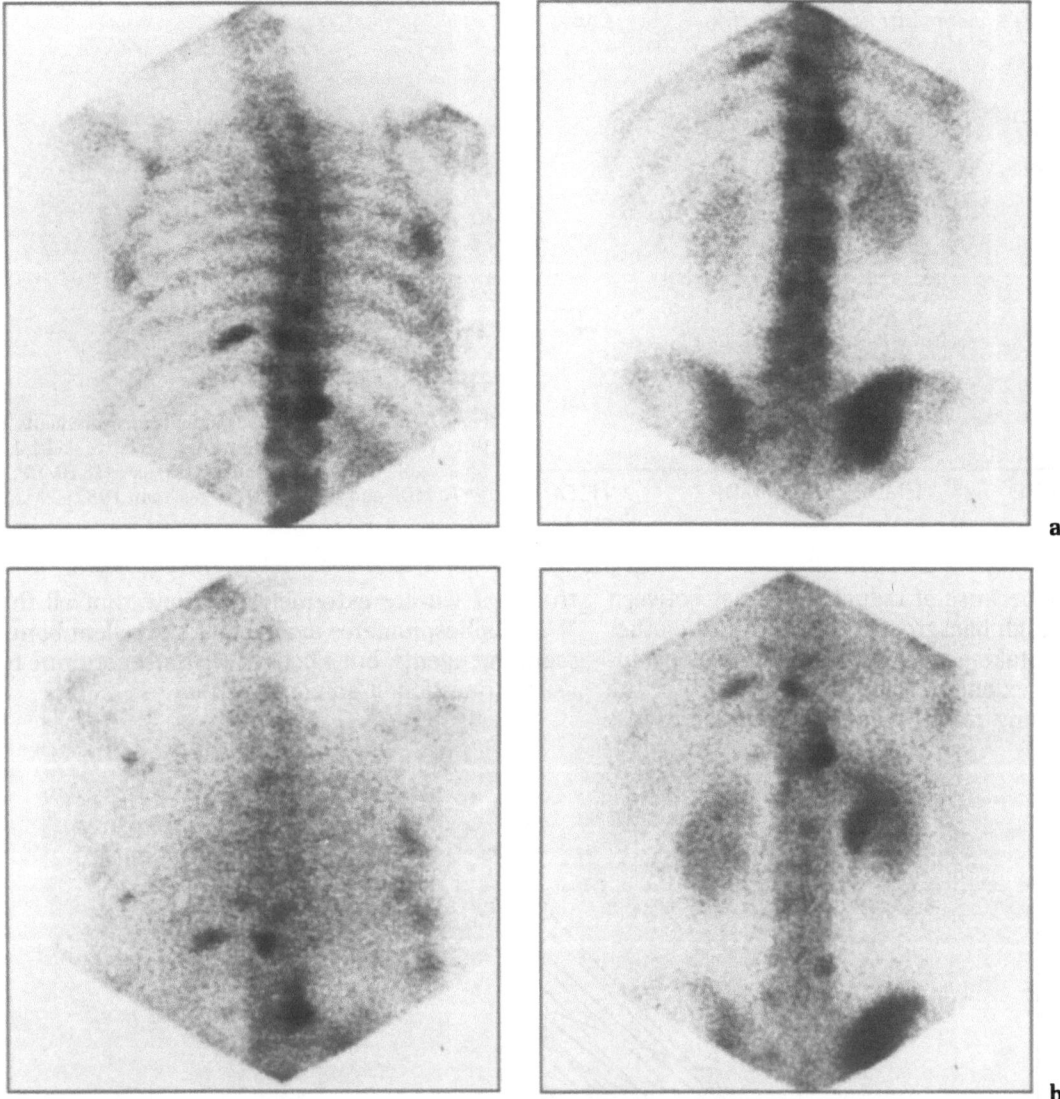

Fig. 4.4a, b. Images of posterior spine. a MDP scan; b DMAD scan. It is apparent that several lesions are seen on b but not on a.

suggested that ^{99m}Tc-HEDP with its tighter normal range and lower absolute skeletal uptake may show advantages over higher uptake agents as it provides a wider range in which to detect abnormality with less overlap between normal and abnormal (Fogelman et al. 1981). ^{99m}Tc-DMAD has not been evaluated in this context.

The availability of ^{99m}Tc-labelled diphosphonate for bone scanning has revolutionised our ability to investigate skeletal disease. Uptake of diphosphonate is directly related to skeletal metabolism, and potential uses and applications of bone-scanning and quantitative techniques are only just becoming appreciated by physicians with bone-related interests such as metabolic bone disease,

rheumatology, oncology and orthopaedics. It is now clear that various diphosphonates can have quite different affinities for bone (Fogelman et al. 1981) with different clinical properties. However, at the present time, there has not been found to be any significant difference amongst the commercially available ^{99m}Tc diphosphonates as regards lesion detection, although it has been shown that ^{99m}Tc-DMAD, a low-uptake agent can on occasion visualise lesions that are not detected by other diphosphonates. There does not appear to be any advantage in continuing to develop agents with higher bone uptake, and it is at least theoretically possible that by further increasing bone uptake of tracer a significant reduction in lesion detection

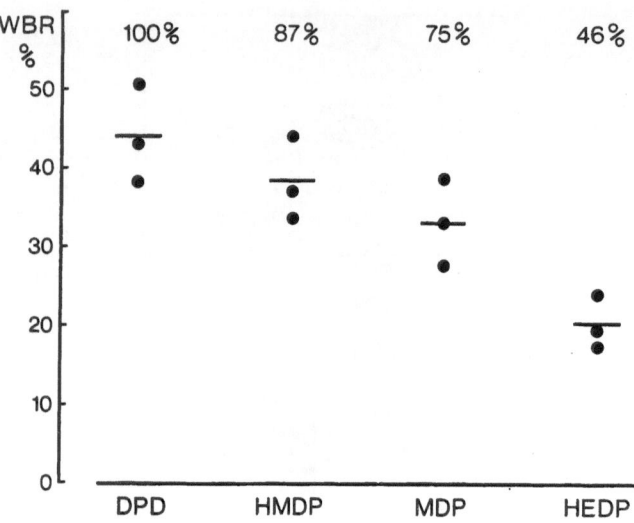

Fig. 4.5. 24-h WBR of diphosphonate measurements in three volunteer subjects showing the relative skeletal uptakes of 99mTc-DPD (taken as 100%), 99mTc-HMDP, 99mTc-MDP and 99mTc-HEDP. (Fogelman 1982)

could occur because of reduced contrast between lesions and high background activity. On the other hand, low-uptake agents should be further evaluated in more extensive trials to assess whether the initial promising results can be substantiated. It is true that we are extremely fortunate that all the 99mTc diphosphonates available are excellent bone-scanning agents, but I believe we must continue to ask the question "Can we do better?"

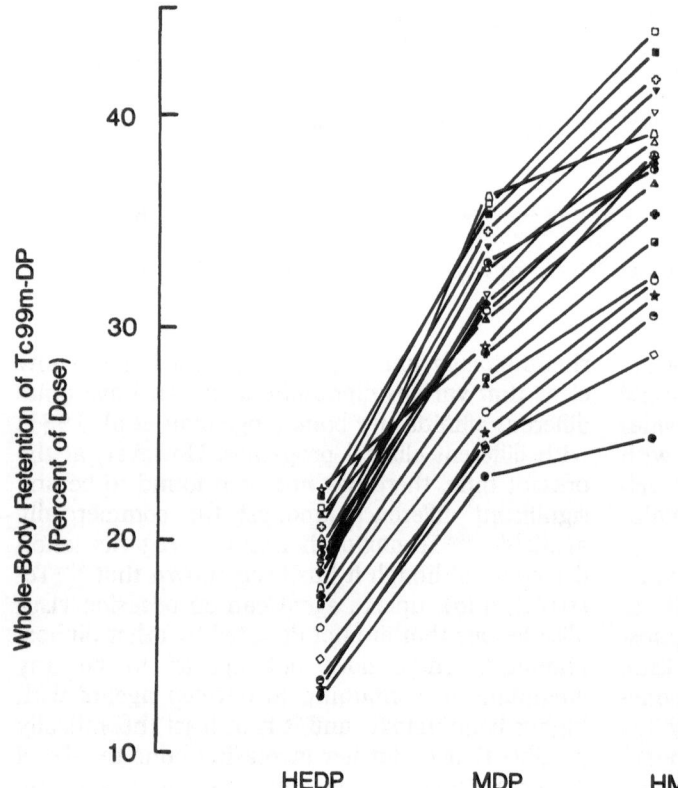

Fig. 4.6. Repeat 24-h WBR measurements using 99mTc-HEDP, 99mTc-MDP, and 99mTc-HMDP in 20 normal subjects. (Fogelman et al. 1981)

References

Ackerhalt RE, Blau M, Bakshi S, Sondel JA (1974) A comparative study of three ^{99m}Tc-labelled phosphorus compounds and ^{18}F-fluoride for skeletal imaging. J Nucl Med 15: 1153–1157

Arnold JS, Barnes WE, Khedkar N, Nelson M (1978) Computerized kinetic analysis of two ^{99m}Tc-Sn-diphosphonates demonstrating different binding characteristics. AJR 131: 553

Bevan JA, Tofe AJ, Benedict JJ, Francis MD, Barnett BL, (1980) Tc-99m HMDP (hydroxymethylene diphosphonate): a radiopharmaceutical for skeletal and acute myocardial infarct imaging. 1. Synthesis and distribution in animals. J Nucl Med 21: 961–966

Buell U, Kleinhans E, Zorn-Bopp E, Reuschel W, Muenzing W, Moser EA, Seiderer M (1982) A comparison of bone imaging with Tc-99m DPD and Tc-99m MDP: concise communication. J Nucl Med 23: 214–217

Castronovo FP, Callahan RJ (1972) New bone scanning agent: ^{99m}Tc labeled 1-hydroxyethylidene-1, 1-disodium phosphonate. J Nucl Med 13: 823–827

Citrin DL, Bessent RG, Greig WR (1974) Clinical evaluation of ^{99m}Tc-labeled monofluorophosphate: a comparison with ethane-hydroxy-diphosphonate. J Nucl Med 15: 1110–1112

Citrin DL, Bessent RG, Tuohy JB, Elms ST, McGinley E, Greig WR, Blumgart LH (1975) A comparison of phosphate bone-scanning agents in normal subjects and patients with malignant disease. Br J Radiol 48: 118–121

Davis AG, Jones AG (1976) Comparison of ^{99m}Tc-labeled phosphate and phosphonate agents for skeletal imaging. Semin Nucl Med 6: 19–31

Delaloye B, Delaloye-Bischof A, Dudczak R, Koppenhagen K, Mata F, Penafiel A, Maul FD, Pasquier J (1985) Clinical comparison of ^{99m}Tc-HMDP and ^{99m}Tc-MDP. A multicenter study. Eur J Nucl Med 11: 182–185

Domstad PA, Coupal JJ, Kim EE, Blake JS, DeLand FH (1980) ^{99m}Tc-hydroxymethane diphosphonate: a new bone imaging agent with a low tin content. Radiology 136: 209–211

Dunson GL, Stevenson JS, Cole CM, Mellor MK, Hosain F (1973) Preparation and comparison of technetium-99m diphosphonate, polyphosphate and pyrophosphate in nuclear bone imaging radiopharmaceuticals. Drug Intell Clin Pharmacol 7: 470–474

Fletcher JW, Solaric-George E, Henry RE, Donati RM (1973) Evaluation of ^{99m}Tc-pyrophosphate as a bone imaging agent. Radiology 109: 467–469

Fogelman I (1982) Diphosphonate bone scanning agents—current concepts. Eur J Nucl Med 7: 506–509

Fogelman I, McKillop JH, Citrin DL (1977) A clinical comparison of ^{99m}Tc-hydroxyethylidene diphosphonate (H.E.D.P.) and ^{99m}Tc-pyrophosphate in the detection of bone metastases. Clin Nucl Med 2: 364–367

Fogelman I, Bessent RG, Turner JG, Citrin DL, Boyle IT, Greig WR (1978) The use of whole-body retention of Tc-99m diphosphonate in the diagnosis of metabolic bone disease. J Nucl Med 19: 270–275

Fogelman I, Citrin DL, McKillop JH, Turner JG, Bessent RG (1979) A clinical comparison of ^{99m}Tc-HEDP and ^{99m}Tc-MDP in the detection of bone metastases: concise communication. J Nucl Med 20: 98–101

Fogelman I, Pearson DW, Bessent RG, Tofe AJ, Francis MD (1981) A comparison of skeletal uptake of three diphosphonates by whole-body retention: concise communication. J Nucl Med 22: 880–883

Francis MD, Ferguson DL, Tofe AJ, Bevan JA, Michaels SE (1980) Comparative evaluation of three diphosphonates: in vitro adsorption (C-14 labeled) and in vivo osteogenic uptake (Tc-99m complexed). J Nucl Med 21: 1185–1189

Hale TI, Jucker A, Vgenopoulos K, Sauter B, Wacheck W, Bors L (1981) Clinical experience with a new bone seeking ^{99m}Tc radiopharmaceutical. Nucl Compact 12: 54–55

Hughes SPF, Jeyasingh K, Lavender PJ (1975) Phosphate compounds in bone scanning. J Bone Joint Surg [Br] 57: 214–216

Krishnamurthy GT, Tubis M, Endow JS, Singhi V, Walsh CF, Blahd WH (1974) Clinical comparison of the kinetics of ^{99m}Tc-labeled polyphosphate and diphosphonate. J Nucl Med 15: 848–855

Littlefield JL, Rudd TG (1983) Tc-99m hydroxymethylene diphosphonate and Tc-99m methylene diphosphonate: biological and clinical comparison: concise communication. J Nucl Med 24: 463–466

Lundell G, Marell E, Backstrom A, Casseborn S, Ruden B-I (1975) Bone scanning with ^{99m}Tc compounds in metastasizing mammary carcinoma. Acta Radiol Ther Phys Biol 14: 333–336

Mele M, Conte E, Fratello A, Pasculli D, Pieralice M, D'Addabbo A (1983) Computer analysis of Tc-99m DPD and Tc-99m MDP kinetics in human: concise communication. J Nucl Med 24: 334–338

Nelson MF, McKee LC, Van Wazer JR (1977) Clinical evaluation of some phosphorus bone-imaging agents: concise communication. J Nucl Med 18: 566–569

Pauwels EKJ, Blom J, Camps JAJ, Hermans J, Rijke AM (1983) A comparison between the diagnostic efficacy of ^{99m}Tc-MDP, ^{99m}Tc-DPD and ^{99m}Tc-HDP for the detection of bone metastases. Eur J Nucl Med 25: 166–169

Pendergrass HP, Potsaid MS, Castronovo FP (1973) The clinical use of ^{99m}Tc-diphosphonate (HEDSPA). Radiology 107: 557–562

Rosenthall L, Arzoumanian A, Lisbona R, Itoh K (1977) A longitudinal comparison of the kinetics of ^{99m}Tc-MDP and ^{99m}Tc-HEDP in humans. Clin Nucl Med 2: 232–234

Rosenthall L, Arzoumanian A, Damtew B, Tremblay J (1981) A crossover study comparing Tc-99m-HMDP and MDP in patients. Clin Nucl Med 6: 353–355

Rosenthall L, Stern J, Arzoumanian A (1982) A clinical comparison of MDP and DMAD. Clin Nucl Med 7: 403–406

Rudd TG, Allen DR, Smith FD (1979) Technetium-99m-labeled methylene diphosphonate and hydroxyethylidene diphosphonate—biologic and clinical comparison: concise communication. J Nucl Med 20: 821–826

Schroth H-J, Hausinger F, Garth H, Oberhausen E (1984) Comparison of the kinetics of methylene-diphosphonate (MDP) and dicarboxypropan-diphosphonic acid (DPD), two radiodiagnostics for bone scintigraphy. Eur J Nucl Med 9: 529–532

Schwarz A, Kloss G (1981) Technetium-99m DPD—a new skeletal imaging agent. J Nucl Med 22: 77 (abstract)

Serafini AN, Watson DD, Nelston JP, Smoak WM (1974) Bone scintigraphy—comparison of ^{99m}Tc-polyphosphate and ^{99m}Tc-diphosphonate. J Nucl Med 15: 1101–1104

Silberstein EB (1980) A radiopharmaceutical and clinical comparison of ^{99m}Tc-Sn-hydroxymethylene diphosphonate. Radiology 136: 747–751

Silberstein EB, Saenger EL, Tofe AJ, Alexander GW, Park H-M (1973) Imaging of bone metastases with ^{99m}Tc-Sn-EHDP (diphosphonate), ^{18}F, and skeletal radiography. A comparison of sensitivity. Radiology 107: 551–555

Silberstein EB, Maxon HR, Alexander GW, Rauf C, Bahr GK (1978) Clinical comparison of technetium-99m diphosphonate and pyrophosphate in bone scintigraphy: concise communication. J Nucl Med 19: 161–163

Smith ML, Martin W, McKillop JH, Fogelman I (1984) Improved lesion detection with dimethyl-amino-diphosphonate: a report of two cases. Eur J Nucl Med 9: 519–520

Subramanian G, McAfee JG (1971) A new complex of ^{99m}Tc for skeletal imaging. Radiology 99: 192–196

Subramanian G, McAfee JG, Bell EG, Blair RJ, O'Mara RE, Ralston

PH (1972a) ^{99m}Tc-labeled polyphosphate as a skeletal imaging agent. Radiology 102: 701–704

Subramanian G, McAfee JG, Blair RJ, Mehter A, Connor T (1972b) ^{99m}Tc-EHDP: a potential radiopharmaceutical for skeletal imaging. J Nucl Med 13: 947–950

Subramanian G, McAfee JG, Blair RJ, Kallfelz FA, Thomas FD (1975) Technetium-99m-methylene diphosphonate—a superior agent for skeletal imaging: comparison with other technetium complexes. J Nucl Med 16: 744–755

Subramanian G, McAfee JG, Thomas FD, Feld TA, Zapf-Longo C, Palladino E (1983) New diphosphonate compounds for skeletal imaging: comparison with methylene diphosphonate. Radiology 149: 823–828

Tofe AJ, Francis MD (1972) In vitro optimization and organ distribution studies in animals with the bone scanning agent ^{99m}Tc-Sn-EHDP. J Nucl Med 13: 472 (abstract)

Van Duzee BF, Schaefer JA, Ball JD, Chilton HM, Cowan RJ, Kuni C, Trow R, Watson NE (1984) Relative lesion detection ability of Tc-99m HMDP and Tc-99m MDP: concise communication. J Nucl Med 25: 166–169

Weber DA, Keyes JW, Wilson GA, Landman S (1976) Kinetics and imaging characteristics of ^{99m}Tc-labeled complexes used for bone imaging. Radiology 120: 615–621

Yano Y, McRae J, Van Dyke DC, Anger HO (1973) Technetium-99m-labeled stannous ethane-1-hydroxy-1, 1-diphosphonate: a new bone scanning agent. J Nucl Med 14: 73–78

5 · Bone Scanning in Metastatic Disease

J. H. McKillop

Introduction

The isotope bone scan is now generally accepted as the initial investigation of choice in the search for bone metastases from most tumours. The relative insensitivity of the bone radiograph for the detection of metastases has long been noted (Borak 1942; Shackman and Harrison 1947), and symptoms from bone metastases occur before there is radiographic evidence of abnormality in a sizable minority of patients (Clain 1965).

Uptake of the bone-scanning agents in normal bone is the result of both skeletal blood flow and some aspect of skeletal metabolism, possibly osteoblastic activity (Fogelman 1980). This topic has been extensively covered in Chapter 2. The localisation of bone-scanning agents in areas of abnormal bone is similarly dependent on bone metabolism. The increased sensitivity of the bone scan over the bone radiograph for the detection of metastases is due to the fact that invasion of the skeleton by malignant cells will excite functional (metabolic) changes before there is significant structural change. Bone metastases usually evoke both an increase in local blood flow and reactive new bone formation at a time when no bone destruction or bone reaction can be seen radiographically (Charkes et al. (1968).

Appearance of Metastases on the Bone Scan

Metastases from most tumours will excite some osteoblastic response in the bone, even when apparently lytic on the bone radiograph. The characteristic appearance of a metastasis on the bone scan is thus one of focally increased uptake or a "hot spot". The usual appearance of multiple metastases is of irregularly distributed areas of increased uptake (Fig. 5.1). The site of the primary tumour cannot be inferred from the appearances of the metastases on the scan.

In the patient with extensive bone metastases, the bone scan may resemble the "superscan" appearance of metabolic bone disease. This pattern may occur with any tumour but is most commonly seen in disseminated prostatic cancer. The scan shows generally increased tracer uptake in the skeleton with low background activity and faint or absent renal images (Fig. 5.2). The "metastatic" superscan can usually, though not always, be distinguished from that due to metabolic disease by the slightly irregular uptake of tracer within the skeleton, especially the ribs (Fogelman et al. 1977).

If the metastasis fails to excite an osteoblastic response the bone scan may appear normal. The incidence of false-negative scan results in bone

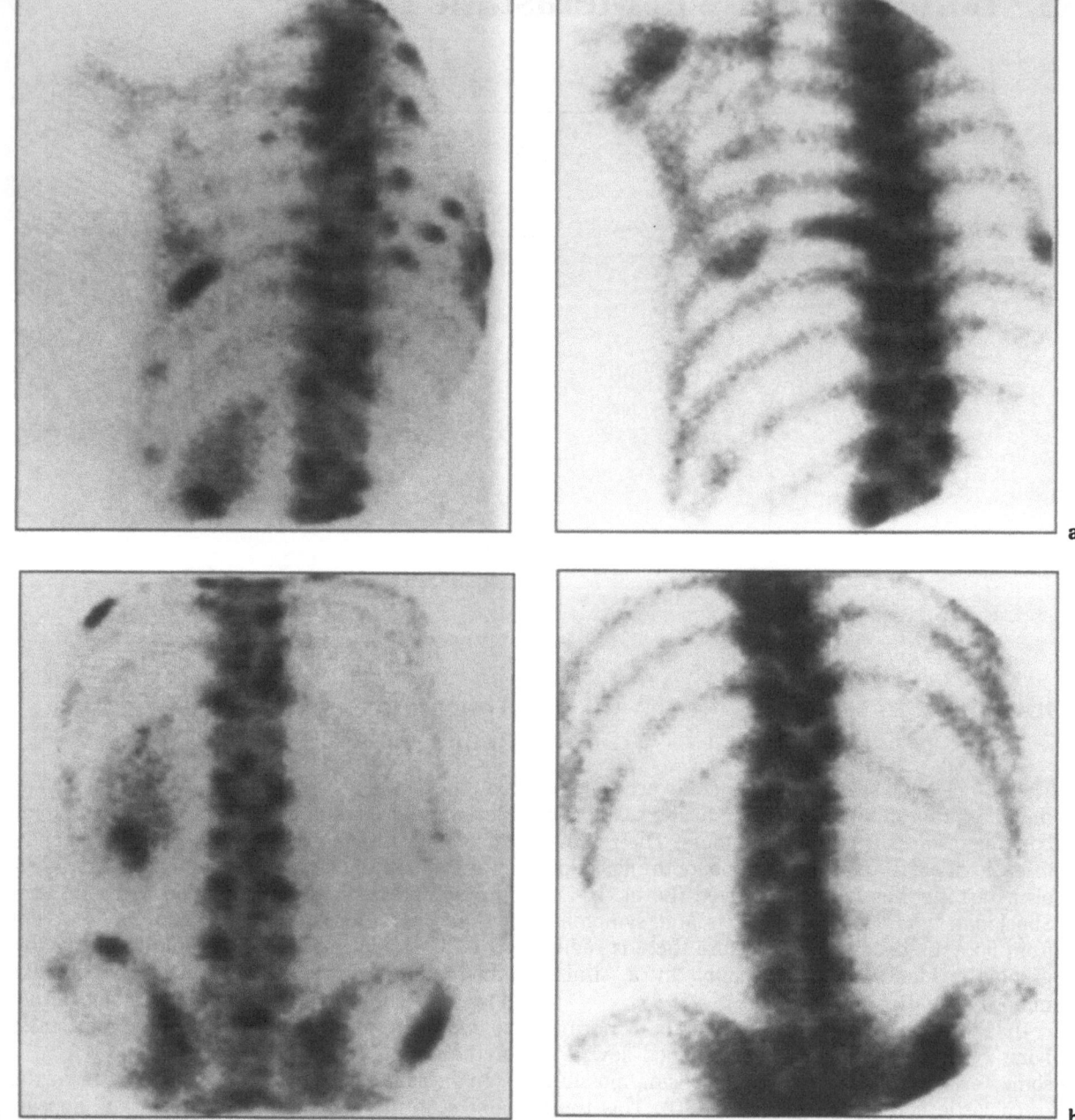

Fig. 5.1a,b. Bone scan of patient with breast carcinoma and bone metastases. Irregular foci of increased tracer uptake throughout the ribs, dorsal and lumbar spine, both sacroiliac joints and both iliac bones. The right kidney is absent (nephrectomy after trauma) and pooling of urine is seen at the lower pole of the left kidney.

Fig. 5.2a,b. Diffusely increased uptake in patient with widespread skeletal metastases from carcinoma of the prostate. The kidneys are not seen. The picture resembles the superscan of metabolic bone disease apart from slight irregularity of tracer uptake in the left ribs.

metastases has been reported to be less than 3% (Pistenma et al. 1975; Citrin and McKillop 1978). In patients with a high suspicion of metastases but a normal bone scan, bone radiographs should be obtained.

In the case of some bone metastases the bone scan may show areas of decreased uptake ("cold spots" or photopaenic lesions; Stadalnik 1979). The lesion may either appear as a central cold area with increased activity around it (Fig. 5.3) or as a purely

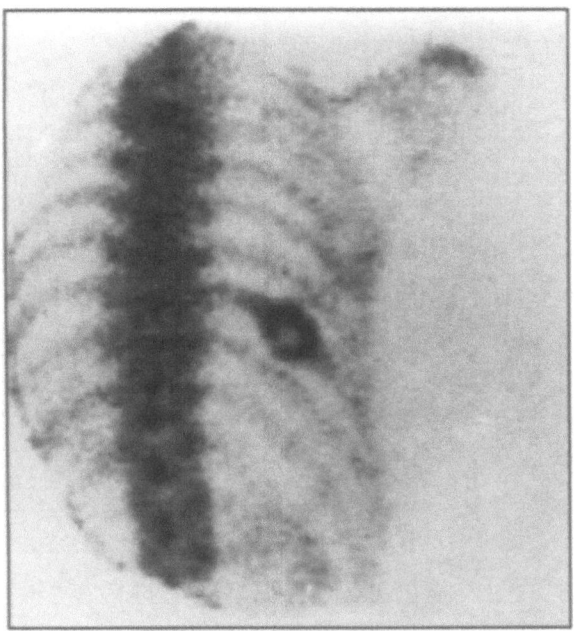

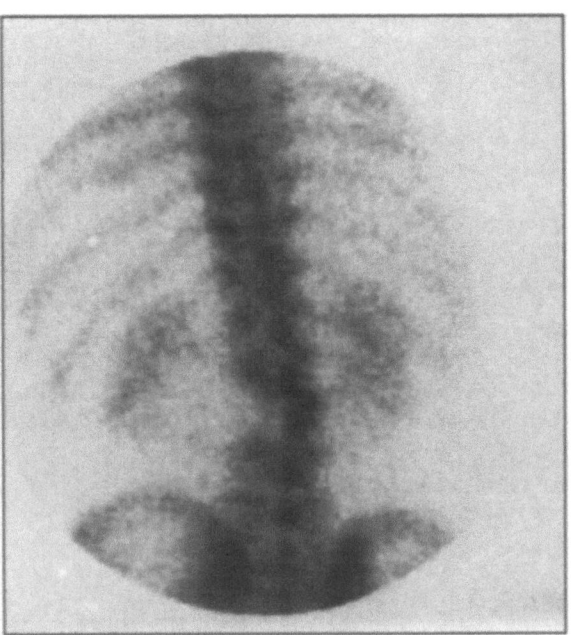

Fig. 5.3. Rib metastasis from carcinoma of prostate showing increased uptake around a cold centre.

Fig. 5.4. Metastasis from anaplastic carcinoma (site unknown) causing a cold spot in the left half of LV-3. There is also some decreased uptake in the lower part of the body of LV-2.

cold lesion (Fig. 5.4). Photopaenic metastases have been reported in many different tumours, including those in children (Weingrad et al. 1984), but are particularly common in myeloma (Wahner et al. 1980) and in renal carcinoma (Kim et al. 1983). The frequency with which cold lesions are recognised may increase in the future as newer gamma cameras with increased resolution become more widely available. Currently, around 2% of metastatic lesions are reported to produce cold spots (Kober et al. 1979).

The scan characteristics of individual metastases may change spontaneously in the course of the disease, either from "hot" to normal (Goergen et al. 1974), from "hot" to "cold" (Makoha and Britton 1980), or from individual "hot spots" to superscan (Manier and van Nostrand 1983). Therapy may produce further changes in scan appearances, but these will be considered separately.

Significance of Bone Scan Abnormalities in the Cancer Patient

The normal bone scan has been discussed in detail in Chapter 3, and the need to recognise areas of the skeleton which normally show increased tracer uptake has been stressed. The periarticular areas represent a common area of potential confusion. Recently it has also been reported that sites of muscle insertion may show some increase in tracer uptake. The deltoid tuberosity may be associated with focally increased uptake which can be misinterpreted as a pathological lesion (Fink-Bennett and Vicuna-Rios 1980). "Stippling" of the ribs at the insertion of the ileocostalis thoracis portion of the erector spinae muscles has been reported to occur as a normal variant in around 7% of patients (Fink-Bennett and Johnson 1985).

The main shortcoming of the bone scan is the non-specificity of a "hot spot" for metastatic disease. Many forms of benign skeletal disease produce a hot spot. There is no way of being absolutely certain from the bone scan alone as to whether the abnormality is due to metastases or some more benign disease.

The *avidity* of uptake of tracer within the lesion does not provide any guide as to its nature—metastases, fractures, osteomyelitis and Paget's disease all commonly cause markedly increased tracer uptake. Some malignant lesions, on the other hand, will cause only slightly increased bone tracer uptake. Some recent work has suggested that benign and malignant lesions within the spine

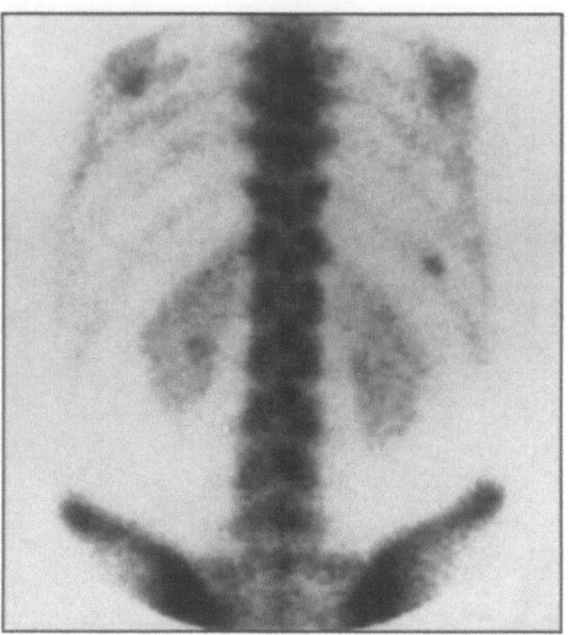

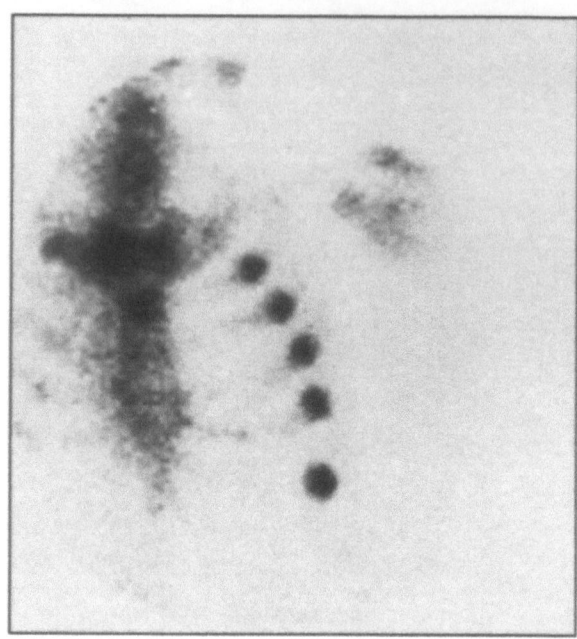

Fig. 5.5. Single hot spot in the right 11th rib of a woman presenting with Stage I breast cancer and no clinical evidence of bone metastases. A bone scan 6 months later was normal.

Fig. 5.6. Multiple anterior rib fractures following a road accident in a man with surgically treated prostatic cancer. The scan was otherwise normal and he had no evidence of metastases 15 months later.

might be differentiated by measuring lesion to non-lesion uptake ratio at 4 and 24 h after injection (Israel et al. 1985). Patients with degenerative disease of the spine in this study showed no significant change in the ratio between 4 and 24 h. Patients with metastases had a higher mean lesion to non-lesion uptake ratio at 4 h, and it increased further at 24 h. This interesting observation requires confirmation.

The *number* of lesions on a bone scan may provide some guide as to the likely cause. The patient who shows multiple areas of increased uptake irregularly scattered through the skeleton, is very likely to have metastatic disease, but other causes such as trauma or Paget's disease cannot be completely excluded. Patients with a primary cancer who have a single bone scan abnormality are an especially difficult group (Fig. 5.5). Around 7% of patients with metastases will present with a single lesion on the bone scan (Corcoran et al. 1976; Rappaport et al. 1978; Brown 1983). A single abnormality, however, has a significant probability of being due to a non-malignant lesion. In the three series cited, 55% of the solitary scan abnormalities were due to neoplastic disease. The remainder were due to trauma (25%), infection (10%) and miscellaneous causes (10%). The probability of a malignant cause for a solitary hot spot in patients with a known pri-

mary cancer also varies with the site of the bone scan abnormality. Tumeh et al. (1985) have reported that solitary rib lesions are rare in cancer patients and, when present, are usually due to benign disease. McNeil (1984) states that in the case of solitary rib lesions the frequency of a malignant cause has been estimated to vary between 1% and 17%, while around 80% of vertebral lesions are malignant. Isolated joint abnormalities are likely to be due to arthritis.

The *location* and *distribution* of multiple bone scan lesions may also help in determining their nature. For example, a linear array of hot spots in the ribs (Fig. 5.6) is probably due to trauma (Schutte 1980; Harbert et al. 1981). In the case of metastatic lesions from breast and lung cancer, thoracic spine or rib lesions are common (more than 80% of the total) and limbs sites uncommon (15% of the total) (Wilson and Calhoun 1981).

The *shape* of a scan abnormality may occasionally be helpful in determining the cause. Thus an elongated rib lesion (Fig. 5.7) is likely to be malignant, while a focal rib lesion is often due to fracture (Matin 1982). The intense uniform involvement, often of a whole bone, in Paget's disease is well recognised (see Chap. 8 p. 90), but similar appearances may occur in metastatic disease, especially in carcinoma of the prostate (Citrin and McKillop 1978).

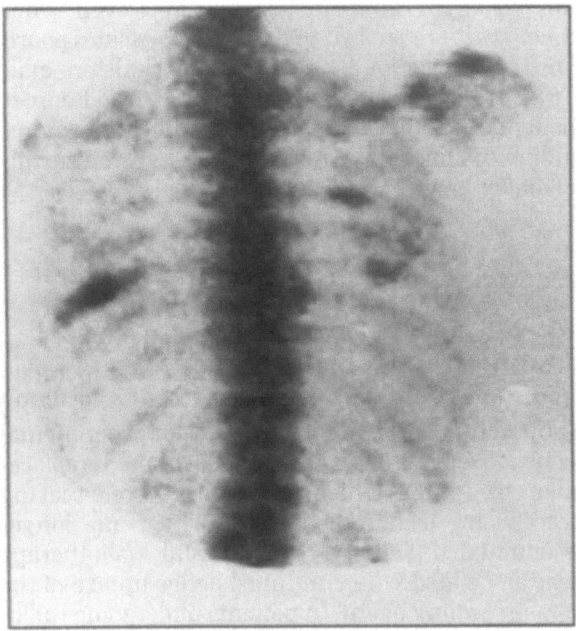

Fig. 5.7. Elongated rib lesions caused by metastatic carcinoma of the breast. Some increased uptake is seen in the right shoulder. The nature of this remains unclear as the radiograph shows only degenerative change.

Single photon emission computed tomography (SPECT) has had a relatively small application so far to bone scintigraphy, but especially in the case of spinal lesions it may be of value in localising more precisely the area of abnormality, thus helping to clarify the likely cause.

All bone scan abnormalities should be correlated with the results of other, more specific investigations. Initially a radiograph of the area showing the hot spot should be obtained. This may either show a benign cause for the scan appearance, confirm the presence of metastases or be normal at the site of scan abnormality. When standard radiographs are normal, computed tomography of bone can be valuable in evaluating the significance of a scan abnormality (Durning et al. 1983; Muindi et al. 1983).

In some patients, especially those with solitary bone scan lesions, bone biopsy may be necessary to establish whether a scan abnormality is due to malignant disease (Collins et al. 1979). The bone scan can be useful in guiding the site for open bone biopsy, either by injecting methylene blue over the site of the abnormality if biopsy is performed within a few hours of the scan, or by inserting a small metal marker if there is to be a longer delay before biopsy (Froelich et al. 1983).

Effects of Surgical Procedures on the Bone Scan

The bone scan is very sensitive to trauma, and surgical procedures in cancer patients may produce bone scan changes. In patients with lung cancer or breast cancer focal rib abnormalities are frequently seen on the side of the operative procedure, caused by surgical trauma. It is important not to attribute such changes to tumour involvement. In the case of mastectomy, the removal of the breast tissue may result in apparent prominence of the underlying ribs on the bone scan caused by reduced tissue attenuation of photons (Citrin and McKillop 1978). Increased activity in the ipsilateral shoulder after mastectomy has also been described (Seo et al. 1981). This appearance has been attributed to a reflex sympathetic dystrophy syndrome. Increased radioisotope uptake in the soft tissue of the arm on the mastectomy side is also common (Bledin et al. 1982).

Patients with malignant disease frequently undergo bone marrow aspiration or bone biopsy. Both sternal and iliac crest marrow aspiration do not usually produce any bone scan abnormality (Tyler and Powers 1982; McKillop et al. 1984). By comparison, a scan abnormality can usually be detected within a few days of transiliac bone biopsy and persists for several months (McKillop et al. 1984).

Indications for Bone Scanning in Extraosseous Malignancy

Pretreatment Staging and Routine Follow-up After Primary Therapy

In the 15 years since the introduction of the ^{99m}Tc-labelled phosphate agents many studies have been performed to assess the value of routine bone scanning in asymptomatic patients with primary tumours which frequently metastasise to bone. The role of the bone scan has been investigated both for pretreatment staging and for the early detection of asymptomatic metastatic disease in patients who have had treatment for the primary neoplasm. In spite of the considerable volume of work in this area, there is still great controversy over the value of routine bone scanning in clinically "early" tumours. This point will be considered further under individual tumour types. Other recent reviews have appeared on aspects of the subject (Harbert 1982; Parbhoo 1983; McNeil 1984).

Investigation of the Patient with a Clinical Suspicion of Bone Metastases

In patients with a clinical suspicion of bone metastases, either because of symptoms or laboratory evidence of bone involvement or because of tumour recurrence elsewhere, the bone scan is generally accepted as the most important initial investigation because of its high sensitivity and the ease with which a whole-body image can be obtained. As noted above, an abnormal bone scan should be followed by more specific investigations directed to the sites of scan abnormality. Even in the patient with radiographic evidence of bone metastases the scan often has value in demonstrating more extensive disease than suspected radiographically. This may have considerable importance, for example when planning radiotherapy fields, or may indicate a more easily accessible site for bone biopsy.

The relationship between bone pain and bone metastases is complex. Patients with malignant disease and a single site of bone pain are found frequently to have multiple metastases, and patients with no bone pain may have metastatic disease (Front et al. 1979). On the other hand, Winchester et al. (1979) found that only 60% of a series of patients with bone pain and breast cancer had demonstrable metastases. Schutte (1979) found a better correlation between bone pain and bone metastases in patients with malignant disease, but noted the absence of pain in 13 (13%) out of 97 patients with metastases and an abnormal bone scan. Of the 13 patients, 10 (77%) showed radiographic evidence of osteoblastic metastases. Patients with breast cancer receiving adjuvant chemotherapy have been suggested to be a group with a high incidence of asymptomatic bone metastases (Hammond et al. 1978).

Schutte and Park (1983) have investigated the role of bone scintigraphy in patients presenting with low back pain. In a group of 38 patients presenting with "non-specific" back pain, only 7 (18%) had bone scans indicative of clinically significant disease. By contrast, in 138 patients with backache and a past history of malignancy nearly 40% had bone scan evidence of a subsequently proven metastasis. A further 14% had scan evidence of traumatic or degenerative lesions, and in half of them it was not possible to exclude malignancy from the bone scan.

Hypercalcaemia is another feature which will suggest the development of bone metastases in patients with known malignancies and is a common indication for a bone scan. Hypercalcaemia may occur from lung, breast or other cancers without any apparent bone metastases, and even when metastases are present their extent correlates poorly with the level of hypercalcaemia (Ralston et al. 1982). These results suggest that, in addition to bone destruction, as yet unidentified hormonal influences may have a role in the hypercalcaemia of malignancy.

Assessment of Response to Therapy

The bone scan has been used by many workers to assess the response of bone metastases to radiotherapy or systemic therapy. Galasko (1975b) showed that effective radiotherapy for experimental bone metastases in an animal model caused replacement of tumour which accumulated bone-seeking tracers by a fibrous stroma which no longer accumulated activity. Unsuccessful radiotherapy was associated with continued active uptake of the bone-scanning agent. In patients undergoing radiotherapy, successful treatment produces a decrease in uptake in the metastases and a return to unity of the tumour to normal bone activity ratio (Castronovo et al. 1973). Normal bone included in the radiation field will also show diminution in tracer uptake compared with untreated bone (Cox 1974; Citrin and McKillop 1978). An example is shown in Fig. 5.8.

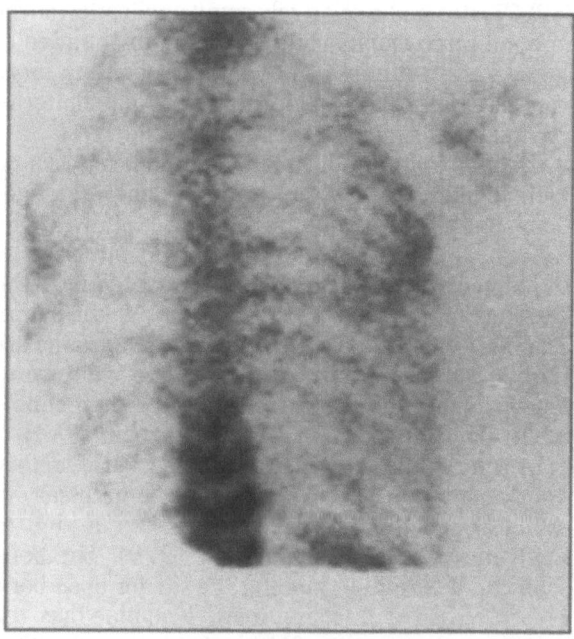

Fig. 5.8. Decreased tracer uptake in the upper thoracic spine of a patient previously treated with mantle irradiation for lymphoma.

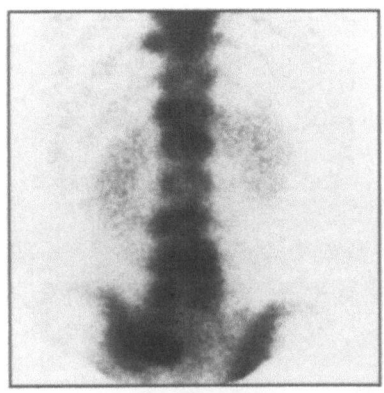 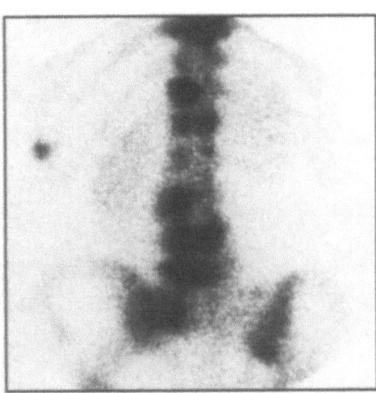 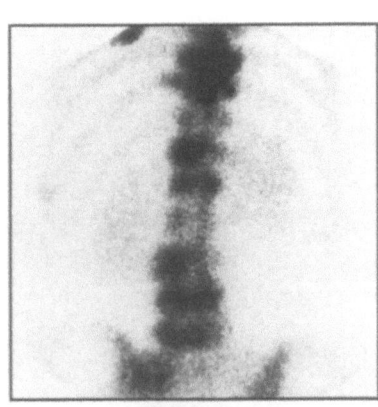

a   b, c

Fig. 5.9. a Bone scan from a woman with multiple metastases from breast carcinoma. b Scan 3 months later, after introduction of systemic chemotherapy, shows increased tracer uptake in previously noted lesions and new areas of increased uptake. c At 6 months after introduction of therapy the uptake in lesions is less and fewer lesions are seen than on the immediate post-treatment scan. The scans demonstrate the flare phenomenon.

In a tumour model showing spontaneous resolution of bone metastases, healing of the lesions was associated with an initial rise in uptake of the bone-scanning agent, followed by a gradual fall to normal. Radiographically this healing was associated with the appearance of large quantities of cortical new bone, which resembled callus (Parbhoo 1983). A similar sequence of changes on the bone scan has been described for bone metastases treated successfully by hormonal therapy or chemotherapy—the so-called flare phenomenon (Gillespie et al. 1975; Alexander et al. 1976). This phenomenon consists of an osteoblastic response which occurs as bone metastases heal (Fig. 5.9). As a result, the existing lesions show increased activity on the scan for a period. In addition, previously undetected lesions may become visible, resulting in abnormalities at new sites in the skeleton (Rossleigh et al. 1982). As healing progresses, the intensity of the lesions decreases and they may disappear. The flare phenomenon is well recognised during treatment of metastases from carcinoma of the breast with systemic therapy (Citrin et al. 1981; Rossleigh et al. 1984). It also occurs during systemic treatment of metastatic carcinoma of the prostate, though there is disagreement as to whether the phenomenon is rare (Pollen et al. 1984) or common (Levenson et al. 1983) in this tumour. The flare phenomenon is maximal in the first few months after starting systemic therapy (Citrin 1980; Drelichman et al. 1984).

The use of serial bone scans to assess the response of skeletal metastases to systemic therapy requires considerable caution. Reproducibility of scan technique is essential. Factors such as time from injec-

tion of tracer to imaging, time of acquisition for individual views and constancy of image contrast must be carefully controlled.

In patients receiving systemic therapy for bone metastases reduction in the number of lesions on the bone scan (Fig. 5.10) usually indicates successful treatment and healing of the metastases (Citrin et al. 1981; Parbhoo 1983; Rossleigh et al. 1984). Conversely, an increase in the number of lesions present on the bone scan more than 6 months after institution of therapy (Fig. 5.11) usually indicates disease progression. Apparent new lesions on the scan earlier than this should be interpreted with care because of the flare phenomenon.

The significance of changes of intensity of uptake in individual lesions during systemic therapy is more controversial. Assessing changes in intensity of uptake can be difficult; Condon et al. (1980) showed that changes in intensity of less than 40% were not likely to be detected by visual interpretation. Various methods have been used in an attempt to quantitate both the intensity of uptake within bone lesions and the degree to which the skeleton is involved (Condon et al. 1980; Citrin et al. 1981). These methods allow more objective assessment of serial changes in lesions uptake (Pitt and Sharp 1985), though it has yet to be shown that they have clinical relevance.

Some workers have used decrease in lesion intensity to represent improvement and increase in intensity to indicate progression and have shown that changes of this type correlate quite well with other markers of changing disease extent and with the clinical course (Citrin et al. 1981; Pollen et al. 1981; Levenson et al. 1983). Other studies have

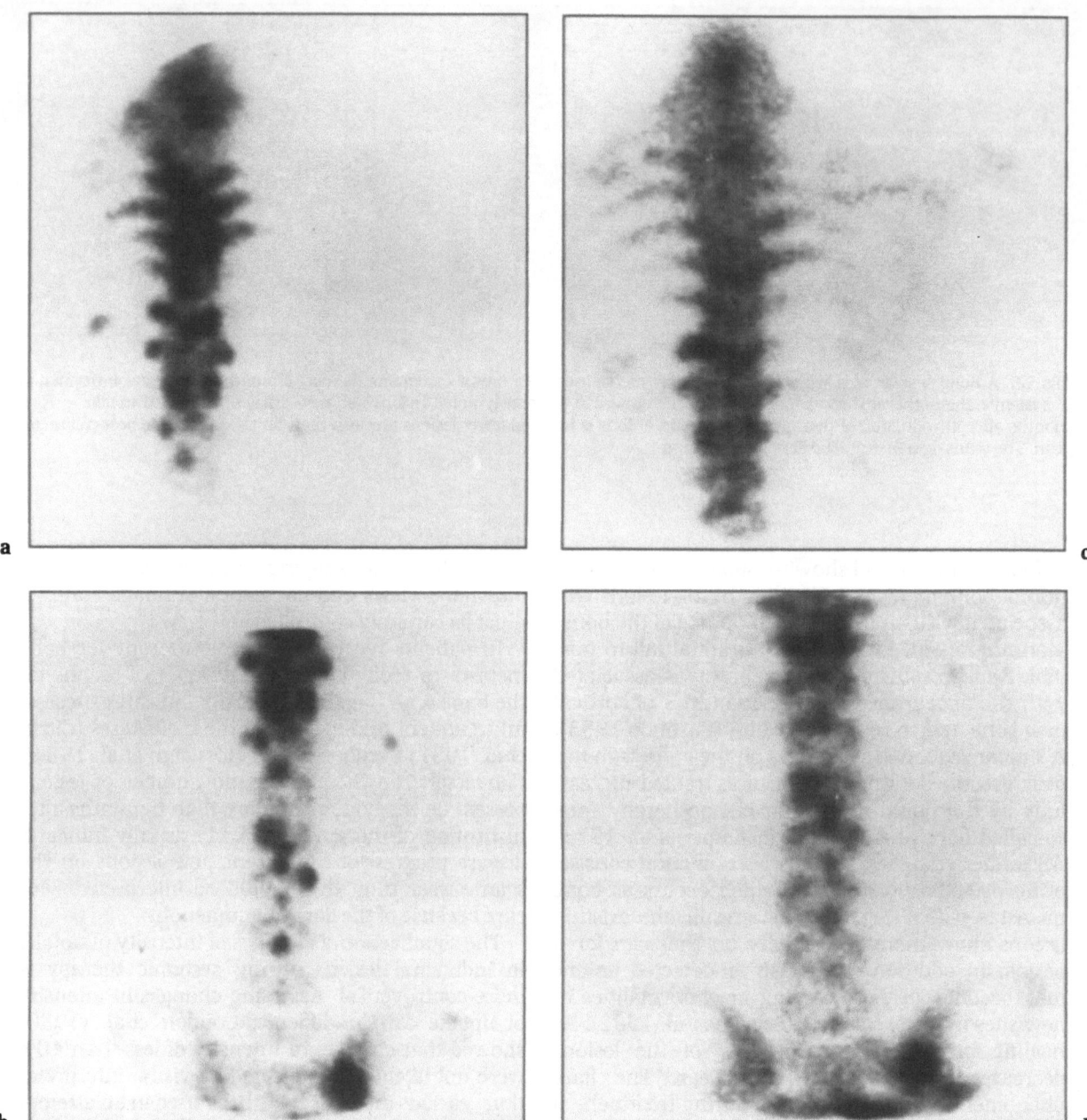

Fig. 5.10. a,b Bone scan of thoracic and lumbar spine showing extensive metastases from prostatic carcinoma. c,d Bone scan 1 year later is still abnormal but shows many fewer lesions as a result of good response to bilateral orchidectomy.

suggested that intensity of uptake is a poor indicator of response to treatment. Condon et al. (1980) found that uptake in some lesions decreased at a time when new lesions were appearing elsewhere. Aggressive lesions, especially those penetrating through the cortex, could show decrease in tracer uptake as the lesion progressed, presumably because the lesion was extending so rapidly that there was no chance for reactive new bone formation.

Bone Scanning in Individual Tumours

Breast Cancer

Breast cancer is the commonest cause of death from cancer in women from the age of 15 to 75 years.

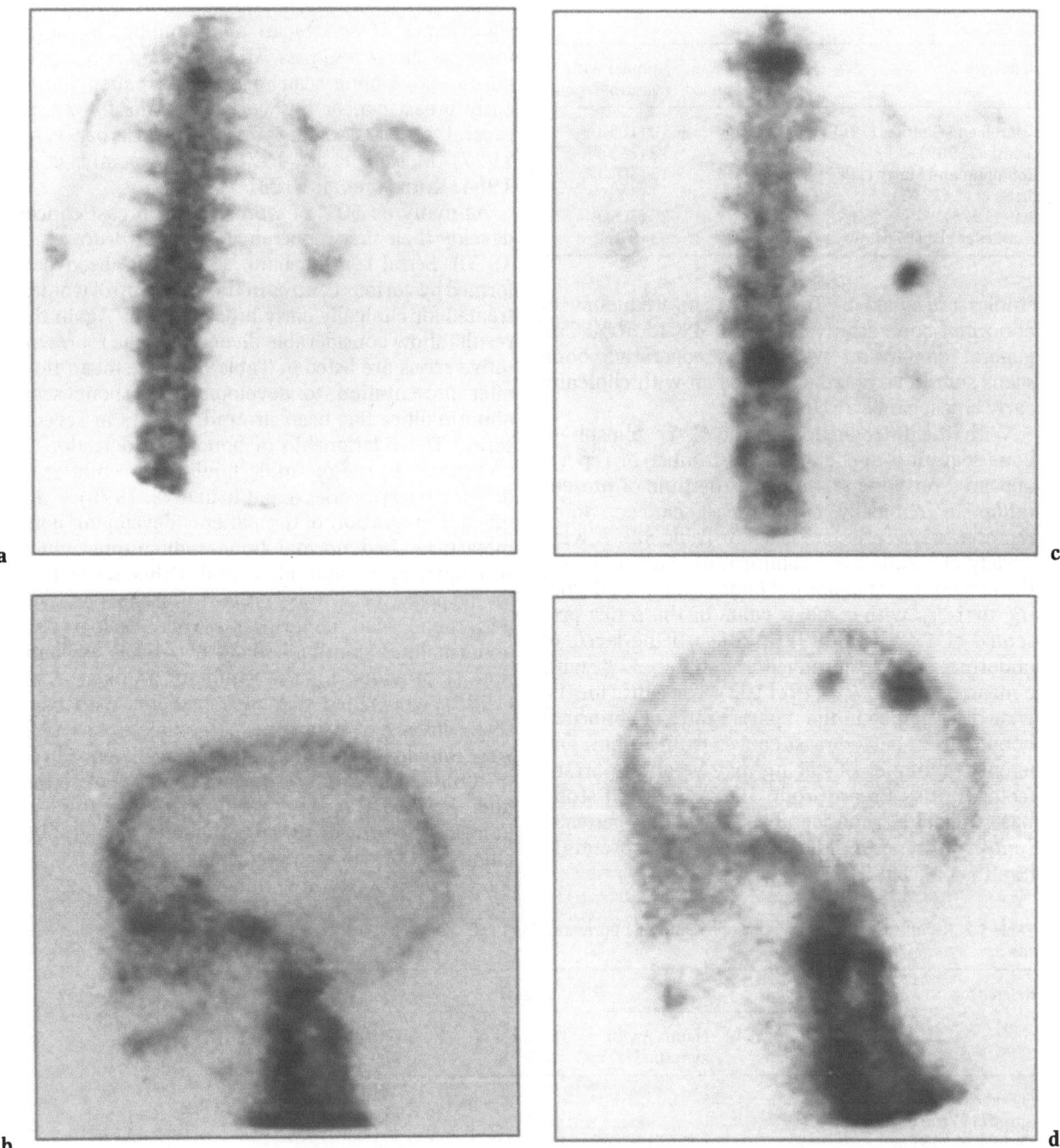

Fig. 5.11. a,b Single bone metastasis in upper thoracic spine of woman with breast carcinoma metastatic to the lung. The skull is normal. c,d Bone scan 10 months later shows progressive bone disease in spite of tamoxifen therapy.

Bone metastases are present in some 50%–85% of women with breast cancer coming to autopsy (Abrams et al. 1950; Gilbert and Kagan 1976; Galasko 1981). Isotope bone scanning has been very extensively applied to patients with breast cancer, but there is still considerable controversy over its role, especially in patients with clinically early breast cancer and no symptoms of bone metastases.

Six studies using early bone-scanning agents (fluorine or strontium radioisotopes) were carried out in patients with clinically localised (Stage I or Stage II) primary breast cancer. The findings of these

Table 5.1. Fluorine and strontium bone scans in "early" breast cancer

Reference	Number of patients studied	Number with abnormal scans
Sklaroff and Charkes (1968)	64	10 (16%)
Galasko (1969)	50	12 (24%)
Hoffmann and Marty (1972)	43	13 (30%)
Green et al. (1973)	69	3 (4%)
Blair (1975)	92	28 (30%)
Charkes et al. (1975)	35	3 (9%)

studies are given in Table 5.1. The frequency of abnormal bone scan varied from 4% to 30%. The general conclusion was that preoperative bone scans should be obtained in women with clinically early breast cancer.

With the introduction of the ^{99m}Tc phosphate bone-scanning agents, a large number of reports appeared on bone scanning at the time of presentation in clinically early breast cancer. Some representative series are listed in Table 5.2. A wide variety of results were obtained. In clinical Stage I the percentage of abnormal bone scans varied from 0% to 18%, with a mean value in the series presented of 4.4% (35/799). In Stage II the levels of abnormal bone scan ranged from 0% to 32%, with a mean value of 7.2% (79/1102). The cause for the wide discrepancy in the reported rates of abnormal bone scan in early breast cancer is uncertain. Different techniques of staging may be an important factor (British Breast Group 1978). A recent study has indicated considerable variation between centres in the criteria for bone scan interpretation (Smith et al. 1985).

As stressed already, it is essential to confirm the significance of bone scan abnormalities by other more specific techniques. The reported frequency of false-positive bone scan evidence in patients with early breast cancer has varied around 1%–2% in several series assessing this point (Gerber et al. 1977; McNeil et al. 1978; Moneypenny et al. 1984; Kunkler et al. 1985).

As many as 50% of women with breast cancer develop their first recurrence in bone (Bruce et al. 1970). Serial routine bone scans have been performed by various centres in the follow-up of women treated for clinically early breast cancer. Again the results show considerable diversity. Some representative series are listed in Table 5.3. The mean time after presentation to development of bone scan abnormalities has been around 2 years in several series. The relationship of bone scan detection of metastases to radiographic findings is a matter of debate. In some series (e.g. Citrin et al. 1976), a significant proportion of the patients developing bone metastases had normal bone radiographs which subsequently became abnormal. Other series (e.g. Moneypenny et al. 1984) report that most patients with bone scan abnormalities had radiographic abnormalities simultaneously. A possible explanation is provided by the study of Kunkler et al. (1985), who noted that most patients with bone scan evidence of metastases had radiographs which were initially interpreted as normal. When reviewed in conjunction with scintigrams, the rate of abnormal bone radiographs increased, because of increased weight being put on subtle radiographic changes at sites of scan abnormality.

Table 5.2. Results of ^{99m}Tc phosphate bone scanning at presentation in clinically early breast cancer

Reference	Stage I		Stage II	
	Number of patients	Number with abnormal scans	Number of patients	Number with abnormal scans
El Domeiri and Shroff (1976)	10	0	14	1 (7%)
Citrin et al. (1976)	49	6 (12%)	26	5 (19%)
Campbell et al. 1976	50	9 (18%)	17	7 (41%)
Baker et al. (1977)	27	1 (4%)	36	0
Gerber et al. (1977)	73	2 (3%)	37	0
Davies et al. (1977)	98	2 (2%)	56	1 (2%)
McNeil et al. (1978)	37	0	85	3 (3.5%)
O'Connell et al. (1978)	30	1 (3%)	42	4 (9%)
Hammond et al. (1978)	1	0	28	3 (11%)
Clark et al. (1978)	71	5 (7%)	99	4 (4%)
Lindholm et al. (1978)	98	3 (3%)	244	15 (6%)
Komaki et al. (1979)	24	4 (17%)	41	13 (32%)
Burkett et al. (1979)	80	1 (1%)	59	2 (4%)
Wilson et al. (1980)	86	0	87	3 (3%)
Kunkler et al. (1985)	65	1 (1.5%)	231	18 (8%)

Table 5.3. Results of follow-up ^{99m}Tc phosphate bone scans in patients with clinically early breast cancer and normal studies at presentation

Reference	Follow-up period	Number developing abnormal scans
Lentle et al. (1975)	12 months (mean)	10/52 (19%)
Citrin et al. (1976)	36 months (mean)	15/64 (23%)
Gerber et al. (1977)	24 months (mean)	12/47 (26%)
Bishop et al. (1979)	24 months	26/278 (9%)
Chaudary et al. (1983)	24 months	24/241 (10%)
Moneypenny et al. (1984)	up to 5 years	37/510 (7%)
Kunkler et al. (1985)	up to 4 years	31/328 (9%)

The frequency of abnormal bone scans at presentation in patients with more advanced breast cancer is generally accepted to be higher. Some representative series for Stage III disease are set out in Table 5.4, with a mean figure of 27.6% (109/394).

The prognostic significance of abnormal bone scans in clinically early breast cancer has been examined by various authors. Some reports, such as those of Sklaroff and Charkes (1968), Perez et al. (1983) and Moneypenny et al. (1984) have found the bone scan to be a poor predictor of subsequent skeletal relapse, because of both false-positive and false-negative results from isotope studies. Other studies have suggested that an abnormal bone scan implies a poor prognosis.

Galasko (1975a) found that all patients with abnormal bone scans had confirmed bone metastases over a 5-year follow-up and had a mortality of 83%, compared with 21% for patients with normal scans. Blair (1975) confirmed an increased mortality in patients with abnormal scans, and Charkes et al. (1975) reported that all patients with abnormal scans developed metastases

Table 5.4. Results of bone scanning at presentation in Stage III breast cancer

Reference	Number of patients	Number with abnormal scans
Hoffmann and Marty (1972)	11	6 (55%)
Lentle et al. (1975)	23	2 (9%)
El Domeiri and Shroff (1976)	31	14 (45%)
Roberts et al. (1976)	20	6 (30%)
Campbell et al. (1976)	13	8 (62%)
Baker et al. (1977)	41	10 (24%)
Gerber et al. (1977)	12	5 (42%)
Davies et al. (1977)	38	6 (16%)
McNeil et al. (1978)	31	5 (16%)
O'Connell et al. (1978)	13	2 (15%)
Hammond et al. (1978)	14	3 (21%)
Clark et al. (1978)	31	12 (39%)
Lindholm et al. (1979)	51	8 (16%)
Komaki et al. (1979)	27	10 (37%)
Wilson et al. (1980)	38	12 (32%)

over follow-up of 20 months. McKillop et al. (1978) found a mortality of 65% in patients with abnormal scans, compared with 10% in those with normal scans over a mean follow-up of 36 months. A similar increase in mortality in patients with abnormal scans was reported by McNeil et al. (1978), Komaki et al. (1979), Roberts and Hayward (1983) and Kunkler et al. (1985).

The role of the bone scan in following the response of breast carcinoma metastases to systemic therapy has already been partly discussed. Galasko (1975a), Alexander et al. (1976), Citrin et al. (1981), Parbhoo (1983) and Rossleigh et al. (1984) all concluded that the changes in the bone scan yielded useful objective evidence on the response to treatment. By contrast, Hortobagyi et al. (1984) found that the bone radiograph showed a better correlation with the response of non-osseous metastases than did the bone scan.

With such conflicting data in the literature it is not surprising that there is still no overall consensus on the role of bone scanning in breast cancer (Harbert 1982; McNeil 1984). In general, although it still has some proponents, the great initial enthusiasm for routine preoperative scanning of all women with clinically early breast cancer has faded somewhat. This is due to acceptance of the fact that the yield of true-positive evidence from bone scans in Stage I and II breast cancer is likely to be small and has to be offset against some false-positive results. Also important in the change of attitude is the trend towards less radical surgery for breast cancer and the realisation that systemic therapies are relatively ineffective in control of metastatic disease. Thus the therapeutic implications of an abnormal bone scan have become less clear cut. For similar reasons routine annual bone scans in asymptomatic patients are no longer performed in many centres (Thomsen et al. 1984; Wickerham et al. 1984).

It is generally accepted that bone scans should be obtained in patients with symptoms of bone metastases, soft tissue metastases and locally advanced disease for prognostic purposes. A bone scan at presentation is indicated in all patients being entered into therapeutic trials, to help to assess adequacy of randomisation of patients to groups. If serial bone scanning during follow-up is being carried out, a study at the time of presentation is useful as a baseline for later comparison.

Lung Cancer

Many patients presenting with lung cancer have multiorgan involvement at the time of presentation (Naruke et al. 1976). Bone metastases are common, being present at autopsy in 30%–50% of patients with lung cancer (Abrams et al. 1950; Gilbert and Kagan 1976). Surgery is inappropriate in patients with disseminated disease, particularly as it has an average operative mortality of 5%–10% (McNeil 1984).

Bone scanning has been used widely in patients with lung cancer. Sauerbrunn (1972) found abnormal strontium bone scans in 29/82 (35%) patients with lung cancer. The presence of bony metastases was confirmed in 18 (22%). Studies by Operchal et al. (1976) and Donato et al. (1979) on unselected patients with bronchial carcinoma showed a frequency of abnormal bone scans of 19/65 (31%) and 20/60 (33%) respectively.

If only patients with operable tumours or who are asymptomatic for metastases are considered, the rate of abnormal scans falls. Kies et al. (1978) demonstrated confirmed bone metastases in 8/42 (19%) patients with no bone symptoms and in 7/9 (78%) symptomatic patients. Similarly, Hooper et al. (1978) found abnormal studies in 4% of asymptomatic patients compared with 36% of those with symptoms. Kelly et al. (1979) obtained abnormal bone scans in 45% of their whole series of lung cancer patients, but in only 8/59 (14%) asymptomatic patients. Ramsdell et al. (1977) studied patients with apparently resectable lung cancer and found a true-positive rate of abnormalities in bone scans of 1/52 (2%). There was also a false-positive rate of 2%. The only conflicting results were from the series reported by Fujimura (1978), in which the rate of abnormal bone scans was similar in patients with surgically treated and inoperable bronchial carcinoma: 9/23 (39%) vs. 27/67 (40%). A high incidence of abnormal bone scans at presentation has been recorded in patients with small cell or anaplastic lung cancer (Bitran et al. 1981; Levenson et al. 1981).

The poor prognosis of an abnormal bone scan in lung cancer was stressed by Gravenstein et al. (1979). In their series, 46 patients had abnormal scans at presentation. Of these, 40 (87%) had died within 6 months and another 4 (10%) by 12 months. By contrast, 50% of the patients with a normal scan at presentation survived more than 6 months. The poor prognosis associated with an abnormal bone scan was confirmed by Levenson et al. (1981).

Little information is available on the use of bone scans in the follow-up after surgery for lung cancer. Donato et al. (1979) reported that of seven patients with resectable lung cancer and normal radiographs and bone scans at presentation, three had abnormal bone scans within 5 months.

Bone scanning at presentation is indicated in all patients with lung cancer who have clinical or biochemical evidence of possible bone metastases. Its use in asymptomatic patients with apparently resectable disease needs further evaluation. It seems reasonable at the moment to obtain bone scans preoperatively in asymptomatic patients to spare morbidity and mortality from surgery which has no hope of being succesful because of skeletal involvement. It is essential, however, that all scan abnormalities are confirmed by other methods to be definitely due to metastases, to ensure that false-positive results do not exclude patients from potentially curative resection.

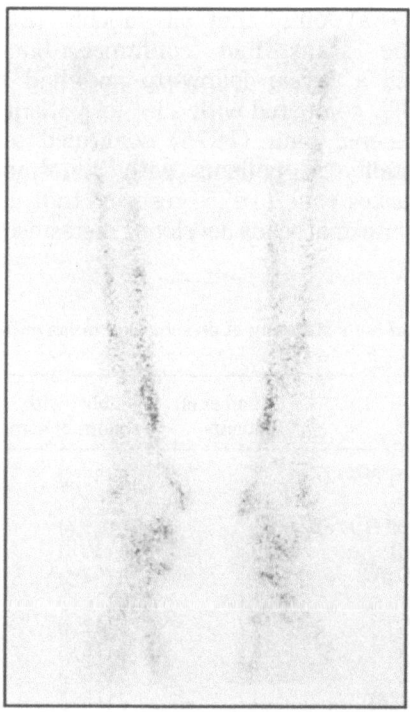

Fig. 5.12. Bone scan image of tibiae from a patient with carcinoma of the lung, showing increased tracer uptake along cortical borders (double stripe sign). Appearances are characteristic of HPOA.

The bone scan will also show abnormalities in patients with hypertrophic pulmonary osteoarthropathy (HPOA), ranging from localised bracelet-like activity in the tibiae and wrists, to generalised uptake in the long bones (Fig. 5.12; Lopez-Majano and Sobti 1984). Within the long bones the scan may show intense pericortical activity, the so-called double stripe or tramline sign (Terry et al. 1975). The scan evidence of HPOA may resolve very quickly after treatment of the primary tumour. Return of the bone scan to normal within 1 month of radiation therapy and surgical resection has been reported, although radiographs showed no change (Freeman and Tonkin 1976). Finger clubbing may produce increased uptake in the distal phalanges (Citrin and McKillop 1978), and bone scan changes may be seen even in patients with no clinical evidence of clubbing (Sy and Seo 1984).

Prostatic Cancer

The reported incidence of bone metastases at autopsy in prostatic cancer is 50%–70% (Abrams et al. 1950; Gilbert and Kagan 1976). Endocrine manipulation of this tumour may be successful either in controlling symptoms of bone metastases or in slowing progression of the lesions.

Bone scans on unselected series of patients with prostatic cancer reveal a high incidence of bone metastases at presentation (Table 5.5). The frequency of abnormal bone scans is related to tumour characteristics. Biersack et al. (1980) reported that the frequency of abnormal bone scans was 7% for T1 tumours, 19% for T2, 49% for T3 and 65% for T4. Similar results were reported by O'Donoghue et al. (1978) and Langhammer et al. (1980). Histological type is also important, with uniform adenocarcinomas showing an increasing rate of metastases with increasing dedifferentiation (Langhammer et al. 1980).

Table 5.5. Frequency of abnormal bone scans at presentation in prostatic cancer

Reference	Number of patients	Number with abnormal scans
Shafer and Reinke (1977)	110	37 (34%)
O'Donoghue et al. (1978)	90	30 (34%)
McGregor et al. (1978)	50	23 (46%)
Paulson and the Uro-Oncology Research Group (1979)	425	145 (34%)
Biersack et al. (1980)	153	46 (30%)
Lund et al. (1984)	128	65 (51%)

Paulson and the Uro-Oncology Research Group (1979) related the frequency of abnormal scans to clinical staging. In this series the rate of abnormal scans was 7/82 (9%) in Stage I, 20/100 (20%) in Stage II 19/79 (24%) in Stage III and 98/163 (60%) in Stage IV. McNeil and Polak (1981), citing the data of Paulson and also unpublished results from the Veterans Administration Co-operative Study on Prostatic Cancer, concluded that the yield of true positive results at presentation in prostatic cancer was around 5% for Stage I, 10% for Stage II and 20% for Stage III.

The extent of bone metastases judged scintigraphically correlates reasonably well with the serum acid phosphatase level (Kida and Higuchi 1983). However, Huben and Schellhammer (1982), summarising the results of four series, commented that of patients with scintigraphically demonstrated bone metastases only 51% had bone pain and only 61% had elevated serum acid phosphatase.

McNeil (1984), using data in the literature, estimated the relative sensitivity of various procedures for prostatic bone metastases to be as follows (assuming a value of 1.0 for scintigraphy): radiographic skeletal surveys 0.68; alkaline phosphatase levels 0.54–0.77; enzymatic assays for serum acid phosphatase 0.5–0.6.

A problem may be encountered in the patients with diffuse osteoblastic metastases from prostatic cancer: The bone scan may not show focal defects but rather have a superscan appearance and thus be interpreted as normal (Paulson and the Uro-Oncology Research Group 1979). The diagnosis can usually be made because of some irregularity of uptake of tracer, especially in the ribs (Fogelman et al. 1977). It has also been suggested that an index of image quantitation related to the ratio of uptake in bone and soft tissue can clearly differentiate these patients from other diagnostic categories (Constable and Cranage 1981).

Lund et al. (1984) have shown that patients with an abnormal bone scan at presentation have a mortality rate of around 45% at 2 years, compared with 20% for those with a normal initial scan. It is recommended that all patients presenting with carcinoma of the prostate should have a bone scan.

Little data is available on the use of routine serial scanning in patients who have normal scan at presentation. Lund et al. (1984) found that around 10% of patients with an initial normal scan had an abnormal study at 1 year and 20% at 2 years. They concluded that annual scans were of value in patients with normal previous scans, to detect occult metastases which require endocrine therapy. By contrast, Huben and Schellhammer (1982), in a study of 100 patients with carcinoma of the prostate and a normal initial scan, reported that only 19% developed abnormal scans during a mean follow-up of 47 months. All patients with abnormal scans had either bone pain or an elevated serum acid or alkaline phosphatase. They concluded that routine follow-up scans were not justifiable.

The use of bone scans to follow the response to treatment has been studied by various groups. Lund et al. (1984) concluded that serial scans during treatment were useful, as patients with scan evidence of remission showed an improved survival rate. Pollen et al. (1981) noted that patients with scan evidence of disease progression had a 41% chance of survival at 6 months and 7% at 12 months. For those without scan evidence of progression the 6 and 12 months' survival figures were 88% and 60%, respectively. Levenson et al. (1983) concluded that both bone scans and bone radiographs were required for full assessment of systematically treated prostatic bone metastases. Sy and colleagues (1981) used the bone scan to study patients who had orchidectomy for bone pain: Complete regression of metastases was seen in 4/24 and an additional 8 had incomplete resolution.

The bone scan can be used to assess response to systemic therapy of bone metastases from prostatic cancer. Further studies are required, however, to establish how much additional information is achieved compared with clinical and other parameters of disease progression.

Urinary Tract Cancers

The frequency of bone metastases at autopsy is around 30%–50% for renal carcinoma and 12%–25% for bladder cancer (Abrams et al. 1950; Gilbert and Kagan 1976). Cole et al. (1975) reported that 5 of 12 patients presenting with renal carcinoma had bone metastases on scintigraphy. Two of the patients with abnormal bone scans had normal skeletal radiographs. The method of selecting patients for study was not discussed. Clyne et al. (1983) found 7 true-positive scan results and 2 false-positive scan results in 32 consecutive patients with renal carcinoma, a true-positive rate of 22%. Five of the patients with true-positive scan results had bone pain. During follow-up a further eight patients showed true-positive bone scan abnormalities, six having bone pain. In this series, bone scans were 100% sensitive and 95% specific for bone metastases, the figures for bone radiographs being 67% sensitivity and 100% specificity. The question of the solitary lesion on the bone scan of patients with genitourinary malignancy has been studied by Robey and Schellhammer (1984), who have recom-

mended following the bone scan by plain radiographs, X-ray tomography, computed tomography and finally biopsy in sequence until the diagnosis of metastatic disease is established or refuted. Rosen and Murphy (1984) found bone scan evidence of metastases at presentation in 3/40 (8%) patients with renal carcinoma. They concluded that routine scintigraphy was unwarranted in the absence of skeletal symptoms before the diagnosis of renal lesions, especially as the presence of an abnormal bone scan did not alter the indication for nephrectomy.

Reddy and Merrick (1983) reported that of 12 patients with known bone metastases from renal carcinoma, 4 (33%) had normal bone scans. They stressed the importance of looking for photopaenic (cold) lesions. This message also emerged from the study of Kim et al. (1983), in which 7/68 (11%) biopsy-proven renal metastases to bone were cold on scan. A further 6 (9%) were associated with a normal scan. The bone scan was more sensitive than bone radiographs.

Parthasarathy et al. (1978), in a retrospective study, reported abnormal bone scans in 13/26 (50%) of patients with bladder cancer. The indications for bone scintigraphy were not specified. Three prospective studies have suggested that the true incidence of metastases at presentation is much lower, probably lying between 2% (Berger et al. 1981; Lindner et al. 1982) and 5% (Davey et al. 1985). Bone scans should be reserved for those bladder cancer patients in whom there is a clinical suspicion of skeletal metastases.

Gynaecological Cancer

Cervical carcinoma does not show a marked predilection to metastasise to bone. Two large series give a total of 140 out of 3452 patients (4%) as having clinical or autopsy evidence of bone involvement (Carlson et al. 1967; Blythe et al. 1975).

Katz et al. (1979) studied 100 women with cervical carcinoma by bone scanning. Of 21 patients with advanced disease (Stage III, IV or recurrent disease), 4 (19%) had definite metastases on scan. All 79 patients with early (Stage I or II) disease had no evidence of bone metastases. Renal asymmetry, suggesting urinary tract obstruction, was seen in 11 patients, 7 of whom had advanced disease. They concluded that bone scanning was not warranted as a routine test in asymptomatic patients with Stage 0, I or II carcinoma, but that if carried out renal asymmetry should be carefully evaluated (Fig. 5.13). Similar findings were obtained from the study by Kamath et al. (1983). Bassan and Glaser

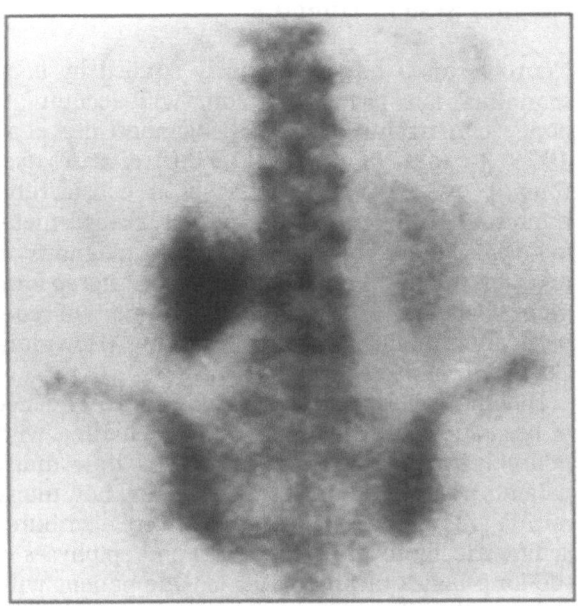

Fig. 5.13. Clinically unsuspected left hydronephrosis demonstrated on the bone scan of a woman with locally recurrent carcinoma of the uterine cervix.

(1982) reached a different conclusion. They found that abnormal bone scans were obtained in 14/148 (10%) of their patients, including 12 positive results in patients with Stage I or Stage II disease. Histological type of the tumour was paramount in their study, with 13/19 (68%) of patients with poorly differentiated primaries having bone metastases. They concluded that bone scans were mandatory for all patients with poorly differentiated tumours, whatever the clinical stage.

Photopulos et al. (1977) performed a variety of investigations including bone scanning in 73 patients being followed up after surgery for cervical cancer. The yield of the various procedures was low, and they stated that specialised investigations should be reserved for patients with a clinical suspicion of metastases.

In three series investigating patients with endometrial cancer at the time of presentation, only 1/111 had an abnormal bone scan (Mettler et al. 1981; Kamath et al. 1982; Harbert et al. 1982). Kamath et al. (1982) reported that of 77 patients with recurrent disease, 4 (5%) had bone metastases demonstrated by bone scanning.

In patients with Stage I or II ovarian cancer, 0/43 (Mettler et al. 1982) and 0/6 patients (Harbert et al. 1982) had positive bone scans. Mettler et al. (1982) reported that 3/40 (8%) patients with Stage III disease had bone metastases, all having grade III lesions histologically.

Alimentary Cancer

Little information is available on bone scanning in patients with alimentary tumours. Vider et al. (1977) found abnormal bone scans in 3/6 (50%) patients presenting with colorectal cancer but did not comment on the stage of the patients or on whether they were symptomatic for metastases. Antoniades et al. (1976) reported that none of three patients presenting with colorectal cancer had abnormal bone scans.

Hatfield et al. (1976) carried out bone scans in 16 patients with pancreatic cancer and found 1 abnormal study (rate of 6%). From a review of the literature on radiographic and autopsy findings they concluded that the true incidence of bone metastases in this tumour might be as high as 20%.

Melanoma

There is considerable variation in the reported rate of skeletal metastases from melanoma. In a review of the literature in 1949, Wilmer and Breckenridge recorded a range of 0.9%–18.6%. Autopsy series have suggested figures as high as 49% (Selby et al. 1956).

A number of studies have been performed on the role of bone scintigraphy in melanoma. Roth et al. (1975) found abnormal bone scans in 1/51 (2%) patients with Stage I or II disease and in 2/13 (15%) with Stage IV disease. Thomas et al. (1979) had similar results with no abnormal bone scans in 79 patients with Stage I or II disease and true-positive scan evidence in 10/57 (18%) patients with Stage III disease. Aranha et al. (1979) found no abnormal studies in 50 patients with Stage I disease. Au et al. (1984) reported abnormal scans in 5/112 (4%) patients with Stage I disease. All proved to be false-positive results on follow-up.

Fon et al. (1981) studied 50 patients at presentation, of whom 26 (52%) had bone scan evidence of metastases, confirmed in "most cases" by bone biopsy. In 12, bone was the only metastatic site at presentation. The precise staging of the patients is not given but it is stated that "most were symptomatic or Stage III". Five patients had radiographic evidence of osteolytic lesions but normal scans. Muss et al. (1979) found 14/49 (30%) patients with advanced melanoma had true-positive bone scan abnormalities, and one had a false-positive result. All had bone pain. No cases of false-negative scan results were found in this series: Of 13 patients with bone pain but normal scans, none had clinical evidence of bone metastases on follow-up. Pecking et al. (1981) found 22/96 (24%) true-positive and

6/96 (7%) false-positive results in Stage III disease. By comparison, Doiron and Bernardino (1981) found that all 8 abnormal bone scans in 38 patients with Stage III disease were false-positive results.

Bone scans are not indicated for asymptomatic patients with Stage I or II melanoma, but should be part of the initial evaluation of all patients with more advanced disease and of all symptomatic patients. All bone scan abnormalities should be confirmed by radiographs or biopsy. Radiographs should be obtained of all symptomatc sites shown as normal on bone scan to exclude osteolytic lesions.

Thyroid Cancer

Differentiated thyroid cancer, especially of the follicular variety, has a propensity to spread to bone, as do anaplastic tumours. An overall incidence of bone metastases of over 30% has been quoted for thyroid cancer patients (Eddleston 1980). The lesions are predominantly osteolytic, though osteoblastic metastases do occur (Bhushan et al. 1985). Metastases from well-differentiated tumours frequently retain the ability to trap iodine and can often be demonstrated by ^{131}I imaging.

Early studies with ^{85}Sr suggested that bone scanning was poor in detecting thyroid cancer bone metastases (Charkes and O'Mara 1969). Castillo et al. (1980) also found bone scans to be unsatisfactory, with only 41% of 37 bone lesions in 8 patients being shown on ^{18}F or ^{99m}Tc phosphate studies. Whole-body ^{131}I scans demonstrated 89% of the lesions. Dewan (1979) reported a closer correlation between bone scan and ^{131}I scan findings, although the latter delineated the metastases more clearly.

De Groot and Reilly (1984) compared a variety of investigative techniques in 108 patients with thyroid cancer, 29 of whom were known to have metastases. Bone scans were more sensitive than skeletal radiographs for bone metastases, but a combination of physical examination, chest radiograph and ^{131}I whole-body scans detected all cases of metastatic carcinoma. They concluded that bone scans were useful in the evaluation of patients with known metastatic disease but were not cost or time effective in the routine follow-up of asymptomatic patients previously treated for thyroid cancer.

A recent study (Hoefnagel et al. 1985) has suggested that whole-body imaging with the potassium analogue ^{201}Tl may be superior to ^{131}I imaging in the follow-up of thyroid cancer patients.

In medullary cancer of the thyroid, bone scanning has been reported to be effective in demonstrating bone metastases in patients with elevated serum calcitonin levels (Johnson et al. 1984).

Nervous System Tumours

Neuroblastoma has been widely studied by bone scanning. The primary tumour will accumulate bone scan agents in 35% (Howman-Giles et al. 1979) to 60% (Smith et al. 1980) of cases (see Chap. 15, p. 214). There has been considerable interest recently in the use of ^{131}I-labelled meta-iodobenzylguanidine (MIBG) for the diagnosis of neuroblastoma (Kimmig et al. 1984). Children with neuroblastoma show a significant number of renal tract abnormalities on bone scanning (Howman-Giles et al. 1979).

Howman-Giles et al. (1979) found scan evidence of bone metastases in 29/59 (49%) children with neuroblastoma. They did not specify how many patients were studied at presentation and how many during follow-up. Bone metastases were distributed symmetrically in the metaphyses and epiphyses of the long bones in nine patients. One patient with radiographically apparent metastases had a scan interpreted as normal. Kaufman et al. (1978) reported a 22% false-negative rate caused by metastases to the ends of long bones. Podarsky et al. (1983) reported 21 abnormal studies from 42 scans in 35 children with neuroblastoma. The false-positive rate for the bone scan in this series was 4.8% and the false-negative rate 9.5%.

At present, bone scanning and bone radiographs are complementary in neuroblastoma and both are required for adequate staging. On the scan careful attention must be paid to the metaphyseal areas, with the knowledge that osteolytic (cold) or bilateral lesions may occur. The role of ^{131}I-MIBG has still to be defined, though initial reports are encouraging (Shapiro et al. 1985).

There are a few reports in the literature of bone scan demonstration of skeletal involvement by intracranial malignancy (Schatzki et al. 1976; Booher and Schmidtknecht 1977; Cagnoni et al. 1977).

Head and Neck Tumours

Head and neck tumours may invade bone locally or metastasise to distant sites in the skeleton. Wolfe et al. (1979) found only one abnormal bone scan in 105 patients, many of whom had advanced disease. They concluded that bone scans were of no value in the routine work-up of this group of patients, as did Belson et al. (1980).

Front et al. (1978) reported on the usefulness of the bone scan in defining local bony involvement, scintigraphy being superior to conventional radiographs. The use of special views (Gates and Goris 1976) and SPECT (Brown et al. 1977) may further increase the diagnostic yield. A recent study (Gray and Souttar 1985) has found bone scan to be superior to oral pan tomography (OPT) for the demonstration of bony involvement by intraoral cancers.

References

Abrams HL, Spiro R, Goldstein N (1950) Metastases in carcinoma; analysis of 1000 autopsied cases. Cancer 3: 74–85

Alexander JL, Gillespie PJ, Edelstyn GA (1976) Serial bone scanning using technetium 99m diphosphonate in patients undergoing cyclical combination chemotherapy for advanced breast cancer. Clin Nucl Med 1: 13–17

Antoniades J, Croll MN, Walner RJ, Brady LW, McKhann CB (1976) Bone scanning in carcinoma of the colon and rectum. Dis Colon Rectum 19: 139–143

Aranha GV, Simmons RL, Gunnarsson A, Grage TB (1979) The value of preoperative screening procedures in Stage I and II malignant melanoma. J Surg Oncol 11: 1–6

Au FC, Maier WP, Malmud LS, Goldman LI, Clark WH (1984) Preoperative nuclear scans in patients with melanoma. Cancer 53: 2095–2097

Baker FR, Holmes ER, Alderson PO, Khouri NF, Wagner HN (1977) An evaluation of bone scans as screening procedures for occult metastases in primary breast cancer. Ann Surg 186: 363–368

Bassan JS, Glaser MG (1982) Bony metastases in carcinoma of the uterine cervix. Clin Radiol 33: 623–625

Belson TP, Lehman RH, Chobanian SL, Malin TC (1980) Bone and liver scans in patients with head and neck carcinoma. Laryngoscope 90: 1291–1296

Berger GL, Sadlowski RW, Sharpe JR, Finney RP (1981) Lack of value of routine preoperative bone and liver scans in cystectomy candidates. J Urol 125: 637–639

Bhushan B, Vashist GP, Prasad K, Kaul V, Pathania AGS (1985) Osteoblastic metastases from thyroid carcinoma. Br J Radiol 58: 563–565

Biersack HJ, Wegner G, Distelmaier W, Krause U (1980) Ossare Metastasierung des Prostatakerzinoms in Abhangigkeit von Tumorgrosse und Geschwulstdifferenzienung. Nuklearmedizin 19: 29–32

Bishop HM, Blamey RW, Morris AH et al. (1979) Bone scanning: its lack of value in the follow up of patients with breast cancer. Br J Surg 66: 752–754

Bitran JD, Beukerman C, Pinsky S (1981 Sequential scintigraphic staging of small cell carcinoma. Cancer 47: 1971–1975

Blair JS (1975) Does early detection of bone metastases by scanning improve prognosis in breast cancer? Clin Oncol 1: 185–190

Bledin AG, Kim EE, Haynie TP (1982) Bone scintigraphic findings related to unilateral mastectomy. Clin Nucl Med 7: P20 (abstract)

Blythe JG, Cohen MH, Buchsbaum HJ et al. (1975) Bony metastases from carcinoma of the cervix. Occurrence, diagnosis and treatment. Cancer 36: 475–484

Booher KR, Schmidtknecht TM (1977) Cerebellar medulloblastoma with skeletal metastases. Case report and review of the literature. J Bone Joint Surg [Am] 59: 684–686

Borak J (1942) Relationship between the clinical and roentgenological findings in bone metastases. Surg Gynecol Obstet 75: 599–604

British Breast Group (1978) Bone scanning in breast cancer. Br Med J II: 180–181

Brown ML (1983) Significance of the solitary lesion in pediatric bone scanning. J Nucl Med 24: 114–115

Brown ML, Keyes JW, Leonard PF, Thrall JH, Kircos LT (1977) Facial bone scanning by emission tomography. J Nucl Med 18: 1184–1188

Bruce J, Carter DC, Fraser J (1970) Patterns of recurrent disease in breast cancer. Lancet I: 433–435

Burkett ME, Scanlon EC, Garces RF, Khandekar JD (1979) The value of bone scans in the management of patients with carcinoma of the breast. Surg Gynecol Obstet 149: 523–535

Cagnoni G, Pupi A, Bisi G et al. (1977) Bone scan of the skull in neurosurgery. Acta Neurochir (Wien) 38: 150 (abstract)

Campbell DJ, Banks AJ, Davis GD (1976) The value of preliminary bone scanning in staging and assessing the prognosis of breast cancer. Br J Surg 63: 811–816

Carlson V, Declos L, Fletcher GH (1967) Distant metastases in squamous cell carcinoma of the cervix. Radiology 88: 961–966

Castillo LA, Yeh SDJ, Leeper RD, Benua RS (1980) Bone scans in bone metastases from functioning thyroid carcinoma. Clin Nucl Med 5: 200–209

Castronovo FP, Potsaid MS, Pendergrass HP (1973) Effects of radiation therapy on bone lesions as measured by ^{99m}Tc-diphosphonate. J Nucl Med 14: 604–605

Charkes ND, O'Mara RM (1969) The osseous system. In: Freeman LM, Johnson PM (eds) Clinical scintillation imaging. Harper and Row, New York, pp 326–383

Charkes DM, Young I, Sklaroff (1968) The pathological basis of the strontium bone scan. JAMA 206: 2482–2488

Charkes ND, Malmud LS, Caswell T et al. (1975) Preoperative bone scans: use in women with early breast cancer. JAMA 233: 516–518

Chaudary MA, Maisey MN, Shaw PJ, Rubens RD, Hayward JL (1983) Sequential bone scanning and chest radiographs in the postoperative management of early breast cancer. Br J Surg 70: 517–518

Citrin DL (1980) The role of the bone scan in the investigation and treatment of breast cancer. CRC Crit Rev Diagn Imaging 16: 39–55

Citrin DL, McKillop JH (1978) Atlas of technetium bone scans. Saunders, Philadelphia

Citrin DL, Furnival CM, Bessent RG, Greig WR, Bell G, Blumgart LH (1976) Radioactive technetium phosphate bone scanning in preoperative assessment and follow up study of patients with primary cancer of the breast. Surg Gynecol Obstet 143: 360–364

Citrin DL, Hougen C, Zweibel W et al. (1981) Use of serial bone scans in assessing response of bone metastases to systemic treatment. Cancer 47: 680–685

Clain A (1965) Secondary malignant disease of bone. Br J Cancer 19: 15–29

Clark DG, Painter RW, Sziklas JJ (1978) Indications for bone scans in preoperative evaluation of breast cancer. Am J Surg 135: 667–670

Clyne CAC, Frank JW, Jenkins JD, Smart CJ (1983) The place of ^{99m}Tc-polyphosphonate bone scan in renal carcinoma. Br J Urol 55: 174–175

Cole AT, Mandell J, Fried FA, Staab EV (1975) The place of bone scan in the diagnosis of renal cell carcinoma. J Urol 114: 364–365

Collins JD, Bassett L, Main GD, Kagan C (1979) Percutaneous biopsy following positive bone scans. Radiology 132: 439–442

Condon BR, Buchanan R, Garvie NR et al. (1980) Assessment of progression or secondary bone lesions following cancer of the breast or prostate using serial radionuclide imaging. Br J Radiol 54: 18–23

Constable AR, Cranage RW (1981) Recognition of the superscan in prostatic bone scintigraphy. Br J Radiol 54: 122–125

Corcoran RJ, Thrall JH, Kyle RW (1976) Solitary abnormalities in bone scans of patients with extraosseous malignancies. Radiology 121: 663–667

Cox PH (1974) Abnormalities in skeletal uptake of ^{99m}Tc polyphosphate complexes in areas of bone associated with tissues which have been subjected to radiation therapy. Br J Radiol 47: 851–855

Davey P, Merrick MV, Duncan W, Redpath AT (1985) Bladder cancer: the value of routine bone scintigraphy. Clin Radiol 36: 77–79

Davies CJ, Griffiths PA, Preston BJ, Morris AH, Elston CW, Blamey RW (1977) Staging breast cancer. Role of scanning. Br Med J II: 603–605

DeGroot LJ, Reilly M (1984) Use of isotope bone scans and skeletal survey x-rays in the follow up of patients with thyroid carcinoma. J Endocrinol Invest 7: 175–179

Dewan SS (1979) The bone scan in thyroid cancer. J Nucl Med 20: 271–272 (letter)

Doiron MJ, Bernardino ME (1981) A comparison of non invasive imaging modalities in the melanoma patient. Cancer 47: 2581–2584

Donato AT, Ammerman EG, Sullesta O (1979) Bone scanning in the evaluation of patients with lung cancer. Ann Thorac Surg 27: 300–304

Drelichman A, Decker A, Al-Sarraf M, Vaitkevicius VK, Muz J (1984) Computerized bone scan. A potentially useful technique to measure response in prostatic carcinoma. Cancer 53: 1061–1065

Durning P, Best JJK, Sellwood RA (1983) Recognition of metastatic bone disease in cancer of the breast by computed tomography. Clin Oncol 9: 943–946

Eddleston B (1980) Radiological assessment. In: Duncan W (ed) Thyroid cancer. Springer, Berlin Heidelberg New York, pp 93–97

El Domeiri AA, Shroff S (1976) Role of preoperative bone scan in carcinoma of the breast. Surg Gynecol Obstet 142: 722–724

Fink-Bennett D, Johnson J (1985) Stippled ribs—a potential pit fall in bone scan interpretation. J Nucl Med 26: P82 (abstract)

Fink-Bennett D, Vicuna-Rios J (1980) The deltoid tuberosity—a potential pit fall ('the delta sign') in bone scan interpretation. J Nucl Med 21: 211–212

Fogelman I (1980) Skeletal uptake of diphosphonate: a review. Eur J Nucl Med 5: 473–476

Fogelman I, McKillop JH, Greig WR, Boyle IT (1977) Absent kidney sign associated with symmetrical and uniformly increased uptake of tracer by the skeleton. Eur J Nucl Med 2: 257–260

Fon GT, Wong WS, Gold RH, Kaiser LR (1981) Skeletal metastases of melanoma. AJR 137: 103–108

Forrest APM, Cant ELM, Roberts MM et al. (1979) Is investigation of patients with breast cancer for occult metastatic disease worthwhile? Br J Surg 66: 749–751

Freeman MH, Tonkin AK (1976) Manifestations of hypertrophic pulmonary osteoarthropathy in patients with carcinoma of the lung. Demonstration by ^{99m}Tc pyrophosphate bone scans. Radiology 120: 363–365

Froelich JW, McKusick KA, Strauss HW et al. (1983) Localisation of bone lesions for open biopsy. Radiology 146: 549–550

Front D, Hardoff R, Robinson E (1978) Bone scintigraphy in primary tumours of the head and neck. Cancer 42: 111–117

Front D, Schneck SO, Frankel A, Robinson E (1979) Bone metastases and bone pain in breast cancer. Are they closely related? JAMA 242: 1747–1748

Fujimura N (1978) Detection of bone metastases from bronchogenic carcinoma by bone scintigraphy with ^{99m}Tc-phosphorus compounds. I. Incidence of bone metastases from bronchogenic carcinoma and their prognosis. Nippon Acta Radiol 38: 1054–1063

Galasko CSB (1969) The detection of skeletal metastases from mammary cancer by gamma camera scintigraphy. Br J Surg 56: 757–760

Galasko CSB (1975a) The significance of occult metastases detected by scintigraphy in patients with otherwise apparently "early" mammary cancer. Br J Surg 62: 649–696

Galasko CSB (1975b) The pathological basis for skeletal scintigraphy. J Bone Joint Surg [Br] 57: 353–357

Galasko CSB (1981) Anatomy and pathways for skeletal metastases. In: Weiss L, Gilbert HA (eds) Bone metastases. Hall, Boston, pp 49–63

Gates GF, Goris ML (1976) Maxillary-facial abnormalities assessed by bone imaging. Radiology 121: 677–682

Gerber FH, Goodreau JJ, Kirchner PT, Fonty WJ (1977) Efficacy of preoperative and postoperative bone scanning in the management of breast carcinoma. N Engl J Med 297: 300–303

Gilbert HA, Kagan AR (1976) Metastases: incidence, detection and evaluation. In: Weiss L (ed) Fundamental aspects of metastases. North Holland Elsevier, Excerpta Medica, Amsterdam, pp 385–405

Gillespie PJ, Alexander JL, Edelstyn GA (1975) Changes in ^{87m}Sr concentrations in skeletal metastases in patients responding to cyclical combination chemotherapy for advanced breast cancer. J Nucl Med 16: 191–193

Goergen TG, Alazraki NP, Halpern SE, Heath V, Ashburn WL (1974) "Cold" bone lesions: a newly recognised phenomenon on bone imaging. J Nucl Med 15: 1120–1124

Gravenstein S, Peltz MA, Poreis W (1979) How ominous is an abnormal scan in bronchogenic carcinoma? JAMA 241: 2523–2524

Gray HW, Souttar DS (1985) Bone scanning in the demonstration of local bony involvement by intra-oral tumours. Eur J Nucl Med 11: A20 (abstract)

Green D, Jeremy R, Towson J, Morris J (1973) The role of fluorine 18 scanning in the detection of skeletal metastases in early breast cancer. Aust NZ J Surg 43: 251–257

Hammond N, Jones SE, Salmon SE, Paton D, Woolfenden J (1978) Predictive value of bone scans in an adjuvant breast cancer program. Cancer 41: 138–142

Harbert JC (1982) Efficacy of bone and liver scanning in malignant diseases: facts and opinions. In: Freeman LM, Weissmann HS (eds) Nuclear medicine annual 1982. Raven, New York, pp 373–402

Harbert JC, George FY, Kerner ML (1981) Differentiation of rib fractures from metastases by bone scanning. Clin Nucl Med 6: 359–361

Harbert JC, Rocha L, Smith FO, Delgado G (1982) The efficacy of radionuclide bone scans in the evaluation of gynecological cancers. Cancer 49: 1040–1042

Hatfield DR, Deland FH, Maruyama Y (1976) Skeletal metastases in pancreatic cancer: study by isotopic bone scanning. Oncology 33: 44–47

Hoefnagel CA, Delprat CC, Marcuse HR (1985) The role of Tl 201 total body scintigraphy in the follow up of thyroid carcinoma. J Nucl Med 26: P31 (abstract)

Hoffman HC, Marty R (1972) Bone scanning. Its value in the preoperative evaluation of patients with suspicious breast masses. Am J Surg 124: 194–199

Hooper RG, Beechler CR, Johnson MC (1978) Radioisotope scanning in the intitial staging of bronchogenic carcinoma. Am Rev Resp Dis 118: 279–286

Hortobagyi GN, Libshitz HI, Seabold JE (1984) Osseous metastases of breast cancer: clinical, biochemical, radiographic and scintigraphic evaluation of response to therapy. Cancer 53: 577–582

Howman-Giles RB, Gilday DL, Ash JM (1979) Radionuclide skeletal survey in neuroblastoma. Radiology 131: 497–502

Huben RP, Schellhammer PF (1982) The role of routine follow up bone scans after definitive therapy of localised prostatic cancer. J Urol 128: 510–512

Israel O, Front D, Frenkel A, Kleinhaus U (1985) 24 hour/4 hour ratio of technetium-^{99m} methylene diphosphonate uptake in patients with bone metastases and degenerative bone changes. J Nucl Med 26: 237–240

Johnson DG, Coleman RE, McCook TA, Dale JK, Wells SA (1984) Bone and liver images in medullary carcinoma of the thyroid. J Nucl Med 25: 419–422

Kamath CRV, Maruyama Y, De Land FH, van Nagell JR (1982) Value of bone scanning in detecting occult skeletal metastases from adenocarcinoma of the endometrium. Diagn Gynecol Obstet 4: 155–158

Kamath CRV, Maruyama Y, De Land FH, van Nagell JR (1983) Role of bone scanning for evaluation of carcinoma of the cervix. Gynecol Oncol 15: 171–185

Katz RD, Alderson PO, Rosenhein NB, Bowerman JW, Wagner HN Jr (1979) Utility of bone scanning in detecting occult metastases from cervical carcinoma. Radiology 133: 469–472

Kaufman RA, Thrall JH, Keyes JW, Brown ML, Zaken JF (1978) False negative bone scans in neuroblastoma metastatic to the ends of long bones. Am J Roentgenol Radium Ther Nucl Med 130: 131–135

Kelly RJ, Cason RJ, Ferrie CB (1979) Efficacy of radionuclide scanning in patients with lung cancer. JAMA 242: 2855–2857

Kida T, Higuchi Y (1983) Correlation between extent of metastatic lesions in whole body bone scintigraphy of patients with prostatic cancer and prostatic acid phosphatase in serum with Eiken PAP RIA kit. Oncology 40: 346–350

Kies MS, Baker AW, Kennedy PS (1978) Radionuclide scans in staging of carcinoma of the lung. Surg Gynecol Obstet 147: 175–176

Kim EE, Bledin AG, Gutierrez C, Haynie TP (1983) Comparison of radionuclide images and radiographs for skeletal metastases from renal cell carcinoma. Oncology 40: 284–286

Kimmig B, Brandeis WE, Eisenhut M, Bubeck B, Hermann HJ, zum Winkel K (1984) Scintigraphy of a neuroblastoma with I-131 meta-iodobenzylguanidine. J Nucl Med 25: 773–775

Kober B, Hermann HJ, Wetzel E (1979) "Cold lesions" in bone scintigraphy. Fortschr Rontgenstr 131 545–551

Komaki R, Donegan W, Manoli R, Teh EL (1979) Prognostic value of pretreatment bone scans in breast carcinoma. Am J Roentgenol Radium Ther Nucl Med 132: 877–881

Kunkler IH, Merrick MV, Rodger A (1985) Bone scintigraphy in breast cancer: a nine year follow up. Clin Radiol 36: 279–282

Langhammer H, Steuer G, Gradinger R et al. (1980) Skeletal metastases from prostatic carcinoma; consideration of histological type and local tumour stage. Schweiz Med Wochenschr 110: 11–15

Lentle BS, Burns PE, Dierich H et al. (1975) Bone scintiscanning in the initial assessment of carcinoma of the breast. Surg Gynecol Obstet 141: 43–47

Levenson RM, Sauerbrunn BJL, Ihde DC et al. (1981) Small cell cancer: radionuclide bone scans for assessment of tumour extent and response. Am J Roentgenol Radium Ther Nucl Med 137: 31–35

Levenson RM, Sauerbrunn BJL, Bates HR, Newman RD, Eddy JL, Ihde DC (1983) Comparative value of bone scintigraphy and radiography in monitoring tumor response in systemically treated prostatic cancer. Radiology 146: 513–518

Lindholm A, Lundell L, Martenson B, Thulin A (1979) Skeletal scintigraphy in the initial assessment of women with breast cancer. Acta Chir Scand 145: 65–71

Lindner A, Dekernion JB (1982) Cost effectiveness of pre cycstectomy radioisotopic scans. J Urol 128: 1181–1182

Lopez-Majano V, Sobti P (1984) Early diagnosis of pulmonary osteoarthropathy in neoplastic disease. J Nucl Med Allied Sci 28: 69–76

Lund F, Smith PH, Suciu S (1984) Do bone scans predict prognosis in prostatic cancer? Br J Urol 56: 58–63

Makoha FW, Britton KE (1980) Reversion of a "hot" spot to a "cold" spot in untreated metastatic disease. Nucl Med Comm 1: 233–238

Manier SM, van Nostrand D (1983) From "hot spots" to "superscan". Clin Nucl Med 8: 626–627

Matin P (1982) Bone scanning of trauma and benign conditions. In: Freeman LM, Weissmann HS (eds) Nuclear medicine annual 1982. Raven, New York, pp 81–118

McGregor B, Tulloh AGS, Quinlan MF, Lovegrove F (1978) The role of bone scanning in the assessment of prostatic carcinoma. Br J Urol 50: 178–181

McKillop JH, Blumgart LH, Wood CB et al. (1978) The prognostic and therapeutic implications of the positive radionuclide bone scan in clinically early breast cancer. Br J Surg 65: 649–652

McKillop JH, Maharaj D, Boyce BF, Fogelman I (1984) Bone scan appearances following biopsy of bone and bone marrow. Radiology 153: 241–242

McNeil BJ (1984) Value of bone scanning and malignant disease. Semin Nucl Med 14: 277–286

McNeil BJ, Polak JF (1981) An update on the rationale for the use of bone scans in selected metastatic and primary bone tumours. In: Pauwels EKJ, Schutte HE, Taconis WK (eds) Bone scintigraphy. University Press, Leiden, pp 187–208

McNeil BJ, Pace PD, Gray EB, Adelstein SJ, Wilson RE (1978) Preoperative and follow up bone scans in patients with primary carcinoma of the breast. Surg Gynecol Obstet 147: 745–748

Mettler FA, Christie JH, Garcia JF, Baldwin MH, Wicks JD, Barstow SA (1981) Radionuclide liver and bone scanning in the evaluation of patients with endometrial carcinoma. Radiology 141: 777–780

Mettler FA, Christie JH, Crow NE, Garcia JF, Wicks JD, Barstow SA (1982) Radionuclide bone scan, radiographic bone survey and alkaline phosphatase—studies of limited value in asymptomatic patients with ovarian carcinoma. Cancer 50: 1483–1485

Moneypenny IJ, Grieve RJ, Howell A, Morrison JM (1984) The value of serial bone scanning in operable breast cancer. Br J Surg 71: 466–468

Muindi J, Coombes RC, Golding S, Parboo TJ, Khan O, Husband J (1983) The role of computed tomography in the detection of bone metastases in breast cancer patients. Br J Radiol 56: 233—236

Muss HB, Richards F, Barnes PL, Willand VV, Cowan RJ (1979) Radionuclide scanning in patients with advanced malignant melanoma. Clin Nucl Med 4: 516–518

Naruke T, Seumasu K, Ishikawa S (1976) Surgical treatment of lung cancer with metastasis to mediastinal nodes. J Thorac Cardiovasc Surg 71: 279–285

O'Connell MJ, Wahner HJ, Ahmann DL, Edis AJ, Silvers A (1978) Value of preoperative radionuclide bone scans in suspected primary breast carcinoma. Mayo Clin Proc 53: 221–226

O'Donoghue EP, Constable AR, Sherwood T, Stevenson JJ, Chisholm GD (1978) Bone scanning and plasma phosphatases in carcinoma of the prostate. Br J Urol 50: 172–177

Operchal JA, Bowen RD, Grove RB (1976) Efficacy of radionuclide procedures in the staging of bronchogenic carcinoma. J Nucl Med 17: 530 (abstract)

Parbhoo S (1983) Serial scintiscans in monitoring patients with bone metastases. In: Stoll BA, Parbhoo S (eds) Bone metastases: monitoring and treatment. Raven, New York, pp 201–240

Parthasarathy KL, Lansberg R, Bakshi SP, Donoghue G, Merrin C (1978) Detection of bone metastases in urological malignancies utilising ^{99m}Tc-labelled phosphate compounds. Urology 11: 99–102

Paulson DF and the Uro-Oncology Research Group (1979) The impact of current staging procedures in assessing disease extent of prostatic adenocarcinoma. J Urol 121: 300–302

Pecking A, Najean Y, Renault P (1981) Detection of malignant melanoma metastases: value of radio isotope methods. Nouv Presse Med 10: 885–892

Perez DJ, Powles RJ, Milan J et al. (1983) Detection of breast carcinoma metastases in bone: relative merits of x-rays and skeletal scintigraphy. Lancet II: 613–616

Photopulos GJ, Shirley RE, Ansbacher R (1977) Evaluation of conventional diagnostic tests for detection of recurrent carcinoma of the cervix. Am J Obstet Gynecol 129: 533–535

Pistenma DA, McDougall IR, Kriss JP (1975) Screening for bone metastases—are only scans necessary? JAMA 231: 46–50

Pitt WR, Sharp PF (1985) Comparison of quantitative and visual detection of new focal bone lesions. J Nucl Med 26: 230–236

Podarsky AER, Stark DD, Hattner RS, Gooding GA, Moss AA (1983) Radionuclide bone scanning in neuroblastoma: skeletal metastases and primary tumor localisation of ^{99m}Tc-MDP. AJR 141: 469–472

Pollen JJ, Gerber K, Ashburn WL, Schmidt JD (1981) Nuclear bone imaging in metastatic cancer of the prostate. Cancer 47: 2585–2594

Pollen JJ, Witztum KF, Ashburn WL (1984) The flare phenomenon on radionuclide bone scan in metastatic prostate cancer. AJR 142: 773–776

Ralston S, Fogelman I, Gardner MD, Boyle IT (1982) Hypercalcaemia and metastatic bone disease: is there a casual link? Lancet II: 903–905

Ramsdell JW, Peters RM, Taylor AT, Alazraki NP, Tisi GM (1977) Multiorgan scans for staging of lung cancer: correlation with clinical evaluation. J Thorac Cardiovasc Surg 73: 653–659

Rappaport AH, Hoffer PB, Genant HK (1978) Unifocal bone findings by scintigraphy. Clinical significance in patients with known primary cancer. West J Med 129: 188–192

Reddy PS, Merrick MV (1983) Skeletal scintigraphy in carcinoma of the kidney. Br J Urol 55: 171–173

Roberts JG, Gravelle IH, Baum M et al. (1976) Evaluation of radiography and isotope scintigraphy for detecting skeletal metastases in breast cancer. Lancet II: 237–239

Roberts MM, Hayward JL (1983) Bone scanning and early breast cancer: five year follow up. Lancet I: 997–998

Robey EL, Schellhammer PF (1984) Solitary lesions on bone scan in genito-urinary malignancy. J Urol 132: 1000–1002

Rosen PR, Murphy KG (1984) Bone scintigraphy in the initial staging of patients with renal cell carcinoma. J Nucl Med 25: 289–291

Rossleigh MA, Lovegrove FTA, Reynolds PM, Byrne MJ (1982) Serial bone scans in the assessment of response to therapy in advanced breast carcinoma. Clin Nucl Med 7: 397–402

Rossleigh MA, Lovegrove FTA, Reynolds PM, Byrne MJ, Whitney BP (1984) The assessment of response to therapy of bone metastases in breast cancer. Aust NZ J Med 14: 19–22

Roth JA, Eilber FR, Bennett LR, Morton DL (1975) Radionuclide photoscanning. Usefulness in preoperative evaluation of melanoma. Arch Surg 110: 1211–1212

Sauerbrunn BJL, Hansen M, Napoli L (1972) Strontium bone scans in carcinoma of the lung: a comparative, prospective study. J Nucl Med 13: 465–466

Schatzki DC, McIlmoyle G, Lowis S (1976) Diffuse osteoblastic metastases from an intracranial glioma. Am J Roentgenol Radium Ther Nucl Med 128: 321–323

Schutte HE (1979) The influence of bone pain on the results of bone scans. Cancer 44: 2039–2043

Schutte HE (1980) Some special views in bone scanning. Clin Nucl Med 5: 172–173

Schutte HE, Park WM (1983) The diagnostic value of bone scintigraphy in patients with low back pain. Skeletal Radiol 10: 1–4

Selby HM, Sherman RS, Pack GT (1956) A roentgen study of bone metastases from melanoma. Radiology 67: 224–228

Seo IS, Sy WM, Chiarello S (1981) Ipsilateral activity in the shoulder area on bone image after mastectomy: its significance. J Nucl Med 22: P78–79 (abstract)

Shackman R, Harrison CV (1947) Occult bone metastases. Br J Surg 35: 385–389

Shafer RB, Reinke DB (1977) Contribution of the bone scan, serum acid and alkaline phosphatase and radiographic bone survey to the management of newly diagnosed carcinoma of the prostate. Clin Nucl Med 2: 200–203

Shapiro B, Copp JE, Sisson JC, Eyre PL, Wallis J, Beierwaltes WH (1985) Iodine-131 meta iodobenzylguanidine for the location of suspected pheochromocytoma: experience in 400 cases. J Nucl Med 26: 576–585

Sklaroff DM, Charkes ND (1968) Bone metastases from breast cancer at the time of radical mastectomy. Surg Gynecol Obstet 127: 763–767

Smith FW, Gilday DL, Ash JM, Reid RH (1980) Primary neuroblastoma uptake of ^{99m} technetium methylene diphosphonate. Radiology 137: 501–504

Smith ML, Martin W, McKillop JH et al. (1985). Bone scan interpretation: a multicentre analysis. In: Proceedings of the European congress of nuclear medicine, London, 1985 (in press)

Stadalnik RC (1979) "Cold spot"—bone imaging. Semin Nucl Med 9: 2–3

Sy WM, Seo IS (1984) Subclinical clubbing of fingers and toes on bone scintigraph. J Nucl Med 25: P25 (abstract)

Sy WM, Finkelstein P, Seo IS, Combs A (1981) Serial bone scans in orchidectomized men with prostatic bone metastases. Clin Nucl Med 6: 456 (abstract)

Terry DW, Isitman AI, Holmes RA (1975) Radionuclide bone images in hypertrophic pulmonary osteoarthropathy. Am J Roentgenol Radium Ther Nucl Med 124: 571–576

Thomas JH, Panoussopoulus D, Liesmann GE, Jewell WR, Preston DF (1979) Scintiscans in the evaluation of patients with malignant melanoma. Surg Gynecol Obstet 149: 574–576

Thomsen HS, Lund JO, Munck O, Andersen KW, Stockel M, Rossing N (1984) Bone metastases in primary operable breast cancer. The role of serial scintigraphy. Eur J Cancer Clin Oncol 20: 1019–1023

Tumeh SS, Beadle G, Kaplan WD (1985) Clinical significance of solitary rib lesions in patients with extraskeletal malignancy. J Nucl Med 26: 1140–1143

Tyler JL, Powers TA (1982) Bone scanning after marrow biopsy. J Nucl Med 23: 1085–1087

Vider M, Maruyama Y, Narvaez R (1977) Significance of the vertebral venous (Batson's) plexus in metastatic spread in colorectal cancer. Cancer 40: 67–71

Wahner HW, Kyle RA, Beabout JW (1980) Scintigraphic evaluation of the skeleton in multiple myeloma. Mayo Clinic Proc 55: 739–746

Weingrad T, Heyman S, Alavi A (1984) Cold lesions on bone scan in pediatric neoplasms. Clin Nucl Med 9: 125–130

Wickerham L, Fisher B, Cronin W et al. (1984) The efficacy of bone scanning in the follow up of patients with operable breast cancer. Breast Cancer Res Treat 4: 303–307

Wilmer D, Breckenridge RL (1949) Bone metastases in malignant melanoma. Am J Roentgenol 62: 388–394

Wilson GS, Rich MA, Brennan MJ (1980) Evaluation of bone scan in preoperative clinical staging of breast cancer. Arch Surg 115: 415–419

Wilson MA, Calhoun FW (1981) The distribution of skeletal metastases in breast and pulmonary cancer. J Nucl Med 22: 594–597

Winchester DP, Sewer SF, Khandekar JD et al. (1979) Symptomatology as an indicator of recurrent or metastatic breast cancer. Cancer 43: 956–960

Wolfe JA, Rowe LD, Lowry LD (1979) Value of radionuclide scanning in the staging of head and neck carcinoma. Ann Otol Rhinol Laryngol 88: 832–836

6 · The Bone Scan in Primary Bone Tumours and Marrow Disorders

J. H. McKillop

Introduction

Skeletal radiography and bone biopsy are the main investigations in patients with suspected primary bone tumours. The bone scan can be helpful when results of radiography are equivocal or negative and can be used to demonstrate distant metastases from malignant bone tumours, both at presentation and during follow-up.

Primary Bone Tumours

Isotope Bone Scanning in the Differential Diagnosis of a Primary Bone Tumour

In a recent study, Goodgold and colleagues (1983) evaluated the use of bone scans in differentiating between benign and malignant bone tumours in a series of 78 patients. Intensity of uptake alone did not differentiate between malignant primary bone tumours (21 cases) and benign bone tumours (57 cases). Using a combination of shape and size of the tumour on bone scan and the pattern of tracer uptake, they correctly classified 70 patients as having either a benign or malignant lesion. Unfortunately, this study appeared in abstract form only, and the precise criteria adopted for the classification of the tumours is not specified.

Most other workers have found the bone scan to be less useful in the differential diagnosis of primary bone tumours. Lesions which do not cause any abnormality on the bone scan are unlikely to be malignant, and enhanced blood pool activity and markedly increased bone tracer uptake are more common with a malignant lesion. However, there is considerable overlap in the scintigraphic appearances of benign and malignant tumours so that the bone scan is generally considered to be unreliable in distinguishing between them (Rosenthall and Lisbona 1980; Simon and Kirchner 1980). ^{67}Ga imaging may be more helpful in distinguishing benign from malignant bone lesions in that lack of ^{67}Ga uptake usually indicates a benign lesion, though some benign tumours will show ^{67}Ga uptake (Kirchner and Simon 1981).

Some similarities also exist in the scintigraphic appearance of different malignant bone tumours. This question has recently been addressed by Murray and McLean, studying three of the more common primary bone malignancies (Murray 1980; McLean and Murray 1984). Over a 9-year period they obtained bone scans from 22 patients with osteogenic sarcoma, 16 with Ewing's sarcoma and 14 with chondrosarcoma. Lesions were assessed for intensity of uptake, tracer distribution within the tumour (patchy or homogeneous), degree of distortion of the bony outline, definition of the scintigraphic margin and, where this information was available, vascularity of the lesion on blood pool images. No unique scintigraphic pattern was found,

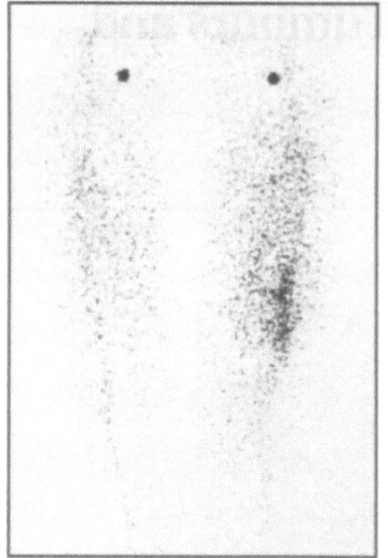 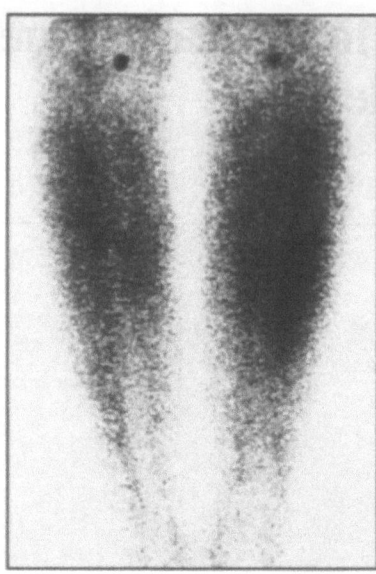 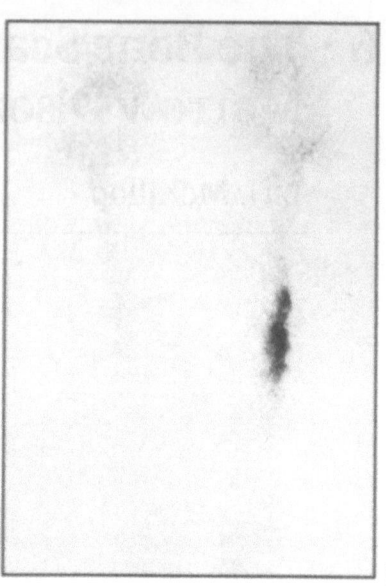

a   b, c

Fig. 6.1. Three-phase bone scan from a 30-year-old woman with Ewing's sarcoma of the mid-shaft of the left femur. The dynamic flow study obtained in the first 40 s after tracer injection (**a**), the blood pool equilibrium image 5 min after injection (**b**) and the standard static images 3 h after injection (**c**) all show increased activity in the tumour. Hot markers indicate position of the knees in the flow and blood pool images.

but each tumour type had a number of commonly recurring features. Osteogenic sarcoma typically showed markedly increased tracer uptake, patchy tracer distribution within the lesion (with areas of decreased activity being seen against a generally increased uptake compared with normal bone), marked distortion of the bony outline and a moderately well-defined margin. In paraosteal osteosarcoma tracer distribution was more uniform within the lesion. In Ewing's sarcoma, the usual appearance was of markedly increased uptake, homogeneous tracer distribution within the tumour, a moderately distorted bony outline and a poorly defined tumour margin. In patients with chondroscarcoma the bone scan usually showed moderately increased tracer uptake in the lesion, with areas of increased activity being seen against a background of decreased activity compared with

normal bone, only slight distortion of the bone outline and a well-defined tumour margin. Vascularity was increased in each tumour type (Fig. 6.1), though blood pool images were available in only 18 patients (4 osteogenic sarcoma, 6 Ewing's sarcoma and 8 chondrosarcoma). The findings of this study are summarised in Table 6.1. The authors concluded that the scintigraphic appearances could be useful in helping to classify the tumour in those patients in whom the radiographic and histological appearances are atypical.

The use of dynamic (three-phase) bone scanning to differentiate between osteomyelitis, Paget's disease and primary bone tumours has been evaluated (Gandsman et al. 1983). In osteomyelitis blood flow was increased both in the lesion and in bone above and below the lesion. The increase was especially marked in the blood pool (second) phase. In

Table 6.1. A comparison of the characteristic bone scan appearance of osteosarcoma, Ewing's sarcoma and chondrosarcoma (adapted from McLean and Murray 1984)

Bone scan appearance	Osteogenic sarcoma	Ewing's sarcoma	Chondrosarcoma
Tracer uptake	Markedly increased	Markedly increased	Moderately increased
Tracer distribution within lesion	"Cold areas on "hot" background	Homogeneous	"Hot" areas on a cold background
Distortion of bony outline	Marked	Moderate	Mild
Tumour margin	Moderately defined	Poorly defined	Well defined

bone tumours the flow increase was more localised to the lesion and was especially significant in the arterial (first) phase. In early Paget's disease only a mild, local increase in flow was seen, but in advanced Paget's disease the pattern observed was very similar to that seen in primary bone tumours.

Osteogenic Sarcoma

Osteogenic sarcoma may occur at any age but most commonly occurs in childhood or in early adulthood. It is probably the most frequently encountered primary bone tumour. The tumour may arise at any site in the skeleton, but about 90% occur in the long bones of the limbs (Lichtenstein 1977). Osteogenic sarcoma may show the presence of "skip" lesions proximally in the affected bone, sometimes confined to the medullary cavity. Treatment consists of excision of the tumour whenever possible. In the case of limb tumours this requires either amputation or en bloc excision of the bone and prosthetic reconstruction of the excised length of bone. Excision of the tumour is now usually followed by adjuvant chemotherapy. The 5-year survival rates from osteogenic sarcoma were previously around 10%–20% (Cade 1955), but higher survival rates are now achieved. It is possible, but by no means established, that this is due to the introduction of adjuvant chemotherapy (Frei et al. 1979).

The bone scan is markedly abnormal in osteogenic sarcoma. The primary tumour usually shows intense tracer uptake and expansion of the bone (Fig. 6.2). Areas of decreased tracer uptake may be seen within the tumour, probably caused by localised necrosis. As noted above, the tumour is hypervascular.

Several studies have assessed the ability of the isotope bone scan to demonstrate the extent of the primary tumour and thus assist in deciding the level of amputation. Goldmann et al. (1975) compared bone scan appearances with pathological evidence and standard radiography in 13 patients. In 12 cases the bone scan and radiographic findings correlated well with one another and with the tumour extent found pathologically in the excised specimen. In the remaining patient an area of increased uptake proximally on the bone scan was normal on the radiograph and did not show any evidence of tumour cells histologically. More recently, Papanicolaou et al. (1982), reporting on 20 consecutive cases of osteogenic sarcoma, concluded that the ^{99m}Tc-MDP bone scan allowed preoperative determination of the extent of osteosarcoma of the long bones with a high degree of accuracy. Other groups have been less impressed on the value of the

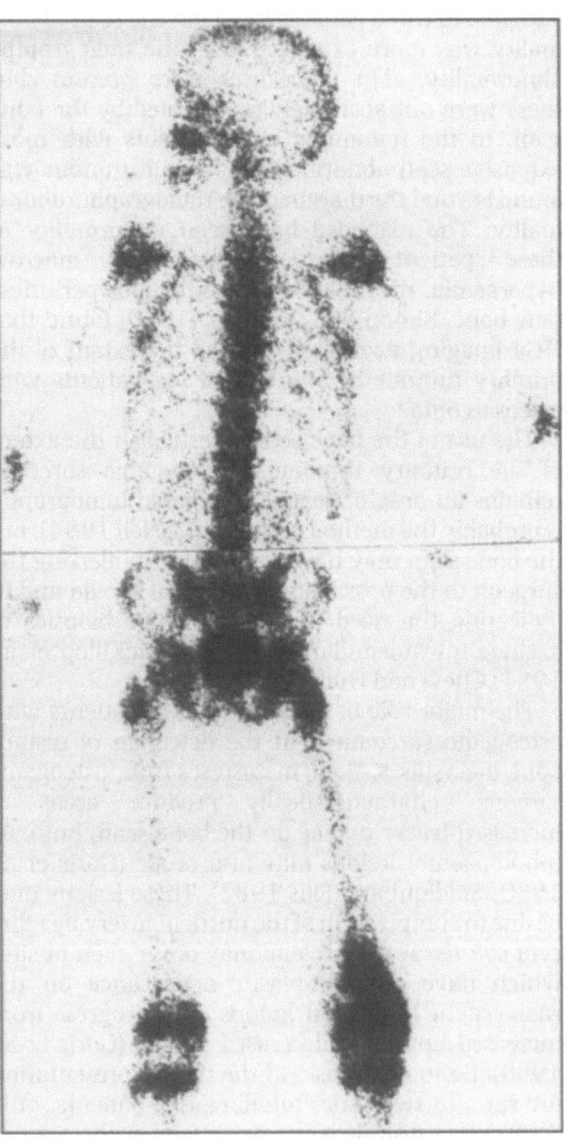

Fig. 6.2. Posterior bone scan from a 17-year-old boy with osteogenic sarcoma of the lower end of the right femur. The tumour shows markedly increased tracer uptake with a localised area of decreased uptake medially. The remainder of the right femur shows increased activity compared with the left. This is due to increased blood flow as there was no evidence of proximal tumour spread.

bone scan in this context. Generally increased uptake in the limb bearing the osteosarcoma is well documented (Goldmann and Braunstein 1975) and may lead to appearances similar to those seen in proximal tumour spread (McKillop et al. 1981). Falsely extended uptake in osteogenic sarcoma was also reported by Chew and Hudson (1982), who found that the scan accurately represented the extent of the primary tumour in only 7 out of 18 patients. In three patients in whom the scan abnormality was more extensive than the radiographic abnormality, skip metastases were present, but these were not accurately represented by the bone scan. In the remaining eight patients with more extensive scan abnormality no occult tumour was found beyond the margin of the radiographic abnormality. The extended bone scan abnormality in these patients was attributed to marrow hyperaemia, medullary reactive bone or periosteal new bone. Simon and Kirchner (1980) found that ^{67}Ga imaging accurately defined the extent of the primary tumour in nine out of ten patients with osteosarcoma.

The use of the bone scan to establish the extent of the primary tumour in osteogenic sarcoma remains an area of debate. Computed tomography is probably the method of choice (McNeil 1984), but the bone scan may have some value in alerting the surgeon to the possibility of proximal spread and in indicating the need for intraoperative biopsies to exclude intramedullary extension (McKillop et al. 1981; Chew and Hudson 1982).

The major role of the bone scan in patients with osteogenic sarcoma is in the detection of distant bone metastases. Bone metastases from osteogenic sarcoma characteristically produce areas of increased tracer uptake on the bone scan, but cold (photopaenic) lesions may also occur (Goris et al. 1980; Siddiqui and Ellis 1982). These lesions may be due to compression of the nutrient artery by adjacent soft tissue disease and may occur even at sites which have an osteoblastic appearance on the radiograph. Individual lesions may progress from increased uptake to decreased uptake (Goris et al. 1980). Bone metastases at the time of presentation are rare. In two series totalling 107 patients, only 3 (3%) had distant bone metastases at the time of presentation (Goldstein et al. 1980a; McKillop et al. 1981). Though the incidence of metastases is low, their presence radically alters the treatment of the patient, as amputation is no longer appropriate. A bone scan at presentation is therefore indicated to detect occult bony metastases (McNeil 1984).

The lungs are the most common site of metastases in osteogenic sarcoma, and more than 90% of patients with this disease die with pulmonary metastases (Jeffree et al. 1975). Recurrent disease in the past almost always first occurred in the lungs, with bone metastases being a late complication (Moore et al. 1973). For this reason, McNeil et al. (1973) recommended that in patients being followed up after primary therapy for osteosarcoma bone scanning should be reserved for those who had developed lung metastases or had symptoms of bone metastases.

Three recent studies, however, have suggested that a different pattern of metastatic disease may be emerging. Goldstein et al. (1980a) reported on serial bone scans in 56 patients with osteogenic sarcoma receiving adjuvant chemotherapy. In this group of patients 16% had distant bone metastases as their first site of tumour recurrence. McKillop et al. (1981), in a similar study of serial routine bone scans, found that bone was the first site of tumour recurrence in 7/47 (15%) patients receiving adjuvant chemotherapy. Similar results have also been reported by Giuliano et al. (1984), who found an increase in frequency of initial recurrence at sites other than the lungs. It is unclear whether this apparent change in the pattern of metastases from osteosarcoma is due solely to the introduction of adjuvant chemotherapy (Giuliano et al. 1984).

The apparent change in the pattern of metastatic disease from osteosarcoma means that a case can now be made for routine bone scanning in patients who have undergone primary therapy for osteosarcoma. McNeil and Hanley (1980), using actuarial techniques, concluded that approximately 1% per month of patients receiving adjuvant chemotherapy for osteosarcoma developed bone metastases in the period from 5 to 29 months after presentation. Thereafter, the rate of development of bone metastases declined. Routine bone scanning every 6 or 12 months in these patients may yield useful prognostic information, though it is dubious whether this has any therapeutic implications for the individual patient (McNeil 1984). In trials of adjuvant chemotherapy serial bone scans should be obtained to yield information on the pattern of recurrent disease in patients in whom the treatment fails. In patients not receiving adjuvant therapy bone scans should only be obtained when bone metastases are discovered or when there are symptoms to indicate bone metastases.

The use of bone scanning for demonstrating local bone recurrence has also been considered. McNeil et al. (1973), using ^{18}F scintigrams, studied patients undergoing radiotherapy for osteosarcoma. Decreased uptake in the region of the primary tumour occurred within 3 or 4 months in the case of successful treatment. Persistence of intense focal uptake at the primary site beyond this time was associated with local recurrence, though infection and pathological fracture produced a similar appearance. McKillop et al. (1981) reported that in patients treated by amputation intense focal uptake in the bone stump at 6 months or more postoperatively was associated with local recurrence.

The accumulation of bone-scanning agents in lung metastases from osteosarcoma has been recognised for some time, the first description being by McNeil et al. (1973) using ^{18}F imaging. Subsequent investigations have confirmed that lung metastases may also take up ^{99m}Tc-labelled phosphate agents (Ghaed et al. 1974). Other soft tissue lesions such as lymph node, renal, hepatic and chest wall metastases have been detected on the bone scan (Teates et al. 1977; Heyman 1980; McKillop et al. 1981). Only a minority of soft tissue metastases, however, will show accumulation of bone-scanning agents (Goldstein et al. 1980a; McKillop et al. 1981).

Vanel et al. (1984) have compared X-ray computed tomography (CT), standard radiography, chest tomography, scintigraphy and bone single photon emission computed tomography (SPECT) in 32 patients being screened for lung metastases from osteosarcoma. Using CT as the reference technique, the sensitivity of the techniques for detecting patients with metastases was pulmonary tomography 88%, standard radiography 57%, scintigraphy 21% and SPECT 41%. In identification of individual metastatic lesions the figures were pulmonary tomography 48%, standard radiography 32%, scintigraphy 5% and SPECT 8%. They concluded that chest radiography and CT should be used for screening for pulmonary metastases from osteosarcoma.

Bone scans from patients with osteosarcoma should be carefully inspected for soft tissue uptake as this may be the first indication of disease recurrence. The bone scan, however, cannot be relied upon as a primary method of detecting extraosseous metastases.

Paget's Sarcoma

In a proportion of patients with Paget's disease a sarcoma may develop in an area of affected bone. The frequency of this complication is unclear, but it is uncommon and probably does not exceed 1% (Hamdy 1981).

Active Paget's disease produces increased uptake of tracer on the bone scan and this has led to difficulty in identifying the presence of a superimposed osteosarcoma (McKillop et al. 1977). Yeh et al. (1982) reported on the bone scan appearances in 12 patients with Paget's sarcoma. The tumour characteristically showed less uptake of ^{99m}Tc-MDP than benign pagetic bone. The tumour concentration of ^{67}Ga uptake was irregular. A temporary clinical response to chemotherapy was associated with decreased ^{67}Ga uptake.

Smith et al. (1984) described a series of 85 patients with Paget's sarcoma seen over a 50-year period. A variety of imaging tests were performed in these patients, including ^{99m}Tc-MDP bone scans in 17 and ^{67}Ga scans in 16. Decreased ^{99m}Tc-MDP uptake at the tumour site was common. This appearance occurred more often in lesions that were lytic on radiographs but was also seen in some sclerotic tumours. Sudden interruption of the diffusely increased uptake of Paget's disease by a cold area occurred at the tumour site in 13 of the 17 patients and was most apparent in lesions in the long bones. ^{67}Ga imaging shows a slight increase in tracer uptake in benign pagetic bone compared with normal bone; however, in the presence of a sarcoma there was a marked increase of ^{67}Ga uptake, especially in the region of a soft tissue mass, the area where MDP was cold being replaced by intense gallium uptake (Smith et al. 1984).

In patients with Paget's disease the development of a sarcoma can often be confirmed by standard radiography, CT and biopsy. In equivocal cases the combination of bone scanning and ^{67}Ga scanning may be a useful prelude to biopsy and may help in identifying the most appropriate site for biopsy.

Ewing's Sarcoma

Ewing's sarcoma is a malignant tumour of bone which most often occurs in the age range 10–25 years. The cell of origin is uncertain but is thought to be of mesenchymal derivation (Lichtenstein 1977). Recent management of the patients with megavoltage therapy and adjuvant chemotherapy has resulted in improved survival and disease-free intervals.

The characteristic bone scan appearance of the primary Ewing's sarcoma is of intense tracer uptake, with homogenous distribution of tracer within the tumour, moderate distortion of the bone outline and poor definition of the tumour margin (McLean and Murray 1984). The ability of the bone scan to define the margin of the primary tumour has not been studied to the same extent as in osteosarcoma, because of the infrequency of amputation as a treatment. Frankel et al. (1974) compared bone scintigraphy, ^{67}Ga imaging and bone radiography in 27 patients with Ewing's sarcoma and concluded that all were of equal usefulness in detecting the primary tumour, though the ^{67}Ga study sometimes suggested a more extensive primary lesion than the other two investigations. McNeil et al. (1973) reported that high-dose radiation therapy to the primary tumour produced a marked diminution in ^{67}Ga uptake in the primary tumour within 3–4 months in uncomplicated cases.

The incidence of bone metastases at presentation in Ewing's sarcoma is higher than is found for osteosarcoma. Goldstein et al. (1980b) reviewed bone scans in 28 patients with osteosarcoma and found bone metastases at presentation in 3 (11%). Nair (1985) collated the results of bone scans at presentation or within 6 months of presentation in 53 patients with Ewing's sarcoma and found distant bone metastases in 25 (47%). In 20 of these patients the bone metastases were not suspected clinically. Bone metastases at presentation were associated with a poor prognosis (Nair 1985).

The occurrence of bone metastases as the first site of tumour recurrence during follow-up of patients with Ewing's sarcoma was first reported by McNeil et al. (1973). Goldstein et al. (1980b) found that bone metastases occurred during follow-up in 10/22 (45%) patients free of metastases at presentation; this was the first site of metastases in 6 patients (27%). Nair (1985) also found the bone scan useful in demonstrating the presence of bone metastases during follow-up, either by showing lesions not suspected on clinical or radiographic grounds or by demonstrating much more extensive metastases than were apparent on radiographs.

Unlike osteosarcoma, extraskeletal metastases from Ewing's sarcoma will not accumulate bone-scanning agents (McNeil et al. 1973; Frankel et al. 1974). Soft tissue metastases, however, may be detected by ^{67}Ga imaging in some cases (Frankel et al. 1974).

Because of the high incidence of occult bony metastases at presentation a bone scan should be part of the initial work-up of all patients with Ewing's sarcoma. The frequency with which bone metastases are the first site of recurrence during follow-up has led to the recommendation that routine follow-up studies should be obtained at 1 and 2 years after presentation (McNeil 1984).

Chondrosarcoma

Chondrosarcoma is a malignant tumour arising from cartilaginous tissue and may develop either within the medullary cavity of the bone (central) or within the cartilaginous cap of an osteochondroma (peripheral). The central tumours may arise *de novo* but are particularly common in patients with skeletal enchondromatosis (Ollier's disease).

The typical bone scan appearance of a chondrosarcoma is of moderately increased tracer uptake, which shows a patchy appearance with "hot" areas being seen against a cold background. In tumours arising from long bones a preponderance of cortical activity is common. Distortion of the bone outline is usually slight and the scintigraphic margin of the tumours is well defined (McLean and Murray 1984).

The bone scan may prove useful in detecting primary lesions not seen on skeletal radiography. This may be a particular problem in the spinal column, a site which accounts for approximately 6% of the primary lesions (Smith et al. 1982).

Benign enchondromas were reported to show normal or slightly increased uptake on ^{18}F bone scanning (Moon et al. 1968), but a more recent report using ^{99m}Tc phosphate suggests that the intensity and uniformity of uptake of bone-scanning agents within cartilaginous tumours cannot be used to determine whether they are benign or malignant (Pearlman and Steiner 1978).

Osteoid Osteoma

Osteoid osteoma is a relatively common tumour, accounting for approximately 10% of benign bone neoplasia (Swee et al. 1979). The lesion may be seen in young children but is most common in adolescents and young adults, becoming distinctly uncommon after the age of 30 (Lichtenstein 1977). The most common sites are in the tibia or femur, which together account for about 50% of cases, but any bone may be involved. There is some debate as to whether osteoblastoma represents a different tumour or is a variant of osteoid osteoma (Dahlin and Johnson 1954; Lichtenstein 1977).

The usual symptom from osteoid osteoma is pain, which may be severe and often becomes worse at night. Relief of the pain by aspirin is characteristic. The typical radiographic appearance is of a small oval or round focus that is usually radiolucent but may be radiopaque. The central area is usually surrounded by reactive sclerosis. The typical radiographic appearance may not be seen in the spine; the lesion often develops in the vertebral arch rather than the body, and sclerotic reaction around a central nidus may be absent (Smith and Gilday 1980).

The characteristic scan appearance is of a small focus of intense tracer uptake (Fig. 6.3). A central colder area may be seen (Helms et al. 1984). On occasions the radiographic appearances do not allow differentiation between an osteoid osteoma and intracortical abscess or chronic sclerosing osteomyelitis. Poor ^{67}Ga uptake in osteoid osteoma will usually distinguish it from osteomyelitis (Lisbona and Rosenthall 1979).

The sensitivity of standard radiographs to detect osteoid osteoma varies from 50% to over 90% (Swee et al. 1979; Smith and Gilday 1980; Omjola et al. 1981). The bone scan has greater sensitivity and is particularly useful in areas such as the small bones of the foot or the spine where radiographic

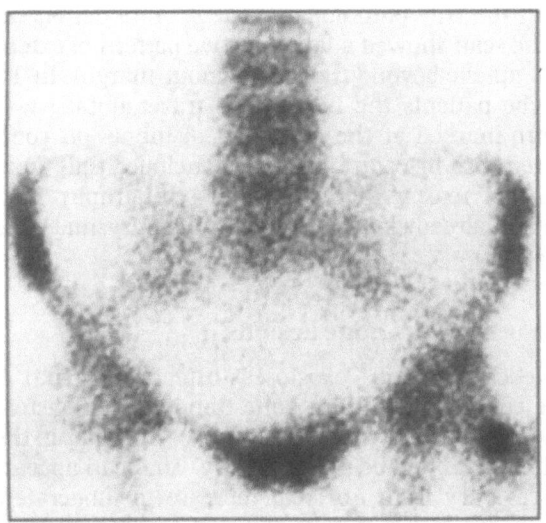 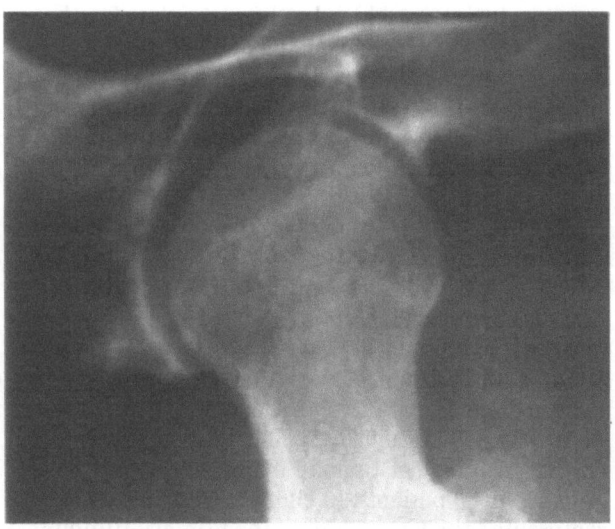

a   b

Fig. 6.3. (a) Bone scan of anterior pelvis and upper femora showing a focus of increased tracer uptake in the left femoral neck caused by an osteoid osteoma. (b) The lesion is just visible as an area of sclerosis on the radiograph.

appearances may be normal. A normal bone scan virtually excludes a diagnosis of osteoid osteoma.

In patients with clinical symptoms suggestive of osteoid osteoma a radiograph of the appropriate area should be obtained first. If this is normal an isotope bone scan should then be performed.

Bone scintigraphy has also been used as an aid in the operative localisation of osteoid osteoma as the tumour may not be easily visible. The patient is injected with a bone-scanning agent some hours prior to surgery and a gamma camera (Rinsky et al. 1980) or a probe (Ghelman et al. 1981) is used in the operating theatre to show that all of the intensely active bone has been removed, indicating complete removal of the tumour. The procedure has recently been described in some detail by O'Brien et al. (1984), who used a probe and a 5 mCi (185 MBq) dose of ^{99m}Tc-MDP injected 2 h preoperatively. A punch biopsy of normal bone is obtained and the activity counted. Repeated biopsies are then obtained from the region of the osteoid osteoma. Affected bone shows increased count rates, which return to normal when the lesion has been completely removed.

Osteoclastoma and Bone Cysts

Osteoclastoma (giant cell tumour) may arise anywhere in the skeleton, but the most common sites are lower end of femur, upper end of tibia and lower end of radius (Lichtenstein 1977). The tumour may be multicentric at presentation, and distinction between malignant and benign lesions is difficult on clinical, radiological or histological grounds (Peimer et al. 1980). Approximately 10% of the tumours are malignant, but in some cases the malignant change may be due to radiotherapy given for a previous benign lesion (Dahlin 1978). Even in benign lesions local recurrence is very common (McGrath 1972).

The scintigraphic appearances of giant cell tumours were described by Peimer et al. (1980), who studied 18 lesions occurring in 5 patients. The characteristic scan appearance was either of intense uptake in the whole tumour or a rim of increased uptake around a cold centre. They also found that the bone scan was useful in detecting local recurrence of the tumour after excision. This scan appearance was confirmed by Levine et al. (1984) in a series of 21 patients: 9 showed uniformly increased tracer uptake within the tumour while 12 had significantly less uptake in the centre of the tumour compared with the periphery.

Goodgold et al. (1984) found that all of a series of six patients with osteoclastoma showed the tumour to have a cold centre and a rim of increased activity on bone scintigraphy. They commented that the scan appearances were very different from those of a simple bone cyst, the most common lesion to mimic osteoclastoma radiologically. Simple (unicameral) bone cysts are often undetectable on scan or show up as a photon-deficient area with a thin rim of peripheral activity (Gooodgold et al. 1984). This description of simple bone cysts corresponds with that given by Moon et al. (1968), who utilised ^{18}F imaging. More intense uptake may be

seen in a bone cyst which has been the site of pathological fracture. Goodgold et al. (1984) claim specificity for the scan appearance of osteoclastoma,
stating that in a series of 100 patients with suspected bone neoplasms only 1 lesion mimicked
osteoclastoma on bone scan. Both Levine et al.
(1984) and Goodgold et al. (1984) found
osteoclastoma to be hypervascular on early (blood
pool) images.

The relationship between the extent of the primary lesion in osteoclastoma and scan appearances
has been evaluated by several groups of workers.
Simon and Kirchner (1980) found bone scan uptake
to be extended beyond the true extent of the tumour
in 2/3 patients studied. Levine et al (1984) correlated histological tumour extent and bone scan
findings in 19 patients. In eight the scan accurately
represented the true extent of the primary tumour;
in one the tumour extent was underestimated on
bone scan because of avascular necrosis. In the
remaining ten the scan overestimated the tumour
extent, though the discrepancy was no greater than
4 cm in any case. Bone scintigraphy did not demonstrate the extraosseous tumour extension found
at surgery in nine patients and identified
preoperatively in all nine by CT or angiography.
They concluded that bone scanning was less useful
than conventional tomography or computed
tomography in planning surgical margins.
Goodgold et al (1984) found extended scan uptake
beyond the margin of the primary tumour in 4/6
patients, but stated that this uptake could not be
easily confused with the tumour margin. They concluded that CT, conventional tomography, plain
radiography and scintigraphy were of equal value
when planning surgery.

Simon and Kirchner (1980) found the ^{67}Ga scan
to be abnormal at the site of the primary tumour
in 2/3 patients with osteoclastoma, and uptake did
not extend beyond the tumour margin. Levine et al,
(1984) obtained ^{67}Ga images in seven patients with
osteoclastoma. The images were normal in three
cases, slightly abnormal in two and definitely abnormal in two. They concluded that ^{67}Ga was of very
limited value in this tumour.

Aneurysmal bone cysts are formed of comunicat-
ing pools of venous blood bordered by connective
tissue septa which show giant cell reaction. They
are regarded as a distinct entity, though similar
lesions may be seen in association with a variety
of benign and malignant osseous tumours (Lichtenstein 1977). Early reports (Gilday and Ash 1976;
Makhija 1981) reported the bone scan to be abnormal in this condition. Hudson (1984) found the
bone scan to be abnormal in all 25 cases he studied.
In 22 cases the bone scan appearances correlated
with the true pathological extent of the lesion; in
3 the scan showed a false-positive pattern of extended uptake beyond the true tumour margin. In 16
of the patients the increase in tracer uptake was
more marked at the periphery of the lesion compared with its centre. Hudson concluded that there
was no reason to recommend scintigraphy in a
patient already known to have an aneurysmal bone
cyst.

Miscellaneous Bone Lesions

Osteocartilaginous exostoses (osteochondroma) is
the commonest benign bone tumour (Lichtenstein
1977). The lesion may be solitary or multiple, in the
latter case often being hereditary. The scan appearances vary from no local increase to moderately
increased tracer uptake (Sy 1981). The multiple
lesion variety may undergo sarcomatous degeneration, but scintigraphy has no value in predicting this
(Goodgold et al. 1983).

Bone islands consist of foci of compact lamellar
bone within normal cancellous bone. Approximately one-half of the lesions cause increased tracer uptake on bone scan, the remainder producing
no abnormality (Hall et al. 1980). The radiographic
appearances of a bone island and an osteoblastic
metastasis may be similar. In this situation a normal
bone scan will exclude the malignant lesion (Go et
al. 1980).

An intraosseous ganglion is a benign cystic lesion
of bone which is subchondral in location and adjacent to but not communicating with the joint. The
lesion may cause pain, which may be interpreted
as being due to joint disease. The bone scan demonstrates focally increased activity in the lesion
(Makhija and Lopano 1983) and saves the patient
from undergoing unnecessary joint investigations.

Chondroblastoma appears as a lytic lesion in the
epiphyseal ossification centre of long bones and may
invade adjacent bone. The bone scan appearances
vary from normal (Bell et al. 1974) to markedly
increased uptake (Humphrey et al. 1980).

Benign cortical irregularity of the distal femur
(BCIDF) is a condition which may mimic the radiographic appearances of malignancy (Barnes and
Gwinn 1974). The bone scan is normal in BCIDF
(Conway et al. 1975; Velchik et al. 1984), thus distinguishing it from primary malignant lesions of
bone.

Increased uptake of bone-scanning agent has also
been described in cholesteatoma (Milstein and
Nusynowitz 1979), ameloblastoma (Olson and
McCombs 1977), periosteal leiomyoma (Conklin et
al. 1981), intracranial osteoma (Karl et al. 1983)
and osteoblastoma (Makhija and Stein 1983).

Marrow Disorders

Multiple Myeloma

Skeletal involvement is a major component of multiple myeloma and is characterised by the lack of an osteoblastic reaction (Lichtenstein 1977). Radiographic changes of osteolytic lesions, fractures and demineralisation can help in making the diagnosis.

A number of studies have compared bone scan and radiographic findings in myeloma. The bone scan is often abnormal in patients with myeloma, but the number of lesions detected is usually many fewer than found by bone radiographs (Wahner et al. 1980; Woolfenden et al. 1980; Waxman et al. 1981). Large osteolytic lesions may be missed completely on the bone scan. The bone scan will identify a number of lesions not visualised radiographically, and this can be of value in the patient with either bone pain or a tissue mass and no radiographic abnormality (Wahner et al. 1980; Woolfenden et al. 1980; Freeman et al. 1984). A "superscan" appearance has been reported in association with myeloma (Anscombe and Walkenden 1983) but this is a very unusual occurrence. Hepatic uptake of bone-scanning agents in myeloma has been reported and has been attributed to the presence of hepatic amyloid resulting from the myelomatosis (Tur-Kaspa et al. 1981).

Waxman et al. (1981) performed both bone scan and gallium imaging in patients with multiple myeloma. In 5 of the 18 patients imaged lesions were demonstrated which showed high gallium uptake and normal or only slightly abnormal bone tracer uptake. The disease had a fulminant course in this subgroup of patients and all died within 3 months. The authors conclude that this combination of scintigraphic findings identifies a subgroup of patients with rapidly progressive disease who may benefit from alternative treatment modalities such as radiation therapy. This interesting observation requires further validation.

Overall the bone scan contributes little to the assessment of the patient with myeloma and bone radiographs should be the primary investigation when looking for evidence of bone involvement. The routine use of the bone scan in this group of patients cannot be justified, either at presentation or during the follow-up, and scintigraphy should be reserved for the patient with bone pain but normal bone radiographs.

Histiocytosis

"Histiocytosis" is a general term used to describe a number of conditions such as eosinophilic granuloma. Hand-Schüller-Christian disease and Letterer-Siwe disease in which the predominant abnormality is proliferation of histiocytes. Skeletal lesions are often prominent in this group of conditions.

Bone scanning has been advocated for the detection of skeletal involvement by histiocytosis by some investigators who concluded that the bone scan is more sensitive than bone radiographs (Gilday and Ash 1976; Schaub et al. 1982). Other series have found the bone scan to be relatively insensitive; Parker et al. (1980), for example, found that the bone scan detected only 35% of the lesions visible on radiographs and did not show any additional lesions. Antonmattei et al. (1979) stressed the importance of looking for photopaenic lesions. Crone-Munzebrock and Brassow (1983) concluded that the radiographic skeletal survey was superior to bone scanning for the primary detection of bony lesions, but the isotope technique was more reliable for follow-up examination and for detection of recurrences. At present the bone scan and skeletal radiography should be regarded as complementary techniques in the assessment of histiocytosis X.

Mastocytosis

Systemic mastocytosis produces mast cell hyperplasia with the clinical syndrome of urticaria pigmentosa. Abnormal new bone formation may occur resulting in radiographic abnormalities. The bone scan may demonstrate diffusely increased bone activity with little or no kidney visualisation—the "superscan" appearance (Ensslen et al. 1983). More focal bone scan abnormalities have also been reported, and the bone scan appears to be more sensitive than either radiography or standard biochemistry in determining the presence of bone involvement (Rosenbaum et al. 1984).

Lymphomas and leukaemias

Ferrant et al. (1975) found abnormal bone scans indicating skeletal involvement in 10 out of 38 patients with Hodgkin's disease. All but one of the patients with an abnormal bone scan had Stage III or Stage IV disease, and four also had abnormal skeletal radiographs. Schechter et al. (1976) described abnormal bone scans in eight patients with

Hodgkin's disease, seven of them having Stage IV disease. Eggenstein et al. (1978) obtained bone scans in 67 patients with Hodgkin's disease. Unsuspected bony involvement was demonstrated by the scan in five patients, but there were nine false-positive results. Details of staging of the patients was not presented. Overall, Eggenstein and his colleagues concluded that bone scintigraphy was more reliable than bone radiography for detection of bone involvement.

Martin and Ash (1977) have commented that the bone scan is very sensitive in detecting skeletal involvement by non-Hodgkin's lymphoma and may show more extensive disease than the radiograph. Schechter et al. (1976) found bone scan abnormalities in 10 out of 16 patients with non-Hodgkin's lymphoma. All but one of the patients imaged had either Stage III or Stage IV disease. Eggenstein et al. (1978) found bone scanning to be less useful than radiographs in non-Hodgkin's lymphoma and attributed this to the fact that the bone involvement was often diffuse and predominantly osteolytic.

There appears to be no place for routine bone scanning in early (Stage I or Stage II) lymphoma. Even in more advanced disease its main use should be in the investigation of patients with bone pain.

Focal abnormalities on the bone scan may be seen in patients with leukaemia (Gilday et al. 1977); Wong et al. 1983). In children with leukaemia the appearances may mimic those seen in disseminated neuroblastoma with diffusely increased uptake in the metaphyses and loss of the accentuation of uptake normally seen in the actively growing epiphyses.

References

Anscombe A, Walkenden SB (1983) An interesting bone scan in multiple myeloma—?myeloma superscan. Br J Radiol: 489–492

Antonmattei S, Tetalman MR, Lloyd TV (1979) The multiscan appearance of eosinophilic granuloma. Clin Nucl Med 4: 53–55

Barnes GR, Gwinn JL (1974) Distal irregularities of the femur simulating malignancy. Am J Roentgenol Radium Ther Nucl Med 122: 180–185

Bell EG. Subramanian G, Blair RJ et al. (1974) Bone scanning in pediatrics. In: James AE, Wagner HN, Cooke RE (eds) Pediatric nuclear medicine. Saunders, Philadelphia, pp 344–368

Cade S (1955) Osteogenic sarcoma. A study based on 133 patients. J R Coll Surg Edinb 1: 79–111

Chew FS, Hudson TM (1982) Radionuclide bone scanning of osteosarcoma: falsely extended uptake patterns. AJR 139: 49–54

Conklin JJ, Camargo EE, Wagner HN (1981) Bone scan detection of peripheral periosteal leiomyoma. J Nucl Med 22: 97

Conway JJ, Gooneratne N, Simon G (1975) Radionuclide evaluation of distal femoral metaphyseal irregularities which simulate neoplasm. J Nucl Med 16: 521–522

Crone-Munzebrock W, Brassow F (1983) A comparison of radiographic and bone scan findings in histiocytosis X. Skeletal Radiol 9: 170–173

Dahlin DC (1978) Giant cell tumours. In: Bone tumours—general aspects and data in 6221 cases, 3rd edn. Thomas, Springfield Ill, pp 99–115

Dahlin DC, Johnson EW (1954) Giant osteoid osteoma. J Bone Joint Surg [Am] 36: 559–570

Eggenstein G, Drochmans A, De Roo M, Wildiers J, Devos P, Van der Schueren G (1978) Bone scintigraphy as detection method for bone and bone marrow involvement in malignant lymphoma with regard to other exploration techniques. J Belge Radiol 61: 471–480

Ensslen RD, Jackson FI, Reid AM (1983) Bone and gallium scans in mastocytosis: correlation with count rates, radiography and microscopy. J Nucl Med 24: 586–588

Ferrant A, Rodhain J, Michaux JL, Piret L, Maldague B, Sokal G (1975) Detection of skeletal involvement in Hodgkin's disease: a comparison of radiography, bone scanning and bone marrow biopsy in 38 patients. Cancer 35: 1346–1353

Frankel RS, Jones AE, Cohen JA, Johnson, KW, Johnston GS, Pomeroy TC (1974) Clinical correlations of ^{67}Ga radionuclide studies with radiography in Ewing's sarcoma. Radiology 110: 597–603

Freeman ML, Van Drunen M, Gergans G, Kaplan E (1984) Accumulation of bone scanning agent in multiple myeloma. Clin Nucl Med 9: 49

Frei E, Jaffe N, Link M, Abelson H (1979) Adjuvant chemotherapy of osteogenic sarcoma: progress, problems and prospects. In: Jones SE, Salmon SE (eds) Adjuvant therapy of Cancer II. Grune and Stratton, New York, pp 355–363

Gandsman EJ, Deutsch SD, Tyson IB (1983) Use of dynamic bone scanning in the differential diagnosis of osteomyelitis, Paget's disease and primary bone tumours, J Nucl Med 24: P83 (abstract)

Ghaed N, Thrall JH, Pinsky SM, Johnson MC (1974) Detection of extraosseous metastases from osteosarcoma with ^{99m}Tc-polyphosphate bone scanning. Radiology 112: 373–375

Ghelman B, Thompson FM, Arnold WD (1981) Intraoperative localisation of an osteoid osteoma. J Bone Joint Surg [Am] 63: 826–827

Gilday DL, Ash JM (1976) Benign bone tumours. Semin Nucl Med 6: 33–46

Gilday DL, Ash JM, Reilly BJ (1977) Radionuclide skeletal survey for paediatric neoplasm. Radiology 123: 399–406

Giuliano AE, Feig S, Eilber FR (1984) Changing metastatic patterns of osteosarcoma. Cancer 54: 2160–2164

Go RT, El-Khoury GY, Wehbe MA (1980) Radionuclide bone image in growing and stable bone island. Skeletal Radiol 5: 15–18

Goldmann AB, Braunstein P (1975) Augmented radioactivity on bone scans of limbs bearing osteosarcoma. J Nucl Med 16: 423–424

Goldmann AB, Becker MH, Braunstein P, Francis KC, Genieser NB, Firooznia H (1975) Bone scanning—osteogenic sarcoma. Correlation with surgical pathology. Radiology 124: 83–90

Goldstein H, McNeil BJ, Zufall E, Jaffe N, Treves S (1980a) Changing indications for bone scintigraphy in patients with osteosarcoma. Radiology 135: 177–180

Goldstein H, McNeil BJ, Zufall E, Treves S (1980b) Is there still a place for bone scanning in Ewing's sarcoma? J Nucl Med 21: 10–12

Goodgold HM, Chen DC, Majd M, Nolan NG (1983) Scintigraphy of primary bone neoplasia. J Nucl Med 24: P57 (abstract)

Goodgold HM, Chen DP, Majd M, Nolan NG, Malawer M (1984) Scintigraphic features of giant cell tumour. Clin Nucl Med 9: 526–530

Goris ML, Basso LV, Etcubanas E (1980) Photopenic lesions in bone scintigraphy. Clin Nucl Med 5: 299–301

Hall FM, Goldberg RP, Davies JAK, Fainsinger MH (1980) Scintigraphic assessment of bone islands. Radiology 135: 737–742

Hamdy RC (1981) Paget's disease of bone. Assessment and management. Praeger Scientific, Eastbourne

Helms CA, Hattner RS, Vogler JB (1984) Osteoid osteoma: radionuclide diagnosis. Radiology 151: 779–784

Heyman S (1980) The lymphatic spread of osteosarcoma shown by Tc-99m-MDP scintigraphy. Clin Nucl Med 5: 543–545

Hudson TM (1984) Scintigraphy of aneurysmal bone cysts. AJR 142: 761–765

Humphrey A, Gilday DL, Brown RG (1980) Bone scintigraphy in chondroblastoma. Radiology 137: 497–499

Jeffree GM, Price HG, Sissons HA (1975) The metastatic patterns of osteosarcoma. Cancer 32: 87–107

Karl RD, Hartshorne MF, Cawthorn MA et al. (1983) Skull scintigraphy: intracranial osteoma. Clin Nucl Med 8: 626–627

Kirchner PT, Simon MA (1981) Radioisotope evaluation of skeletal disease. J Bone Joint Surg [Am] 63: 673–681

Levine E, De Smet AA, Neff JR, Martin NL (1984) Scintigraphic evaluation of giant cell tumour of bone. AJR 143: 343–348

Lichtenstein L (1977) Bone tumours, 5th edn. Mosby, St Louis

Lisbona R, Rosenthall L (1979) Role of radionuclide imaging in osteoid osteoma. Am J Roentgenol Radium Ther Nucl Med 132: 77–80

Makhija MC (1981) Bone scanning in aneurysmal bone cyst. Clin Nucl Med 6: 500–501

Makhija MC, Lopano AJ (1983) Intra-osseous ganglion: bone imaging with Tc 99m-MDP. Clin Nucl Med 8: 54–55

Makhija MC, Stein IH (1983) Bone imaging in osteoblastoma. Clin Nucl Med 8: 141

Martin DJ, Ash JM (1977) Diagnostic radiology in non-Hodgkin's lymphoma. Semin Oncol 4: 297–309

McGrath PJ (1972) Giant cell tumour of bone: an analysis of fifty two cases. J Bone Joint Surg [Br] 54: 216–229

McKillop JH, Fogelman I, Boyle IT, Greig WR (1977) Bone scan appearance of a Paget's osteosarcoma: failure to concentrate HEDP. J Nucl Med 18: 1039–1040

McKillop JH, Etcubanas, E, Goris ML (1981) The indications for and limitations of bone scintigraphy in osteogenic sarcoma: a review of 55 patients. Cancer 48: 1133–1138

McLean RG, Murray IPC (1984) Scintigraphic patterns in certain primary malignant bone tumours. Clin Radiol 35: 379–383

McNeil BJ (1984) Value of bone scanning in neoplastic disease. Semin Nucl Med 14: 277–286

McNeil BJ, Cassady JR, Geiser, CF, Jaffe N, Traggis D, Treves S (1973) Fluorine-18 bone scintigraphy in children with osteosarcoma or Ewing's sarcoma. Radiology 109: 627–631

McNeil NJ, Hanley J (1980) Analysis of serial radionuclide bone images in osteosarcoma and breast carcinoma. Radiology 135: 171–176

Milstein DM, Nusynowitz ML (1979) Cranial cholesteatoma: unusual ^{99m}Tc-Sn polyphosphate and ^{99m}Tc pertechnetate scintiphotos. Clin Nucl Med 4: 240–241

Moon NF, Dworkin HJ, La Fleur PD (1968) The clinical use of sodium fluoride F18 in bone photoscanning. JAMA 204: 116–122

Moore GE, Gerner RE, Brugarolas A (1973) Osteogenic sarcoma. Surg Gynecol Obstet 136: 359–366

Murray IPC (1980) Bone scanning in the child and young adult. Skeletal Radiol 5: 1–14

Nair N (1985) Bone scanning in Ewing's sarcoma. J Nucl Med 26: 349–352

O'Brien TM, Murray TE, Malone LA et al. (1984) Osteoid

osteoma: excision with scintimetric guidance. Radiology 153: 543–544

Olson WH, McCombs RK (1977) Positive (^{99m}Tc) diphosphonate and ^{67}Ga-citrate scans in ameloblastoma. J Nucl Med 13: 348–349

Omjola MF, Cockshott WP, Beatty EG (1981) Osteoid osteoma: an evaluation of diagnostic modalities. Clin Radiol 132: 199–204

Papanicolaou N, Kozakewich H, Treves S, Goorin A, Emans J (1982) Comparison of the extent of osteosarcoma between surgical pathology and skeletal scintigraphy. J Nucl Med 23: P7 (abstract)

Parker BR, Pinckney L, Etcubanas E (1980) Relative efficacy of radiographic and radionuclide bone surveys in the detection of the skeletal lesions of histiocytosis X. Radiology 134: 377–380

Pearlman RJ, Steiner CE (1978) Chondrosarcoma—correlative study of nuclear imaging and histology. Bull Hosp Jt Dis Orthop Inst 39: 153–164

Peimer CA, Schuller AL, Mankin HJ (1980) Multicentric giant-cell tumour of bone. J Bone Joint Surg [Am] 62: 642–656

Rinsky LA, Goris M, Bleck EE, Halpern A, Hirshman P (1980) Intraoperative skeletal scintigraphy for localisation of osteoid osteoma of the spine. J Bone Joint Surg [Am] 62: 143–144

Rosenbaum RC, Frieri M, Metcalfe DD (1984) Patterns of skeletal scintigraphy and their relationship to plasma and urinary histamine levels in systemic mastocytosis. J Nucl Med 25: 859–864

Rosenthall L, Lisbona R (1980) Role of radionuclide imaging in benign bone and joint disease of orthopedic interest. In: Freeman LM, Weissmann HS (eds) Nuclear medicine annual 1980. Raven, New York, pp 267–302

Schaub T, Eissner D, Hahn K, Greinacher I (1982) Bone scanning and follow up of skeletal lesions in histiocytosis X. In: Raynaud C (ed) Proceedings of the 3rd world congress on nuclear medicine and biology, vol 1, Pergamon, Paris, pp 849–850

Schechter JP, Jones SE, Woolfenden JM, Lilien DL, O'Mara RE (1976) Bone scanning in lymphoma. Cancer 38: 1142–1148

Siddiqui AR, Ellis JH (1982) "Cold spots" on bone scan at the site of osteosarcoma. Eur J Nucl Med 7: 480–481

Simon MA, Kirchner PT (1980) Scintigraphic evaluation of primary bone tumours. J Bone Joint Surg [Am] 62: 758–764

Smith FW, Gilday DL (1980) Scintigraphic appearances of osteoid osteoma. Radiology 137: 191–195

Smith FW, Nandi SC, Mills K (1982) Spinal chondrosarcoma demonstrated by Tc 99m-MDP bone scan. Clin Nucl Med 7: 111–112

Smith J, Botet JF, Yeh SDJ (1984) Bone sarcomas in Paget's disease: a study of 85 patients. Radiology 152: 583–590

Swee RG, McLeod RA, Beabout JW (1979) Osteoid osteoma: detection, diagnosis and localisation. Radiology 132: 117–123

Sy WM (1981) Benign bone tumours. In: Sy WM (ed) Gamma images in benign and metabolic bone diseases, vol 1. CRC Press, Boca Raton, Fla, pp 127–150

Teates CD, Brower AC, Williamson BR (1977) Osteosarcoma extraosseous metastases demonstrated on bone scans and radiographs. Clin Nucl Med 2: 298–302

Tur-Kaspa R, Samuels LD, Levo Y (1981) Detection of hepatic amyloidosis by technetium labelled pyrophosphate scan in primary and secondary amyloidosis and in multiple myeloma. Nucl Med Comm 2: 4–8

Vanel D, Henry-Amar M, Lumbroso J et al. (1984) Pulmonary evaluation of patients with osteosarcoma: roles of standard radiography, tomography, CT, scintigraphy and tomoscintigraphy. AJR 143: 519–523

Velchik MG, Heyman S, Todd Makler P, Goldstein HA, Alavi A (1984) Bone scintigraphy: differentiating benign cortical irregularity of the distal femur from malignancy. J Nucl Med 25: 72–74

Wahner HW, Kyle RA, Beabout JW (1980) Scintigraphic evaluation of the skeleton in multiple myeloma. Mayo Clinic Proc 55: 739–746

Waxman AD, Siemsen JK, Levine AM et al. (1981) Radiographic and radionuclide imaging in multiple myeloma: the role of gallium scintigraphy. J Nucl Med 22: 232–236

Wong K-Y, Benton C, Gelfand MJ, Aron BS, Lampkin BC, Bore KE (1983) Isolated bone relapse in long term survivors of acute lymphoblastic leukaemia. J Pediatr 102: 92–94

Wollfenden JM, Pitt MJ, Durie BGM, Moon TE (1980) Comparison of bone scintigraphy and radiology in multiple myeloma. Radiology 134: 723–728

Yeh SDJ, Rosen G, Benua RS (1982) Gallium scans in Paget's sarcoma. Clin Nucl Med 7: 546–552

7 · The Bone Scan in Metabolic Bone Disease

I. Fogelman

Introduction

Skeletal uptake of ^{99m}Tc-labelled diphosphonate depends primarily upon osteoblastic activity and, to a lesser extent, skeletal vascularity (Fogelman 1980). A bone scan image therefore presents a functional display of total skeletal metabolism and as such has a potentially valuable role to play in the assessment of patients with metabolic bone disorders. However, the bone scan appearances in metabolic bone disease are often non-specific, and their recognition depends upon a subjective impression of increased tracer uptake throughout the whole skeleton (Fogelman and Citrin 1981). This may be particularly difficult to detect when dealing with mild disease. It is the presence of focal lesions, as in metastatic disease, that makes a bone scan appear obviously abnormal. While focal lesions are easily identified, slightly increased tracer uptake throughout the whole skeleton may be virtually impossible to detect by visual inspection alone. Thus inevitably there will be difficulty in evaluating the bone scans from many patients with metabolic bone disease. However, in the more severe cases scan appearances can be quite striking and virtually diagnostic.

Why is the Bone Scan Abnormal?

Many of the metabolic bone diseases, with the exception of osteoporosis, are characterised by high bone turnover and are often associated with elevated levels of serum parathyroid hormone which causes increased bone resorption. As there is direct coupling between bone resorption and formation, an osteoblastic response follows osteoclastic activity leading to new bone formation (Frost 1963). It is recognised that bone-seeking radiopharmaceuticals adsorb onto bone at sites of new bone formation, with particular affinity for areas where active mineralisation is occurring. A comprehensive review of bone-seeking radiopharmaceutical uptake mechanisms is given in Chapter 2. While it has previously been suggested that tracer uptake may be associated with immature collagen (Rosenthall and Kaye 1976), it has been shown that if mineral and immature collagen are present together there is marked preferential uptake of tracer by mineral (Francis et al. 1981). Nevertheless, in situations where there is considerable excess of osteoid, it is uncertain what contribution this may make to total uptake of radiopharmaceutical.

Osteomalacia presents something of a paradox. This condition results from vitamin D deficiency, which produces a profound mineralisation defect. In severe cases there is a massive excess of osteoid present with markedly reduced mineralisation. Yet in this situation there is extremely high affinity for bone-seeking tracers—a fact which has been known for many years; in the early 1960s it was shown that patients with osteomalacia had increased radiocalcium accretion rates (Heaney 1963). The explanation presented was that although there is excess osteoid with reduced mineralisation, there is so much osteoid which is mineralising, albeit slowly, that the total area of mineralisation in the skeleton is in fact increased, even though the rate at any individual site is reduced (Nordin et al. 1976). This explanation is not totally convincing, and the reason why increased bone uptake of tracer should occur in osteomalacia is not yet fully understood. It may even be that in osteomalacia high tracer uptake is to some extent artefactual, with increased diffusion in an extremely large "osteoid pool".

Nevertheless, the bulk of evidence to date does suggest that bone uptake of tracer reflects skeletal metabolism and that this is likely to be primarily due to parathyroid hormone effect. Certainly, from clinical experience, one has a strong impression that the bone scan appearances in metabolic bone disease reflect the degree of hyperparathyroidism that is present.

Bone Scan Appearances

It is now recognised that in metabolic bone disease certain patterns of bone scan abnormality are commonly seen. Fogelman et al. (1979) previously described seven metabolic features that are characteristic of metabolic bone disorders in general:

1. Increased tracer uptake in axial skeleton
2. Increased tracer uptake in long bones
3. Increased tracer uptake in periarticular areas
4. Faint or absent kidney images

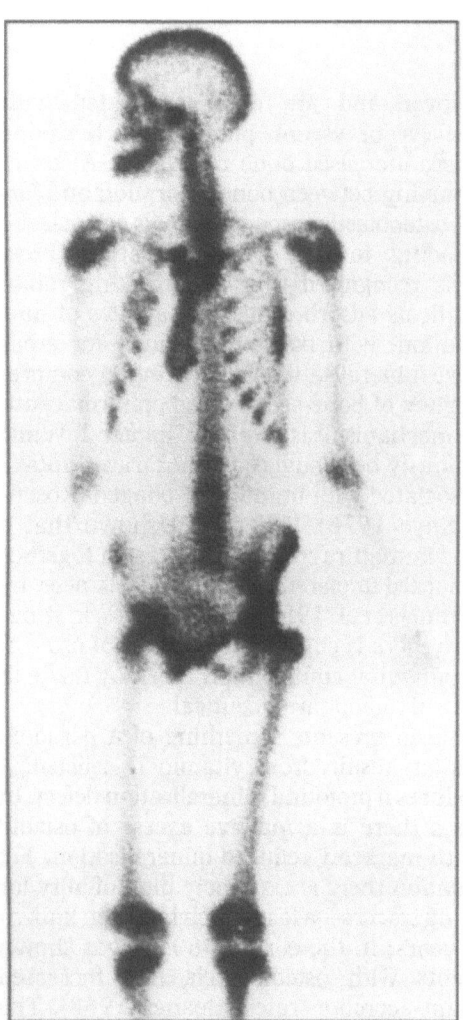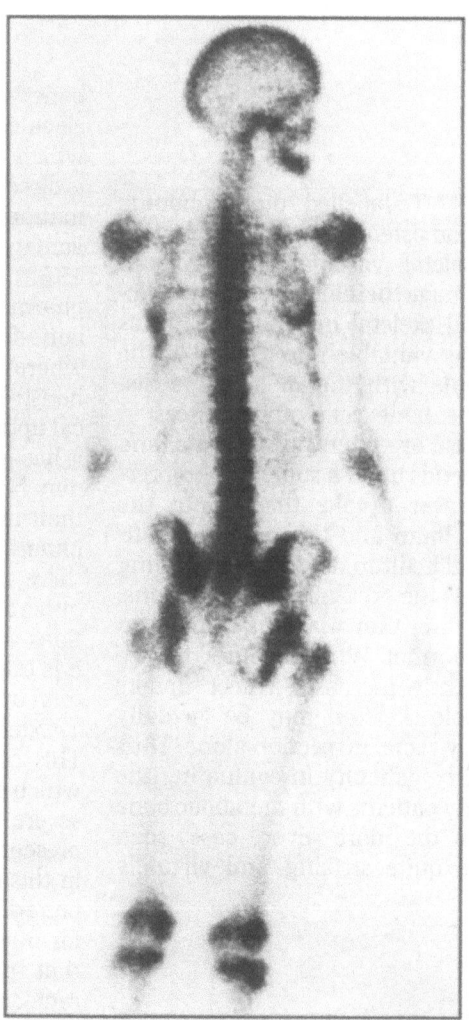

Fig. 7.1a,b. Bone scan anterior (a) and posterior (b) views from a patient with osteomalacia. There is high uptake of tracer throughout skeleton with extremely good contrast between bone and soft tissue. Note, in particular, high uptake in calvaria and mandible typical of hyperparathyroidism, "beading" of costochondral junctions, "tie sternum" and extremely faint renal images. In addition, there are several focal abnormalities in ribs caused by pseudofractures.

5. Prominent calvaria and mandible
6. Beading of the costochondral junctions
7. "Tie sternum"

However, it must be emphasised that these features are non-specific and, with the exception of absent kidney images, can all be seen in normal subjects. Indeed, these features are frequently seen in adolescents, in whom the growing skeleton is metabolically active.

The "classic" bone scan appearance in metabolic bone disease is an image that strikes one immediately as being of such excellent quality that it is almost too good to be true (Fig. 7.1). There is extremely high contrast between bone and adjacent soft tissue, and the individual metabolic features described reflect increased tracer uptake at various sites throughout the skeleton. The features listed include increased tracer uptake in the axial skeleton, long bones and periarticular areas. In these cases increased uptake is a matter of subjective judgement. However, increased tracer uptake in the calvaria and mandible may on occasion be particularly prominent and produce striking images which are clearly recognisable as abnormal. Indeed, in its extreme form, increased uptake in calvaria and mandible may be virtually pathognomonic of hyperparathyroidism (Fig. 7.2). When there is increased skeletal avidity for tracer, renal images may appear faint or even be absent (Fig. 7.3) as a result of less tracer being available for excretion, with resulting heightened contrast between bone

and kidneys. The costochondral junctions may be prominent (Fig. 7.4), and this appearance has been referred to as "beading" or the "rosary bead" appearance. In the sternum, characteristic appearances may often be seen, with a general increase

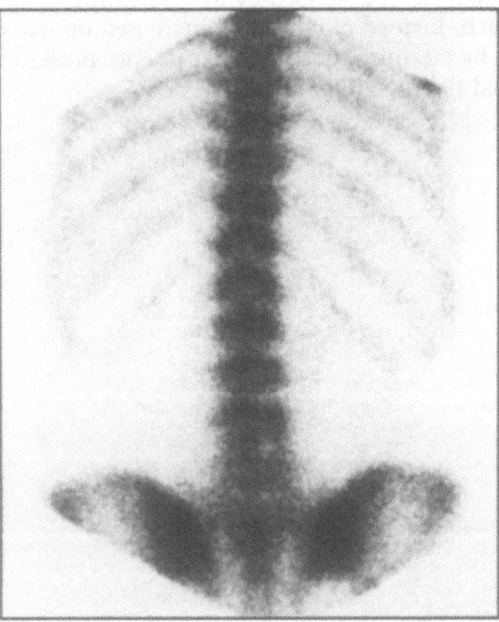

Fig. 7.3. High uptake of tracer throughout spine with kidneys not visualised.

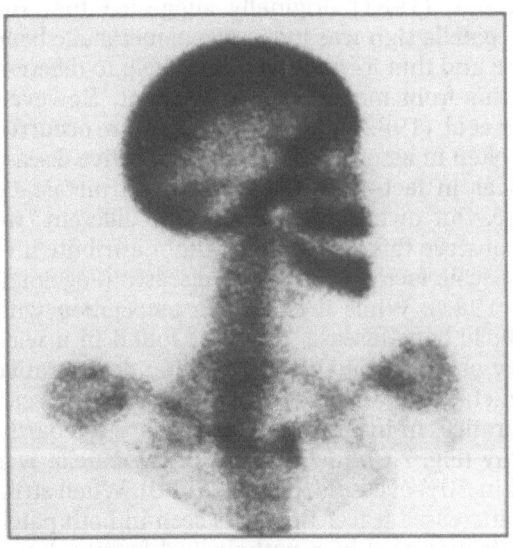

Fig. 7.2. Extremely high uptake of tracer throughout calvaria and mandible. This patient has renal osteodystrophy and severe secondary hyperparathyroidism.

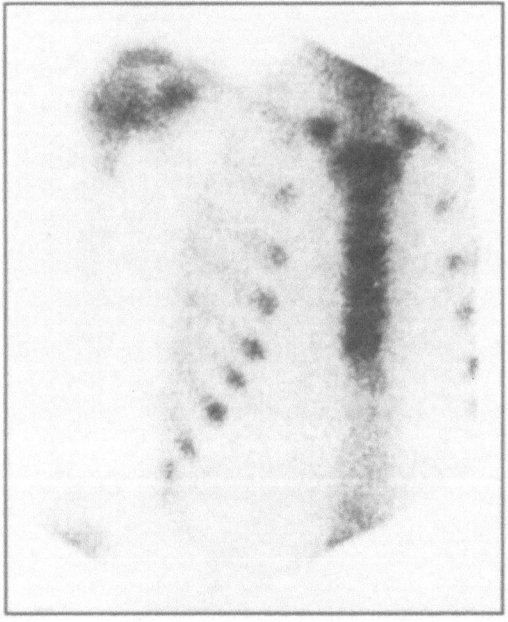

Fig. 7.4. "Beading" of costochondral junctions.

of tracer uptake by the manubrium and, in particular, the lateral borders of the body (Fig. 7.5). Because of its anatomical position and its often striking appearance, with flared lower portion and narrowing of the junction between manubrium and body, the descriptive term "tie sternum" has been applied (Fogelman et al. 1978a). A variation on this theme has been described by Sy and Smith (1981) in which, instead of uniformly increased uptake of tracer by sternum, horizontal stripes are present—"striped-tie" sign (Fig. 7.5b).

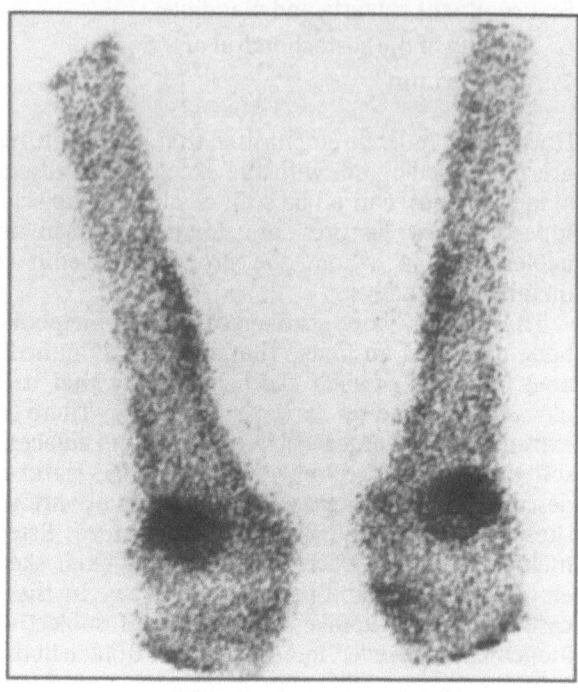

Fig. 7.6. "Hot" patella sign. Note also patchy increased tracer uptake along cortical borders of the femora, appearances characteristic of hypertrophic pulmonary osteoarthropathy.

a

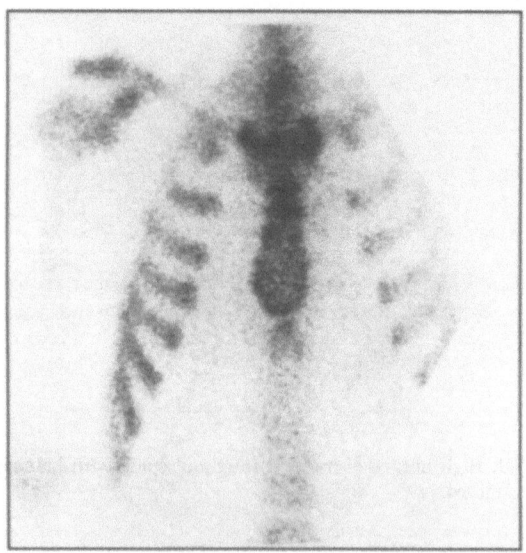

b

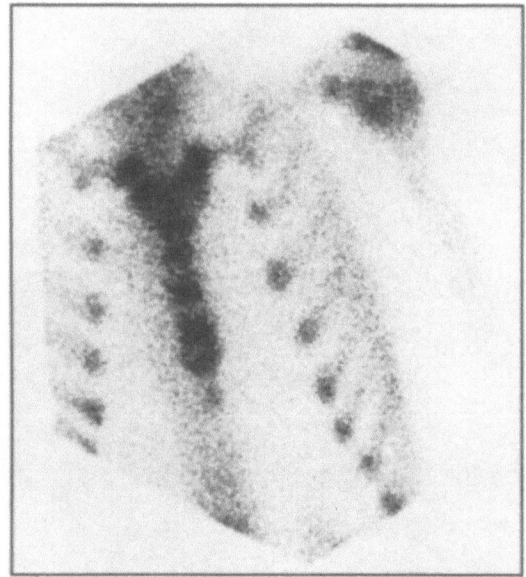

Fig. 7.5. a Increased uptake of tracer in sternum—"tie" sign; b striped "tie" sign. Note also the costochondral "beading".

There has been some controversy as to whether or not the "hot" patella sign is indicative of metabolic bone disease. A hot patella on the bone scan is defined as uptake of tracer in the patella greater than that by the distal femur or proximal tibia of the ipsilateral leg (Kipper et al. 1982; Fig. 7.6). Sy and Smith (1981) originally suggested that the "hot" patella sign was indicative of metabolic bone disease and that its presence could help to differentiate this from metastatic involvement. However, Kipper et al. (1982) found that this feature occurred most often in association with degenerative disease and was in fact seen in patients with metastatic disease. Our own experience is quite different; we often observe this feature but cannot attribute it to any specific factor or group of diseases (Fogelman et al. 1983). While it is seen in association with metabolic bone disease, it can be found in a wide variety of other conditions, including degenerative and metastatic disease. In a report of bone scan appearances in hypertrophic pulmonary osteoarthropathy (Fig. 7.6), involvement of the patella was noted in 50% of cases (Ali et al. 1980). When strikingly increased tracer uptake is seen in both patellae, this may well be a pathological feature, but it has no differential diagnostic value. My own view is that the patellae should be ignored in the context of metabolic bone disease.

Another relevant aspect, provoking some controversy, is the question of the effect of age on bone scan appearances. There is no doubt that in the growing skeleton there is high affinity for tracer, and it should be remembered that many chronic diseases may delay maturation of the skeleton; thus the finding of increased uptake may persist into the early 20s. It is widely believed that the quality of bone scan images deteriorates with advancing age (Wilson 1981). While this may be true of extreme old age, for practical purposes it is not relevant in the age group 20–60 years, and perhaps even somewhat older. However, other factors which may be found with advancing age such as obesity and cardiac failure may have a detrimental affect on bone scan quality.

Essentially, the recognition of metabolic bone disease on a bone scan depends upon the detection of increased tracer uptake throughout the skeleton. While this remains subjective, I believe that the concept of metabolic features is a useful one as it heightens awareness as to the possibility of metabolic bone disease being present. A further refinement is to obtain a semi-quantitative score (metabolic index) from the bone scan image (Fogelman et al. 1979); however, skeletal uptake of tracer can be quantitated much more accurately by measurement of 24-h whole-body retention of ^{99m}Tc-diphosphonate, which has been shown to provide a sensitive means of identifying patients with increased bone turnover (Fogelman et al. 1978b). All aspects of bone scan quantitation and skeletal retention of ^{99m}Tc diphosphonate are discussed in Chapter 16.

Renal Osteodystrophy

In patients with severe renal osteodystrophy one may see the most striking bone scan appearances found in the various metabolic bone disorders. There is markedly increased tracer uptake throughout the axial and peripheral skeleton and, in keeping with this, the kidneys appear faint and are frequently not visualised. There is extremely high contrast between bone and soft tissues, and the overall effect is to produce a so-called superscan image (Sy and Mittal 1975; Lien et al. 1976; Olgaard et al. 1976). The skull appearances may be virtually pathognomonic of severe hyperparathyroidism, with marked increased uptake throughout the calvaria and mandible. Beading of the costochondral junctions and a "tie sternum" are also commonly seen. It is probable that most of the scan findings are due to increased bone turnover result-

ing from secondary hyperparathyroidism, but coexistent osteomalacia may contribute in some cases. The bladder may not be visualised because of failure to excrete tracer. Absence of the bladder helps to differentiate the bone scan in renal osteodystrophy from that in other metabolic disorders.

Alberts et al. (1981) evaluated eight patients with symptomatic renal osteodystrophy and found the bone scan and derived metabolic index to be of value in assessing the extent of skeletal disease. Seven of the eight patients had abnormal bone scans, and in addition the scans were of value in the identification of fractures and pseudofractures when present. De Graaf et al. (1984) quantitated skeletal uptake of tracer on the basis of computer analysis of bone scan images in 30 patients with histological evidence of renal osteodystrophy. Bone scan images were obtained 5 h after injection and following haemodialysis in an attempt to reduce soft tissue activity. However, it was found that soft tissue activity could not be normalised in patients with minimal bone disease, and images were generally of poor quality. However, in all cases total skeletal quantitation from bone scan images differentiated patients from normal controls, and it was suggested that the technique provided a reliable method for identifying metabolic bone disease. The results of quantitation were correlated with several histological parameters, but no significant correlation was found with either osteoid volume or osteoid surface. The authors suggested that this provides further evidence that hyperparathyroidism and not the amount of osteoid is the more important factor with regard to tracer uptake on bone.

While there are relatively few reports of direct comparisons between radiography and bone scanning in metabolic bone disease, renal osteodystrophy has been extensively studied. Sy and Mittal (1975) evaluated 14 chronic dialysis patients and found the bone scan to be abnormal in 93% of patients, while radiography showed changes in only 29%. Olgaard et al. (1976) studied 30 patients on haemodialysis and classified their bone scans into four groups, according to the degree of increased tracer uptake in the lower limbs. On this basis, they found that 90% of the scans but only 33% of the radiographs were abnormal. The same group later reported their experience of 51 non-dialysed patients with advanced renal failure and found that the bone scans were suggestive of renal osteodystrophy in 66% of cases, while changes were detected by radiography in 25% of cases (Olgaard et al. 1979). Cavalli et al. (1976) studied 43 patients with chronic renal disease (34 on dialysis) and found that the bone scan indicated that 88% had skeletal disease, while radiographs were abnormal in 50%. DeGraaf et al. (1978) studied 30 dialysis patients and found the bone scan was abnormal in 83%, while radiographs showed skeletal disease in 46%. Therefore, it seems clear that in chronic renal failure the bone scan is more sensitive than radiography for detecting skeletal disease.

Osteosclerosis may occasionally be seen on radiographs of the spine in patients with renal osteodystrophy; the bone scan equivalent is linear areas of increased tracer uptake corresponding to the cortical borders of vertebrae, against a background of generalised high uptake in the spine (Fogelman and Citrin 1981). Sites of ectopic calcification may be recognised, and the bone scan is more sensitive than routine radiography in identifying pulmonary calcification (Devacaanthan et al. 1976; De Graaf et al. 1979). The bone scan is also of value in the assessment of renal transplant patients complaining of bone pain. These patients may develop avascular necrosis, which is usually related to corticosteroid therapy. Weight-bearing areas such as the femoral head, femoral condyle, or talus are most often affected and involved sites are seen on the scan

as focal areas of increased tracer uptake (Dumler et al. 1977). The other important differential diagnosis of bone pain in this immunosuppressed group is osteomyelitis, which also appears strongly positive on the bone scan (Fogelman and Boyle 1980). The possibility of aluminium-induced bone disease should always be considered. However, as will be discussed later, the scan appearances in this condition are quite different and generally of extremely poor quality.

Primary Hyperparathyroidism

Primary hyperparathyroidism is a common disorder which is now being diagnosed with increasing frequency and at an earlier stage because of the availability of routine calcium estimations and parathyroid hormone assay. The degree of bone scan abnormality generally reflects the amount of skeletal involvement, and there is thus a wide range of scan appearances from normal to, occasionally, those mimicking severe renal osteodystrophy (Sy 1974; Weigmann et al. 1977). However, it should

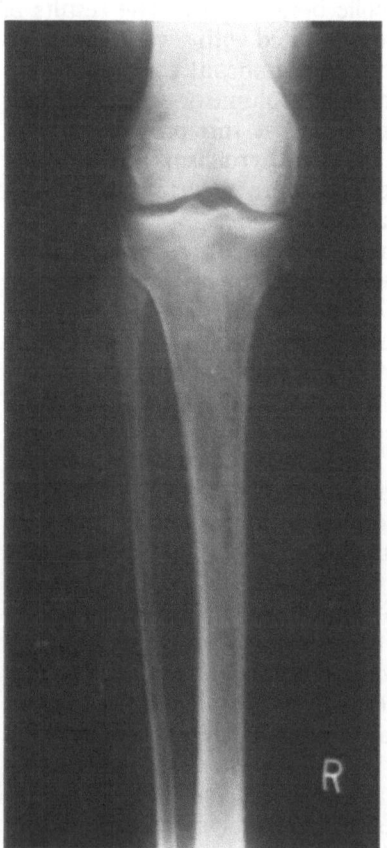
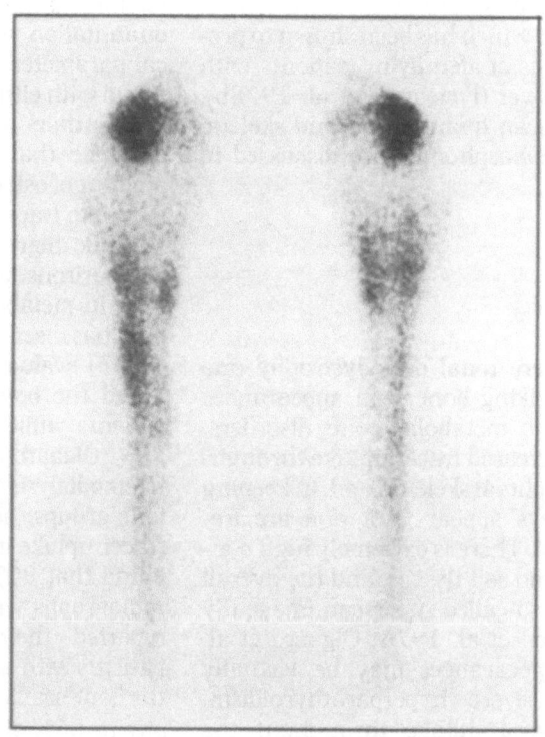

a

b

Fig. 7.7. a Radiograph of right tibia shows several Brown tumours. b These sites show increased uptake on scan, and lesions are also apparent in left tibia. Note also "hot" patellae.

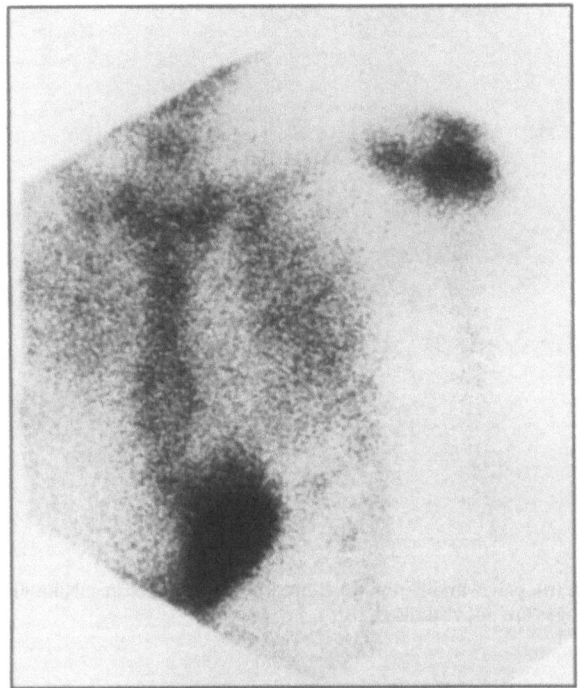 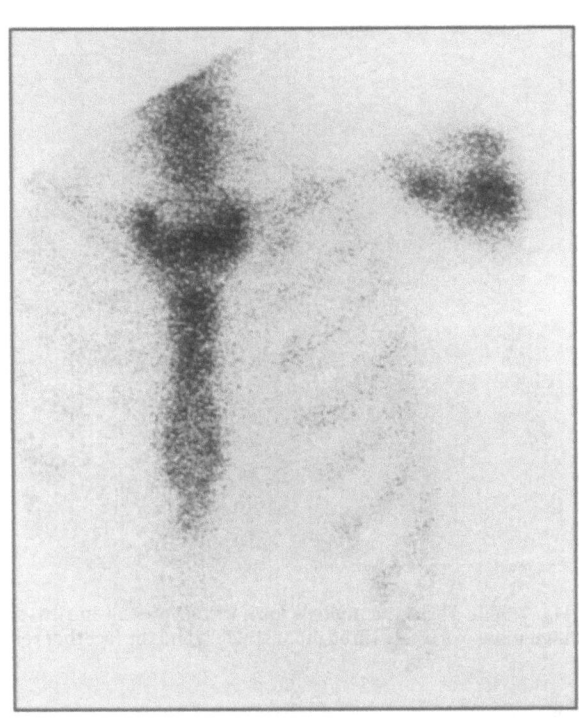

a   b

Fig. 7.8. a Anterior view of chest from patient presenting with acute renal failure and severe hypercalcaemia. Note tracer uptake in stomach and lungs caused by ectopic calcification. b Repeat study 1 month later following rehydration and initial dialysis shows return to normal. This patient had milk-alkali syndrome, but similar findings are seen on occasion with primary hyperparathyroidism.

be emphasised that the bone scan usually appears normal and thus has no clear diagnostic role to play in the routine evaluation of patients with suspected primary hyperparathyroidism. Radiographic skeletal surveys are also normal in most cases, but specific changes such as subperiosteal erosions can occasionally be seen. The bone scan is the more sensitive of the two investigations (Fogelman and Carr 1980), and if scan appearances are not suggestive of metabolic bone disease then radiographs will invariably be normal. Despite apparently normal diphosphonate uptake on the bone scan by visual assessment, quantitative measurements (e.g. 24-h whole-body retention of diphosphonate) are frequently elevated (Fogelman et al. 1980a) as a result of mild diffuse increase in skeletal metabolism.

The presence of focal abnormalities on the bone scan in primary hyperparathyroidism are uncommon but may be seen when Brown tumours are present (Evens et al. 1969; Fogelman and Citrin 1981; Fig. 7.7), with chondrocalcinosis (Sy et al. 1977), or following vertebral collapse. In addition, in rare instances when a patient presents with aggressive, rapidly advancing primary hyperparathyroidism, multiple sites of ectopic calcification may be seen on the bone scan (Fig. 7.8).

Osteomalacia

The bone scan appearances in osteomalacia are usually abnormal and will often suggest the presence of metabolic bone disease (Fogelman et al. 1978a). The scan findings, however, are non-specific and all the metabolic features listed on p. 74 may be seen. Focal abnormalities cannot be considered to be metabolic features, but their presence, when the scan appears characteristic of metabolic bone disease, is suggestive of pseudofractures (Fig. 7.9). The bone scan provides a sensitive means of identifying pseudofractures, particularly in the ribs, and may detect lesions which are not visualised with conventional radiology (Fogelman et al. 1977a; Singh et al. 1977). However, lesions in the pelvis can on occasion be missed on the bone scan because of their symmetrical nature, or if they are obscured by bladder activity (Fogelman et al. 1978a). Pseudofractures are most often seen in the ribs, and in our experience 90% of patients who have such lesions will have rib involvement. Thus it is uncommon to see pseudofractures in isololation at other sites such as femoral neck or pelvis.

Fogelman et al. (1978a) evaluated 60 bone scans for the presence of metabolic features from 10

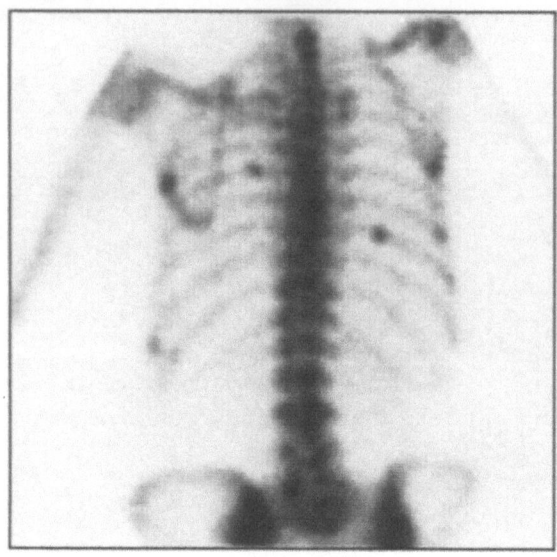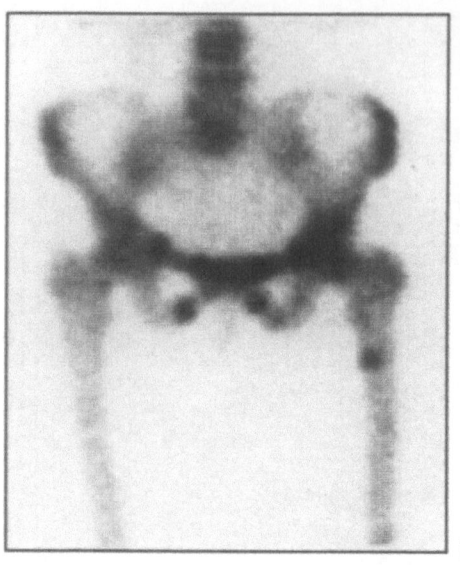

a
b

Fig. 7.9a,b. There are multiple focal lesions present in ribs, scapula (a), pelvis and femur (b) caused by pseudofractures. Note also high uptake of tracer throughout skeleton and the fact that renal images are not visualised.

patients with osteomalacia, 20 with metastatic disease and 30 normal subjects. In this study, nine of the ten patients with osteomalacia were correctly identified by two independent observers. Wilkins et al. (1983) used the bone scan to evaluate 17 elderly subjects with equivocal biochemical evidence of osteomalacia. Once again the scans were evaluated for the presence of metabolic features and it was considered that 10 of the 17 studies were abnormal. Histological studies were made of bone in all subjects, and the presence of excess osteoid was found in the ten patients whose scans were suggestive of metabolic bone disease. In addition, two other patients were found to have abnormal bone histology. It was considered that the bone scan provided the most practical, non-invasive means of detecting osteomalacia in the elderly.

Recently, the entity of aluminium-induced osteomalacia has been recognised in uraemic patients on haemodialysis (Parkinson et al. 1981). This disorder is characterised by bone pain, fractures, osteomalacia with little elevation of either serum alkaline phosphatase or parathyroid hormone levels, raised serum calcium values and general resistance to vitamin D treatment. Osteomalacia occurs because aluminium is deposited at the calcification front and blocks mineralisation. Thus, aluminium essentially acts as a bone "poison", which is quite different from the vitamin D deficiency state normally found in osteomalacia. Vanherweghem et al. (1984) have assessed the value of bone scan imaging in aluminium bone disease in a group of

33 dialysis patients. They presented scan images from patients with this disorder showing very poor quality images with high background activity (Fig. 7.10a) resulting from the relative failure of tracer to be taken up by bone. The quality of the scan images was dramatically improved following treatment with desferrioxamine (Fig. 7.10b). In this study patients were dialysed between injection and imaging, and scans were later given a semi-quantitative score based on metabolic features. Patients were divided into group A—those who developed hypercalcaemia while on vitamin D therapy (10 patients)—and group B—those who tolerated the treatment well (23 patients). Group A (aluminium bone disease) had lower values for bone scan quantitation, and it was suggested that the metabolic index could be of value in detecting uraemic patients at risk of vitamin D intoxication. Furthermore, 24 patients were studied before and after desferrioxamine administration, and it was observed that the 7 with lower values for scan quantitation had larger increases in serum aluminium following treatment than the 17 with an initially higher score. In 11 patients calcium accretion rates were calculated on the basis of radiocalcium retention and serum-specific activity for 10 days after an intravenous injection of 50 μCi (1850 kBq) of [47]Ca chloride. Those subjects with low values for scan quantitation had significantly lower values for calcium accretion (1.7 cf. 10.6 mg/day/cm, $P < 0.001$).

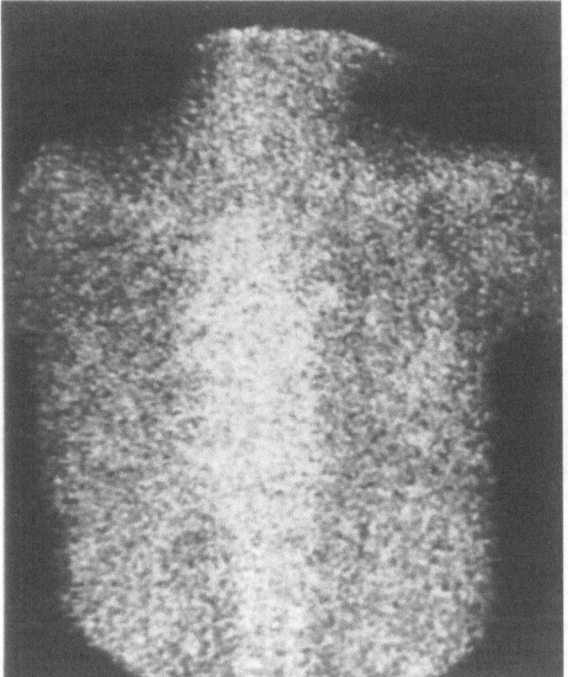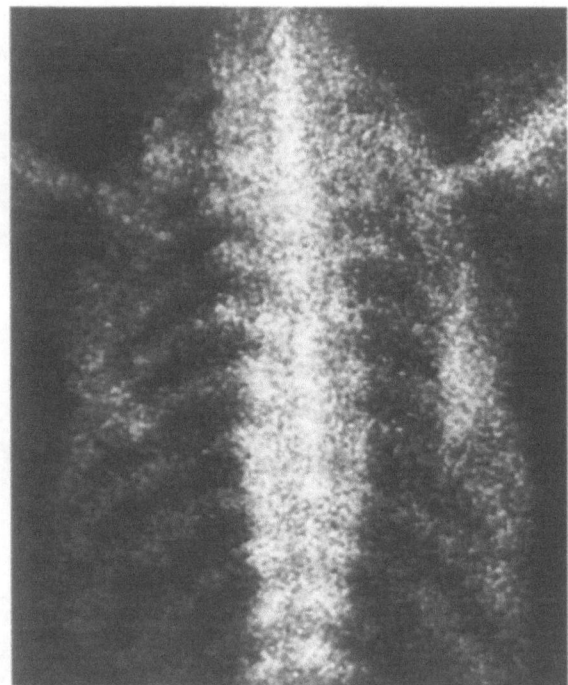

a   b

Fig. 7.10. a Posterior view of thoracic spine from a patient with aluminium bone disease. There is a "block" to mineralisation, tracer is not taken up at bone surfaces and there is high background activity. b Following desferrioxamine treatment there is dramatic improvement in scan appearances. (Vanherweghem et al. 1984)

Osteoporosis

The bone scan has not been found to have an important role to play in the diagnosis of osteoporosis (Fogelman and Carr 1980). This is a disorder where gradual change in bone mass may occur over many years, and, in keeping with the relatively minor imbalance in skeletal metabolism which is often present, the bone scan appearances are usually normal. However, the scan images may on occasion appear poor in quality because of relatively low bone uptake of tracer with a "washed-out" pattern of activity in the axial and appendicular bones. It has been suggested that this occurs in severe or "end-stage" osteoporosis caused by markedly reduced or even absent osteoblastic activity (Levine et al. 1977). Sy (1981) has observed these features in 72% of his patients with osteoporosis. We do not see this scan pattern as often, although poor definition of individual vertebrae is frequently noted (Fig. 7.11). When kyphoscoliosis is observed on the bone scan, or if there appears to be loss of spinal height with proximity of ribs to each other, or increased closeness of rib cage to pelvis, such appearances suggest vertebral collapse (Sy 1981) and would be in keep-ing with a diagnosis of osteoporosis. However, such evidence is indirect, and in practice the bone scan provides a less reliable means of diagnosing osteoporosis than radiography (Fogelman and Carr 1980).

Osteoporotic bones are abnormally brittle and fractures may occur. These are easily recognisable on the bone scan and are seen as focal areas of increased tracer uptake (Matin 1979). If vertebral collapse is present, scan appearances are characteristic with intense linear increase in tracer uptake (Fig. 7.11) corresponding to the site or sites of fracture. This intense uptake usually fades over a period of 1–2 years following collapse (Fig. 7.11), and thus the scan is of value in assessing the age of the vertebral collapse (Fogelman and Carr 1980). Even when scan appearances are quite typical of benign vertebral collapse, tumour cannot definitely be excluded and radiographs should be obtained. In the situation of a patient known to have osteoporosis and vertebral collapse who presents with back pain, the scan may be helpful in evaluating symptomatology. A normal scan would exclude recent fracture, and other causes for back pain should then be considered.

Schulz et al. (1984) have recently described the use of bone scanning to evaluate the skeletal

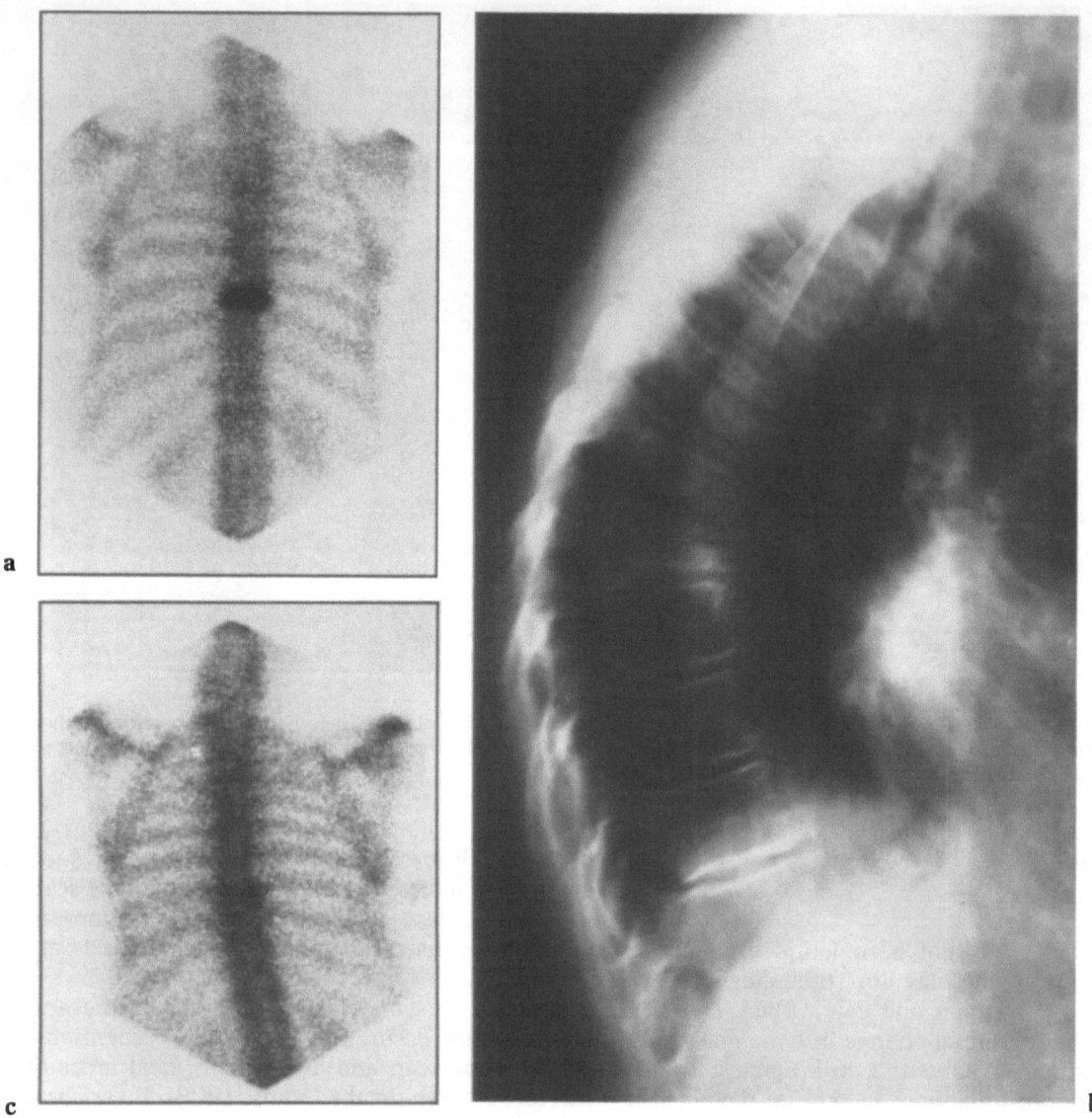

Fig. 7.11.a,b Intense linear increased tracer uptake seen in dorsal vertebra 8 (a) corresponding to vertebral collapse present on radiograph (b). c Repeat scan 8 months later shows considerable resolution.

response to sodium fluoride, a drug which stimulates osteoblastic activity. Studies were obtained in 12 women with osteoporosis before and after 6 months' treatment. All the pre-treatment bone scans were abnormal, but many of these findings may have represented degenerative change. Patients received a relatively large amount of fluoride (80 mg) together with 1500 mg calcium per day. In all cases images following treatment showed new areas of increased tracer uptake, primarily at sites in the peripheral skeleton where trabecular bone was present, such as metaphyses of long bones. Previous studies of bone mass with single photon absorptiometry suggested that sodium fluoride had no effect on the appendicular skeleton (Briancon and Meunier 1981) and thus the recent findings are rather unexpected. However, it is well known that approximately 40%–50% of patients receiving sodium fluoride will develop "rheumatic" pains which have been attributed to new or activated degenerative joint disease (Riggs et al. 1982). Schulz has suggested that the pain may in most instances be due to metaphyseal periostitis. O'Duffy et al. (1986) studied 11 osteoporotic women who had developed lower extremity pain while taking sodium fluoride (60–90 mg/day). Bone scans from these patients revealed an increased number of focal lesions when compared with asymptomatic osteoporotic women receiving sodium fluoride or those treated with oral calcium. Furthermore, serial radiographs demonstrated stress microfractures in 5 of the 11 symptomatic subjects, and lesions were present on the bone scan at these sites. However, many other lesions were present on the scans, and it is clear that microfractures are not the sole cause of painful bones. It was postulated that pain usually results from intense regional bone remodelling which may be complicated by stress microfracture. While the conclusions drawn as to the cause of pain associated with sodium fluoride therapy are somewhat different in the above studies, it is nevertheless apparent that the bone scan provides a sensitive means of monitoring the peripheral skeletal response to this drug.

While the bone scan has an extremely limited role to play in the diagnosis of osteoporosis, it may nevertheless occasionally provide valuable information in osteoporotic subjects. When patients present with severe back pain and vertebral collapse, it may not always be apparent that osteoporosis is the diagnosis and one may be concerned as to the possibility of coexistent disease, such as metastases or infection. In this situation the bone scan provides the most sensitive means of evaluating the skeleton.

Reflex Sympathetic Dystrophy Syndrome and Migratory Osteolysis

In the reflex sympathetic dystrophy syndrome (RSDS) rapid loss of bone may occur in a limb causing severe demineralisation. The aetiology of RSDS is not known, although trauma appears to be a contributing factor in many cases. The syndrome has certain similarities to disuse osteoporosis but is generally more severe, may occur in the presence of only moderate motor dysfunction and is not reversed by exercise. The bone scan has been found to provide a sensitive means of identifying RSDS, and this is discussed further in Chapter 11 (see p. 145).

Miscellaneous Conditions

There are many other conditions that can be considered under the heading of metabolic bone disease. Some of these are extremely uncommon, while others are of little clinical relevance. In the majority of cases there is only limited experience with bone scanning. For the purpose of describing the bone

scan appearances, these conditions can be divided into two broad groups: (1) those that cause a generalised alteration in skeletal metabolism, and (2) those that affect the skeleton in a more focal way.

Generalised Skeletal Involvement

Whenever there is generalised increase in bone turnover, there will be increased tracer uptake throughout the whole skeleton and the bone scan appearances may be indistinguishable from those found in conditions such as osteomalacia or renal osteodystrophy. Clearly, the degree of scan abnormality will depend upon the extent of skeletal involvement.

The most common and important condition in this section is thyrotoxicosis. The severity of associated skeletal disease is generally less than with primary hyperparathyroidism, probably because thyroxine is a less potent stimulator of bone resorption than parathyroid hormone and also because thyrotoxicosis is likely to be detected earlier because of its well-recognised clinical presentation. Surprisingly, there is relatively little information available regarding the bone scan appearance in this common condition. However, Kukar and Sy (1981) have reported that when skeletal involvement is present, the axial and appendicular bones may show symmetrically increased tracer uptake, and all the previously described metabolic features may be present.

We have previously reported the bone scan findings in acromegaly (Fogelman et al. 1980b), where generalised increased tracer uptake throughout the skeleton with metabolic features may be found associated with active disease (Fig. 7.12). In this condition, prognathism could often be detected on the scan, which helped to differentiate acromegaly from other diseases. In addition, the bone scan appeared to be a valuable means of identifying the degenerative changes that commonly occur.

Other conditions that have been reported to show the bone scan appearance of diffusely increased tracer uptake with metabolic features include hypervitaminosis D (Fogelman et al. 1977b) and mastocytosis (Sy et al. 1976). More recently, Rosenbaum et al. (1984) reported that various bone scan patterns could be found in systemic mastocytosis and they classified these into normal, unifocal, multifocal and diffuse. Patients with diffuse disease had the highest plasma and urinary histamine levels, and it was suggested that the bone scan might be of value in assessing the overall severity of disease.

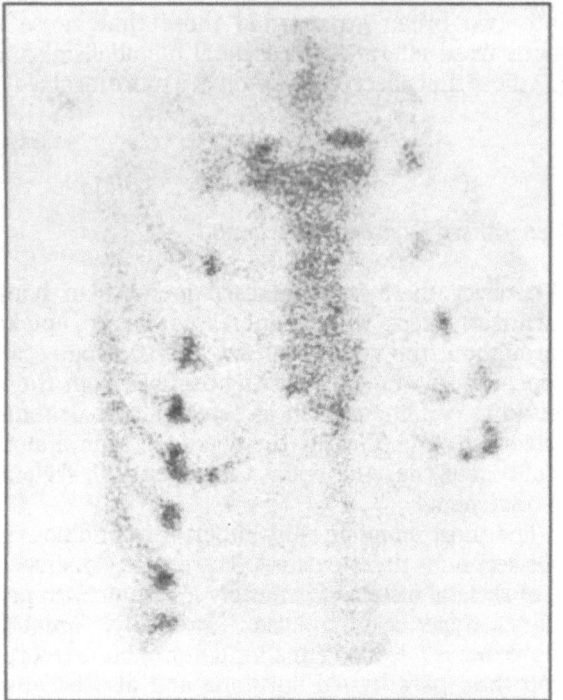
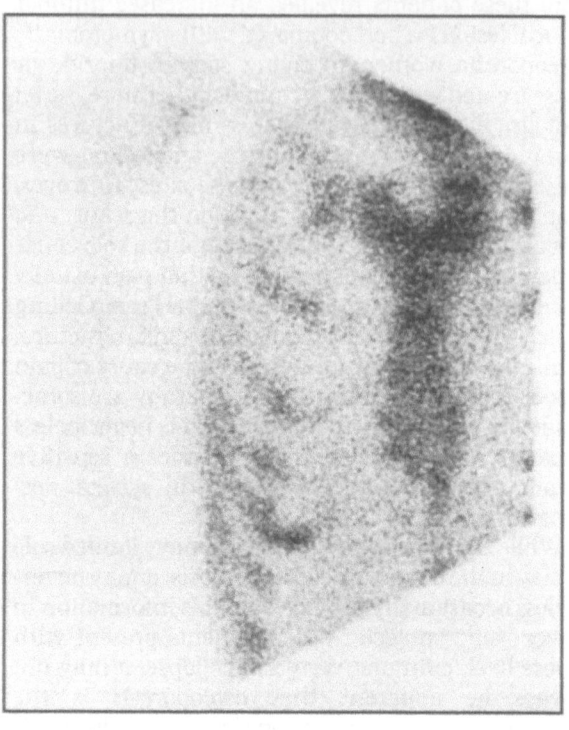

Fig. 7.12. a Costochondral beading seen in acromegalic patient. **b** Following removal of pituitary tumour, however, this is no longer apparent, suggesting reduction in skeletal metabolism, in keeping with good clinical and biochemical response.

We have experience of bone scanning in one patient with adult hypophosphatasia—a rare cause of osteomalacia which is associated with extremely low serum alkaline phosphatase activity—and skeletal uptake of tracer appeared normal. However, focal abnormalities were seen in both femora at the site of pseudofractures.

In osteopetrosis there is generalised osteosclerosis, and the basic defect is thought to be osteoclastic dysfunction. Park and Lambertus (1977) have reported bone scan findings in two adult cases and they did not find any increase of tracer uptake in the axial skeleton. However, there was dense increased tracer uptake in the metaphyseal

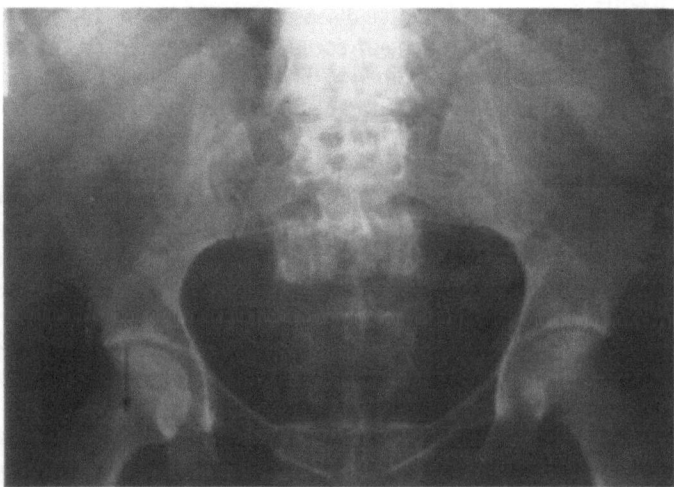
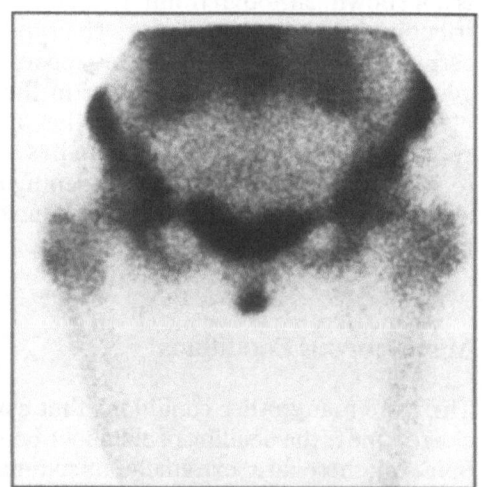

Fig. 7.13. (a) Bone island is seen on radiograph of right femoral neck. **b** No abnormality is present on scan, however, indicating that lesion is not metabolically active.

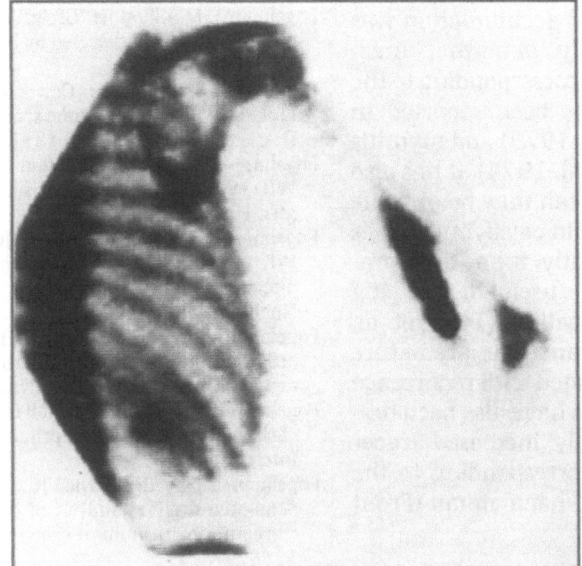

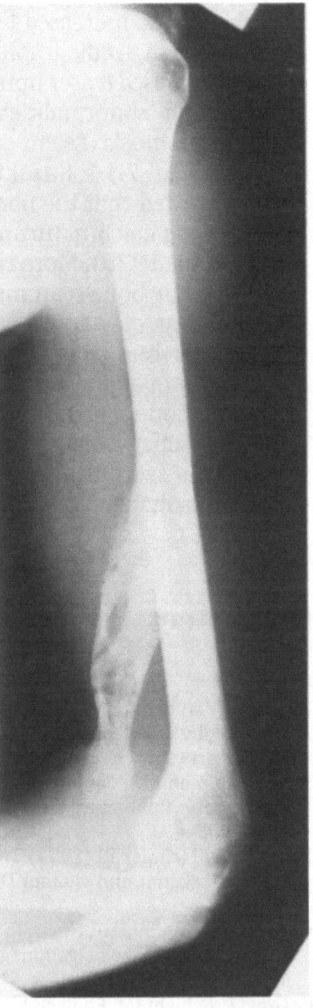

Fig. 7.14a,b. Bone scan view of right posterior thorax and arm (a) shows increased tracer accumulation lying within the brachialis muscle corresponding to soft tissue calcification seen on radiograph (b). Scan appearances represent continuing active bone turnover associated with myositis ossificans.

regions of most of the long bones and the tubular bones of the hand, with more generalised diffuse uptake in the cranial and facial bones. It was considered that the scan was particularly helpful in identifying complications associated with osteopetrosis, such as fracture or osteomyelitis.

It has been suggested that there is a generalised reduction in tracer uptake by the skeleton in both hypothyroidism and Cushing's syndrome (Kukar and Sy 1981).

Focal Skeletal Involvement

Many conditions may cause a local alteration in skeletal metabolism and therefore will be seen as focal abnormalities on the bone scan. It is possible to mention only some of these disorders in the present review, and it should be kept in mind that

occasionally sclerotic lesions that are no longer metabolically active may be seen on the radiograph but not on the bone scan. Bone islands, for example, are often not seen on a bone scan (Fig. 7.13; Hall et al. 1980).

Engelmann's disease (progressive diaphyseal dysplasia) and fibrous dysplasia are both disorders that may produce striking focal abnormalities on the bone scan with intense increased uptake of tracer. Essentially, the scan appearances are similar to those found in Paget's disease, and there may be difficulty in differentiating these conditions on the basis of the scan findings alone. Osteopoikilosis, osteopathia striata, and melorheostosis are unusual benign sclerotic dysplasias, each with striking characteristic radiographic appearances. Whyte et al. (1978) have reported, however, that the bone scan appearances are normal in osteopoikilosis and osteopathia striata, suggesting that these disorders may not be metabolically active. However, in melorheostosis, increased tracer accumulation was seen in each radiographically abnormal area. Focally increased tracer uptake corresponding to the radiographic abnormalities has been reported in tumoral calcinosis (Leicht et al. 1979) and myositis ossificans (Fig. 7.14; Suzuki et al. 1974). It has also been suggested that the bone scan may be of value in estimating calcium turnover in calcifying masses (Leicht et al. 1979). More recently, it has been proposed that the bone scan may be useful in assessing the maturity of ectopic ossification (Tyler et al. 1984); this has clinical relevance, as premature surgical removal may be associated with recurrence of disease. Bone scan alterations have also been described in scurvy, where focally increased tracer uptake was seen in a femur corresponding to the site of a resolving subperiosteal haematoma (Front et al. 1978).

References

Alberts C, Van der Schoot JB, Busemann-Sokole E (1981) Bone scintigraphy and densitometry in symptomatic haemodialysis bone disease. Eur J Nucl Med 6: 505–509

Ali A, Tetalman MR, Fordham EW et al. (1980) Distribution of hypertrophic pulmonary osteoarthropathy. Am J Radiol 134: 771–780

Briancon D, Meunier PJ (1981) Treatment of osteoporosis with fluoride, calcium and vitamin D. Orthop Clin North Am 12: 629–648

Cavalli PL, Camuzzini GF, Ghezzi P, Palanca R, Rovere A, Tortore P (1976) Total body gammagraphy in uraemic patients. Minerva Nefrol 23: 142–148

de Graaf P, Schicht IM, Pauwels EK, te Velde J, de Graeff J (1978) Bone scintigraphy in renal osteodystrophy. J Nucl Med 19: 1289–1296

de Graaf P, Schicht IM, Pauwels EKJ, Souverijn JHM, de Graeff J (1979) Bone scintigraphy in uremic pulmonary calcification. J Nucl Med 20: 201–206

de Graaf P, Pauwels EKJ, Vos PH, Schicht IM, te Velde J, de Graeff J (1984) Observations on computerized quantitative bone scintigraphy in renal osteodystrophy. Eur J Nucl Med 9: 419–425

Devacaanthan K, Yap AU, Chayes Z, Stein RM (1976) Pulmonary calcification in chronic renal failure; use of diphosphonate scintiscan as a diagnostic tool. Clin Nephrol 6: 488–491

Dumler F, Vulpetti AT, Guise ER, Levin NM (1977) ^{18}F –scintigraphy in the early diagnosis of osteonecrosis of the femoral head in chronic haemodialysis and transplantation. Clin Nephrol 8: 349–353

Evens RG, Ashburn W, Bartter FC (1969) Strontium 85 scanning of a "brown tumour" in a patient with parathyroid carcinoma. Br J Radiol 42: 224–225

Fogelman I (1980) Skeletal uptake of diphosphonate: a review. Eur J Nucl Med 3: 473–476

Fogelman I, Boyle IT (1980) Bone scanning in clinical practice. Scott Med J 25: 45–49

Fogelman I, Carr D (1980) A comparison of bone scanning and radiology in the evaluation of patients with metabolic bone disease. Clin Radiol 31: 321–326

Fogelman I, Citrin DL (1981) Bone scanning in metabolic bone disease: a review. Appl Radiol 10: 158–166

Fogelman I, McKillop JH, Greig WR, Boyle IT (1977a) Pseudofracture of the ribs detected by bone scanning. J Nucl Med 18: 1236–1237

Fogelman I, McKillop JH, Cowden EA, Fine A, Boyce B, Boyle IT, Greig WR (1977b) Bone scan findings in hypervitaminosis D: case report. J Nucl Med 18: 1205–1207

Fogelman I, McKillop JH, Bessent RG, Boyle IT, Turner JG, Greig WR (1978a) The role of bone scanning in osteomalacia. J Nucl Med 19: 245–248

Fogelman I, Bessent RG, Turner JG, Citrin DL, Boyle IT, Greig WR (1978b) The use of whole-body retention of Tc-99m diphosphonate in the diagnosis of metabolic bone disease. J Nucl Med 19: 270–275

Fogelman I, Citrin DL, Turner JG, Hay ID, Bessent RG, Boyle IT (1979) Semi-quantitative interpretation of the bone scan in metabolic bone disease. Eur J Nucl Med 4: 287–289

Fogelman I, Bessent RG, Beastall G, Boyle IT (1980a) Estimation of skeletal involvement in primary hyperparathyroidism. Ann Intern Med 92: 65–67

Fogelman I, Hay ID, Turner JG, Citrin DL, Greig WR (1980b) Semi-quantitative analysis of the bone scan in acromegaly: correlation with human growth hormone values. Br J Radiol 53: 874–877

Fogelman I, McKillop JH, Gray HW (1983) The 'hot' patella sign—is it of any clinical significance? J Nucl Med 24: 312–315

Francis MD, Horn PA, Tofe AJ (1981) Controversial mechanism of technetium-99m deposition on bone. J Nucl Med 22: 72 (abstract)

Front D, Hardaoff R, Levy J, Benderly A (1978) Bone scintigraphy in scurvy. J Nucl Med 19: 916–917

Frost HM (1963) Bone remodelling dynamics. Thomas, Springfield, Ill

Hall FM, Goldberg RP, Davies JAK, Fainsinger MH (1980) Scintigraphic assessment of bone islands. Radiology 135: 737–742

Heaney RP (1963) Evaluation and interpretation of calcium-kinetic data in man. Clin Orthop 31: 153–183

Kipper MS, Alazraki NP, Feiglin DH (1982) The "hot" patella. Clin Nucl Med 7: 28–32

Kukar N, Sy WM (1981) Selected endocrine disorders. In: Sy WM (ed) Gamma images in benign and metabolic bone diseases, vol II. CRC Press, Boca Raton, Fla, pp 1–21

Leicht E, Berberich R, Lauffenburger T, Haas HG (1979) Tumoral calcinosis: accumulation of bone-seeking tracers in the calcium deposits. Eur J Nucl Med 4: 419–421

Levine SB, Haines JE, Larson SM, Andrews TM (1977) Reduced skeletal localization of 99m-Tc-diphosphonate in two cases of severe osteoporosis. Clin Nucl Med 2: 318–321

Lien JW, Wiegmann T, Rosenthall L, Kaye M (1976) Abnormal ^{99m}technetium-tin-pyrophosphate bone scans in chronic renal failure. Clin Nephrol 6: 509–512

Matin P (1979) The appearance of bone scans following fractures, including immediate and long-term studies. J Nucl Med 20: 1227–1231

Nordin BEC, Horsman A, Aaron J (1976) Diagnostic procedures. In: Nordin BEC (ed) Calcium, phosphate and magnesium metabolism. Churchill Livingstone, Edinburgh, pp 469–524

O'Duffy JD, Wahner HW, O'Fallon WM, Johnson KA, Mulis J, Riggs BL (1986). Mechanism of acute lower extremity pain syndrome in fluoride-treated osteoporotic patients. Am J Med 80: 561–566

Olgaard K, Heerfordt J, Madsen S (1976) Scintigraphic skeletal changes in uraemic patients on regular haemodialysis. Nephron 17: 325–334

Olgaard K, Madsen S, Heerfordt J, Hammer M, Jensen H (1979) Scintigraphic skeletal changes in non-dialyzed patients with advanced renal failure. Clin Nephrol 12: 273–278

Park H-M, Lambertus J (1977) Skeletal and reticuloendothelial imaging in osteopetrosis: case report. J Nucl Med 18: 1091–1095

Parkinson IS, Ward MK, Kerr DNS (1981) Dialysis encephalopathy, bone disease and anaemia: the aluminium intoxication syndrome during regular haemodialysis. J Clin Pathol 34: 1285–1294

Riggs BL, Seeman E, Hodgson SF, Taves DR, O'Fallon WM (1982) Effect of the fluoride/calcium regimen on vertebral fracture occurrence in postmenopausal osteoporosis. New Engl J Med 306: 446–450

Rosenbaum RC, Frieri M, Metcalfe DD (1984) Patterns of skeletal scintigraphy and their relationship to plasma and urinary histamine levels in systemic mastocytosis. J Nucl Med 25: 859–864

Rosenthall L, Kaye M (1976) Observations on the mechanisms of ^{99m}Tc-labelled phosphate complex uptake in metabolic bone disease. Semin Nucl Med 6: 59–67

Schulz EE, Libanati CR, Farley SM, Kirk GA, Baylink DJ (1984) Skeletal scintigraphic changes in osteoporosis treated with sodium fluoride: concise communication. J Nucl Med 25: 651–655

Singh BN, Kesala BA, Mehta SP, Quinn JL (1977) Osteomalacia on bone scan simulating skeletal metastases. Clin Nucl Med 2: 181–183

Suzuki Y, Hisada K, Takeda M (1974) Demonstration of myositis ossificans by ^{99m}Tc pyrophosphate bone scanning. Radiology 111: 663–664

Sy WM (1974) Bone scan in primary hyperparathyroidism. J Nucl Med 15: 1089–1091

Sy WM (ed) (1981) Osteoporosis. In: Gamma images in benign and metabolic bone diseases. CRC Press, Boca Raton, Fla, pp 223–239

Sy WM, Mittal AK (1975) Bone scan in chronic dialysis patients with evidence of secondary hyperparathyroidism and renal osteodystrophy. Br J Radiol 48: 878–884

Sy WM, Smith AJ (1981) Chronic renal dialysis. In: Sy WM (ed) Gamma images in benign and metabolic bone diseases. CRC Press, Boca Raton, Fla, pp 151–186

Sy WM, Bonventure MV, Camera A (1976) Bone scan in mastocytosis: case report. J Nucl Med 17: 699–701

Sy WM, Mottola O, Lao RS, Smith A, Freund HR (1977) Unusual bone images in hyperparathyroidism. Br J Radiol 50: 740–744

Tyler JL, Derbekyan V, Lisbona R (1984) Early diagnosis of myositis ossificans with Tc-99m diphosphonate imaging. Clin Nucl Med 9: 256–258

Vanherweghem JL, Schoutens A, Bergmann P, Stolear J–C, Abramowicz D, Dhaene M, Smeyers J, Verbeelen D, Fuss M, Kinneart P (1984) Usefulness of ^{99m}Tc-pyrophosphate bone scintigraphy in aluminium bone disease. Trace Elements in Medicine 1: 80–83

Whyte MP, Murphy WA, Siegel BA (1978) ^{99m}Tc-pyrophosphate bone imaging in osteopoikilosis, osteopathia striata and melorheostosis. Radiology 127: 439–443

Wiegmann T, Rosenthall L, Kaye M (1977) Technetium 99m-pyrophosphate bone scans in hyperparathyroidism. J Nucl Med 18: 231–235

Wilkins WE, Chalmers A, Sanerkin NG, Rowe MJ (1983) Osteomalacia in the elderly: the value of radio-isotope bone scanning in patients with equivocal biochemistry. Age Ageing 12: 195–200

Wilson MA (1981) The effect of age on the quality of bone scans using technetium-99m pyrophosphate. Radiology 139: 703–705

8 · The Bone Scan in Paget's Disease

I. Fogelman

Introduction

Paget's disease of bone is a common disorder in the elderly in which excessive production of structurally abnormal bone occurs. It has a reported incidence of around 4% (Hamdy 1981), and is often observed as an incidental finding on radiographic skeletal surveys or bone scans.

The aetiology of Paget's disease remains unknown. In recent years, however, the presence of inclusion bodies in the nuclei of osteoclasts has been noted, and this has led to the proposal that Paget's disease may be viral in origin (Mills and Singer 1976; Rebel et al. 1981). Nevertheless, some controversy exists with regard to this finding (Hamdy 1981). There is an increased incidence of Paget's disease in families (Galbraith 1954; Singer et al. 1978), and it has been recognised for some time that there are marked geographical differences in prevalence. While Paget's disease is common in the UK, the USA, Europe, Australia and New Zealand, it is rare in Scandinavia, Africa and the Middle and Far East (Hamdy 1981). Even within the UK there are considerable regional variations in its incidence (Barker et al. 1977). These observations would seem to favour the view that environmental and hereditary factors are relevant in its development. There may also be a degenerative component in view of the increasing incidence with age (Pygott 1957).

Paget's disease is usually polyostotic, but may be monostotic; it is characterised in its initial phase by excess resorption of bone, which is followed by an intense osteoblastic response, with deposition of collagen in a mosaic pattern (woven bone) rather than the lamellar arrangement seen in normal bone (Alexandre et al. 1981). Thus skeletal architecture becomes disorganised, and coexisting areas of rarifaction and sclerosis may be seen on radiographs. There appears to be an imbalance of bone remodelling in favour of formation, and overall the size of affected bones tends to increase. Cortical thickening and bony expansion are important features when considering the differential diagnosis of sclerotic lesions seen on radiographs. Pagetic bone is extremely vascular (Wootton et al. 1978), and it has been suggested that this contributes to the bone pain which can be so problematic in this condition (Hamdy 1981).

The clinical features of Paget's disease are well known and pain is the commonest presenting complaint. However, coexistent arthritis in weight-bearing areas is frequently present and should always be considered as a possible explanation for pain, particularly when there is poor response to specific therapy for Paget's disease. Less often, pain may be due to fracture and rarely is due to nerve entrapment syndromes or sarcomatous change. Considerable bone enlargement may occur in Paget's disease, with quite striking deformity. However, this is relatively uncommon. Since many patients with Paget's disease are asymptomatic, it is clear that not all will require treatment. Nevertheless, in appropriate cases there can be dramatic relief of bone pain with therapy and currently there are three effective drugs available: mithramycin (Ryan 1977), calcitonin (Avramides 1977) and diphosphonate (Russell et al. 1974). In practice only the latter two are commonly used. Calcitonin is given by injection and may cause troublesome nausea, vomiting and flushing episodes. There is thus an increasing tendency to treat Paget's disease with diphosphonate as it is taken orally and is well tolerated by most patients. However, diphosphonate can cause a significant mineralisation defect in bone and may on occasion be associated with fracture (Boyce et al. 1984). It should therefore be used with caution in patients who have extensive lytic disease, particularly in a weight-bearing bone.

Bone Scan Appearances

Sites of bone which are involved with Paget's disease show both a striking increase in skeletal metabolism and an increase in blood flow, and there is thus high avidity for bone-seeking radiopharmaceuticals. The amount of tracer uptake in bone appears to be directly related to the degree of activity of the disease process (Shirazi et al. 1974). The bone scan appearances in Paget's disease are often characteristic (Serafini 1976), with the predominant feature being markedly increased uptake of tracer, which is usually distributed evenly throughout most or all of the affected bone (Figs. 8.1–8.4). A common exception to this general rule is seen in osteoporosis circumscripta (lytic disease involving the skull), where

tracer uptake is most intense at the margins of the lesion (Fig. 8.5; Rausch et al. 1977). Paget's disease, unlike most other skeletal abnormalities, tends to preserve and even enhance the normal anatomical configuration of bone. Expansion and, on occasion, distortion of involved bones may be seen. The appearances of individual lesions are often striking and pagetic bone seems to be "picked out", as the borders between normal and abnormal bone are well delineated (see Fig. 8.3). When the appendicular skeleton is involved, lesions generally commence at the articular end of the bone and progress into the shaft. The distal aspect of the lesion may be seen to have a sharp edge and this corresponds to the flame-shaped resorption front seen on radiographs (Fig. 8.6). There have been occasional reports of pagetic lesions confined to the diaphyseal area but this appears to be extremely uncommon (Frank 1981; Schubert et al. 1984).

Differential Diagnosis

The scan appearances in Paget's disease are generally characteristic, and when polyostotic disease is present there is seldom any doubt as to the diagnosis. Indeed, it is usually possible to differentiate between Paget's disease and metastatic disease even when they coexist (Fig. 8.7) (Citrin and McKillop 1978). However, both are common conditions

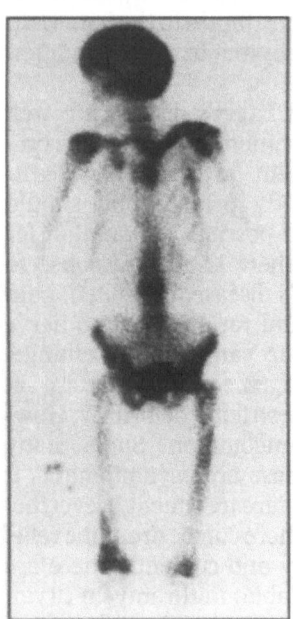 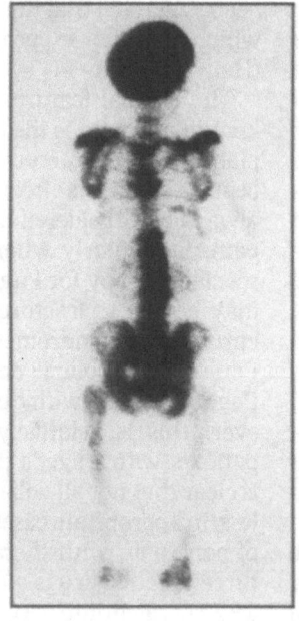

a   b

Fig. 8.1a, b. Whole-body scan anterior (a) and posterior (b) views showing extensive Paget's disease involving skull, left clavicle, spine, pelvis, scapulae and femora.

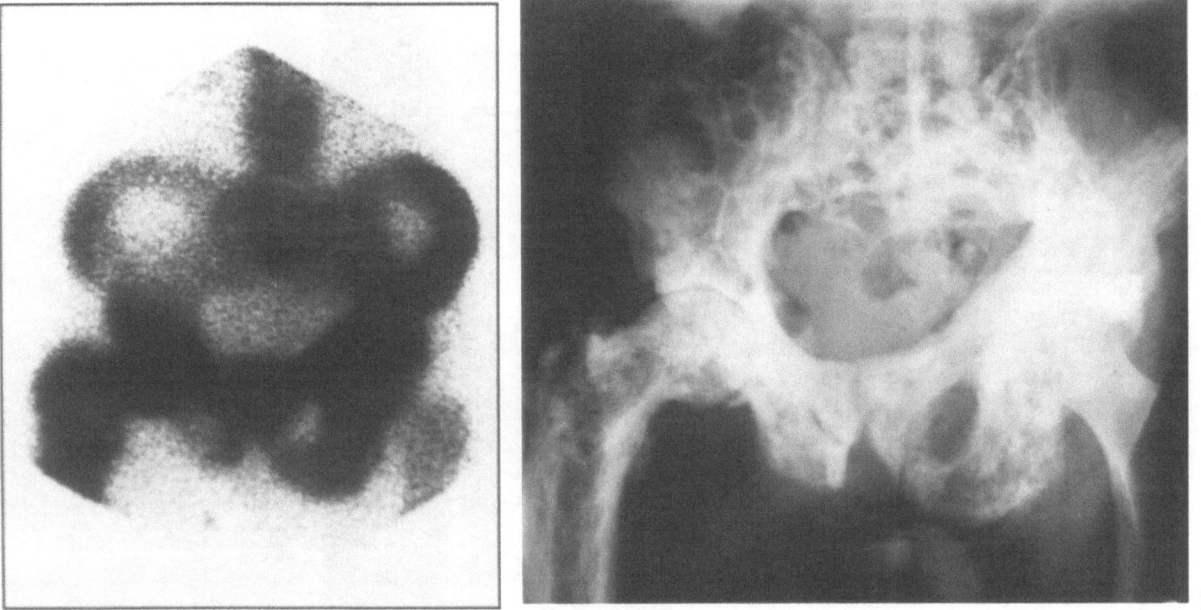

a   b

Fig. 8.2. a Typical scan appearances of Paget's disease involving left hemipelvis, lower right pelvis and right femur. b Radiograph confirms these appearances.

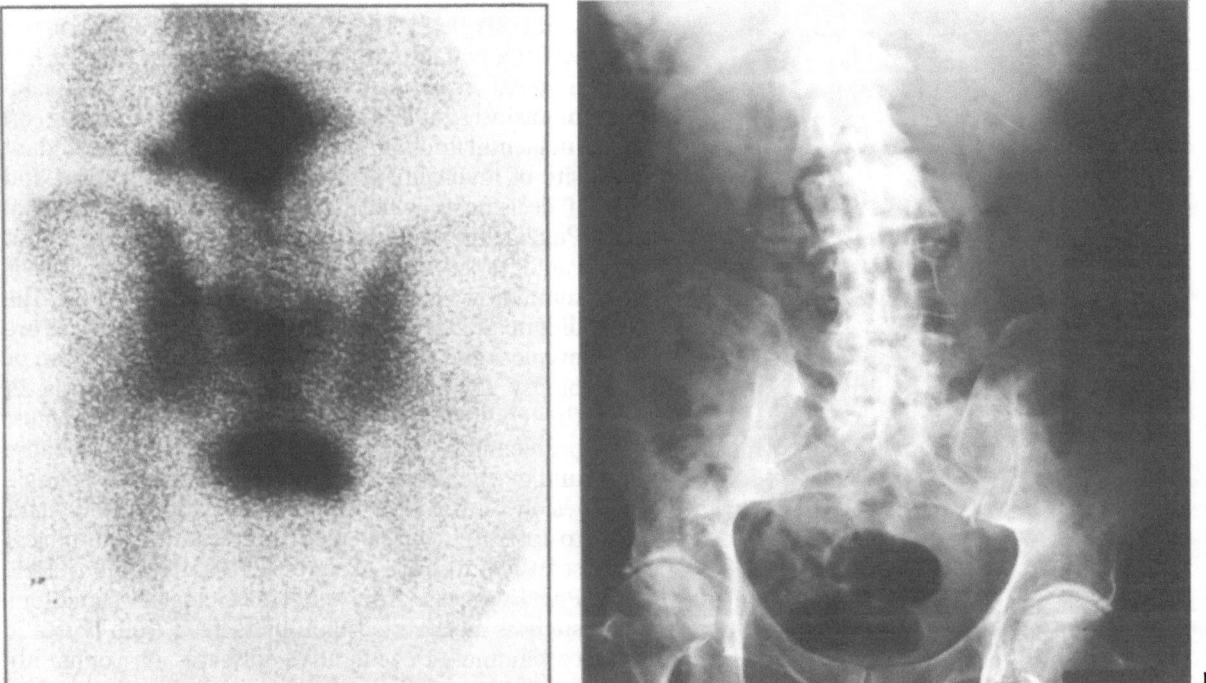

a   b

Fig. 8.3. a On scan there is intense uptake of tracer throughout body of lumbar vertebra 3. Vertebra appears expanded and note transverse processes are involved. This appearance corresponds to changes of Paget's disease seen on radiograph (b). However, there is also increased tracer uptake present in sacrum, presumably reflecting pagetic involvement, although this was not confirmed on the radiograph.

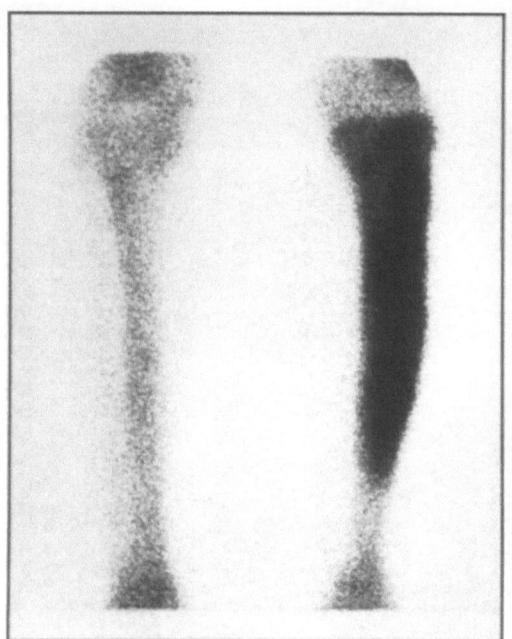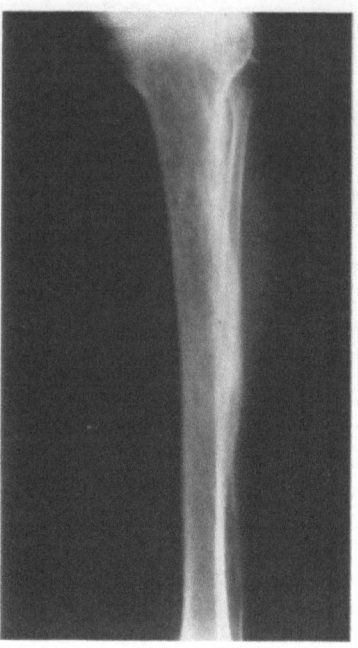

a   b

Fig. 8.4a, b. Paget's disease involving tibia. a Scan; b radiograph.

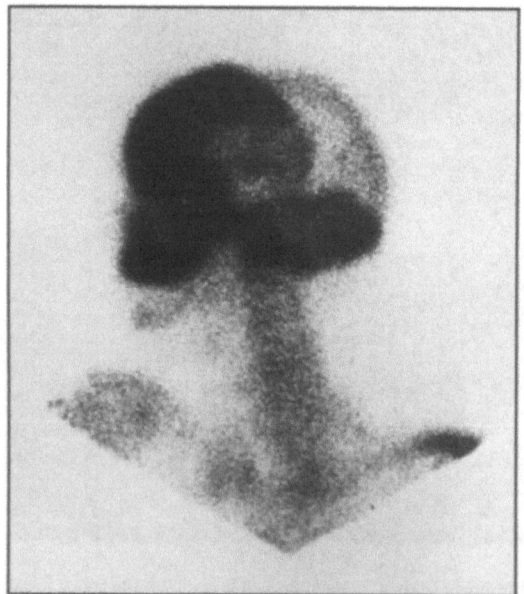

Fig. 8.5. Paget's disease of skull. There is intense uptake of tracer at margins of lytic front.

and inevitably some diagnostic difficulty can arise, particularly when the scan appearances are somewhat atypical. The most difficult problem arises when a patient with a known primary tumour has a bone scan performed to screen for skeletal metastases and Paget's disease is found as an incidental finding. In this situation, each individual site of involvement must be carefully studied and a decision reached as to whether it is typical of Paget's disease or not. It is generally best to obtain radiographs of all "abnormal" areas and this is mandatory where any doubt exists as to the diagnosis. Rarely, when bone scan appearances are atypical and radiography is unhelpful, a CT scan or biopsy will be required to establish a diagnosis. In this context, lesions involving the spine are most problematic, particularly when vertebral collapse and degenerative change are also present. A single lesion on the bone scan is generally more difficult to interpret, but even in this situation the typical scan features are likely to differentiate monostotic Paget's disease from other pathological conditions such as a sclerotic spinal metastasis from prostatic carcinoma. Degenerative disease is commonly found in any elderly population, and while this may present some difficulty in the differential diagnosis of metastatic disease, it is unlikely to cause any confusion as regards the diagnosis of Paget's disease (Fig. 8.8).

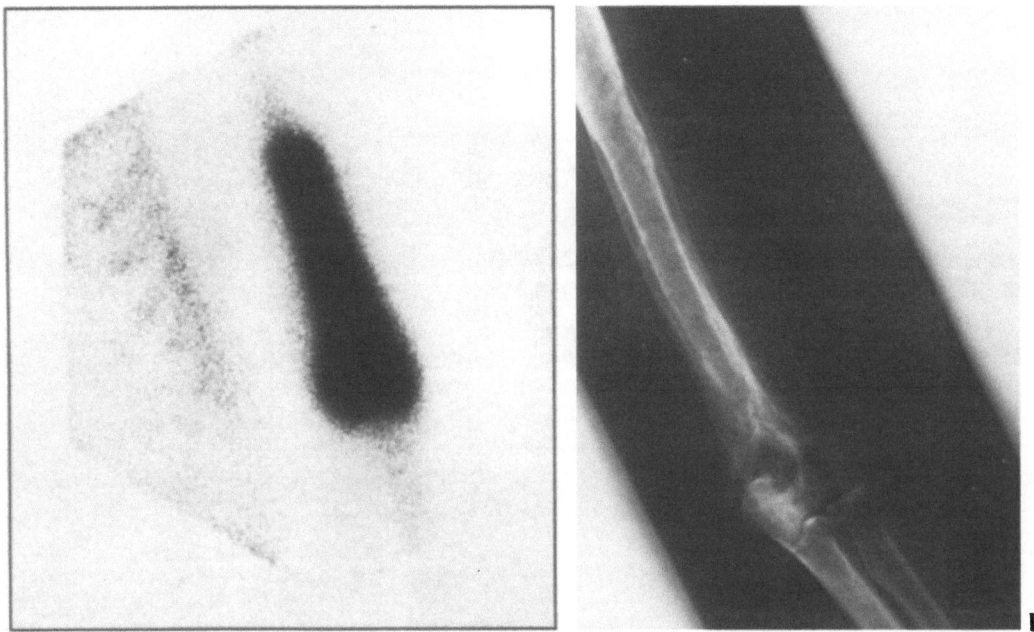

Fig. 8.6. a On scan there is intense uptake of tracer seen in lower left humerus with apparent expansion of bone. b Radiograph confirms Paget's disease. Note cortical resorption and flame-shaped resorption front in shaft of humerus.

Comparison of Bone Scanning and Radiography

It has now been convincingly shown that bone scanning is more sensitive than radiography for detecting sites of Paget's disease throughout the skeleton (Khairi et al. 1974; Shirazi et al. 1974; Serafini, 1976; Vellenga et al. 1976). Fogelman and Carr (1980) studied 23 patients with symptomatic disease with radiographic skeletal surveys and bone scans, and found that of 127 sites of pagetoid involvement, 120 (94.5%) were detected by bone scan, while only 94 (74%) were seen radiographically (Table 8.1). In addition, in six patients the extent of the disease involving a long bone was underestimated by radiography. In this study 33 individual sites were not visualised on radiographs, but it was noted that one-third of these involved areas which are difficult to evaluate with standard radiographic views, e.g. scapulae (Fig. 8.9), ribs and sternum (Milstein et al. 1974). It is apparent that in addition to increased sensitivity for lesion detection further advantages of bone scanning over radiography are clear visualisation, with ease and rapidity of evaluation of the whole skeleton. Recently, Vellenga et al. (1984a) have carried out a bone scan evaluation of a large series of patients with Paget's disease. They found that 59 of 373 lesions (16%) did not show any radiographic abnormality. This group did not obtain routine radiographic skeletal surveys but chose to study only those areas already shown to be abnormal on bone scan. Therefore, compared with most previous studies, there was an inbuilt bias in favour of radiography and yet a clear 16% difference in sensitivity was obtained. The bone scan is thus able to detect areas of pagetoid involvement which are not seen on radiographs. The ability of the scan to visualise some bones that are radiographically difficult is a partial explanation, but more important is the ability of the bone scan to detect physiological rather than structural change. It is probable that most radiographically normal lesions represent early Paget's disease. However, there is very little literature regarding this, and the possibility of other pathological conditions being present must be considered. While coexistent disease such as osteoarthritis is commonly found, one would expect to see evidence of this radiographically, and the scan appearances are usually quite different. Furthermore, in Paget's disease sites of involvement on the bone scan have the same characteristic appearance whether detected by radiography or not. It will be of considerable interest to learn of the eventual outcome of these lesions which appear normal radiographically but abnormal on the bone scan, and sequential studies of such patients are required.

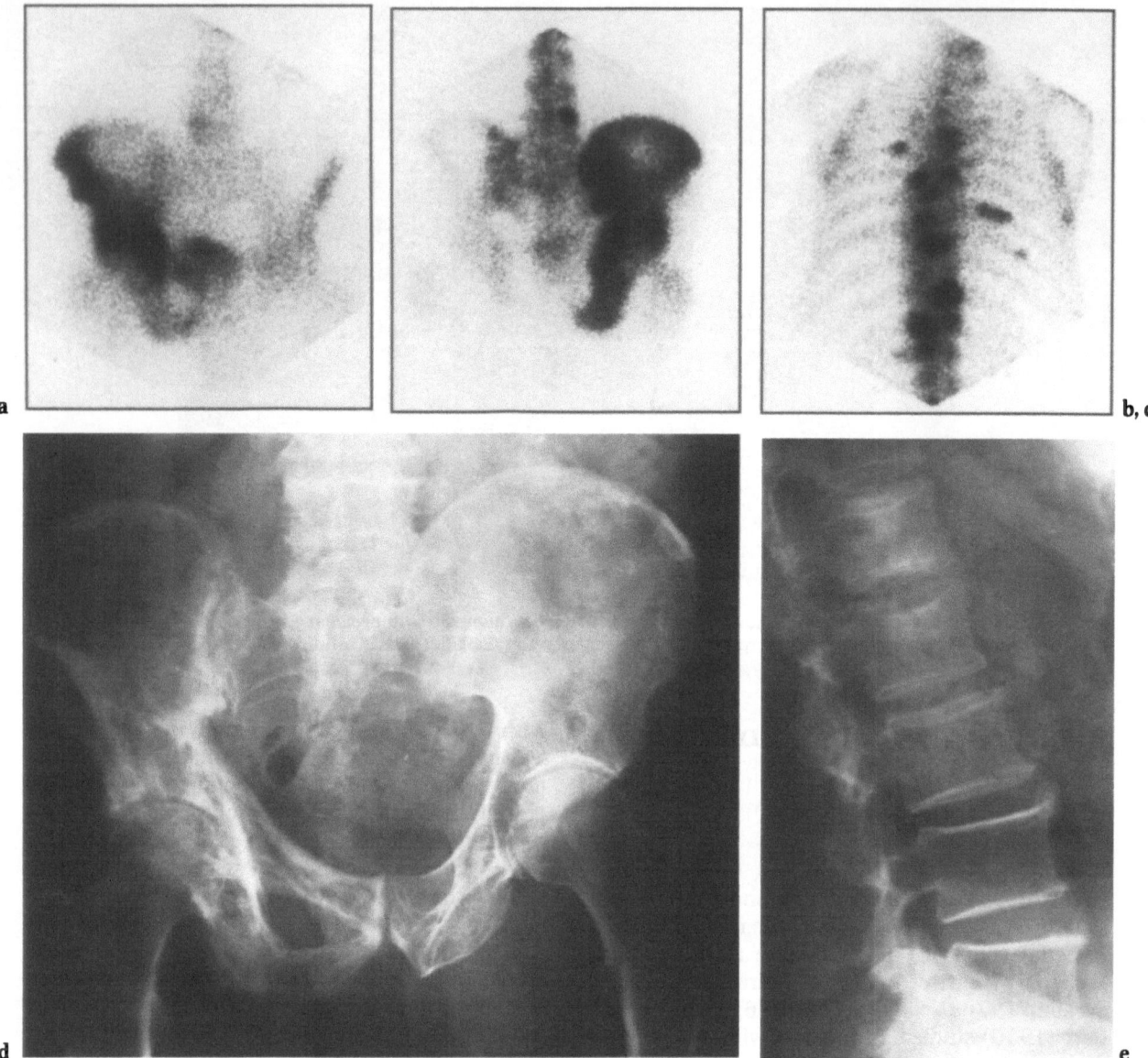

Fig. 8.7. a, b Anterior (a) and posterior (b) views of pelvis show typical appearances of Paget's disease involving right hemipelvis. There is also scan evidence of metastases in spine and ribs (b, c). d, e Radiographs confirm both Paget's disease (d) and metastases (e).

On occasion, areas of pagetoid involvement may be detected by radiograph but not bone scan. Until recently it was thought that such an occurrence was rare and limited to sites that were sclerotic on the radiograph (Fig. 8.10) (Khairi et al. 1973; Shirazi et al. 1974; Fogelman and Carr 1980). It was argued that these were areas of "burnt-out" activity in bone which were no longer metabolically active (Khairi et al. 1973; Shirazi et al. 1974), in keeping with the view that the bone scan presents a functional image of skeletal metabolic activity. However, Vellenga et al. (1984a) have reported finding a small number of lesions radiographically that were not visible on the bone scan, and of the nine such lesions radiographs indicated that two were osteolytic, two were sclerotic and five were mixed. These lesions which appeared normal on bone scan but abnormal on radiograph were essentially found by accident, as radiographs were limited to those areas already shown to be abnormal on bone scans. Although the authors did not specifically make the point, the question must arise as to whether other lesions appearing normal on bone scan but abnormal on radiograph would have been detected if full radio-

Table 8.1: Comparison of sites of involvement on bone scan and radiograph in Paget's disease (Fogelman and Carr 1980)

	Skull	Spine[a] C	D	L	S	Pelvis[b]	Femur	Tibia	Scapula	Humerus	Miscellaneous	Total
Lesions seen on radiograph	6	—	7	15	1	27	22	9	—	4	3	94
Lesions seen on bone scan	9	1	12	17	2	25	22	10	7	5	10	120
Lesions seen on radiograph only	—	—	—	—	1	4	2	—	—	—	—	7
Lesions seen on bone scan only	3	1	5	2	2	2	2	1	7	1	7	33
Patients with symptomatic sites	1	—	2	12	2	8	8	9	—	1	3	46

Lesions in the long bones and scapula are counted as two when bilateral.
[a]Involvement of any area of spine in a single subject is counted as one lesion, while the number of affected vertebrae in that area is not considered.
[b]The pelvis is considered as two separate areas, i.e. right and left hemipelvis.

Table 8.2: Anatomical distribution of Paget's disease, expressed as percentage (adapted from Vellenga et al. 1984a)

Site	Vellenga et al. (1974): Bone scan; 107 patients	Shirazi et al. (1984): Bone scan; 135 patients	Dickson et al. (1945): Radiograph; 367 patients	Guyer and Clough (1978): Radiograph; 1225 patients	Schmorl (1932): Autopsy; 138 patients
Pelvis	65	78	66	76	22
Spine:	42	63	—	—	50
lumbar	33	40	28	31	26
thoracic	25	34	14	26	17
cervical	12	8	2	11	7
Sacrum	30	28	—	31	57
Femur	37	48	47	26	46
Tibia	37	22	35	14	8
Skull	29	48	42	29	28
Humerus	13	17	5	9	4
Scapula	12	37	2	11	—
Foot	9	3	1	8	—
Rib	8	5	3	4	7
Sternum	7	4	—	3	23
Forearm/hand	5	9	3	4	—
Clavicle	5	3	9	7	13

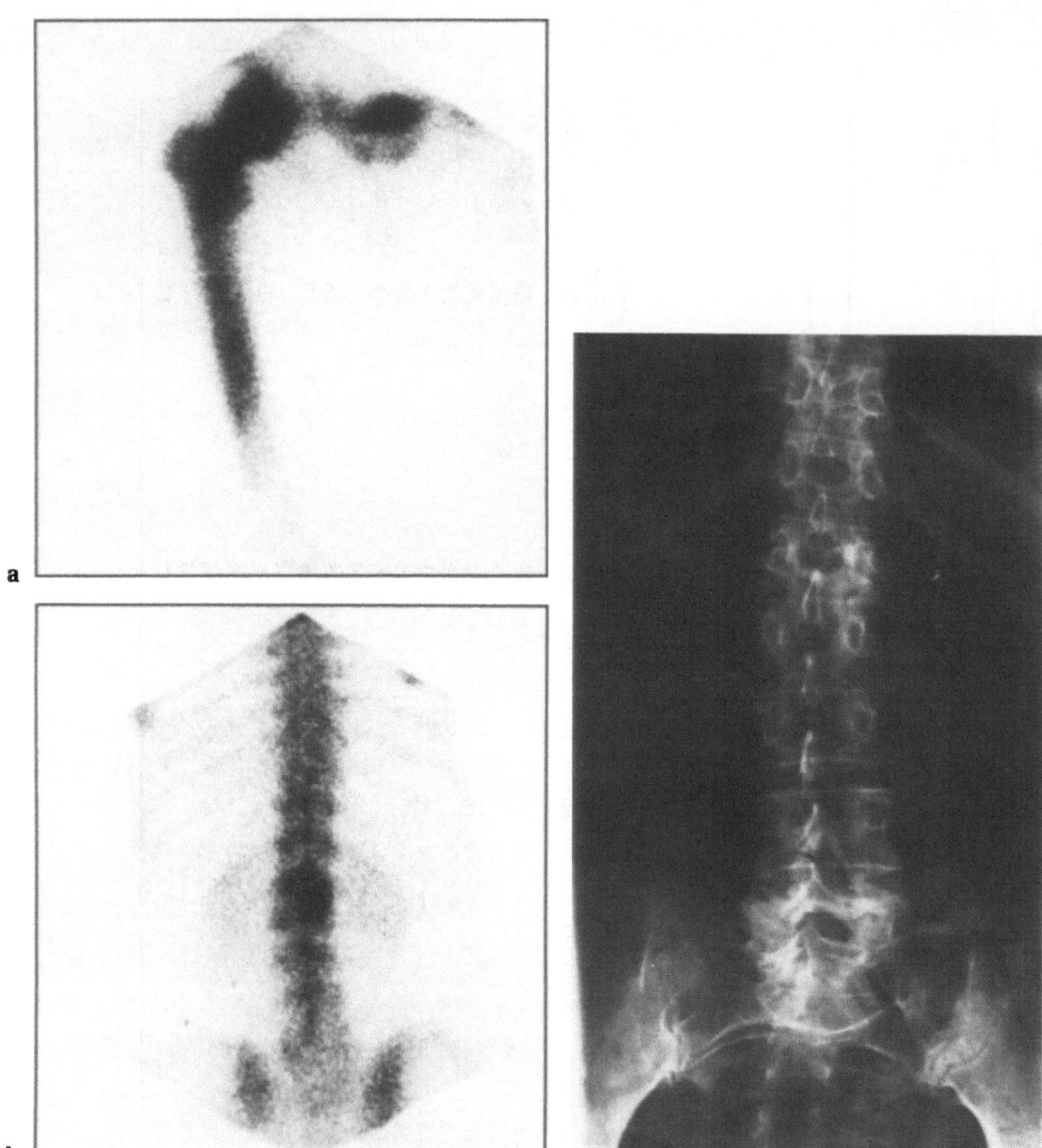

Fig. 8.8. a Bone scan from an elderly patient with Paget's disease in right femur. **b** Scan revealed lesion at right border lumbar vertebrae 1/2. Appearances are non-specific but were thought most likely to represent degenerative disease, which was confirmed on radiograph (c).

graphic skeletal surveys had been obtained. However, it seems improbable that a significant number of such lesions would have been found as all previous series have shown them to be extremely uncommon. Vellenga et al. (1984a) also reported a case where Paget's disease was seen in a histological specimen from the pelvis while both bone scan and radiographs of that site were normal. This indicates that there is a stage of disease where histomorphometric abnormalities may be detected but alterations in skeletal metabolism or structural change are not yet of such a magnitude that they can be detected by imaging techniques.

The bone scan is generally of value in detecting fracture (Marty et al. 1976); when this occurs at a site of pagetic involvement, it may be seen as focally increased tracer uptake superimposed on generalised high uptake. However, it should be recognised that there may be difficulty in diagnosing a fracture in pagetic bone as differentiation of a focal increase in tracer uptake from high background activity may not always be possible. This may be a particular problem when stress fractures are present (Fig. 8.11). Similarly, if osteosarcoma develops at a site of pagetic involvement it may be difficult to recognise on the scan. One should always

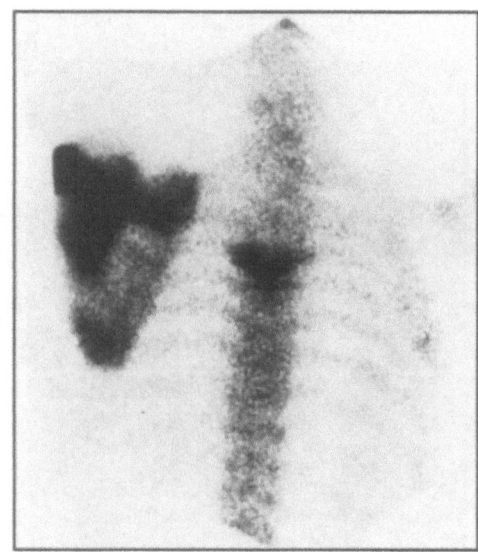

Fig. 8.9. Paget's disease involving left scapula and an upper thoracic vertebra.

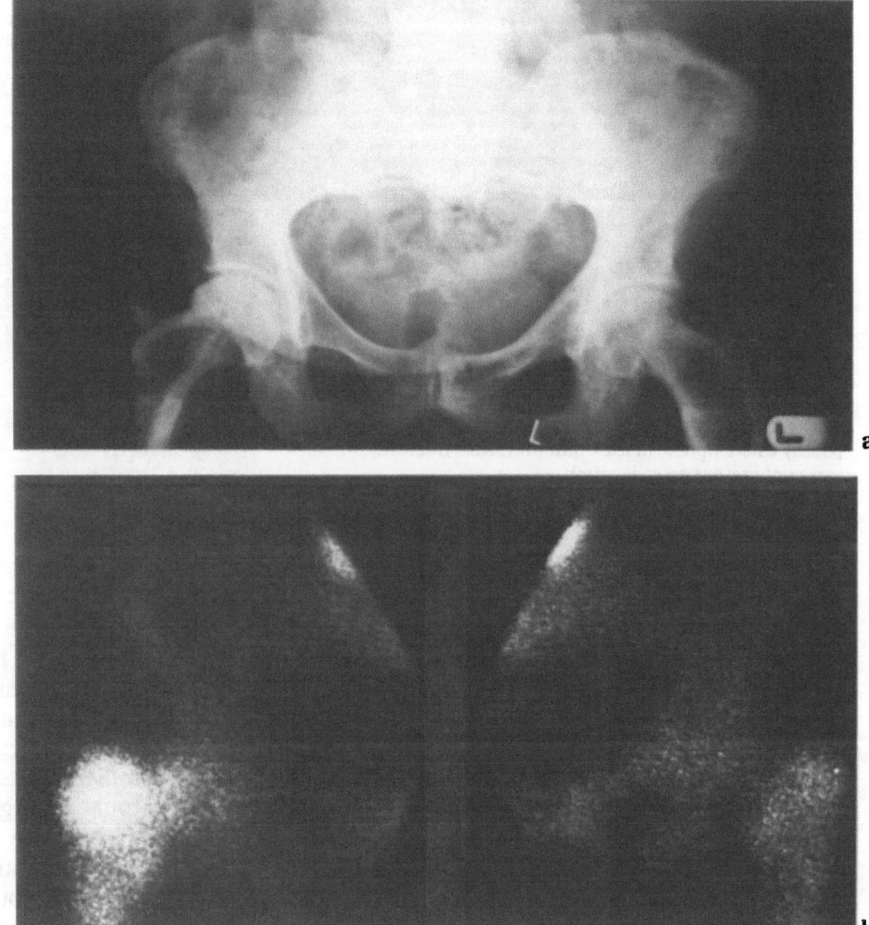

Fig. 8.10a, b. Extensive Paget's disease involving pelvis seen on radiograph (**a**) but not apparent on scan (**b**). (Fogelman and Carr 1980)

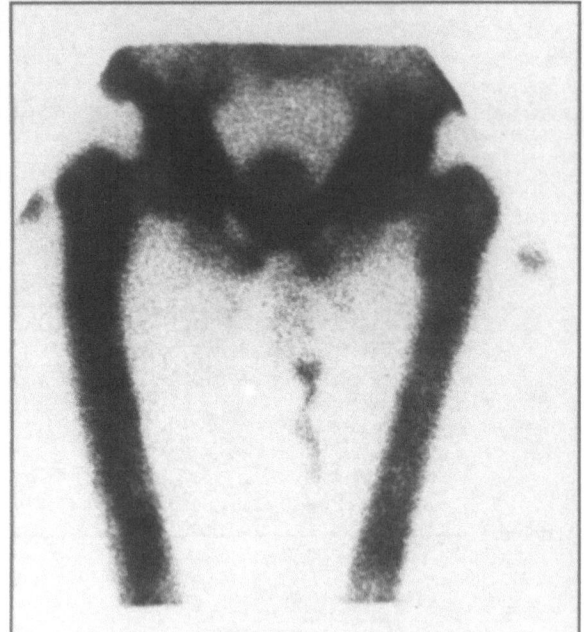

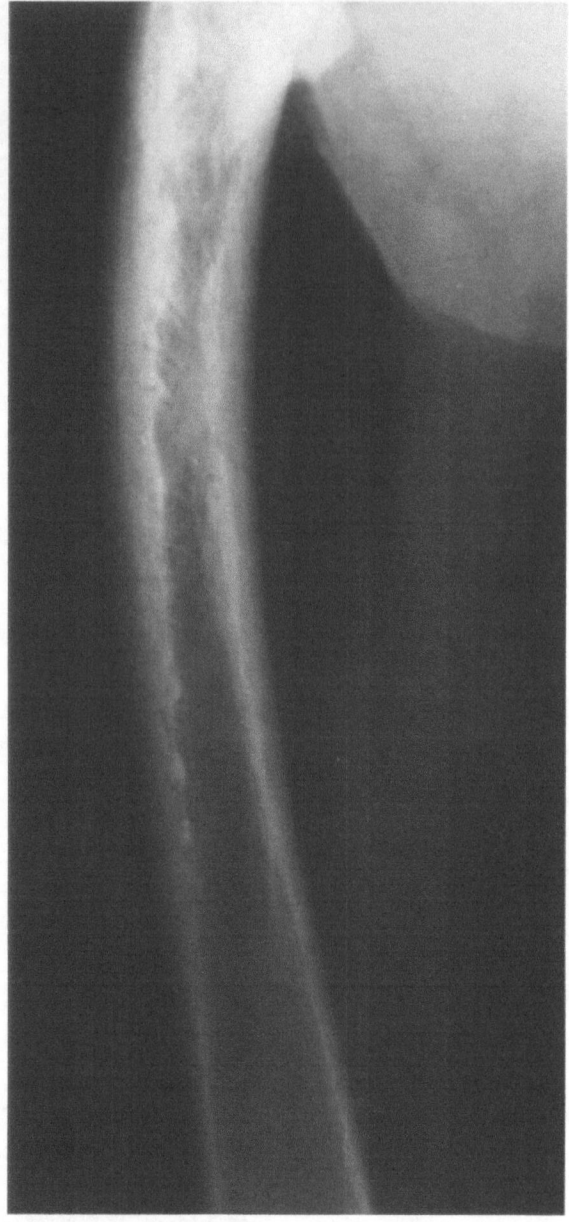

Fig. 8.11a, b. Paget's disease involving femora and pelvis. Scan (**a**) shows patchy uptake of tracer in femora, more marked on right. Radiograph of right femur (**b**) reveals multiple stress fractures, which were not suspected from scan findings. Furthermore, there is patchy tracer uptake in left femur and stress fractures were not present on radiograph.

be concerned about the possibility of sarcomatous change when expansion of a lesion outside normal anatomical borders occurs (Fig. 8.12). While most previously reported cases have indicated that osteosarcoma shows increased tracer uptake (Shirazi et al. 1974), McKillop et al. (1977) reported a case where a large lytic area was present radiographically with a photon-deficient area on the corresponding scan image. Subsequently, there have been other reports of photon-deficient areas occurring in association with sarcomatous change. Yeh et al. (1982) obtained bone and ^{67}Ga scans in 12

patients with Paget's sarcoma. It was found that ^{67}Ga uptake at the site of sarcoma was always greater than the relative ^{99m}Tc diphosphonate uptake and it was suggested that ^{67}Ga was useful in confirming a diagnosis of sarcoma. However, overall it would appear that the bone scan is a somewhat unreliable means of detecting fracture and sarcomatous change in patients with Paget's disease; therefore conventional radiography together with computed tomography and biopsy in cases where tumour is suspected, remain the investigations of choice.

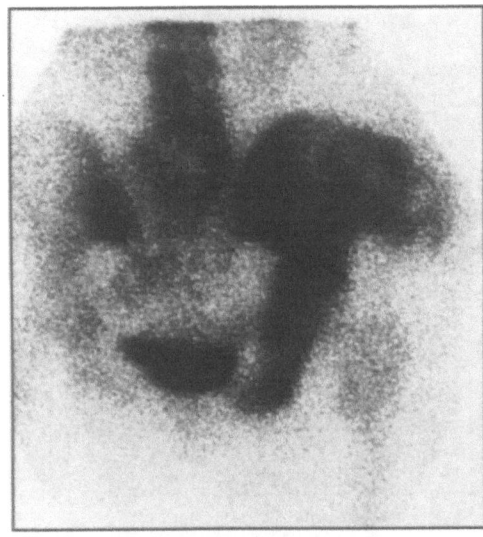 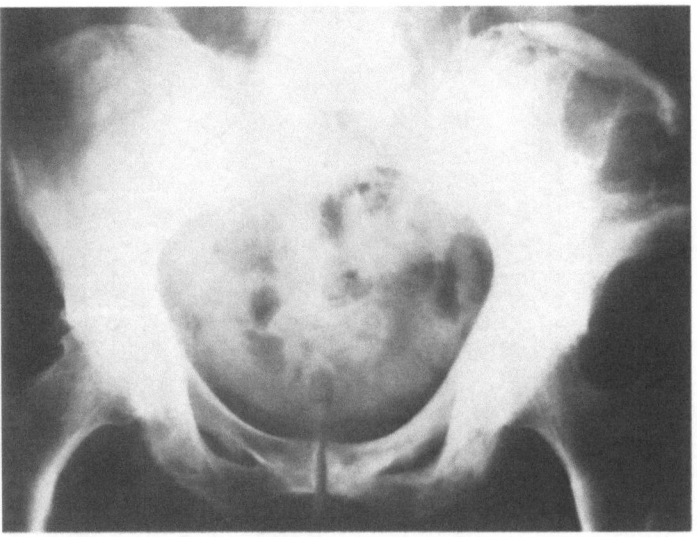

Fig. 8.12a, b. Paget's osteosarcoma. On scan (a) there is pagetic involvement of right hemipelvis with gross disruption of anatomical borders in lateral aspect of iliac wing. On radiograph (b) there is destruction of bone seen at that site.

Anatomical Distribution of Lesions

The anatomical distribution of lesions in Paget's disease was previously assessed by either skeletal radiography (Dickson et al. 1945; Guyer and Clough 1978) or autopsy examination (Schmorl 1932). Considerable experience with bone scanning has now accumulated which allows both good visualisation of the whole skeleton and early detection of disease activity. Table 8.2 lists the frequency of involvement of the various parts of the skeleton from two bone scan series and from three other series where disease was evaluated by other methods. The scatter of lesions seen on the bone scan in Paget's disease differs little from that found radiographically, and spine, pelvis, femur, tibia and skull are the most frequently involved sites. The autopsy series found a surprisingly low incidence of pelvic involvement and high incidence for sternum, but is otherwise in keeping with the other series. The bone scan has, however, identified the scapula and humerus as sites which are more often involved by Paget's disease than had previously been recognised from other studies. It is likely that this is because these sites are seldom symptomatic and may often be missed on routine radiology (Miller et al. 1974).

Monostotic Paget's disease is clearly common (10%–25% of cases) (Shirazi et al. 1974; Wellman et al. 1977; Vellenga et al. 1984a) and may on occasion provide dramatic findings on the bone scan (Fig. 8.13). However, it is of interest that when a patient is suspected of having monostotic Paget's disease on routine radiography, a bone scan will often identify further sites of involvement (Shirazi et al. 1974).

Correlation of Symptoms with Sites of Activity on Bone Scan

It has been suggested that Paget's disease may be classified into lytic, blastic and sclerotic phases on the basis of radiographic appearances (Khairi et al. 1973). In practice, it is often difficult to classify cases accurately in this way as there is usually a mixed picture present in any patient and occasionally even in the same bone. Although the amount of tracer uptake at an involved site is probably influenced by the phase of disease activity, this is generally thought to be of little clinical significance. However, it has been recently suggested that symptoms may correlate with the degree of severity of individual lesions (Vellenga et al. 1984a). It may well be correct that the most metabolically active lesions (and hence those with the highest tracer uptake) are more likely to give rise to symptoms. Certainly, it seems that symptomatic lesions appear markedly abnormal on the bone scan (Shirazi et al. 1974; Fogelman and Carr 1980). However, only a minority of all pagetoid lesions are symptomatic and it is therefore difficult to demonstrate a clear relationship between tracer avidity and symptoms. The

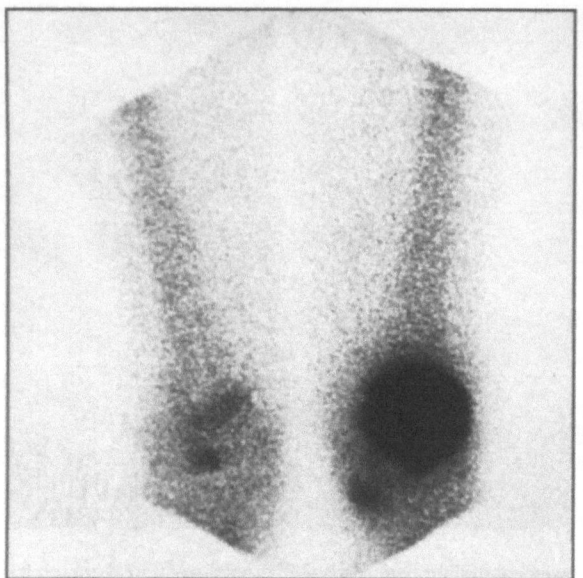
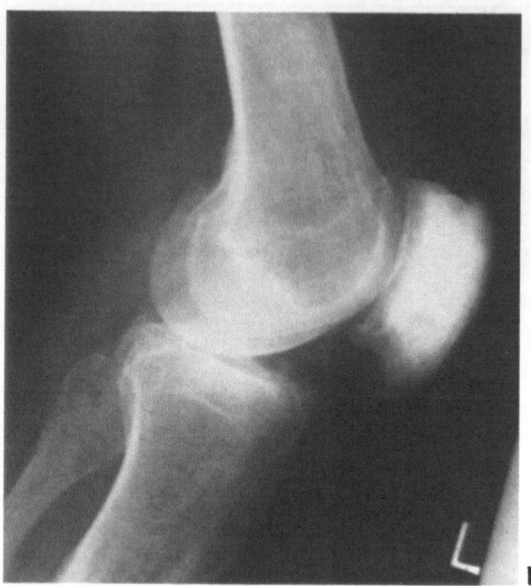

Fig. 8.13. a There is striking increased tracer uptake in left patella. b Radiograph confirms Paget's disease. This patient had monostotic disease involving patella.

relationship between pagetoid lesions and patients' symptoms found by Fogelman and Carr (1980) is summarised in Table 8.1. The most frequently involved sites were spine in 57%, tibia in 39%, and pelvis and femur both in 35% of cases. Thus the weight-bearing bones were most often symptomatic. It has been suggested that headaches are a characteristic feature of Paget's disease (Ibbertson et al. 1979), but Fogelman and Carr (1980) observed that of nine cases with skull involvement only one complained of headache. Thus the skull is a site where there is no direct relationship between tracer uptake and symptoms, as tracer uptake is often intense yet patients seldom have symptoms. Clearly factors other than alterations in skeletal metabolism are important with regard to the development of symptoms, and these may include skeletal vascularity, whether a bone is weight bearing or not, and whether there is deformity of bone with stretching of the periosteum. In general there does not appear to be any clear correlation between the radiographic appearance of individual lesions and either the intensity of tracer uptake at that site or the incidence of symptoms (Vellenga et al. 1984a). However, lesions which appear normal radiographically but abnormal on the bone scan are generally asymptomatic (Fogelman and Carr 1980; Vellenga et al. 1984a).

Evaluation of Treatment

Several studies have now shown that changes in disease activity can be documented on the bone scans of patients with Paget's disease receiving therapy with either calcitonin (Lavender et al. 1977) or diphosphonate (Fig. 8.14) (Stein et al. 1977). While bone scan features generally correspond to biochemical findings, changes on the scan occur relatively slowly and may lag behind biochemistry by several months (Waxman et al. 1977). Thus early in the course of treatment alterations in urinary hydroxyproline and serum alkaline phosphatase, and perhaps even the clinical response, are better prognostic indicators. However, Bourdreau et al. (1983) have found that the scan evaluation of response to treatment can be improved by obtaining radionuclide blood flow studies. In 24 patients serial flow studies generally were in good agreement with alkaline phosphatase results (in 72%) and in the remaining cases were equally split in terms of which test preceded the other. Thus it would appear that, overall, radionuclide blood flow studies and alkaline phosphatase are approximately equally sensitive in terms of monitoring change in disease activity. However, blood flow studies have the limitation that the technique is largely restricted to the appendicular skeleton and to the extent of disease that can be included in the gamma camera field of view. Waxman et al. (1980), in a small study of five patients with Paget's disease, compared scans

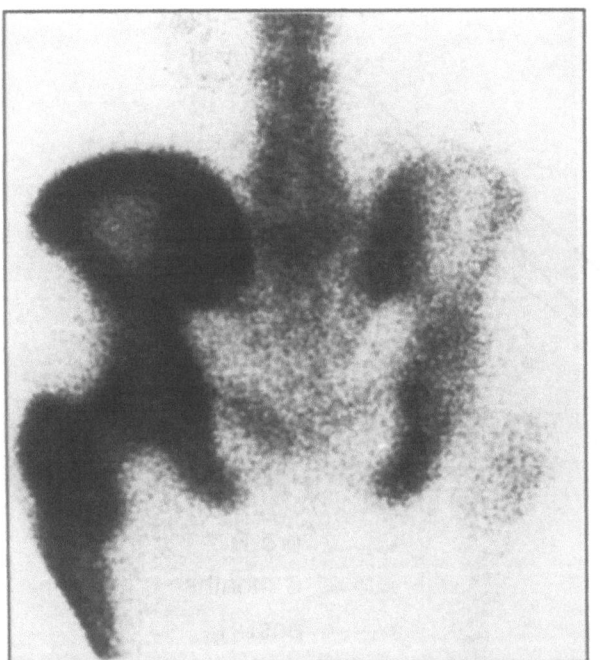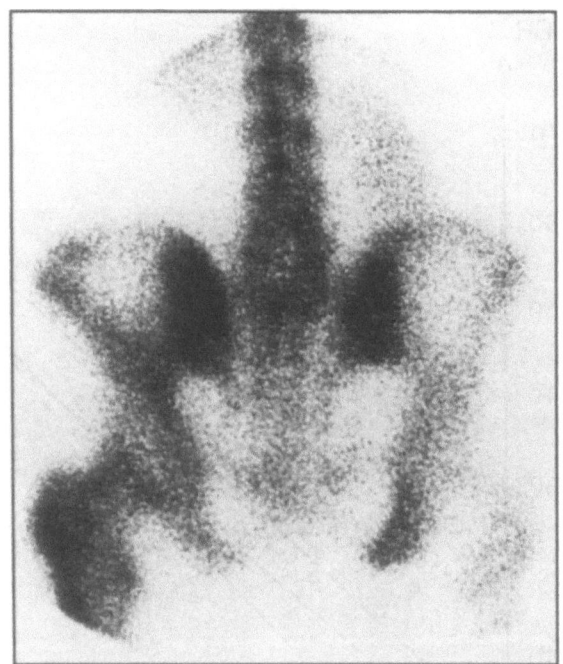

a

b

Fig. 8.14. a Paget's disease involving pelvis and left femur. b Following 9 months' therapy with oral diphosphonate, there has been marked improvement.

obtained with ^{67}Ga and ^{99m}Tc diphosphonate following calcitonin therapy. It was considered that ^{67}Ga reflected biochemical changes more accurately than disphosphonate as uptake of tracer was dependent upon cellular activity rather than available bone surfaces. While this is certainly an interesting observation, it does not appear to have any clinical relevance. However, the bone scan can be used to reassess disease activity from 3 to 6 months following initiation of therapy. A visual display of activity in individual lesions is obtained, while radiographs often remain unchanged over this period. Furthermore, quantitation of tracer uptake by bone can be carried out (Goldman et al. 1975; Lentle et al. 1976; Lurye et al. 1977; Vattimo et al. 1981), thus avoiding the need for subjective evaluation of scan images and providing increased sensitivity for alteration in disease activity. Vellenga et al. (1984b) recently studied 42 patients with pagetic lesions and compared visual assessment of bone scans, using a six-point qualitative score, with computer quantitation, obtaining the ratio of counts in involved bone to those in comparable normal bone. It was concluded that visual assessment generally correlated well with quantitative results. However, 27 of these patients had bone scan studies before and after diphosphonate therapy and there it was found that in 14% of lesions, significant alterations were detected by quantitation alone.

The bone scan appears to provide a sensitive means of anticipating the recurrence of Paget's disease during clinical remission, and in one series approximately one-third of patients with recurrent disease were identified prior to changes in biochemistry (Vellenga et al. 1982). However, the predictive value of a stable bone scan is poor; there seems little justification in obtaining serial bone scans in any pagetic population simply to anticipate relapse.

A more global assessment of skeletal metabolism can be obtained with 24-h whole-body retention of ^{99m}Tc diphosphonate measurements (Vattimo et al. 1981; Smith et al. 1984). This technique can also be used to monitor response to therapy. An interesting point, however, arises as to whether a ^{99m}Tc diphosphonate bone scan with or without quantitation is a valid means of assessing response to treatment with diphosphonate, as it is at least theoretically possible that skeletal affinity for radiolabelled diphosphonate could be altered in the presence of an oral diphosphonate load. Wellman et al. (1977) obtained paired ^{18}F and ^{99m}Tc diphosphonate studies in 15 patients with Paget's disease receiving diphosphonate therapy. Studies were evaluated qualitatively, and it was felt that the same information was obtained with both sets of images. It was concluded that oral diphosphonate did not interfere with interpretation of ^{99m}Tc diphosphonate

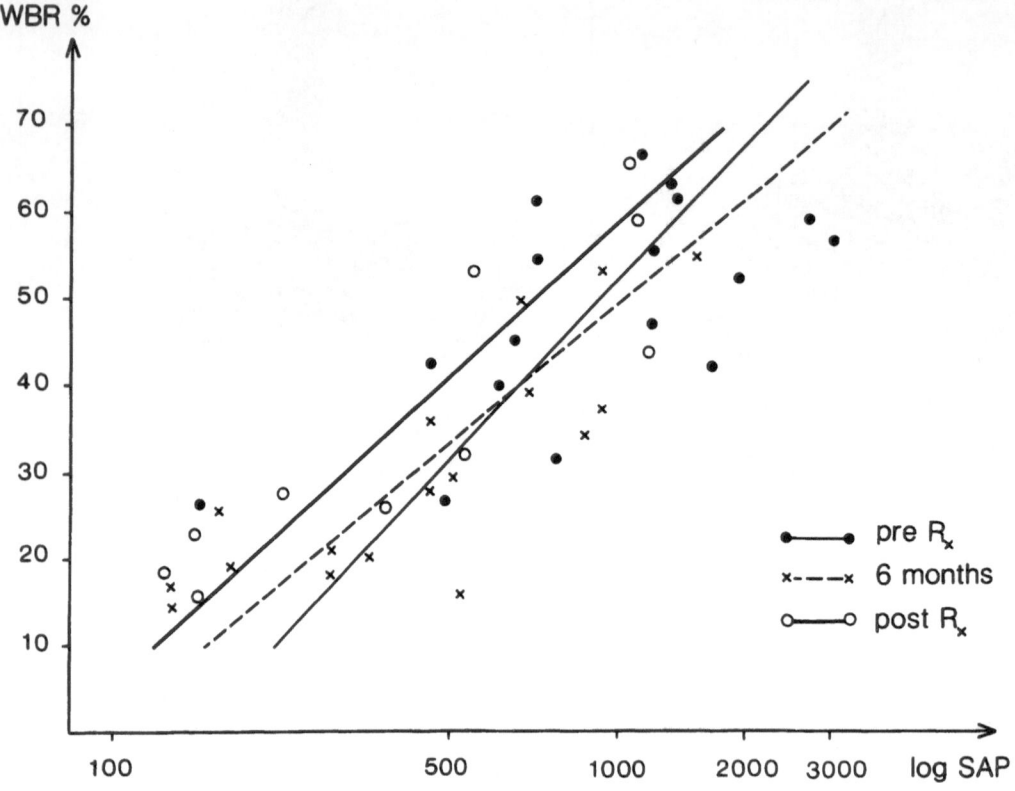

Fig. 8.15. Whole-body retention (*WBR*) of ^{99m}Tc-HEDP vs. log serum alkaline phosphatase (*log SAP*) over course of oral diphosphonate therapy. (Smith et al. 1984)

scans, and it was suggested that even when patients received a significant diphosphonate load the potential binding sites in the skeleton were so numerous that there was no effect with regard to affinity for the bone-scanning agents. Smith et al. (1984) studied 18 patients receiving diphosphonate therapy by obtaining 24-h whole-body retention (WBR) of ^{99m}Tc diphosphonate, serum alkaline phosphatase and urinary hydroxyproline measurements before, during and after 6 months' treatment. The measurements of 24-h WBR of ^{99m}Tc diphosphonate correlated well with both biochemical measurements throughout the treatment period, and the relationship was maintained after cessation of diphosphonate therapy (Fig. 8.15). It was concluded that the measurements of 24-h WBR of ^{99m}Tc diphosphonate accurately reflected disease activity, even in the presence of an oral diphosphonate load.

Although of considerable academic interest, there does not appear to be any clinical indication at the present time for sequential bone scanning in Paget's disease as the patient's response can be gauged more simply and accurately by routine biochemical measurements.

Clinical Use of Bone Scanning

In Paget's disease neither radiograph nor bone scan will identify all sites of involvement, but it is clear that the bone scan is the more sensitive technique. In addition, most authors believe that those sites which are occasionally missed by the bone scan are metabolically inactive. Therefore, it seems reasonable to suggest that the bone scan should be the imaging technique of choice in Paget's disease and radiography should be used to provide supplementary information whenever required.

A bone scan is an ideal screening test in cases of suspected Paget's disease, for example in elderly patients with unexplained bone pain, bony deformity, or those found to have an elevated serum alkaline phosphatase value. In addition to being more sensitive than radiography, the bone scan provides good visualisation of the whole skeleton, allowing accurate assessment of the extent of disease (Merrick and Merrick 1985). Furthermore, the bone scan is simple to perform and much more straightforward and rapid to evaluate than a full radiographic skeletal survey. Paget's disease generally affects an elderly population and patients may have bone symptoms related to other diseases such as osteoarthritis, rheumatoid arthritis or coexistent metastatic disease. A bone scan should be obtained as a baseline investigation, not only to monitor progression of Paget's disease if this is felt necessary, but also for evaluation of new symptoms that may be related to other pathological conditions of bone.

References

Alexandre C, Meunier PJ, Edouard C, Khairi RA, Johnston CC (1981) Effects of EHDP (5 mg/kg/day dose) on quantitative bone histology in Paget's disease of bone. Metab Bone Dis Rel Res 23: 309–315

Avramides A (1977) Salmon and porcine calcitonin treatment of Paget's disease of bone. Clin Orthop 127: 78–85

Barker DJP, Clough PWL, Guyer PB, Gardner MJ (1977) Paget's disease of bone in 14 British towns. Br Med J I: 1181–1183

Bourdreau RJ, Lisbona R, Hadjipavlou A (1983) Observations on serial radionuclide blood-flow studies in Paget's disease: concise communication. J Nucl Med 24: 880–885

Boyce BF, Smith L. Fogelman I, Johnstone E, Ralston S, Boyle IT (1984) Focal osteomalacia due to low-dose diphosphonate therapy in Paget's disease. Lancet I: 821–824

Citrin DL, McKillop JH (eds) (1978) Paget's disease. In: Atlas of technetium bone scans. Saunders, Philadelphia, p 126

Dickson DD, Camp JD, Ghormley RK (1945) Osteitis deformans: Paget's disease of the bone. Radiology 44: 449–470

Fogelman I, Carr D (1980) A comparison of bone scanning and radiology in the assessment of patients with symptomatic Paget's disease. Eur J Nucl Med 5: 417–421

Frank JW (1981) The value of radionuclide bone imaging in atypical Paget's disease. Nucl Med Comm 2: 302–306

Galbraith HJ (1954) Familial Paget's disease of bone. Br Med J II: 29

Goldman AB, Braunstein P, Wilkinson D, Kammerman S (1975) Radionuclide uptake studies of bone: a quantitative method of evaluating the response of patients with Paget's disease to diphosphonate therapy. Radiology 117: 365–369

Guyer PB, Clough PWL (1978) Paget's disease of bone: some observations on the relation of the skeletal distribution to pathogenesis. Clin Radiol 29: 421–426

Hamdy RC (1981) Paget's disease of bone. Praeger, Eastbourne, pp 13–21, 37–46

Ibbertson, HK, Henley JW, Fraser TR, Tait B, Stephens EJ, Scot DJ (1979) Paget's disease of bone—clinical evaluation and treatment with diphosphonates. Aust NZ J Med 9: 31–35

Khairi MR, Wellman HN, Robb JA, Johnston CC (1973) Paget's disease of bone (osteitis deformans): symptomatic lesions and bone scan. Ann Intern Med 79: 348–351

Khairi MRA, Robb JA, Wellman HN, Johnston CC (1974) Radiographs and scans in diagnosing symptomatic lesions of Paget's disease of bone (osteitis deformans). Geriatrics 29: 49–54

Lavender JP, Evans IM, Arnot R, Bowring S, Doyle FH, Joplin GF, MacIntyre I (1977) A comparison of radiography and radioisotope scanning in the detection of Paget's disease and in the assessment of response to human calcitonin. Br J Radiol 50: 243–250

Lentle BC, Russell AS, Heslip PG, Percy JS (1976) The scintigraphic findings in Paget's disease of bone. Clin Radiol 17: 129–135

Lurye DR, Castronovo FP, Potsaid MS (1977) An improved method for quantitative bone scanning. J Nucl Med 18: 1069–1073

Marty R, Denney JD, McKamey MR, Rowley MJ (1976) Bone trauma and related benign disease: assessment by bone scanning. Semin Nucl Med 6: 107–120

McKillop JH, Fogelman I, Boyle IT, Greig WR (1977) Bone scan appearance of a Paget's osteosarcoma: failure to concentrate HEDP. J Nucl Med 18: 1039–1040

Merrick MV, Merrick JM (1985) Observations on the natural history of Paget's disease. Clin Radiol 36: 169–174

Miller SW, Castronovo FP Jr, Pendergrass HR, Potsaid MS (1974) Technetium 99m-labelled diphosphonate bone scanning in Paget's disease. Am J Roentgenol Radium Ther Nucl Med 121: 177–183

Mills BG, Singer FR (1976) Nuclear inclusions in Paget's disease of bone. Science 194: 201–202

Milstein D, Nusynowitz ML, Lull RJ (1974) Radionuclide diagnosis in chest disease resulting from trauma. Semin Nucl Med 4: 339–355

Pygott F (1957) Paget's disease of bone, the radiological incidence. Lancet I: 1170–1171

Rausch JM, Resnick D, Goergen TG, Taylor A (1977) Bone scanning in osteolytic Paget's disease: case report. J Nucl Med 18: 699–701

Rebel A, Basle M, Pouplard A, Malkani K, Filmon R, Lepatazour A (1981) Towards a viral etiology for Paget's disease of bone. Metab Bone Dis Rel Res 3: 235–238

Russell RGG, Smith R, Preston C, Walton RJ, Woods CG (1974) Diphosphonates in Paget's disease. Lancet I: 894–898

Ryan WG (1977) Treatment of Paget's disease of bone with mithramycin. Clin Orthop 127: 106–110

Schmorl G (1932) Veber osteitis deformans Paget. Virchows Arch [Pathol Anat] 283: 694–751

Schubert F, Siddle KJ, Harper JS (1984) Diaphyseal Paget's disease: an unusual finding in the tibia. Clin Radiol 35: 71–74

Serafini AN (1976) Paget's disease of the bone. Semin Nucl Med 6: 47–58

Shirazi PH, Ryan WG, Fordham EW (1974) Bone scanning in evaluation of Paget's disease of bone. CRC Crit Rev Clin Radiol Nucl Med 5: 523–558

Singer FR, Schiller AI, Pyle EB, Krane SM (1978) Paget's disease of bone. In: Aviol L, Krane S (eds) Metabolic bone disease, vol 2. Academic, London, pp 489–575

Smith ML, Fogelman I, Ralston S, Boyce BF, Boyle IT (1984) Correlation of skeletal uptake of ^{99m}Tc-diphosphonate and alkaline phosphatase before and after oral diphosphonate therapy in Paget's disease. Metab Bone Dis Rel Res 5: 167–170

Stein I, Shapiro B, Ostrum B, Beller ML (1977) Evaluation of sodium etidronate in the treatment of Paget's disease of bone. Clin Orthop 122: 347–358

Vattimo A, Cantalupi D, Righi G, Martini G, Nuti R, Turchetti V (1981) Whole-body retention of ^{99m}Tc-MPD in Paget's disease. J Nucl Med Allied Sci 25: 5–10

Vellenga CJ, Pauwels EKJ, Bijvoet OL, Hosking DJ (1976) Evaluation of scintigraphic and roentgenologic studies in Paget's disease under treatment. Radiol Clin (Basel) 45: 292–301

Vellenga CJLR, Pauwels EKJ, Bijvoet OLM, Hosking DJ, Frijlink WB (1982) Bone scintigraphy in Paget's disease treated with combined calcitonin and diphosphonate (EHDP). Metab Bone Dis Rel Res 4: 103–111

Vellenga CJLR, Pauwels EKJ, Bijvoet OLM, Frijlink WB, Mulder JD, Hermans J (1984a) Untreated Paget disease of bone studied by scintigraphy. Radiology 153: 799–805

Vellenga CJLR, Pauwels EKJ, Bijvoet OLM (1984b)) Comparison

between visual assessment and quantitative measurement of radioactivity on the bone scintigram in Paget's disease of bone. Eur J Nucl Med 9: 533–537

Waxman AD, Ducker S, McKee D, Siemsen JK, Singer FR (1977) Evaluation of ^{99m}Tc diphosphonate kinetics and bone scans in patients with Paget's disease before and after calcitonin treatment. Radiology 125: 761–764

Waxman AD, McKee D, Siemsen JK, Singer FR (1980) Gallium scanning in Paget's disease of bone: effect of calcitonin. Am J Radiol 134: 303–306

Wellman HN, Schauwecker D, Robb JA, Khairi MR, Johnston CC (1977) Skeletal scintimaging and radiography in the diagnosis and management of Paget's disease. Clin Orthop 127: 55–62

Wootton R, Reeve J, Spellacy E, Tellez-Yudilevich M (1978) Skeletal blood flow in Paget's disease of bone and its response to calcitonin therapy. Clin Sci 54: 69–74

Yeh SDJ, Rosen G, Benua RS (1982) Gallium scans in Paget's sarcoma. Clin Nucl Med 7: 546–552

9 · The Role of Bone Scanning, Gallium and Indium Imaging in Infection

K. Mido, D. A. Navarro, G. M. Segall and I. R. McDougall

Introduction

Nuclear medicine studies have considerable value in diagnosing infectious conditions in the skeleton. In this chapter we will discuss acute infections of bone and joints separately. The section on acute osteomyelitis will cover radiopharmaceuticals, methods, experimental models and the results of clinical series. Acute infections of joints will be discussed with attention to radiopharmaceuticals, methods and results. The diagnosis of acute infection in prosthetic joints is treated separately. The evaluation of chronic bone infections is described briefly.

Radiopharmaceuticals and Methods

^{99m}Tc phosphate and diphosphonate compounds show increased uptake in sites where there is more blood flow or metabolic bone activity (Siegel et al. 1976). Since both of these are common in acute infections of bones and since these agents are available at all times, a bone scan is frequently the first, or at least an early, study. The dose will depend on the weight of the patient, since most acute bone infections are in children; the standard dose in adults is 15–20 mCi (555–740MBq), in children 25 μCi (925 kBq) per kg.

It is advisable to perform a flow study of the suspected area obtaining images at 3–4 s intervals. If possible, normal bone on the opposite side should be studied simultaneously. This is made easier by using a camera with a large field of view. In the spine adjacent normal bones can be used for comparison. Most acute bone infections have increased blood flow. A blood pool study is obtained 5–10 min after injection. We usually obtain a spot view of 10^6 counts from a camera with a large field of view. Thirdly, static pictures of the entire skeleton are obtained. Figure 9.1 shows a three-phase bone scan in acute osteomyelitis. Because many of the patients are young and bone uptake of the radiopharmaceutical is avid, a delay of 2–3 h is usually sufficient. In older patients it can be necessary to delay 3 or even 4 h before imaging. It is important that meticulous attention is paid to detail. Since the site of osteomyelitis is usually adjacent to hot growth plates, lesions can be masked if only whole-body images are obtained. Spot views and frequently pin-hole views are necessary. Pin-hole spots take a long time to obtain, and, since movement must be avoided, it may be necessary to restrain the areas of interest or even sedate restless children. Gentle handling, a darkened environment, lack of noise and interruptions, presence of a favourite toy etc, are all helpful. Each child has to be evaluated individually. We have found the presence of a nurse from the children's wards who knows the patients, their parents and our staff and procedures to be most valuable.

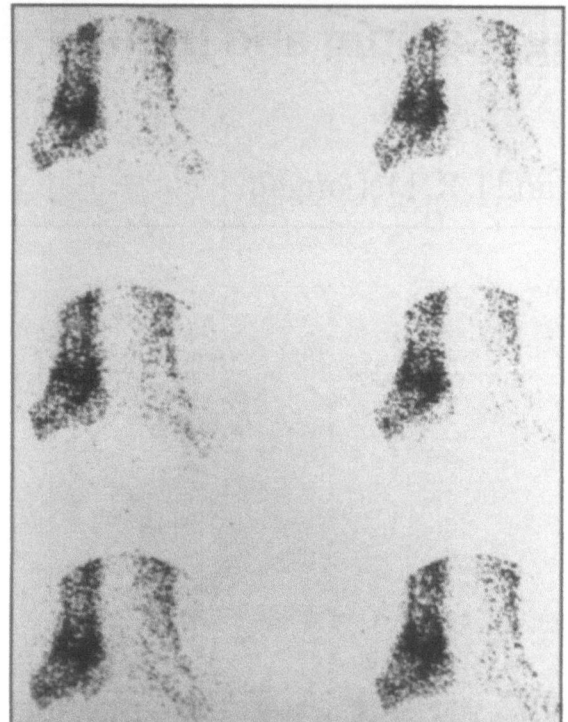

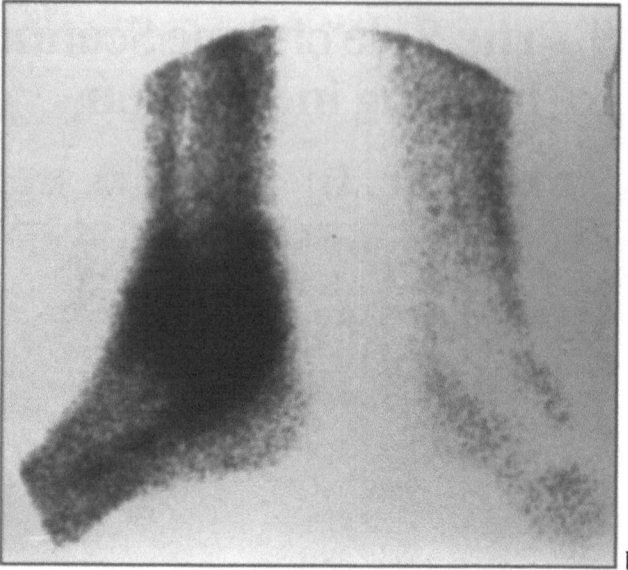

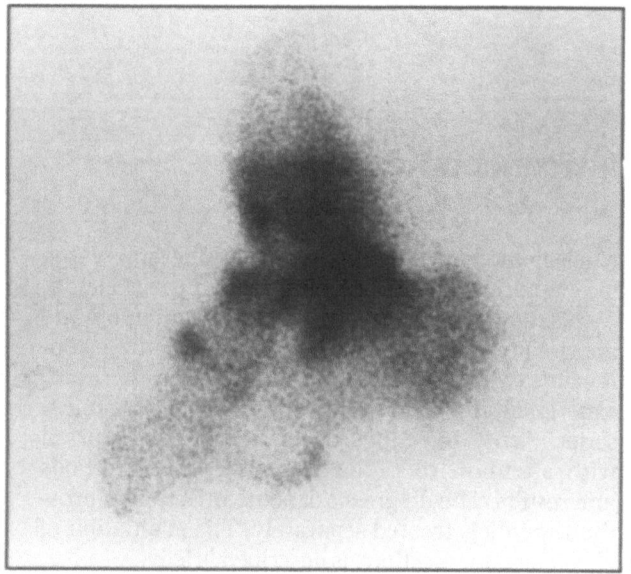

Fig. 9.1a–c. Three-phase bone scan showing increased blood flow, increased blood pool and abnormal focal uptake in ankle, most notably in the talus.

The entire skeleton should be studied since the problem can be multifocal or the location and appearance of other lesions can cause a change in diagnosis. [67]Ga has been used to diagnose acute and chronic inflammation in many sites of the body including the skeleton. The dose used varies from 3–8 mCi (111–296 MBq). We prefer doses in the lower end of the range. Whole-body and spot images are obtained 24 or 48 h after intravenous injection of the radionuclide. [67]Ga emits 4γ rays of energies 93, 186, 298 and 396 keV, and usually the three lowest are used for imaging. In general we have used planar images; however, several groups have shown the value of tomographic studies. If the region of suspected infection is lumbar spine or pelvis, it is important to ensure that ^{67}Ga in the colon superimposed on the spine is not misinterpreted as an abnormality.

[111]In-labelled white cells have been used for diagnosing acute bone and joint infections. The details of cell separation and labelling are beyond the scope of this chapter, but interested readers are referred to Thakur et al. (1976), McDougall et al. (1979).

[111]In as oxine, tropolone or acetylacetone have been used. Our experience is limited to ^{111}In oxine, and, since this preferentially labels granulocytes and our cell separation technique preferentially concentrates granulocytes, our results are based on ^{111}In granulocytes.

Acute Osteomyelitis

Pathology

Haematogenous osteomyelitis is caused most often by *Staphylococcus aureus*. It is most common in children. Osteomyelitis can result from direct penetrating wounds or spread from adjacent soft tissue infection. The consequences can be serious or even fatal, but with early diagnosis and appropriate antibiotics and/or surgery, recovery can be complete and uneventful. Haematogenous osteomyelitis has a predilection for the metaphyses of long bones, which is best understood with knowledge of the vascular supply of bone. In the child, blood supply to the medullary space enters through the nutrient artery and flows through channels towards the growth plate. When these reach the metaphyseal side of the growth plate, they turn back upon themselves in acute loops to empty into a system of large sinusoidal veins where the slow flow of blood provides a favourable medium and opportunity for implantation by bacteria. This vascular partition of the metaphysis from the epiphysis exists from the age of about 1 year until puberty; in both infancy and adulthood, the growth plate does not act as a barrier, and terminal branches of the nutrient artery extend into the epiphysis. Trueta (1959) postulates infectious involvement of the metaphyseal veins in acute osteomyelitis causing early oedema and subsequent expansion of transudates towards the surface of bone across the cortex in the distal metaphyseal region with subsequent elevation of the periosteum. It is this elevation of the periosteum which leads to the formation of an involucrum. An additional consequence is the disruption of the blood supply to the outer portion of the cortex; when this is coupled with deprivation of the blood supply to the inner cortex by thrombosis of the nutrient artery, the consequence is formation of cortical sequestra. Similar microvasculatures exist at equivalent metaphyseal locations such as the ileum, vertebrae, calcaneus, proximal femur adjacent to the greater trochanter and the ischium and predispose these locations to haematogenous osteomyelitis as well (Nixon 1978).

Animal Studies

Given the complex changes that can take place in the microvasculature of bone in acute osteomyelitis, the reactive bony changes in response to the inflammatory process, and the dependence of uptake of technetium radiophosphate compounds on both blood flow and extraction efficiency (Garnett et al. 1975: Lavender et al. 1979; Sagar et al. 1979), it is not easy to predict the temporal course of tracer uptake. In a rabbit model, Dye et al. (1979) found only one out of nine lesions abnormal on bone scan during the first week, with eight out of nine becoming abnormal after that time. Rinsky et al. (1977), also using a rabbit model, found 21 of 23 cases demonstrating either normal or reduced tracer accumulation at 3 days. Subsequently, 15 of 19 (79%) displayed increased uptake by day 10, with no additional hot cases up to 19 days. Norris and Watt (1981), also using rabbits, followed the evolution of experimentally induced acute osteomyelitis with two-phase ^{99m}Tc-MDP scanning and gallium scanning. All cases demonstrated increased activity on the gallium scans and the perfusion phase of the technetium radiophosphate scan, with reduced activity on the delayed radiophosphate scans. Raptopoulos et al. (1982) compared computed tomography, ^{111}In oxine-labelled white blood cells and ^{99m}Tc-MDP, and found that ^{99m}Tc bone scans were positive in only 22% of the animals during the first week but positive in all surviving animals during the second week and thereafter. Both the white blood cell scans and computed tomographic studies disclosed more abnormalities during the first week. Hartshorne et al. (1985) obtained parametric ratio images of ^{67}Ga and ^{99m}Tc-MDP uptake images in a rabbit model of early osteomyelitis. Images obtained during the first 48 h showed preferential gallium accumulation, thought to reflect an initial inflammatory response, while later images at 5–7 days showed a predominance of the radiophosphate agent, indicating the dominant process of osteoblastic repair.

Patient Studies

Earlier series (Duszynski et al. 1975; Gilday et al. 1975) suggested that technetium radiophosphate imaging was very sensitive (95% and 99%, respectively) in diagnosing acute haematogenous osteomyelitis. While Gilday et al. (1975) achieved a 100% specificity by utilising an adjunctive blood pool image in addition to the delayed scan, reliance soley on the delayed scan did not significantly hurt Duszynski's (1975) results as he achieved a 96% specificity. Letts et al. (1975) reported 100% sensitivity and 83% specificity by relying on only the delayed bone scan in a series of 20 children; the single false-positive result was due to a leukaemic bone deposit. Using only delayed scans in a study of nine paediatric patients, Treves et al. (1976) correctly identified all eight cases of osteomyelitis; the single case of cellulitis had a normal bone scan. Majd and Frankel (1976), utilising a two-phase combined blood pool and delayed scan technique in a series of 65 paediatric patients, correctly identified all 20 cases of acute osteomyelitis, although in one case a follow-up bone scan obtained 1 week after the onset of symptoms was required to make the diagnosis. There is insufficient information to calculate the specificity in this series. Gelfand and Silberstein (1977) were able to achieve an 84% sensitivity and 92% specificity in a series of 44 paediatric patients; however, some of his cases had chronic osteomyelitis or osteomyelitis secondary to penetrating trauma in contiguous infection. When analysis is restricted to those patients considered to have acute haematogenous osteomyelitis, 10 of 13 were correctly identified for a sensitivity of 77%.

Sullivan et al. (1980) reviewed 21 paediatric cases of proven osteomyelitis in which the patients had scintigraphy prior to diagnosis. Fourteen of the 21 cases (67%) were initially reported as osteomyelitis. Retrospectively it was thought that 11 of these 14 cases had characteristic and unequivocal abnormalities and that the remaining 3 had subtle asymmetries of the metaphyses. They thought that an additional case, though interpreted as normal in prospect, was abnormal, although subtly so. An additional case that was prospectively thought to represent a joint abnormality only, was noted upon retrospective scrutiny to have an additional focus of increased activity suggesting osteomyelitis. Four of their 21 cases were considered normal both prospectively and retrospectively. However, Gilday (1980) takes exception to their findings and suggests that the poor sensitivity was due to a lack of high-quality gamma camera images and good photographic technique and a failure to interpret subtle changes adjacent to the growth zone of the metaphysis.

Maurer et al. (1981) studied the contribution of the blood pool and radionuclide angiogram portions of a three-phase bone scan in the diagnosis of osteomyelitis. A sensitivity of 92% and specificity of 75% was achieved using the delayed study only. Addition of the blood pool or the blood pool and perfusion did not alter the sensitivity but improved the specificity to 89% and 94%, respectively. However, it should be noted that this study is not directly comparable with those previously described in that the mean age was 42 years and only 28 of the 98 patients were 18 years or younger. The three-phase bone scan may improve the specificity of the technique in an adult population, but it is not clear that such expectations should be held for paediatric applications.

Sfakianakis et al. (1978) performed a prospective study of 25 children with osteomyelitis and performed ^{99m}Tc diphosphonate scans at 8-day intervals. In virulent disease characterised by an acute onset, short history and severe symptoms, the first scan visualised the lesion faintly, while the second study showed a dramatic increase in activity, at which time radiographs became positive.

Rosenthall et al. (1982) demonstrated a sensitivity of delayed bone scanning of 91% in the diagnosis of osteomyelitis in non-violated bone. Howie et al. (1983) applied two-phase combined blood pool and delayed bone scanning in a group of 290 paediatric patients and achieved a sensitivity of 89% and specificity of 94%. It is noteworthy that in three instances, a photopaenic area was correctly interpreted as representing osteomyelitis and that six of the seven false-negative scan results showed increased uptake in the area of subsequently proven osteomyelitis. The hot spots were initially misinterpreted as representing septic arthritis in two cases, soft tissue infection in three cases and non-specific increased activity in one case. Of additional interest are the scan results from 36 sites in 33 patients with a diagnosis proved by a positive culture of pus: The scan result was negative at four of the 21 sites of subperiosteal abscess but at only one of the 15 sites of intramedullary abscess; furthermore, all examples of photopaenic defects occurred at the site of a subperiosteal abscess. Fihn et al. (1984) studied the records of 69 patients who had a total of 86 delayed static bone scans performed for suspected osteomyelitis. Images were interpreted as "definite" or "equivocal" osteomyelitis and as "osteomyelitis absent", also in definite and equivocal categories. When the data was analysed in binary fashion a sensitivity of 79% and specificity of 93% were obtained. However, an image interpretation of osteomyelitis definitely absent was obtained in only one of 19 cases of osteomyelitis. While the results are in general not as good as those of several previously reported series, the patient population is somewhat different in that of the 14 patients with osteomyelitis the youngest was 17 years and only 3 had acute haematogenous osteomyelitis. Indeed, if an image interpretation of "equivocally absent" is considered to be positive for osteomyelitis and a sensitivity of 95% and specificity of 67% are achieved, such results would not be too dissimilar from those obtained by Maurer et al. (1981) employing the delayed scan only.

Handmaker and Giammona (1984) obtained positive results for osteomyelitis in 12 out of 17 paediatric cases on bone scan for a sensitivity of 71%; 13 of these children scanned with gallium all had abnormal sites of uptake corresponding to the site of osteomyelitis. However, four of the five patients with initially negative bone scan results had a positive bone scan result later in their illness.

Some authors have questioned the value of ^{99m}Tc radiophosphate bone scanning in the evaluation of neonatal osteomyelitis. Ash and Gilday (1980) studied 21 neonates suspected of having acute osteomyelitis. Ten infants ranging in age from 7 to 42 days at the time of the first scan were proven to have osteomyelitis in 20 sites, but only 6 (31.5%) were abnormal by bone imaging, 58% were normal and 10.5% equivocal. This was in contradistinction to their positive bone scan results in all 19 of the infants ranging in age from 40 days to 1 year who were subsequently proven to have osteomyelitis and were scanned during the same 4-year period of the study. They found that plain film radiographs demonstrated destruction, and in some cases periosteal new bone was more sensitive. In a retrospective study from the same institution but covering a greater number of years (1970–1979), 19 of the 22 infants (86·4%) had abnormalities on their initial radiographs, but 7 of the 10 patients had bone scan abnormalities (Mok et al. 1982). A more recent study by Bressler et al. (1984) of 33 infants less than 6 weeks of age with suspected osteomyelitis identified 15 individuals with 25 sites of proved osteomyelitis, all of which had abnormal radionuclide localisation. Ten additional sites were identified on bone scan that were radiographically normal. The majority of abnormal sites were hot but two were cold. Of the 25 scintigraphically demonstrated cases of osteomyelitis 23 had radiographic abnormalities at about the same time. It is proposed that the routine use of magnification techniques on more modern equipment accounts for the higher sensitivity achieved compared with that obtained by Ash and Gilday (1980).

Osteomyelitis in Diabetic Patients

The evaluation of the diabetic foot for potential osteomyelitis presents a problem because of associated osteoarthropathy and soft tissue infection. Park et al. (1982) studied the value of three-phase bone scanning in this situation. Four patterns of activity were observed. Moderate to marked increased activity in all three phases of the study was felt to be diagnostic of acute osteomyelitis, while moderate or marked increased activity on only the first two phases indicated cellulitis. Moderate or marked increased activity on only the delayed phase tended to indicate osteoarthropathy or degenerative bony disease. A fourth category displaying reduced activity in all three phases was found in two patients

with acute osteomyelitis and in one normal patient. Excluding the cases with absent flow, the technique had a sensitivity of 95% for acute osteomyelitis. Seldin et al. (1982) obtained similar results in a series of 16 patients; 9 of 10 patients with acute osteomyelitis had intense focal hyperaemia during the arterial phase of the three-phase bone scan. Two of six patients (specificity of 67%) without osteomyelitis also showed focal hyperaemic changes. Although 12 of the 16 patients had foot ulcers, in only one instance did ulcer hyperaemia give a false-positive result on the three-phase bone scan.

Summary of Evidence for Application of Bone Scanning

Theory and experimental evidence suggests a spectrum of scintigraphic presentation of acute haematogenous osteomyelitis, ranging from photopaenic lesions when ischaemic changes predominate to hot lesions when the reparative processes of bony healing predominate, with a middle ground of normal uptake in instances in which the degree of bony reaction is minimal or increased extraction associated with osteoblastic proliferation is offset by focal ischaemia (Berkowitz and Wenzel 1980). Indeed, there are many reports of photopaenic lesions on bone scanning in cases of haematogenous osteomyelitis (Russin and Staab 1976; Trackler et al. 1976; Raghavendra and Braunstein 1977; Teates and Williamson 1977; Berkowitz and Wenzel 1980; Jones and Cady 1981; Barron and Dhekne 1982; Murray 1982; Patel et al. 1983). Given the pre-eminence of soft tissue factors early in the process and the relative insensitivity of radiographic techniques to subtle changes in bone mineralisation, it is not surprising that classic patterns of bone destruction and periosteal new bone are not usually seen (on radiograph) until 10 or 12 days after the onset of symptoms (Capitanio and Kirkpatrick 1970).

In the child suspected of having acute haematogenous osteomyelitis, plain films of the bone in question should be the initial imaging procedure; these may demonstrate a clinically congruent noninfectious lesion or the typical skeletal change of osteomyelitis. The next step should be bone scanning with a technetium phosphate compound. Blood pool or perfusion imaging may be employed adjunctively; however, it should be realised that sensitivity and specificity of the technique are not substantially improved in the paediatric population, although these adjuncts may aid in making a positive diagnosis of a non-osteomyelitic process such as septic arthritis or cellulitis. While there is some controversy in the literature, the bone scan is a very sensitive technique in this context, although false-negative results are certainly to be expected. In the presence of a normal bone scan and persistent clinical suspicion, the next step could be follow-up bone scan (Dye et al. 1979), gallium scanning (Handmaker and Giammona 1984), ^{111}In white cell scan or needle aspiration of the site of maximal suspicion (Kasser 1984). Although some controversy exists as to the sensitivity of radiophosphate bone scanning in neonatal osteomyelitis, the sensitivity of plain film radiographs and the availability of needle aspiration biopsy serve to limit its application in this situation. Evaluation of the diabetic foot for possible osteomyelitis is best approached with the three-phase bone scan, which serves to improve the specificity of the technique. However, caution must be exercised because of the high incidence of coexisting soft tissue infection and non-infectious skeletal abnormalities.

Role of Radiolabelled Leukocytes in Diagnosis of Acute Osteomyelitis

In most of the reports of radiolabelled leucocytes, ^{111}In has been the radionuclide used. Most investigators have used ^{111}In oxine or tropolone, fewer ^{111}In acetylacetone. ^{67}Ga-labelled leucocytes and ^{99m}Tc stannous colloid-labelled leucocytes have been used rarely. As a result, most of the statements which follow are related to [111]In. Table 9.1 gives an analysis of sensitivity and specificity of seven series. While the majority give both a high sensitivity and specificity, there are exceptions. Factors which can influence results include not only the methods of cell separation and labelling but the type of disease being evaluated. Since the methods most widely used preferentially label granulocytes, it should be expected that only those diseases associated with granulocytic infiltration will be imaged successfully. Chronic bone infections will generally *not* give a positive white cell scan result. Fractures which are non-infected give negative white cell scan results.

Several authorities have found that non-infectious arthritis gave false-positive results (Ehrlich et al. 1984), but since several non-infectious arthritides like gout and rheumatoid arthritis are associated with an intense inflammatory infiltrate in the affected joint, this is to be expected. There is one report of a necrotic bone cancer giving a false-positive white cell scan result (Sfakianakis et al. 1982). We have seen a potential false-positive result in the skull caused simply by hyperostosis frontalis. Bone marrow uptake of ^{111}In leucocytes is a normal finding. In adults this is restricted to axial skeleton but in children and

Table 9.1 Analysis of results from seven series using radiolabelled leucocyte imaging

Radiopharmaceutical	Number of patients	Sensitivity	Specificity	Comments
[111]In oxine (Ehrlich et al. 1984)	51 patients (52 scans)	84%	82%	False-positive results in inflammatory arthritis False-negative results when overlying tissue is inflamed
[111]In acetylacetone (Schauwecker et al. 1983)	20 patients (20 scans)	90%	—	Screened first with bone scan
[111]In acetylacetone (Schauweker et al. 1985) vs.	76	100% in acute osteomyelitis	91%	Tropolone gives better early images (4 h) than acetylacetone
tropolone	105	73% in chronic osteomyelitis	100%	
[111]In acetylacetone 3 mCi (111MBq) (Wellman et al. 1981)	79	50%	92%	Screened with bone scan prior to test
[111]In oxine 700 μCi (25 900 kBq) (Fernandez et al. 1982)	53	62%	71%	Non-infectious arthritis gives false-positive results Closed fractures give negative results Open fractures give false-positive results
[111]In oxine (Al-Sheikh et al. 1982)	20	75%	69%	Bone scans are more sensitive (87%) but less specific 23%
[111]In oxine 500 μCi (18 500 kBq) (Propst-Proctor et al. 1982)	80 patients (97 scans)	98%	89%	Not useful for chronic osteomyelitis Very useful for acute osteomyelitis

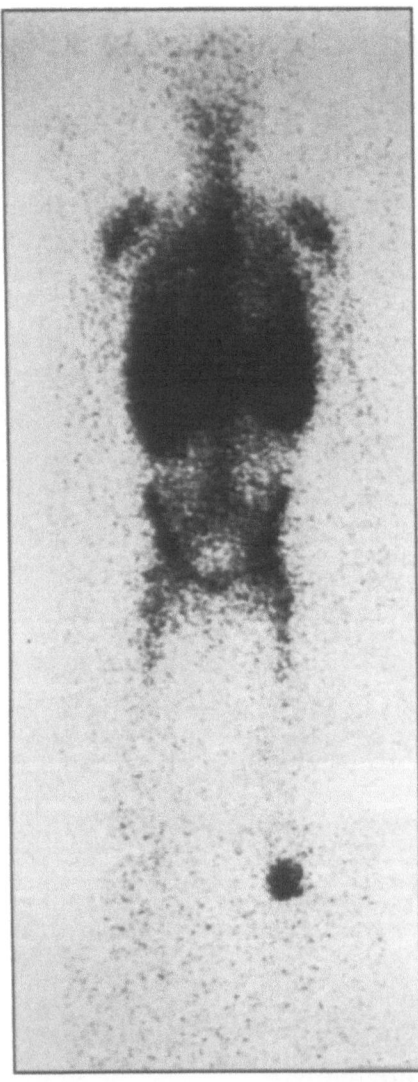

Fig. 9.2. Focal uptake of ^{111}In white cells in tibial plateau in a patient who was suspected of having an abdominal abscess but who was found to have osteomyelitis of the tibia.

certain disease states, the ^{111}In uptake can extend peripherally. Therefore, one can anticipate some uptake of labelled cells in normal skeleton, and nuclear physicians must compare one side with the other, looking for real but subtle differences in uptake. Figure 9.2 shows focal uptake of ^{111}In leucocytes in the tibia; this was quite unexpected since an abdominal problem had been diagnosed clinically.

[111]In white cell scanning is becoming more widely used; ^{111}In oxine white cell scan has recently been approved by the US Food and Drug Administration. The result is usually not available for 20–24 h. The test gives a higher radiation dose than bone scanning. For these reasons we advise that bone scan-

ning be the first nuclear medicine procedure and that white cell scanning be reserved for cases which are difficult to diagnose.

Role of ^{67}Ga in Diagnosis of Acute Osteomyelitis

In 1976 it was suggested that ^{67}Ga was a useful addition to the bone scan to diagnose acute infection (Fig. 9.3; Handmaker and Leonards 1976). As has been pointed out, the bone scan is not always abnormal; normal or cold lesions can be found. If the bone scan does not agree with the clinical impression, ^{67}Ga is a valuable adjunct. The scan is generally more abnormal than the bone scan and this lack of congruency has been used diagnostically. It should be recalled that the mechanisms of uptake are not specific for infection, although they include ^{67}Ga labelling of leucocytes (Burleson et al. 1975), labelling of lactoferrin at the infection site (Weiner et al. 1978), uptake in bacteria, labelling of transferrin (Hoffer 1980) and possibly others. [67]Ga uptake can be expected in benign and malignant tumours, trauma and chronic infection but in these situations the uptake of gallium is usually less intense. In a recent study involving 136 patients with suspected active osteomyelitis, all 12 who had ^{67}Ga uptake greater than ^{99m}Tc-MDP had active osteomyelitis. Where the uptake was equal but distribution different there were 5 false-positive results out of 23; where uptake and distribution were equal there were 4 false-positive results out of 12 (Tumeh et al. 1985). In contrast, Ang and Gelfand (1983) describe a cold lesion on the ^{67}Ga scan in acute osteomyelitis.

Gallium scans revert to normal quickly with successful therapy of osteomyelitis (Namey and Halla 1978), but it is probably better, certainly less expensive and involves less radiation to follow the clinical course with white cell count and sedimentation rate.

Diagnosis of Septic Arthritis

The role of radionuclide imaging in septic arthritis is limited because arthrocentesis and joint fluid culture are relatively easy and diagnostic procedures. However, there are exceptions. The sacroiliac joints are not easily accessible percutaneously. Aspiration can require fluoroscopy and general anaesthesia (Gordon and Kabins 1980). Bacteriological confirmation of intervertebral disc

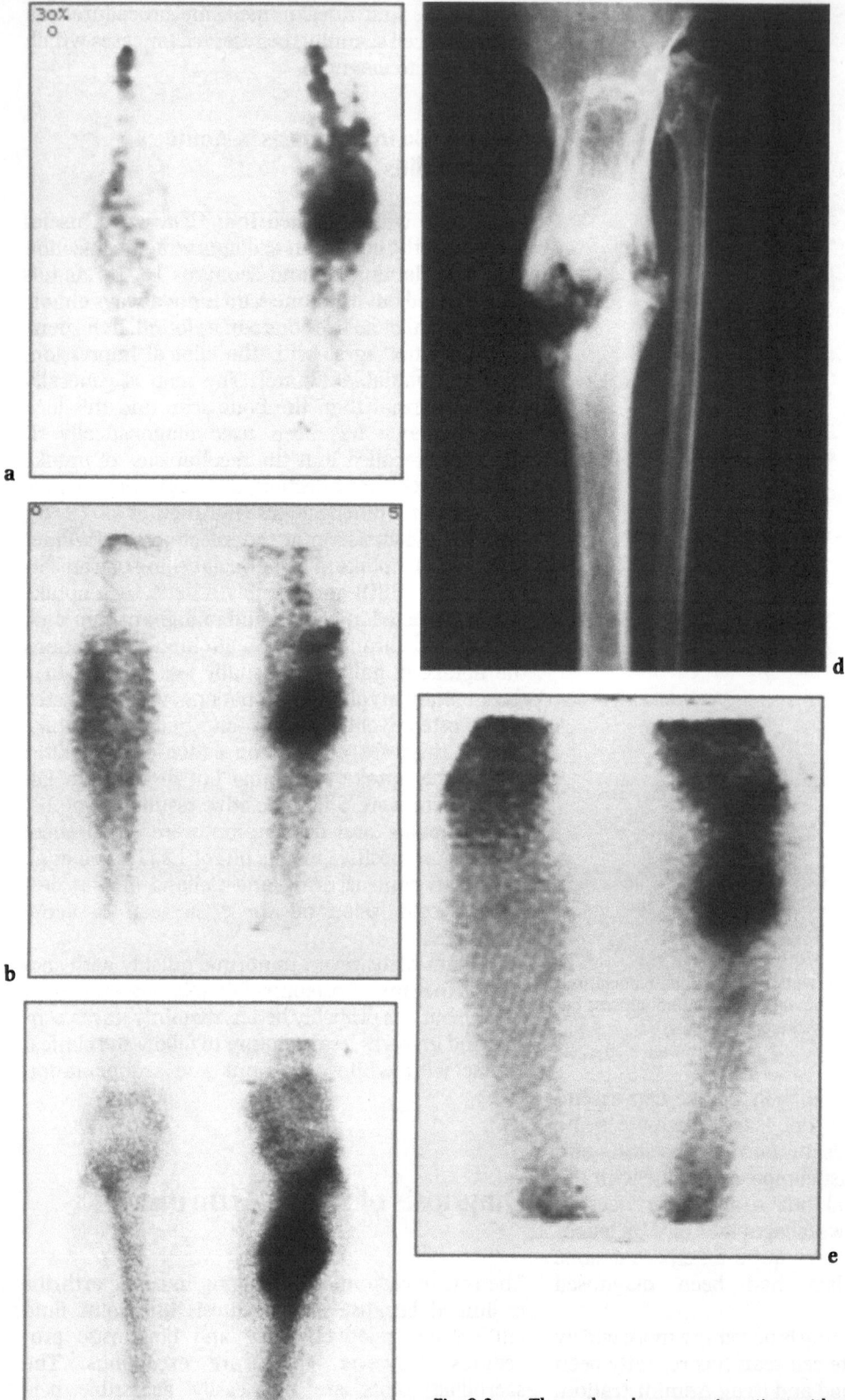

Fig. 9.3a–c. Three-phase bone scan in patient with non-union of left tibial fracture showing increased vascularity and intense uptake, associated with both ends of fracture. d Radiograph. e On gallium scan there is striking increased uptake at fracture site, confirming infection.

infection can be difficult. In one series only 50% of patients with vertebal osteomyelitis had positive cultures (Ambrose et al. 1966). Atcheson et al. (1979) reported two cases of septic arthritis in the foot, in which the bone scan was instrumental in identifying the correct joint for aspiration.

The differentiation of septic arthritis and osteomyelitis from cellulitis on clinical grounds can be difficult. Bone scintigraphy is more sensitive than plain radiography in establishing a diagnosis (Gilday et al. 1975; Majd and Frankel 1976; Gordon and Kabins 1980). There are also reports of the value of radionuclide imaging in differentiating septic arthritis from inflammatory arthritis of other aetiologies (Forrester et al. 1983; Coleman et al. 1982).

Septic arthritis has a characteristic appearance in skeletal scintigraphy employing ^{99m}Tc diphosphonates. The scan shows symmetrical increased activity in the juxta-articular bone on both sides of the involved joint (Majd and Frankel 1976; Rosenthall et al. 1982). The findings are due to increased delivery of tracer from branches of hyperaemic synovial vessels supplying the epiphysis and metaphysis. Osteomyelitis usually has a more focal appearance, although Sullivan et al. (1980) have reported that osteomyelitis involving a single bone can produce similar findings.

Occasionally the scan shows normal or decreased activity (Gilday et al. 1975; Majd and Frankel 1976; Handmaker and Leonards 1976; Maurer et al. 1981; Murray 1982). The diagnosis can be difficult in children because increased activity can be obscured by normal tracer concentration in the growth plates. Decreased blood flow secondary to increased intracapsular pressure plays a probable role. The effect of time in relation to onset of symptoms and antibiotic therapy has not been looked at systematically.

Majd and Frankel (1976) retrospectively studied 65 children in whom skeletal scintigraphy was used to differentiate osteomyelitis from septic arthritis, bone infarction and cellulitis. All seven patients with septic arthritis proven by positive joint culture had abnormal scans with six having the characteristic appearance and one showing decreased activity. There were no false-positive results. In a prospective study of 134 children with a clinical diagnosis of osteomyelitis, 8 of 9 patients with septic arthritis were correctly identified (Gilday et al. 1975). There were no false-positive results and differentiation from cellulitis and osteomyelitis was not difficult. In these two reports immediate blood pool images demonstrated increased blood flow to the joint, and blood pool images were most valuable in identifying patients with cellulitis.

Maurer et al. (1981) advocate the addition of a radionuclide angiogram and blood pool image to the conventional bone scan. In their series of 98 patients with suspected osteomyelitis, 6 patients had isolated septic arthritis. Two patients had normal three-phase studies. The delayed images showed increased uptake on both sides of the joint in four cases. However, an associated osteomyelitis could not be excluded with certainty. The blood pool image was helpful in localising the hyperaemia to the joint in one patient. The radionuclide angiogram showed increased blood flow to the joint in all four cases. However, one case also demonstrated focally increased flow to bone leading to an erroneous diagnosis of an associated osteomyelitis.

There have been several reports comparing the sensitivity and specificity of ^{67}Ga citrate scintigraphy to bone scanning. Gallium has a theoretical advantage over ^{99m}Tc diphosphonates in that it is less dependent on blood flow and does not concentrate as prominently in epiphyseal growth plates. Lisbona and Rosenthall (1977a) studied 11 children with septic arthritis who were scanned with ^{67}Ga citrate one day after a bone scan with ^{99m}Tc-MDP. All 11 patients had abnormal gallium scans, whereas the bone scan was only abnormal in 5 patients. In another report by the same investigators (Lisbona and Rosenthall 1977b), both scans were positive in all six adults with septic arthritis. Rosenthall et al. (1982) reviewed 500 cases of bone, joint and soft tissue infections of which 26 were proven or probable septic arthritis. All patients were first scanned with ^{99m}Tc-MDP followed 24–48 h later by ^{67}Ga citrate. Their results are shown in Table 9.2. In four patients with non-septic synovitis, both scan results were falsely positive. One patient with pigmented villonodular synovitis had an abnormal bone scan and a normal gallium scan. Gordon and Kabins (1980) reported seven definite and three probable cases of pyogenic sacroiliitis. Eight of ten ^{99m}Tc-MDP bone scans in nine patients were positive 2–25 days after the onset of

Table 9.2. Scan results in 26 patients with septic arthritis (Rosenthall et al. 1982)

	MDP+ Ga+	MDP+ Ga−	MDP− Ga+	MDP− Ga−	Total
Proved	6	1	4	2	13
Probable	11	0	0	2	13

	Proved	Probable	Group
Sensitivity of MDP	0.54	0.84	0.69
Sensitivity of Ga	0.77	0.84	0.80
Combined sensitivity	0.84	0.84	0.84

symptoms. Two false-negative scan results were obtained within 4 days of the onset of symptoms. In five cases gallium scans were performed 3–4 days after the bone scan. All were abnormal, including one patient who had a normal bone scan. Horgan et al. (1983) studied three patients with pyogenic sacroiliitis using two-phase bone scans and gallium scintigraphy. ^{99m}Tc-MDP blood pool and ^{67}Ga citrate images were abnormal in all three, but only one patient had an unequivocally abnormal delayed bone scan. The usefulness of ^{67}Ga citrate in 91 patients with vertebral disc space infection was examined by Bruschwein et al. (1980). Sensitivity was 89%, specificity was 85%, positive predictive value was 61% and negative predictive value was 97%.

There have been two studies specifically looking at the ability of bone and gallium scans to distinguish between septic and non-septic arthritis. Coleman et al. (1982) reported 15 cases of rheumatoid arthritis in which there was a suspicion of septic joints. The patients were scanned 2.5 h after receiving 20 mCi (740 MBq) of ^{99m}Tc-MDP and 24 h after receiving ^{67}Ga citrate the next day. Activity over the involved joints and adjacent proximal bone was quantitated. A joint/bone ratio greater than 1.8 was considered abnormal. Eight patients had culture-positive septic arthritis. Six of those eight patients had elevated ^{99m}Tc-MDP ratios and five of eight had elevated ^{67}Ga citrate ratios. Three of seven culture-negative patients also had elevated ^{99m}Tc-MDP ratios and two of seven had elevated ^{67}Ga citrate ratios. When the ^{67}Ga citrate ratio was divided by the ^{99m}Tc-MDP ratio, three of eight patients with septic arthritis had values greater than 1, whereas all culture-negative patients had values less than 1. Forrester et al. (1983) used ^{67}Ga citrate to evaluate 15 cases of inflammatory arthritis of unknown aetiology. Two patients had pure septic arthritis, two had septic arthritis superimposed on rheumatoid arthritis and one had infection superimposed on severe degenerative disease. Gallium uptake was graded on a scale of 0–2+. All infected joints showed 2+ activity, whereas non-infected joints showed 0 or 1+ activity. There has also been one case report of acute rheumatic fever simulating septic arthritis on bone and gallium scanning (Wolff et al. 1980).

The usefulness of white blood cell scans in the diagnosis of septic arthritis has not been fully explored. Using dogs, McAfee et al. (1980) demonstrated that labelled leucocytes localised better than ^{67}Ga citrate in acute inflammatory arthritis induced by injection of sodium urate crystals. Fernandez et al. (1982) reported that non-septic arthritis often gave positive white blood cell scan results. False-

negative scan results in septic arthritis have also been reported (Gainey and McDougall 1984).

Summary

The bone scan with an immediate blood pool image should be the first radionuclide study in the evaluation of septic arthritis. Although the overall sensitivity based on the studies quoted is only 73%, the study can be completed in 2–3 h. If the bone scan is normal and the clinical situation warrants further investigation, a 24-h gallium scan should be performed. The sensitivity of the gallium scan is approximately 80%–90%. Both the bone scan and the gallium scan reliably differentiate bone, joint and soft tissue infection, but the specificity for septic arthritis is low when other inflammatory arthritic conditions are considered.

Diagnosis of Infected Prosthetic Joint

Arthroplasty is a common procedure whose indications include arthritis, trauma, avascular necrosis, congenital dysplasia, and tumours. Complications include loosening, infection, heterotopic bone formation, dislocation, non-union, fracture, synovitis and bursitis. In total hip athroplasty, loosening and infection require removal of the prosthesis in 7.2% and 1.5% of cases, respectively (Tapadiya et al. 1984). Infection can appear months to years after surgery and usually produces no systemic symptoms. If infection is recognised early it may be successfully treated with antibiotics. Late infection requires removal of the prosthesis, whereas loosening can be treated with prompt reimplantation. Infection is usually associated with loosening, whereas the converse is not true. The distinction is often difficult to make. Radiographic signs of infection are an irregular wide area of bone resorption and periosteal new bone formation. Using these criteria Tehranzadeh et al. (1981) found plain radiographs were 53% sensitive and 93% specific. Arthrography occasionally demonstrates abscesses and sinus tracts. Aspiration at the time of arthrography can be diagnostic, but Dussault et al. (1977) reported 4 false-negative culture results in 12 infected hip arthroplasties.

The earliest radionuclide studies were done with strontium. Normal postoperative healing resulted in increased bone activity for 6–10 months (Bauer et al. 1973; Feith et al. 1976). When the ^{99m}Tc-labelled diphosphonates became available, some investigators found that bone activity returned to normal 6–11 months postoperatively (Campeau et al. 1976; Reing et al. 1979). Creutzig (1976) reported that 18 of 22 asymptomatic patients with hip prostheses had normal activity over the femoral component 6 months postoperatively. However, acetabular activity stabilised at 2.7 times normal by 6 months. Utz et al. (1982) studied the normal evolutionary changes in 85 asymptomatic patients with total hip arthroplasties. Activity over the acetabulum, greater trochanter and tip of the femoral component remained markedly elevated in many patients for years, whereas activity over the lesser trochanter and shaft became near normal within 6 months.

Infection and loosening both result in concentration of ^{99m}Tc diphosphonate. Several investigators have looked at the pattern and intensity of activity in an attempt to differentiate between the two. Pearlman (1980) examined 33 patients who complained of pain following total hip replacement. Images were obtained at 30 min and 3 h. Six patients had infection with loosening, three had infection only, and 26 had loosening without infection. All patients in whom infection was present had an expanded vascular pool on the early images as did one-third of those patients in whom infection was absent. However, in the latter group the intesity of this finding was significantly lower. Infection was indistinguishable from loosening on the delayed images. Williams et al. (1981) and McInerney and Hyde (1978) also found that infection and loosening appeared similar on delayed scans.

Rushton et al. (1982) evaluated 19 infected prostheses in 51 patients with painful hips. One patient had a normal bone scan. Most of the cases demonstrated focal activity indistinguishable from loosening. Only some of the grossly infected cases exhibited diffuse uptake. Pederson (1978) evaluated 16 cases with painful hip prostheses and found that heavy diffuse accumulation was seen in six patients with infection, while one showed a focal pattern. However, the diffuse pattern was not specific for infection. It was also seen in one patient with complete loosening, one patient allergic to the metal components and in one patient in whom no cause for pain could be found. The non-specificity of a diffuse pattern was supported by Williamson et al. (1979). In their report of 20 patients with painful hip prostheses, both patients with infection were in this category, as were four with loosening and one with severe synovitis. Tehranzadeh et al. (1981) studied 89 patients with 94 failed total hip prostheses requiring surgery. Twenty-seven patients had bone scans. All nine patients with infection exhibited diffuse high activity around both components, as did two patients in whom only loosening was present.

There have been several reports comparing the accuracy of ^{67}Ga citrate to bone scanning in diagnosing complications of arthroplasty. Reing et al. (1979) evaluated 79 cases involving different kinds of painful prostheses and found that all 19 patients with abnormal gallium scans at 24 h had positive intraoperative cultures. One additional patient with a positive culture had an abnormal bone scan and a normal gallium scan. Rosenthall et al. (1979) studied 46 patients with prostheses or fixing devices who were asymptomatic or had various complications. Twelve patients had normal gallium scans and 16 had mild to moderate gallium uptake in a pattern congruent to the bone scan. None of them were infected. Eighteen patients had abnormal gallium and bone scans with incongruent patterns. Two had non-septic synovitis, while the remaining 16 had osteomyelitis. Horoszowski et al. (1980) studied 14 patients with painful hip prostheses and an abnormal bone scan. Eight patients had an abnormal gallium scan. Six of them had proven infection. In the four patients with a normal gallium scan, pain was due to fracture or heterotopic bone. Two patients had non-diagnostic scans. Williams et al. (1981) found that gallium scanning was 93% sensitive and 91% specific for infection in their study of 30 patients with painful total hip replacement. In contrast to the report of Rosenthall et al. (1979) the bone and gallium scans were congruent in half the cases with proven infection. Rushton et al. (1982) reported 100% accuracy of the gallium scan in 18 patients with non-infected loose prostheses, 13 with infected prostheses, 5 with other complications, and 23 controls.

^{111}In-labelled leucocytes are generally regarded as more specific for infection than gallium. Normal postoperative healing does not give false-positive leucocyte scan results. Mountford et al. (1982) reported two cases of painful hip prostheses less than 6 months after operation. Both patients had abnormal bone scans. The leucocyte scan was correct in identifying infection in one patient and excluding infection in the other. Slight asymmetry of uptake of labelled cells deserves careful evaluation, and abnormalities can be quite subtle. Figure 9.4 shows spot views of ^{111}In white cells in an infected prosthetic shoulder.

Mulamba et al. (1983) studied 30 patients with painful hip arthroplasties. Leucocyte scans were done preoperatively and the results compared with culture taken at the time of surgery. The scan was abnormal in 12 of 13 culture-positive patients. There were no false-positive scan results. McKillop et al. (1984) compared gallium and ^{111}In-labelled leucocytes in 15 patients with painful hip arthroplasties at least 1 year after operation. Of the six patients with infection, five had abnormal gallium scans and three had abnormal leucocyte scans. There were two false-positive gallium scan results, whereas the leucocyte scan was 100% specific.

From the combined data of the reports cited, the sensitivity of ^{99m}Tc diphosphonate (diffuse pattern), ^{67}Ga citrate and ^{111}In-labelled leucocytes in infected arthroplasty is 94%, 96% and 80% respectively. The specificity is 75%, 86% and 100% respectively.

Summary

1. A normal bone or gallium scan makes infection in a prosthetic joint very unlikely.

2. A diffuse pattern on bone scan and an incongruent pattern of ^{99m}Tc diphosphonate and ^{67}Ga citrate with more abnormality on ^{67}Ga is highly suggestive of infection.

3. An abnormal ^{111}In leucocyte scan establishes the diagnosis with reasonable certainty.

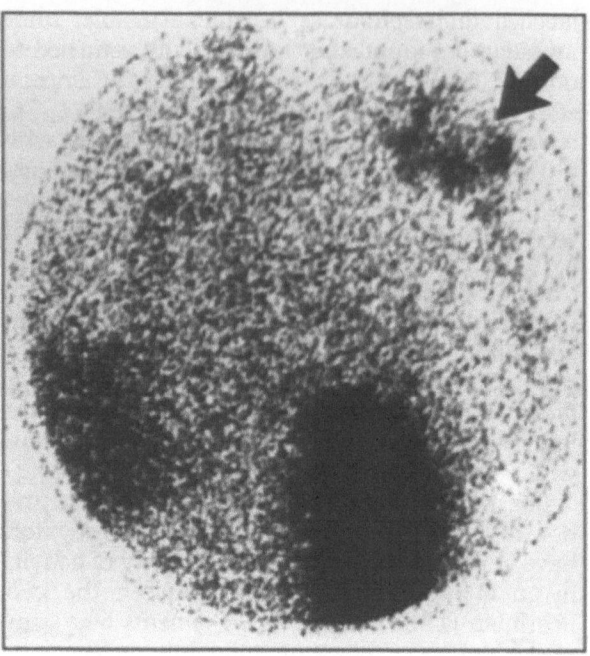

Fig. 9.4. Intense uptake of ^{111}In white cells (*arrow*) in an infected prosthetic shoulder joint.

Chronic Osteomyelitis

The pathological finding in chronic osteomyelitis differs from the acute condition in several ways. The inflammatory cell infiltrate is less marked and lymphocytes and plasma cells predominate, not polymorphonuclears. There can be both destruction and remodelling of bone. As a result of bone repair, the static bone scan is abnormal, although flow and blood pool can be normal. Unfortunately, as discussed above (see p. 109), bone scan remains abnormal for months after successful treatment of acute osteomyelitis. Consequently, it is difficult to determine from scanning alone if one is dealing with healing or chronic disease. If the flow study, blood pool and static images are abnormal, the pattern is suggestive of acute relapse of chronic osteomyelitis (Fig. 9.5) or chronic active osteomyelitis.

The gallium scan is abnormal in chronic osteomyelitis and, depending on the outlook of investigators, this can be interpreted as either beneficial or not. Clearly, if the aim is to differentiate acute from chronic disease, this is not possible. However, if all that is required is to show an abnormality, ^{67}Ga will do this. It has been our experience that the ^{111}In white cell scan, in which the majority of labelled cells are polymorphonuclears, is usually normal in chronic osteomyelitis (Propst-Proctor

et al. 1982). Propst-Proctor et al. (1982) defined chronic infection as being of more than 6 weeks' duration. Goodwin et al. (1980) have shown that ^{111}In-labelled lymphocytes give positive results when the routine white cell scan is normal. Nevertheless, the ^{111}In lymphocyte scan should be considered a research rather than routine clinical procedure, and in most cases of chronic osteomyelitis it will not be necessary. In contrast, Merkel et al. (1985) found the ^{111}In white cell scan was valuable in subacute and chronic musculoskeletal disorders; indeed it was superior to the gallium scan in the same patients. The differences between these studies could be due to selection of patients. In addition, many of the patients studied by Merkel et al. (1985) had undergone surgery, and these authors suggest that they had a significant proportion of lymphocytes (30%) in their white cell preparation which could account for their findings.

Recently, Sayle et al. (1985) reported excellent results in diagnosing chronic osteomyelitis using 2–3 mCi (74–111MBq) ^{111}In chloride and images at 48 or 72 h. In this series there were 54 true-positive, 7 true-negative, 4 false-positive and 3 false-negative results. Because very few "normals" were studied, the specificity was low (64%); however sensitivity was high (95%), leading the authors to conclude that this radiopharmaceutical is the agent of choice for diagnosing chronic osteomyelitis. ^{99m}Tc-MDP

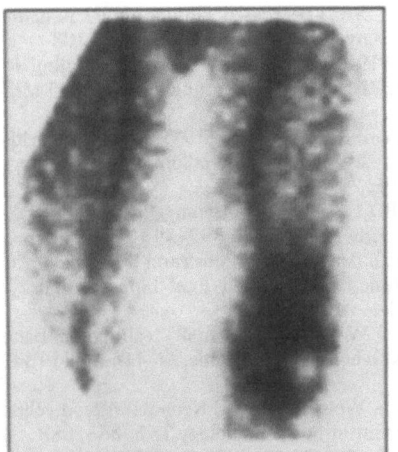

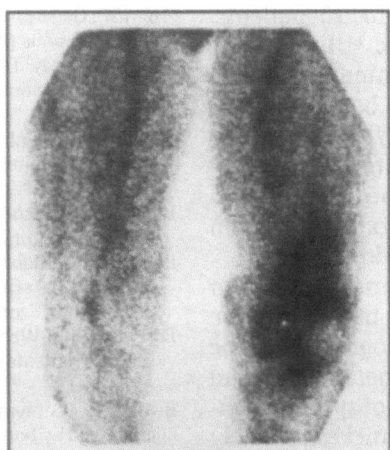

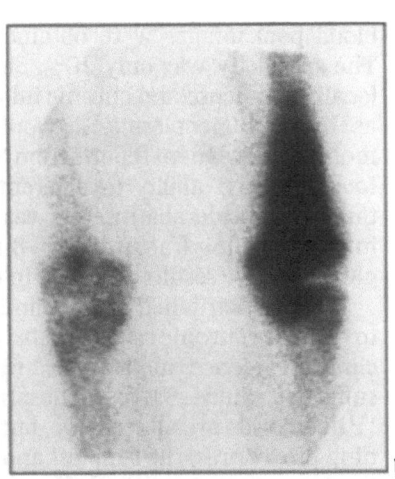

a

b, c

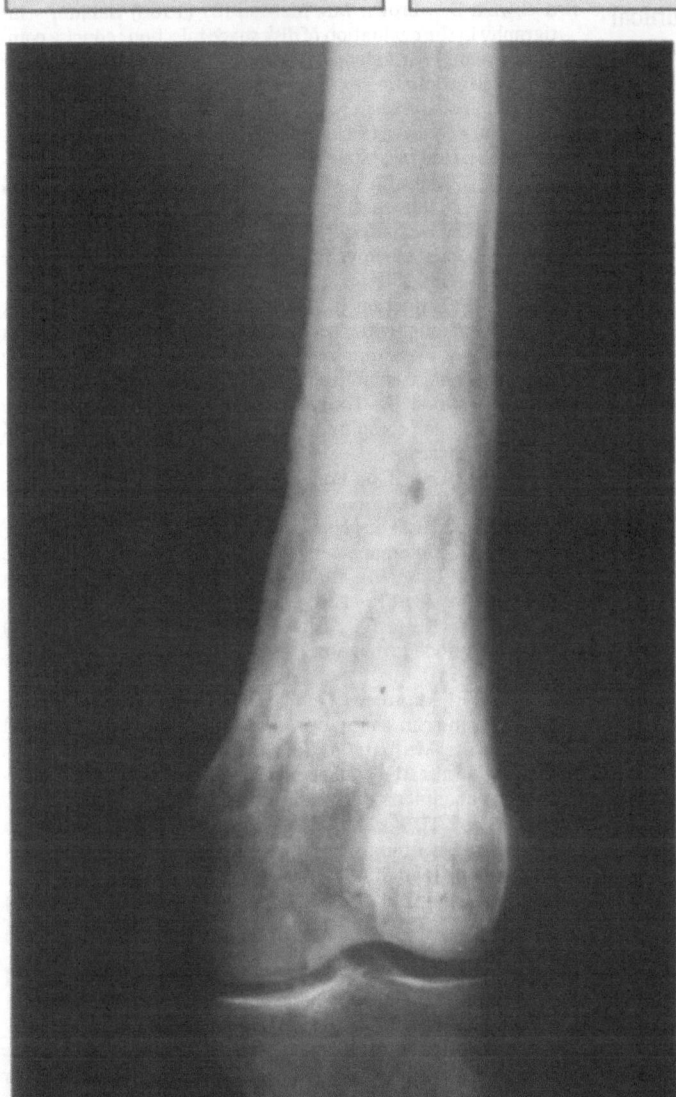

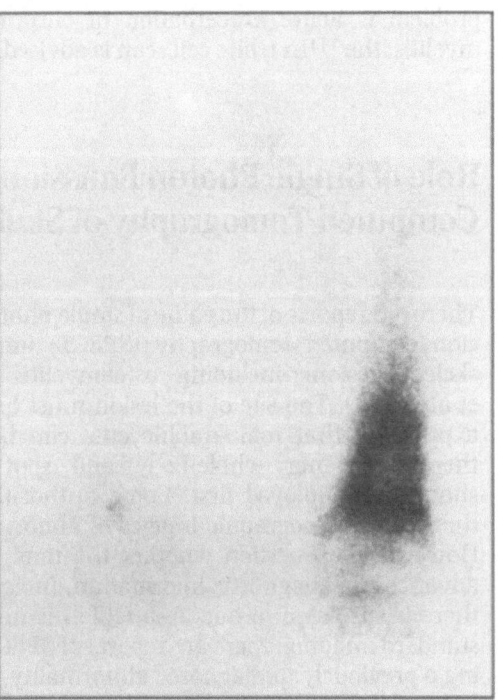

d

e

Fig. 9.5. a–c Three-phase bone scan showing increased vascularity and intense uptake in patient with acute relapse of chronic osteomyelitis in the left femur. d Radiograph. e Following therapy there has been improvement in scan appearances.

blood pool images were obtained in 46 patients. The specificity was only 20%. Since ^{111}In chloride localises in acute and chronic inflammation as well as in some neoplasms, it would be prudent to monitor subsequent reports from Sayle et al. (1985) to judge their ability to differentiate these conditions. Of considerable interest was the fact that non-infected healing fractures of 3–8 months' duration gave negative results on the ^{111}In chloride scan.

We question whether the clinicians need a scan to diagnose chronic osteomyelitis. In many cases the clinical evidence and standard radiographs will be sufficient. Since ^{99m}Tc diphosphonate, ^{67}Ga and ^{111}In chloride are all sensitive, but not specific scanning procedures, the simplest and quickest, namely the bone scan, is advised. However, if the clinical problem is acute exacerbation of chronic osteomyelitis, the ^{111}In white cell scan is advised.

Role of Single Photon Emission Computed Tomography of Skeleton

There are reports of the value of single photon emission computed tomography (SPECT) imaging of skeletal lesions including osteomyelitis (Corbus et al. 1983). The site of the lesion must be known a priori so that tomographic cuts can be made; therefore planar whole-body and spot images should be employed first. Some authorities have then made tomographic images of abnormal sites. However, we question whether the time involved advances the diagnostic information. In contrast, if there is suspicion in one area which is normal on standard imaging, there are reports of SPECT showing a previously undiagnosed abnormality, particularly in the spine and pelvis. SPECT is also helpful when the abnormal region is hidden, for example a pelvic lesion behind a full bladder, although urethral catheterisation or delayed 12–24 h scans will usually suffice.

References

Al-Sheikh W, Sfakianakis GN, Hourani M et al. (1982). A prospective comparative study of the sensitivity and specificity of In-111 leukocyte, gallium 67, and bone scintigraphy and roentgenograms in the diagnosis of osteomyelitis with and without orthopedic prosthesis. J Nucl Med 23: P29

Ambrose GB, Alpert M, Neer CS (1966) Vertebral osteomyelitis. A diagnostic problem. JAMA 197: 101–104

Ang JGP, Gelfand MJ (1983) Decreased gallium uptake in acute hematogenous osteomyelitis. Clin Nucl Med 8: 301–303

Ash JM, Gilday DL (1980) The futility of bone scanning in neonatal osteomyelitis: concise communication. J Nucl Med 21: 417–420

Atcheson SG, Coleman RE, Ward JR (1979) Septic arthritis mimicking cellulitis: distinction using radionuclide bone imaging. Clin Nucl Med 4: 79–81

Barron PJ, Dhekne RD (1984) Cold osteomyelitis radionuclide bone scan findings. Clin Nucl Med 9: 392–393

Bauer GCH, Lindberg L, Naversten Y, Sjöstrand LO (1973) ^{85}Sr radionuclide scintimetry in infected total hip arthroplasty. Acta Orthop Scand 44: 439–450

Berkowitz ID, Wenzel W (1980) "Normal" technetium bone scans in patients with acute osteomyelitis. Am J Dis Child 134: 828–830

Bressler EL, Conway JJ, Weiss SC (1984) Neonatal osteomyelitis examined by bone scintigraphy. Radiology 152: 685–688

Bruschwein DA, Brown ML, McLeod RA (1980) Gallium scintigraphy in the evaluation of disk space infection: concise communication. J Nucl Med 21: 925–927

Burleson RL, Holman BL, Tow DE (1975) Scintigraphic demonstration of abscesses with radioactive gallium labeled leukocytes. Surg Gynecol Obstet 141: 379–382

Campeau RJ, Hall MF, Miale A (1976) Detection of total hip arthroplasty complications with Tc-99m pyrophosphate. J Nucl Med 17: 526 (abstract)

Capitanio MA, Kirkpatrick JA (1970) Early roentgen observations in acute osteomyelitis. Am J Roentgenol Radium Ther Nucl Med 108: 488

Coleman RE, Samuelson Jr CO, Baim S, Christian PE, Ward JR (1982) Imaging with Tc-99m MDP and Ga 67 citrate in patients with rheumatoid arthritis and suspected septic arthritis: concise communication. J Nucl Med 23: 479–482

Corbus HF, Wood JR, Touya JJ (1983) Indications for single photon emission computer tomography of bone. Clin Nucl Med 8: P42 (abstract)

Creutzig H (1976) Bone imaging after total replacement arthroplasty of the hip joint. A follow-up with different radiopharmaceuticals. Eur J Nucl Med 1: 177–180

Dussault RG, Goldman AB, Ghelman B (1977) Radiologic diagnosis of loosening and infection in hip prostheses. J Can Assoc Radiol 28: 119–123

Duszynski DO, Kuhn JP, Afshani E, Riddlesberger MM (1975) Early radionuclide diagnosis of acute osteomyelitis. Radiology 117: 337–340

Dye SF, Lull RJ, McAuley RJ et al. (1979) Time sequence of bone and gallium scan changes in acute osteomyelitis: an animal model. J Nucl Med 20: 647 (abstract)

Ehrlich L, Martin RH, Saliken J (1984) Indium-111 WBC scintigraphy in adult osteomyelitis. J Nucl Med 25: P42

Feith R, Slooff TJ, Kazem I, van Rens ThJG (1976) Strontium ^{87m}Sr bone scanning for the evaluation of total hip replacement. J Bone Joint Surg [Br] 58: 79–83

Fernandez M, Stern PJ, Volarich DT, Cline J, Hanslits ML (1982) Evaluations of In-111 white blood cells in the detection of skeletal disease. J Nucl Med 23: P29

Fihn SD, Larson EB, Nelp WB, Rudd TG, Gerber FH (1984) Should single phase radionuclide bone imaging be used in suspected osteomyelitis? J Nucl Med 25: 1080–1088

Forrester DM, Hensel AL, Brown JC (1983) The use of gallium-67 citrate to distinguish between infectious and non-infectious arthritis. Clin Rheum Dis 9: 333–345

Gainey MA, McDougall IR (1984) Diagnosis of acute inflammatory conditions in children and adolescents using In-111 oxine white blood cells. Clin Nucl Med 9: 71–74

Garnett ES, Bowen BM, Coates G, Nahmias L (1975) An analysis of factors which influence the local accumulation of bone-seeking radiopharmaceuticals. Invest Radiol 10: 564–568

Gelfand MJ, Silberstein EB (1977) Radionuclide imaging. Use in diagnosis of osteomyelitis in children. JAMA 237: 245–247

Gilday DL (1980) Problems in the scintigraphic detection of osteomyelitis. Radiology 135: 791

Gilday DL, Eng B, Paul DJ, Paterson J (1975) Diagnosis of osteomyelitis in children by combined blood pool and bone imaging. Radiology 117: 331–335

Goodwin DA, Hickman JR, Fajardo LF et al. (1980) Migratory patterns of In-111 labeled human lymphocytes in chronic inflammatory disease. J Nucl Med 21: P43

Gordon G, Kabins SA (1980) Pyogenic sacroiliitis. Am J Med 69: 50–56

Handmaker H, Giammona ST (1984) Improved early diagnosis of acute inflammatory skeletal-articular diseases in children: a two-radiopharmaceutical approach. Pediatrics 73: 661–669

Handmaker H, Leonards R (1976) The bone scan in inflammatory osseous disease. Semin Nucl Med 6: 95–105

Hartshorne MF, Graham G, Lancaster J, Berger D (1985) Gallium-67/technetium-99m methylene diphosphonate ratio imaging: early rabbit osteomyelitis and fracture. J Nucl Med 26: 272–277

Hoffer P (1980) Gallium: mechanisms. J Nucl Med 21: 282–285

Horgan JG, Walker M, Newman JH, Watt I (1983) Scintigraphy in the diagnosis and management of septic sacro-iliitis. Clin Radiol 34: 337–346

Horoszowski H, Ganel A, Kamhin M, Zaltman S, Farine I (1980) Sequential use of technetium 99m MDP and gallium 67 citrate imaging in the evaluation of painful total hip replacement. Br J Radiol 53: 1169–1173

Howie DW, Savage JP, Wilson TG, Paterson D (1983) The technetium phosphate bone scan in the diagnosis of osteomyelitis in childhood. J Bone Joint Surg [Am] 65: 431–437

Jones DC, Cady RB (1981) "Cold" bone scans in acute osteomyelitis. J Bone Joint Surg [Br] 63: 376–378

Kasser JR (1984) Hematogenous osteomyelitis: untangling the diagnostic confusion. Postgrad Med 76: 4, 79–86

Lavender JP, Khan RAA, Hughes SPF (1979) Blood flow and tracer uptake in normal and abnormal canine bone: comparisons with Sr-85 microspheres, Kr-81m, and Tc-99m MDP. J Nucl Med 20: 413–418

Letts RM, Afifi A, Sutherland JB (1975) Technetium bone scanning as an aid in the diagnosis of atypical acute osteomyelitis in children. Surg Gynecol Obstet 140: 899–902

Lisbona R, Rosenthall L (1977a) Observations on the sequential use of ^{99m}Tc phosphate complex and ^{67}Ga imaging in osteomyelitis, cellulitis, and septic arthritis. Radiology 123: 123–129

Lisbona R, Rosenthall L (1977b) Radionuclide imaging of septic joints and their differentiation from periarticular osteomyelitis and cellulitis in pediatrics. Clin Nucl Med 2: 337–343

Majd M, Frankel RS (1976) Radionuclide imaging in skeletal inflammatory and ischemic disease in children. Am J Roentgenol Radium Ther Nucl Med 126: 832–841

Maurer AH, Chen DCP, Camargo EE, Wong DF, Wagner HN, Alderson PO (1981) Utility of three-phase skeletal scintigraphy in suspected osteomyelitis: concise communication. J Nucl Med 22: 941–949

McAfee JG, Gagne GM, Grossman ZD, Thomas FD, Roskopf ML, Fernandes P, Lyons BJ (1980) Distribution of leukocytes labeled with In-111 oxine in dogs with acute inflammatory lesions. J Nucl Med 21: 1059–1068

McDougall IR, Baumert JE, Lantieri RL (1979) Evaluation of In-111 leukocyte-whole body scanning. Am J Roentgenol Radium Ther Nucl Med 133: 849–854

McInerney DP, Hyde ID (1978) Technetium ^{99m}Tc pyrophosphate scanning in the assessment of painful hip prosthesis. Clin Radiol 29: 513–517

McKillop JH, McKay I, Cuthbert GF, Fogelman I, Gray HW, Sturrock RD (1984) Scintigraphic evaluation of the painful prosthetic joint: a comparison of gallium-67 citrate and indium-111 labelled leukocyte imaging. Clin Radiol 35: 239–241

Merkel KD, Brown ML, DeWanjee MK, Fitzgerald RH (1985) Comparison of Indium-labeled-leukocyte imaging with sequential technetium-gallium scanning in the diagnosis of low-grade musculoskeletal sepsis. J Bone Joint Surg [Am] 67: 465–476

Mok PM, Reilly BJ, Ash JM (1982) Osteomyelitis in the neonate: clinical aspects and the role of radiography and scintigraphy in diagnosis and management. Radiology 145: 677–682

Mountford PJ, Hall FM, Coakley AJ, Wells CP (1982) Assessment of the painful hip prosthesis with ^{111}In-labelled leukocyte scans. Br J Radiol 55: 378 (letter)

Mulamba L, Ferrant A, Leners N, de Nayer P, Rombouts JJ, Vincent A (1983) Indium-111 leukocyte scanning in the evaluation of painful hip arthroplasty. Acta Orthop Scand 54: 695–697

Murray IPC (1982) Photopenia in skeletal scintigraphy of suspected bone and joint infection. Clin Nucl Med 7: 13–20

Namey TC, Halla JT (1978) Radiographic and nucleographic techniques. Clin Rheum Dis 4: 95–132

Nixon GW (1978) Hematogenous osteomyelitis of metaphyseal-equivalent locations. Am J Roentgenol Radium Ther Nucl Med 130: 123–129

Norris SH, Watt I (1981) Radionuclide uptake during the evolution of experimental acute osteomyelitis. Br J Radiol 54: 207–211

Park H, Wheat LJ, Siddiqui AR et al. (1982) Scintigraphic evaluation of diabetic osteomyelitis: concise communication. J Nucl Med 23: 569 (abstract)

Patel BR, Seid K, Blumenthal BI, Flower WM (1983) Radiologic Seminar CCXXX: Early osteomyelitis—demonstration of unusual findings on 3-phase bone scan. J Miss State Med Assoc 24: 185–187

Pearlman AW (1980) The painful hip prosthesis: value of nuclear imaging in the diagnosis of late complications. Clin Nucl Med 5: 133–142

Pedersen NT (1978) Evaluation of painful hip arthroplasty. Acta Orthop Scand 49: 384–388

Propst-Proctor SL, Dillingham MF, McDougall IR, Goodwin D (1982) The white blood cell scan in orthopedics. Clin Orthop 168: 157–165

Raghavendra BN, Braunstein P (1977) Acute osteomyelitis presenting as a photon-deficient area on bone scan. Clin Nucl Med 2: 134

Raptopoulos V, Doherty PW, Goss TP, King MA, Johnson K, Gantz NM (1982) Acute osteomyelitis: advantage of white cell scans in early detection. AJR 139: 1077–1082

Reing CM, Richin PF, Kenmore PI (1979) Differential bone scanning in the evaluation of a painful total joint replacement. J Bone Joint Surg [Am] 61: 933–936

Rinsky L, Goris ML, Schurman DJ, Nagel DA (1977) ^{99m}Technetium bone scanning in experimental osteomyelitis. Clin Orthop 128: 361–366

Rosenthall L, Lisbona R, Hernandez M, Hadjipavlou A (1979) ^{99m}Tc-PP and ^{67}Ga imaging following insertion of orthopedic devices. Radiology 133: 717–721

Rosenthall L, Kloiber R, Damteu B, Al-Majid H (1982) Sequential use of radiophosphate and radiogallium imaging in the differential diagnosis of bone, joint, and soft tissue infection: quantitative analysis. Diagn Imaging 51: 249–258

Rushton N, Coakley AJ, Tudor J, Wraight EP (1982) The value of technetium and gallium scanning in assessing pain after total hip replacement. J Bone Joint Surg [Br] 64: 313–318

Russin LD, Staab EV (1976) Unusual bone-scan findings in acute osteomyelitis: case report. J Nucl Med 17: 617–619

Sagar DV, Piccone JM, Charkes ND (1979) Studies of skeletal tracer kinetics. III. Tc-99m (Sn) methylenediphosphonate uptake in the canine tibia as a function of blood flow. J Nucl Med 20: 1257–1261

Sayle BA, Fawcett HD, Wilkey DJ, Ceirny G, Mader JT (1985) Indium-111 chloride imaging in chronic osteomyelitis. J Nucl Med 26: 225–229

Schauwecker DS, Mock BH, Wellman HN et al. (1983) Comparison of In-111 acetyl acetone labeled granulocytes, Ga-67 citrate, and 3-phase MDP skeletal imaging in complicated osteomyelitis. J Nucl Med. 24: P64 (abstract)

Schauwecker DS, Mock BH, Park HM, Burt RW, Wellman HN et al. (1985) Clinical comparison of In-111 acetylacetone and In-111 tropolone labeled granulocytes. J Nucl Med 26: P22 (abstract)

Seldin DW, Heiken J, Feldman F, Alderson PO (1982) Three-phase bone scintigraphy in diabetics with foot disease. J Nucl Med 23: P77 (abstract)

Sfakianakis GN, Scoles P, Welch M et al. (1978) Evolution of the bone imaging findings in osteomyelitis. J Nucl Med 19: 706 (abstract)

Sfakianakis GN, Mnaymneh W, Ghandur-Mnaymneh L, Al-Sheikh W, Hourani M, Heal A (1982) Positive indium-111 leukocyte scintigraphy in a skeletal metastasis. AJR 139: 601–603

Siegel B, Donovan R, Alderson PO, Mack GR (1976) Skeletal uptake of ^{99m}Tc-diphosphonate in relation to local blood flow. Radiology 120: 121–123

Sullivan DC, Rosenfield NS, Ogden J, Gottschalk A (1980) Problems in the scintigraphic detection of osteomyelitis in children. Radiology 135: 731–736

Tapadiya D, Walker RH, Schurman DJ (1984) Prediction of outcome of total hip arthroplasty based on initial postoperative radiographic analysis. Clin Orthop 186: 5–15

Teates CD, Williamson BRJ (1977) "Hot and cold" bone lesion in acute osteomyelitis. Am J Roentgenol Radium Ther Nucl Med 129: 517–518

Tehranzadeh J, Schneider R, Freiberger RH (1981) Radiologic evaluation of painful total hip replacement. Radiology 141: 355–362

Thakur ML, Coleman RE, Mayhall CG, Welch MJ (1976) Preparation and evaluation of ^{111}In-labeled leukocytes as an abscess imaging agent in dogs. Radiology 119: 731–732

Trackler RT, Miller KE, Sutherland DH, Chadwick DL (1976) Childhood pelvic osteomyelitis presenting as a "cold" lesion on bone scan: case report. J Nucl Med 17: 620–622

Treves S, Khettry J, Broker FH, Wilkinson RH, Watts H (1976) Osteomyelitis: early scintigraphic detection in children. Pediatrics 57: 173–186

Trueta J (1959) The three types of acute haematogenous osteomyelitis. J Bone Joint Surg [Br] 41: 671–680

Tumeh SS, Aliabadi P, Weissman B, McNeil BJ (1985) Abnormal Tc 99m-MDP/Ga-67 scan patterns in association with active chronic osteomyelitis. J Nucl Med 26: P24

Utz JA, Galvin EG, Lull RJ (1982) Natural history of technetium 99m MDP bone scan in asymptomatic total hip prosthesis. J Nucl Med 23: P28 (abstract)

Weiner RE, Hoffer PB, Thakur ML (1978) Effect of ferric ion on Ga-67 binding to lactoferrin. In: Proceedings of the second international congress of the World Federation of Nuclear Medicine and Biology, Washington DC, 17–21 Sept 1978, P73 (abstract)

Williams F, McCall IW, Park WM, O'Connor BT, Morris V (1981) Gallium-67 scanning in the painful total hip replacement. Clin Radiol 32: 431–439

Williamson BRJ, McLaughlin RE, Wang GJ, Miller CW, Teates CD, Bray ST (1979) Radionuclide bone imaging as a means of differentiating loosening and infection in patients with a painful total hip prosthesis. Radiology 133: 723–725

Wolff JA, Tuomanen EI, Greenberg ID (1980) Radionuclide joint imaging: acute rheumatic fever simulating septic arthritis. Pediatrics 65: 339–341

10 · The Bone Scan in Traumatic and Sports Injuries

P. Matin

Introduction

With the increasing emphasis on fitness and exercise in our society, we are seeing an ever-increasing incidence of athletically related bone and soft tissue injuries. Although radiography is the primary diagnostic modality for detection of skeletal trauma, there are many occasions when radiographs may initially fail to diagnose an injury. Also, there are several types of injuries which are not diagnosable by routine radiographic methods but can be detected easily by nuclear medicine techniques.

There are four primary categories of injury where nuclear medicine techniques may be of use. These include (1) stress fracture and periosteal injury; (2) covert fractures; (3) joint abnormalities and injuries to connective tissues, especially where they attach to bone; and (4) acute skeletal muscle injury and rhabdomyolysis. One of the most important features of the use of nuclear medicine techniques in the evaluation of sports and traumatic injury is the ability, in most cases, to be able to differentiate among these various categories. Other uses of nuclear medicine techniques discussed in this chapter include the evaluation of the vascularity of the osseous structures in the region of injury, and the evaluation of delayed union and non-union of fracture.

Stress Fractures and Periosteal Injury

Stress fractures result when stresses applied to bone create changes in the bone which are greater than the body's ability to counteract them. The resulting injury is probably due to bone resorption being much greater than bone replacement (Roub et al. 1979). These injuries, also known as fatigue fractures, are frequently seen in runners and other athletes whose training regimen produces unusually large stresses on individual osseous structures. They are also frequently found in military recruits and other athletically untrained individuals who participate in new types of training exercises. Also, persons with biomechanical abnormalities of their walking or running gait may be prone to these types of injuries (Prather et al. 1977; Meurman and Elfving 1980; Norfray et al. 1980; Matin 1982; Brill 1983; Holder and Matthews 1984).

Radiographs are known to be of little use in detecting acute stress fractures; therefore, the diagnosis of these abnormalities has become dependent primarily on nuclear medicine techniques. When the detection of stress fractures by nuclear medicine techniques was first popularised several years ago, it became common practice to call any athletically related skeletal abnormality detected on a bone scan a "stress fracture". However, improvement in the spatial resolution of bone scintigraphs in recent years now allows us to differentiate between varying stages of skeletal injury. An entire spectrum of abnormalities from minimal periosteal reaction to true stress fracture is now appreciated. A minimal periosteal reaction might be seen on a bone scan as a faint linear band of increased radionuclide concentration along the periphery of a bone, while a true stress fracture would be seen as a fusiform abnormality extending throughout the entire cortex of the bone. It is obvious that the differentiation will require at least two views of an individual bone in order to make this analysis. For example, what may appear to be a complete transverse abnormality in the tibia in the anterior view may be seen

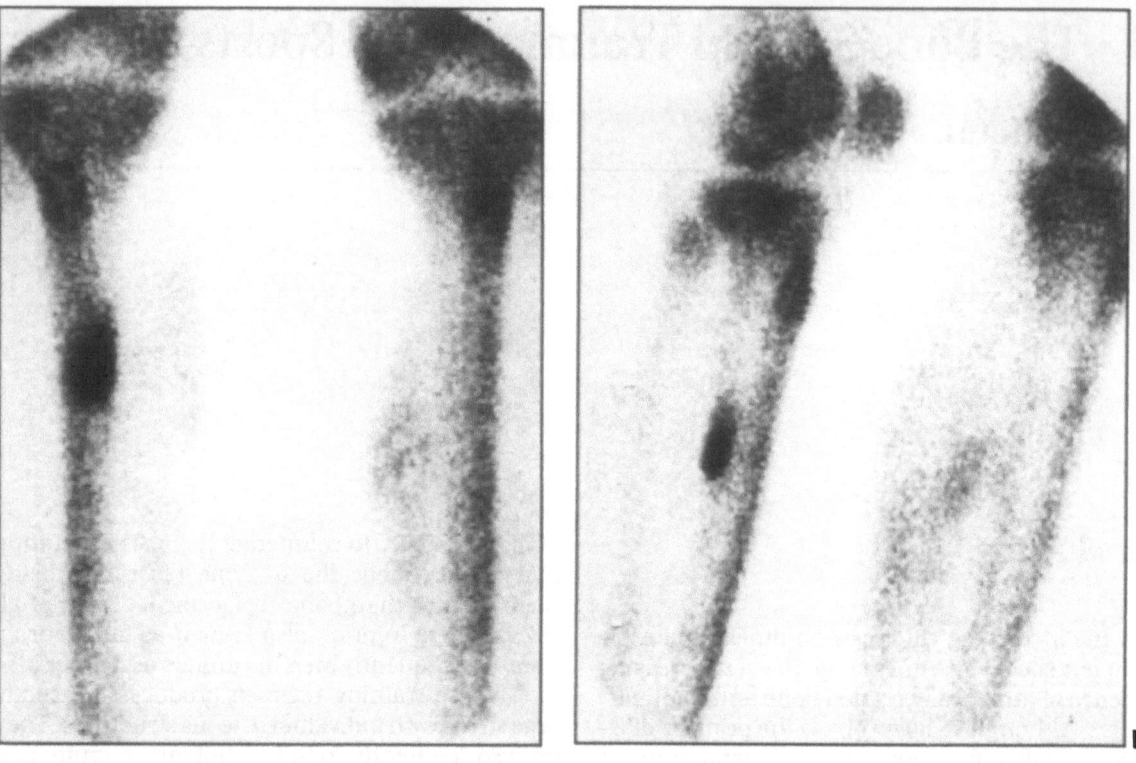

Fig. 10.1a,b. Periosteal reaction in the right tibia of an ultramarathon runner. The anterior view of the tibiae (a) shows what appears to be a full-thickness abnormality in the cortex of the right tibia. This would appear to be a Stage V lesion. However, the lateral view (b) shows that the lesion is superficial and is actually Stage II. An incidental finding in this illustration is increased muscle uptake of the radionuclide, demonstrating rhabdomyolysis, primarily in the calf of the left leg.

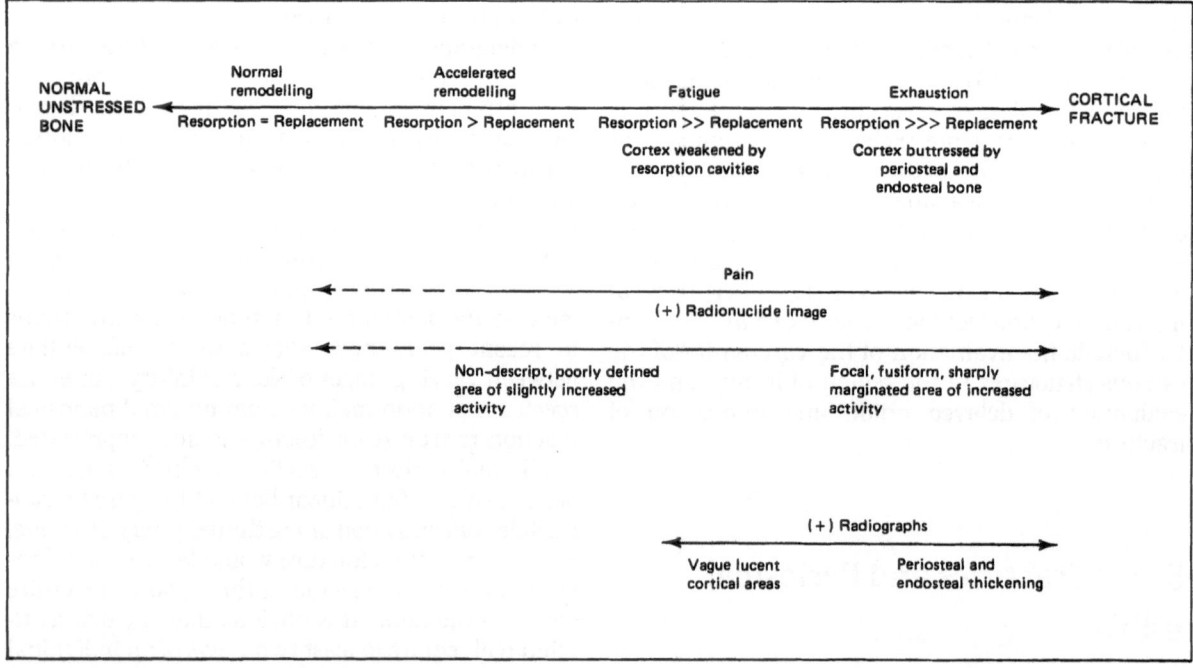

Fig. 10.2. The continuum of bone response to increasing levels of stress and the manner in which factors of pain, radionuclide images and radiographs relate at any given level of stress. (Adapted from Roub et al. 1979)

to be a superficial abnormality in the anterior aspect of the tibia in a lateral view. Figure 10.1 is an example of this type of injury in a young runner. The correct interpretation that the injury was a periosteal reaction rather than a true stress fracture required both the anterior and lateral views.

The treatment of the various types of injuries will differ according to the extent of injury. For example, a true stress fracture of the tibia may require immobilisation, approximately 6 weeks of complete rest, or at least a marked change in regimen so that the tibia is no longer put under stress. However, a minimal periosteal reaction may require only a week or two of rest from the offending activity. Consequently, the differentiation is often very important in the management of the patient. Casts or other immobilisation devices are usually not required in the treatment of periosteal reaction or stress fracture, unless, of course, the athlete would not comply with the physician or trainer's request to discontinue or change his training regimen.

When I first suggested that this differentiation be made, I included two categories—true stress fracture and periosteal reaction (Matin 1982, 1983). Since that time it has been suggested that we utilise additional categories for the description of these types of injuries (Zwas et al. 1985). In actuality, there is probably a continuous spectrum of abnormality which can be explained by the diagram developed by Roub et al. (1979), which is shown as Fig. 10.2. The figure shows that the spectrum of injuries extends from the minimal periosteal injury described above to true stress fractures, according to the amount of stress applied to the bone and the inability of the osseous structure to respond. The figure also shows where nuclear medicine techniques begin to show the abnormality and where radiographs are finally useful in the detection of these injuries.

Although there is a complete spectrum of abnormalities I would suggest that, for simplicity, we use a five-stage description of the abnormalities, such as outlined in Table 10.1. Stage I would represent a very minimal periosteal abnormality with less than 20% of the osseous structure being involved, while Stage V would be a true stress fracture with over 80% of the thickness of the bone being involved. The management of these injuries could probably be handled in a manner similar to that suggested earlier (i.e. the lesser abnormalities would require only a week or two of rest, while the more significant injuries would require the full 6 weeks or so of treatment).

It has been our general experience that the lesser periosteal abnormalities will never show an abnormality on the radiograph, while the more severe injuries, such as the Stage IV or V stress fracture will eventually develop radiographic abnormalities after a week to 10 days following the onset of pain. Of course, many athletes will experience pain and yet continue to carry out their training regimen. This would continue to produce an increasing abnormality in many cases.

Figure 10.3 is an example of periosteal injury and stress fracture in the tibiae of a young runner. The right tibia exhibits a Stage II periosteal reaction. It is interesting that, in the lateral view, the left tibia

Table 10.1. Stages of bone involvement in periosteal reaction/ stress fracture

Stage of injury	Percentage of bone involved	Verbal description
I	0–20	Minimal periosteal reaction
II	20–40	Moderate periosteal reaction
III	40–60	Early stress fracture
IV	60–80	True stress fracture
V	80–100	Full-thickness stress fracture

Suggested relationship of the depth of increased radionuclide concentration in a bone to the descriptive stage of the injury. This is a simplification since there is probably a continuous spectrum of injury from normal to Stage V. Stages I and II will usually not be seen on radiographs, while Stages IV and V will usually be seen eventually on radiographs. At least two views of the bone scan, e.g. anterior and lateral, of the involved bone are required.

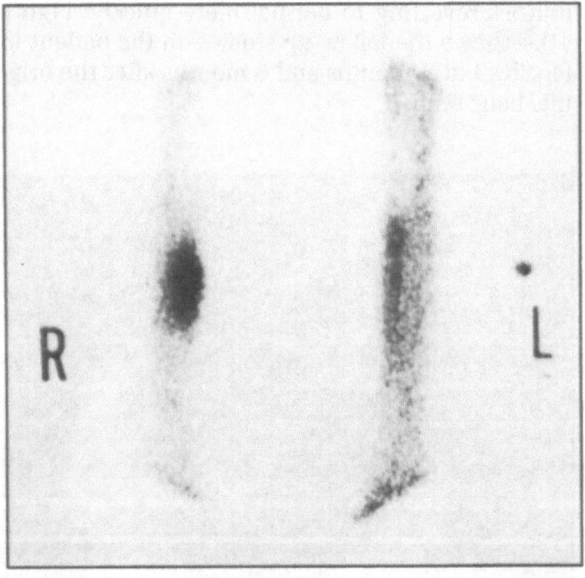

Fig. 10.3. Anterior scintigraph of the lower extremities of a young patient showing a stress fracture (Stage IV) in the right tibia and a periosteal reaction (Stage II) in the left tibia. Only the right tibial lesion eventually demonstrated an abnormality in a radiograph performed approximately a week after the scintigraph. (Matin 1982)

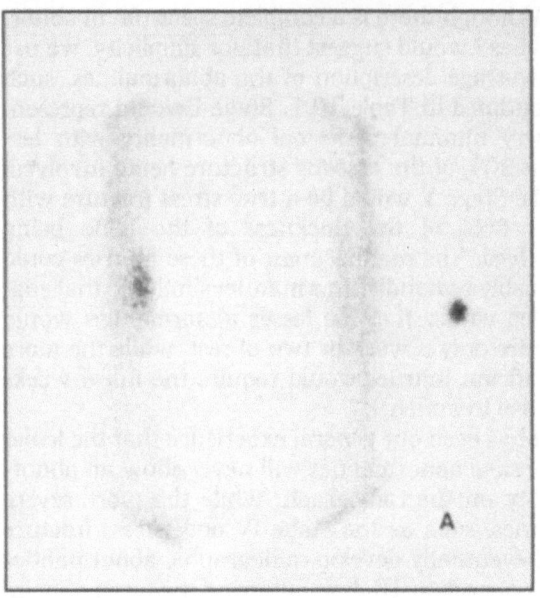
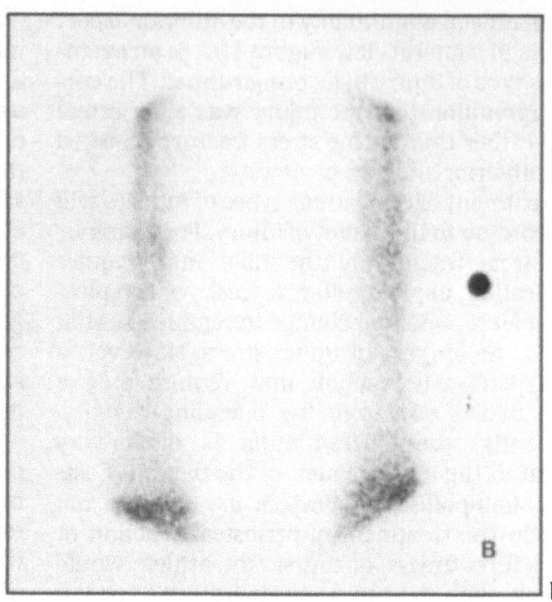

a   b

Fig. 10.4a,b. Healing of the tibial injuries demonstrated in the patient shown in Fig. 10.3. a A scintigraph obtained 3 months after the initial study. The stress fracture in the right tibia is still visualised, but less intensely than on the original study. The periosteal reaction in the left tibia has almost returned to normal. b A follow-up study obtained 6 months after the original scintigraphs. It shows only a trace of increased radionuclide concentration in the right tibia. The *dark dot* in both illustrations is a marker denoting the left tibia. (Matin 1982).

also appeared to be a more extensive abnormality. In addition to the fact that the patients with the more significant injuries require a longer period of rest before returning to their training programmes, the follow-up scintigraphs also show the lesser injuries reverting to normal more quickly. Figure 10.4 shows the follow-up studies on the patient in Fig. 10.3 at 3 months and 6 months after the original bone scan.

Shin splints is an injury discussed in more detail below. However, shin splints can often be detected on bone scintigraphs with the characteristic appearance of an elongated superficial band of increased radionuclide concentration along the posterior medial aspect of the tibia. This may be due to the fact that at least some of the pain is caused by effects of muscle activity upon bone at the sites where the muscle or connective tissues attach to the bone.

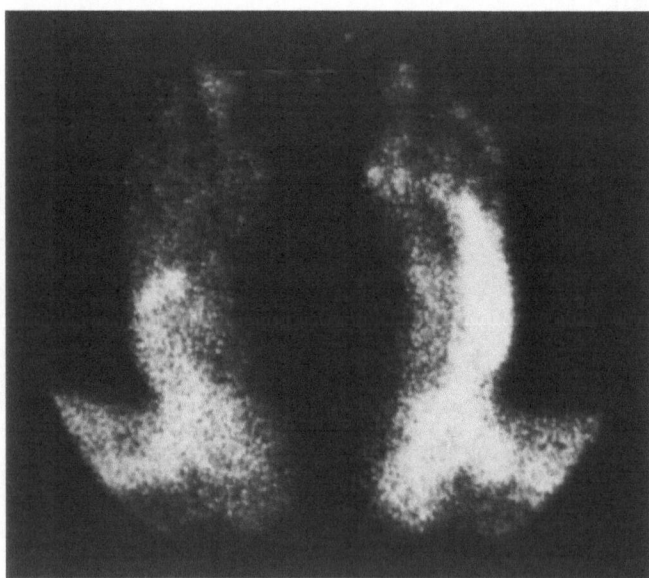

Fig. 10.5. Scintigraphs of the feet in a long-distance hiker. The fourth and fifth metatarsals of the left foot show markedly increased radionuclide concentration indicating "march fractures". The injury occurred approximately 5 days before the scintigraphs were obtained. Radiographs became abnormal approximately a week later. (Matin 1982)

Abnormalities such as this have been called enthesopathies.

Figure 10.5 is an example of a stress fracture in the fourth and fifth metatarsals of a long-distance hiker. These "march fractures" occurred approximately 5 days prior to the scintigraphs. Radiographs became abnormal in this region approximately 1 week later.

Shin Splints and Enthesopathy

As mentioned previously, the term "enthesopathies" refers to an injury where muscles, tendons or other connective tissues attach to bone. Classic "shin splints" is probably at least partially due to this type of injury. Although the term "shin splints" has been used as a generic term for pain involving the lower portions of the legs, the more exact definition refers to the posterior medial aspect of the tibiae. Nuclear medicine studies have shown that patients with true shin splints have the characteristic finding of increased radionuclide concentration along the posterior medial border of the tibia (Brill 1983; Holder and Matthews 1984). A presumed mechanism for this injury is increased

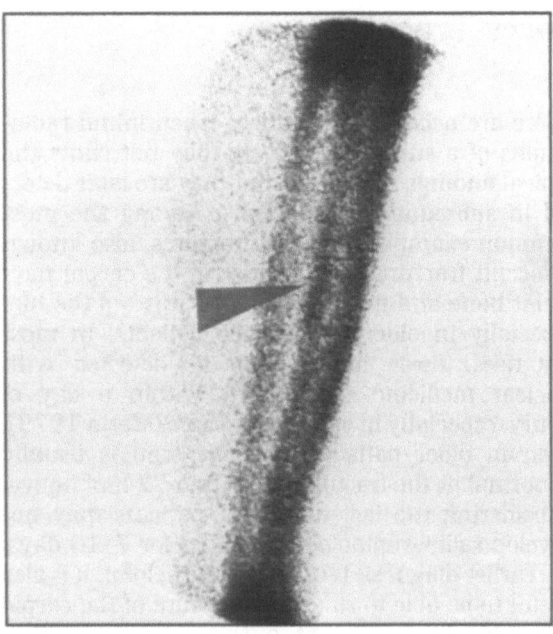

Fig. 10.7. Stage I periosteal reaction in the posterior tibia of a runner. The appearance is similar to that demonstrated in Fig. 10.6, but lesss intensely abnormal. The *marker* points to the abnormality.

stress on the skeletal structures in this region produced by the muscles, or perhaps Sharpey's fibres, pulling upon the periosteum of the bone. This causes an increased metabolic response, with subsequent increased deposition of the radionuclide tracer along the periphery of the bone.

The scintigraphic appearance of this abnormality is very similar to that of periosteal reaction. Figure 10.6 is an example of shin splints in a long-distance runner. The abnormality is seen as an elongated region of slightly increased radionuclide concentration along the posterior medial aspect of the tibiae. Note the similarity in appearance to the patient with a Stage I periosteal reaction of the tibia shown in Fig. 10.7. Other examples of enthesopathy would include inflammation of the pubic symphysis, also known as osteitis pubis, which may be found in athletes who overuse the abdominal or gracilus muscles.

Plantar fasciitis may also be considered an enthesopathy, since the plantar fascia originates from the medial tuberosity of the calcaneus. Increased radionuclide concentration at the region of the medial tuberosity of the calcaneus can help with the diagnosis, although retrocalcaneal bursitis, Achilles tendonitis or a calcaneal stress fracture may also produce a similar appearance. Emission tomography may prove to be useful in the differential diagnosis.

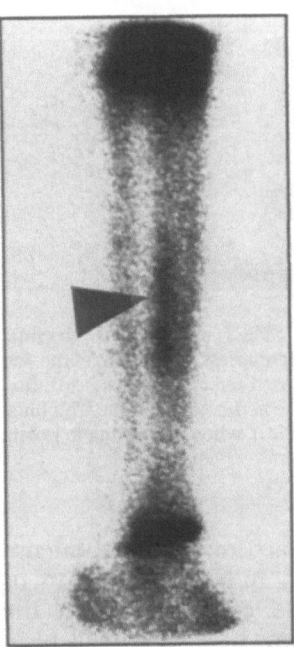

Fig. 10.6. A classic "shin splint" is shown in this lateral view of the right leg. The *marker* points to an elongated region of increased radionuclide concentration in the posterior medial aspect of the tibia.

Covert Fractures

There are occasional instances when initial radiographs of a suspected fracture may not show the typical findings of fracture, but they are later detected in subsequent radiographs. Among the most common examples of covert fractures, also known as occult fractures, are injuries of the carpal navicular bone and non-displaced fractures of the hip, especially in older osteoporotic patients. In most instances, these injuries can be detected with nuclear medicine scintigraphy within a day of injury, especially in younger patients (Matin 1979). Even in older patients the bone scan is usually abnormal at the fracture site within 72 h of injury. Considering the fact that these patients may not develop radiographic abnormalities for 7–10 days, the earlier diagnosis is usually quite helpful. It is also useful to be able to rule out a fracture of the carpal navicular bone so that a splint, cast or other immobilisation device is not used unnecessarily. Figure 10.8 is an example of an acute traumatic fracture of the carpal navicular bone in a 15-year-old youth who fell onto his outstretched hand. The initial radiograph did not demonstrate the fracture, although he had typical pain and swelling usually associated with a fracture of the carpal navicular bone. It is also interesting to note in the illustration

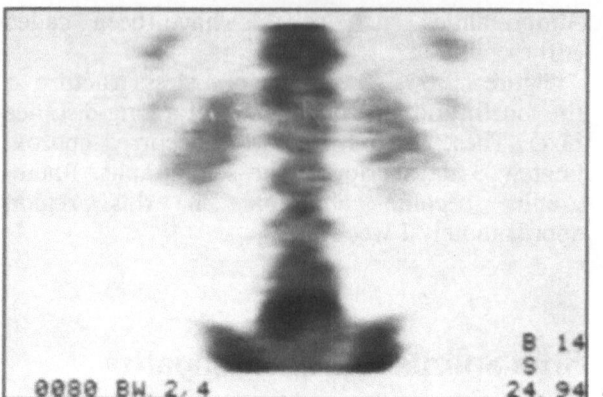

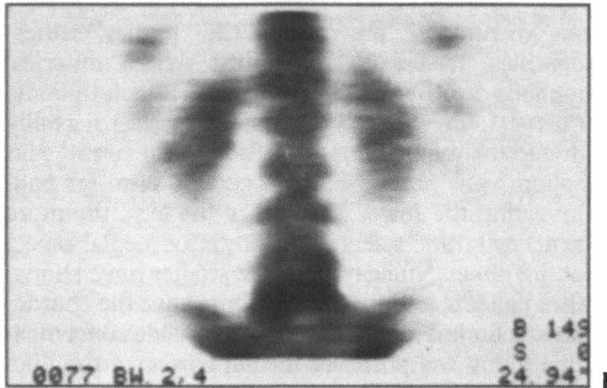

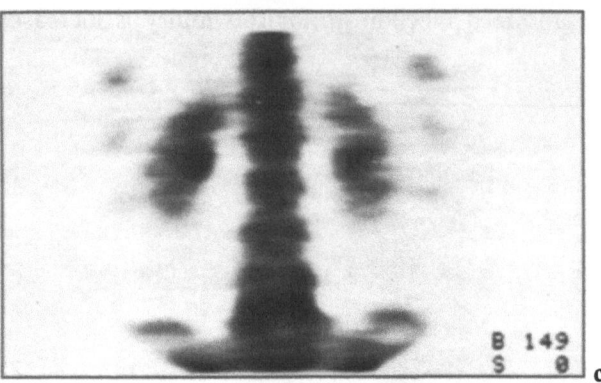

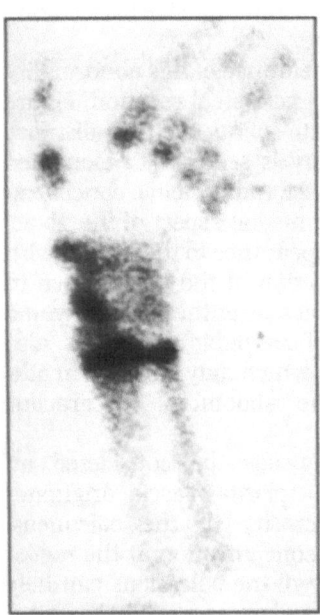

Fig. 10.8. Scintigraph demonstrating a fracture of the carpal navicular bone in a teenage boy imaged approximately 6 h after injury. Increased tracer concentration at the fracture site is equal to that of his epiphyses. (Matin 1982)

Fig. 10.9a–c. Three successive SPECT images in the coronal plane of a patient with a recent compression fracture of the 5th lumbar vertebra. Note the increased radionuclide concentration in L-5 which appears most intense in the middle frame. This illustrates the benefit of the use of SPECT when attempting to isolate an abnormality to a given vertebra.

that the region of the fracture has quite intense uptake of the radionuclide. In fact, it is equal to, or exceeds, the radionuclide concentration in the region of the distal radial and ulnar growth plates.

At times it can be difficult to tell soft tissue trauma from a fracture on the early nuclear medicine images. Typically, the fracture is isolated to skeletal structures, is more discrete in appearance, and is usually more intensely abnormal than soft tissue injuries such as haematomas or sprains. However, at times the differentiation may be difficult and delayed images at 8–24 h after injection may be useful. Experience in the interpretation of these studies, as well as physical examination, usually proves to be a very valuable asset in differentiating soft tissue from skeletal trauma. The development of the nuclear medicine tomographic camera now allows tomographic studies, such as single photon emission computed tomography (SPECT), of regions of suspected fracture. By using localised images in multiple planes the abnormality can be isolated to a single bone, or even a portion of a bone, in many cases. Figure 10.9 is an example of a vertebral fracture in a patient who was involved in an automobile accident. The initial radiographs were suggestive of a fracture, but the use of SPECT helped to confirm the presence of the non-displaced fracture of the vertebral body.

Traumatic Fractures

Several years ago it was believed that traumatic fractures would not appear on a bone scan for several days following the injury. However, improvements in imaging techniques and the use of the newer radiopharmaceuticals available in most nuclear medicine departments allow for the detection of fractures by bone scintigraphy within hours of injury. As shown in Table 10.2, adapted from a study performed a few years ago, fractures were detected within 24 h of an injury in approximately 95% of patients under 65 years old (Matin 1979). In older patients, many of whom were osteoporotic, the detection of the fractures could be delayed by 48–72 h. Since this study was originally published in 1979, we have performed bone scans for suspected fracture in over 1000 patients. In only one instance was the fracture not detected by a bone scan, although delayed radiographs did show a distinct fracture line. This solitary exception to the rule occurred in a young man with a fractured mandible.

Table 10.2. Time after fracture at which bone scan becomes abnormal (Matin 1979)

Time after fracture	Patients studied	Number with abnormal scans	Percentage abnormal	Percentage abnormal under 65 years
1 day	20	16	80	95
3 days	39	37	95	100
1 week	60	59	98	100

It must be emphasised that good-quality images are required for the detection of fractures. We have found that improved quality images can be obtained in most patients if delayed images at 8–24 h after injection are performed. This allows the soft tissue clearance of radionuclide to become maximal and a focal abnormality is often easily detected because of the improved "target/background" ratio.

There are other variations in technique which may be helpful in detecting a covert fracture of the hip in an older patient. We have found that catheterisation of the urinary bladder is useful since many of these patients have a difficult time voiding, and the retained radionuclide in the bladder may obscure or hinder visualisation of the hip regions. Also, views in the posterior or lateral projection, or even oblique views, may be helpful in detecting the fracture. A lead shield over the urinary bladder may also help to improve the quality of the images of the hips.

We have also found that the scintigraphic pattern of fractures changes over a period of time, with three rather distinct stages being apparent. The first phase (acute stage) persists for approximately 2–4 weeks after injury and is characterised by a diffuse region of increased tracer concentration around the fracture site. A distinct fracture line may be seen in this stage, especially in delayed images. The second phase (subacute stage) is characterised by a well-defined linear abnormality at the site of the fracture. This stage lasts approximately 8–12 weeks and shows the most intense uptake at the fracture site. The third phase (healing stage) is characterised by a gradual diminution in the intensity of the abnormality until the bone scan returns to normal. Figure 10.10 demonstrates the three stages in a 29-year-old woman who was thrown from a horse and sustained a compression fracture of the first lumbar vertebra. The first scintigraph, obtained approximately 24 h after injury, shows a rather diffuse area of increased tracer concentration in the superior aspect of L-1. The second scintigraph, obtained approximately 2 months after injury, shows an intense well-defined band of increased tracer concentration at the fracture site. The third scintigraph was obtained approximately 6 months after her accident and shows the gradual decrease in radionuclide concentration typically seen during the healing stage. The final scintigraph was obtained approximately 9 months after her accident and shows no evidence of abnormality.

The time for fractures to return to normal on bone scintigraphs extends well beyond the time for clinical or even radiographic healing. This is because the scintigraph depicts the increased metabolic activity and bone remodelling which usually takes place for

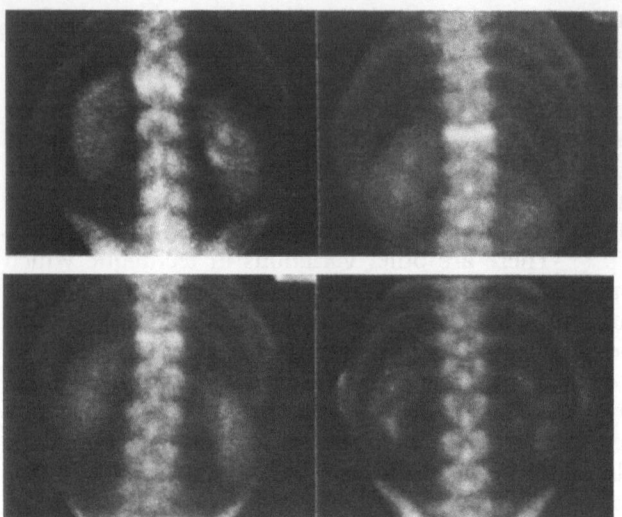

Fig. 10.10. Stages of healing in a 29-year-old female with compression fracture of the first lumbar vertebra. The initial scintigraph was obtained 24 h after injury. The others were obtained at 2 months, 6 months and 9 months after injury. The scintigraph returned to normal by the 9-month study. (Matin 1982)

a considerably longer time than might be expected clinically.

Table 10.3 summarises the time it took for various types of fractures to return to normal on bone scintigraphs. The table only includes non-manipulated closed fractures which were reduced by closed reduction. Compound fractures and fractures which are reduced in open surgery or treated with orthopaedic devices such as rods or screws require a considerably longer time for the bone scan to return to normal. The table shows the percentage of bone scans in patients with closed reductions that had become normal at the fracture site by 1, 2 and 3 years after injury. It also shows the minimum time for fractures to return to normal for various types of bones. As seen in the table, by 2 years after injury approximately 90% of the fractures had returned to normal. By 3 years after injury the percentage approached 100%. Rib fractures showed the most rapid healing, with approximately 80% of the studies being normal by 1 year after injury.

There are rare cases where a patient who had a simple fracture with closed reduction may show increased radionuclide concentration at the fracture site for many years after injury. For some reason, their fractures must have a continuing increase in metabolic activity, increased vascularity or other process at the fracture site. Patients with delayed union or non-union may also show prolonged periods of radionuclide concentration at the fracture site.

Delayed Union and Non-union

A distinction between delayed union and non-union may be difficult both clinically and scintigraphically; however, nuclear medicine procedures may be of assistance in making the differentiation. The bone scan may also help to determine which patients may be aided by the use of percutaneous electrical stimulation (galvanic stimulation) and which patients may eventually need a bone graft or other surgical procedure.

True non-union can be defined as the failure of a fracture site to heal completely by 6–8 months after injury. This entity, which occurs in approximately 5% of all fractures, is more likely when the fracture is open (compound), comminuted, immobilised for an insufficient time, insecurely fixed or kept from healing by improperly placed orthopaedic devices. Physiological factors which

Table 10.3. Normal bone scans at fracture site (Matin 1979)

	Number studied	Normal at 1 year	Normal at 2 years	Normal at 3 years	Minimum time to normal
Vertebrae	32	19 (59%)	29 (90%)	31 (97%)	7 months
Long bones	22	14 (64%)	20 (91%)	21 (95%)	6 months
Ribs	28	22 (79%)	26 (93%)	28 (100%)	5 months
Miscellaneous	20	12 (60%)	18 (90%)	19 (95%)	6 months

may increase the probability of non-union include infection, inadequate blood supply, poor nutritional status, osteoporosis and metabolic abnormalities, especially those which involve bone metabolism such as hyperthyroidism. The incidence of non-union is greatest in the tibia and femur, with a lesser degree in humerus, radius, ulna and clavicle (Gartland 1979). Two types of non-union have been described according to the amount of metabolic activity at the fracture site. The two types are atrophic non-union, in which there is a diminution of radioactivity at the fracture site when compared with the expected intensity of tracer concentration, and reactive non-union, when the tracer concentration is normal or increased (Rosenthall and Lisbona 1980).

Atrophic non-union may be evidenced by a generalised decrease in radionuclide concentration in the region of the bone fragments or by a zone of essentially absent radioactivity at the fracture site. The generalised decrease probably reflects the inability of the bone ends to respond properly to the healing process while the focal "photopaenic" (decreased tracer concentration) area may often be due to pseudoarthrosis, the interposition of soft tissues, the location of an infectious process, or region of interrupted blood supply. True pseudoarthroses may form at the fracture site with the presence of

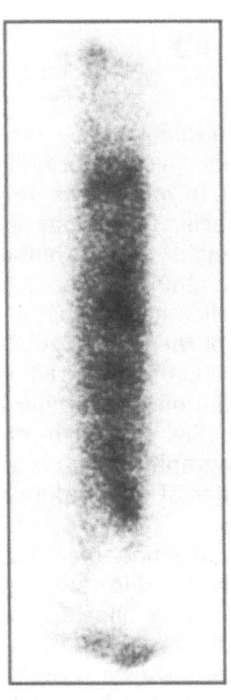

Fig. 10.12. Scintigraph of reactive non-union in the radius of a rodeo cowboy approximately 2 years after fracture. Increased tracer concentration is greater than expected at the fracture site this long after injury. He originally suffered an extensive comminuted fracture. (Matin 1982)

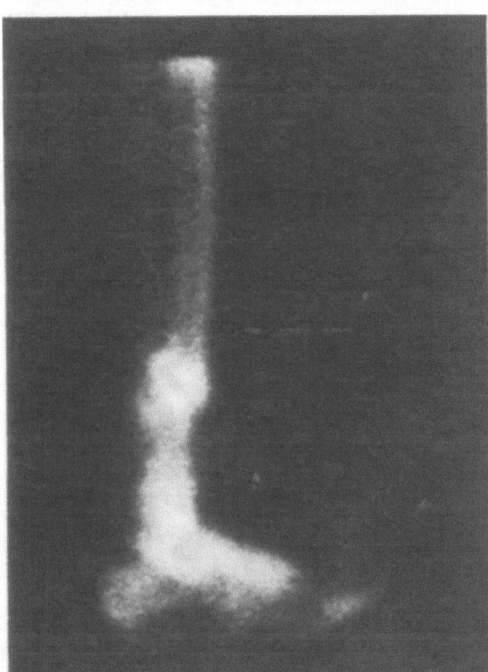

Fig. 10.11. Atrophic non-union in the distal tibia of a young man approximately 1 year after injury. The scintigraph shows a well-pronounced region of decreased radionuclide concentration, surrounded by areas of increased radionuclide uptake in the fracture fragments. (Matin 1982)

an actual joint-like synovial lined cavity containing synovial fluid. In a group of patients with non-union of the atrophic type, the use of percutaneous electrical stimulation did not appear to help stimulate bone healing. However, the patients with reactive non-union showed significant improvement following percutaneous electrical stimulation (Desai et al. 1980). Figure 10.11 is an example of a patient with atrophic non-union. Figure 10.12 demonstrates the appearance of reactive non-union in the forearm of a rodeo cowboy 2 years after his accident.

At this time it is still very difficult, if not impossible, to tell delayed union from reactive non-union in many cases. The fact that there is continued metabolic activity at the fracture site usually means that the fracture fragments are still metabolically active and that percutaneous electrical stimulation may be useful. In patients with atrophic non-union, bone graft or other orthopaedic intervention is usually required.

Delayed union could possibly be diagnosed by comparing the intensity of a fracture site in a suspected case of non-union with studies of patients with fractures of similar osseous structures. A reference file of patients with fractures of various bones at varying times after injury would be useful for making these comparisons.

Radionuclide Arthroscopy

Several institutions have utilised radionuclide arthroscopy for the evaluation of joint space abnormalities (Abdel-Dayem et al. 1981). In most cases, the studies are of maximum benefit when one is attempting to evaluate synovial leaks, bursa enlargement, cysts and similar abnormalities. An example of the use of radionuclide arthroscopy in the diagnosis of a Baker's cyst of the knee is given in Fig. 10.13: Fig. 10.13a depicts a routine radiograph performed after the instillation of a standard contrast agent into the knee; Fig. 10.13b is an example of radionuclide arthrography which was performed following the instillation of ^{99m}Tc sulphur colloid into the joint space.

Although the usefulness of injection of radionuclides into joints has been discussed in the past, it was primarily for the treatment of effusions or other therapeutic purposes. Radionuclide arthrography for diagnostic purposes shows promise because of the very small amount of radionuclide which is required. Only 0.5–1 ml of ^{99m}Tc sulphur colloid is required for good visualisation. The radiation dose is minimal, since only 0.5 mCi (18.5 MBq) of the radiopharmaceutical is required. The benefits of radionuclide arthrography include the very low radiation dose, the minimal volume of injected material and the absence of chemical synovitis or allergenicity. Also, certain abnormalities might be detected more readily, although the procedure will certainly never replace contrast radiography of the knee or arthroscopy.

Detection of Skeletal Muscle Injury

It has been known for many years that nuclear medicine bone-imaging agents will localise in areas of acutely necrotic muscle. This knowledge has been put to practical use for several years by the performance of "myocardial infarct" scans to help detect myocardial infarcts which are difficult to diagnose by electrocardiogram or enzymatic changes (Werner et al. 1977). There were occasional reports of bone-imaging agents localising in areas of idiopathic rhabdomyolysis, electrical burn, excessive exercise and other types of skeletal injuries (Brill 1981).

We were fortunate to participate in the studies involving ultra marathon runners who ran 50 and 100 continuous miles, including the Western States Endurance 100-mile Race. This race involves the running of 100 continuous miles through the pioneer trails of the Sierra Nevada mountains and foothills. From these studies we learned that it is not uncommon to find large amounts of skeletal muscle concentration of bone-seeking radiopharmaceuticals localised to areas of muscle damage (Matin et al. 1983). Interestingly, the amount of muscle damage appears to correlate with the degree of the enzyme creatinine kinase (CPK or CK) in the blood stream. Also, the concentration of the MB isoenzyme of creatinine kinase, which was thought to be solely of cardiac muscle origin, was also found in large concentrations in blood samples obtained from the runners who demonstrated rhabdomyolysis on their bone scans. Figure 10.14 is an

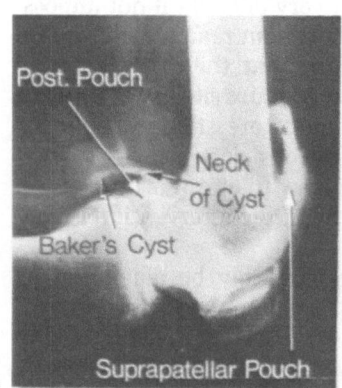
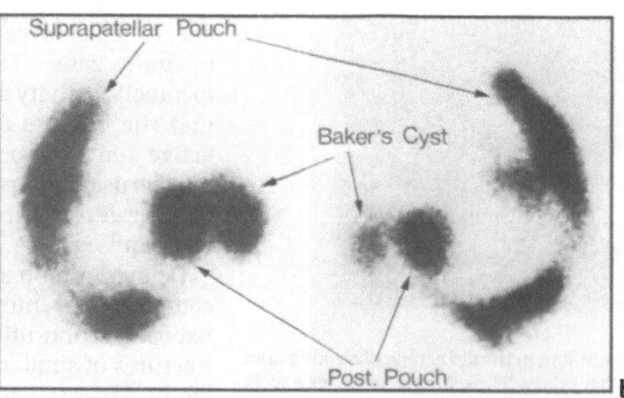

Fig. 10.13a,b. Scintigraphic arthrography of a knee joint showing a Baker's cyst located behind a normal-appearing subpatellar pouch. a Contrast radiograph; b lateral and medial scintigraphs. (Abdel-Dayem et al. 1981)

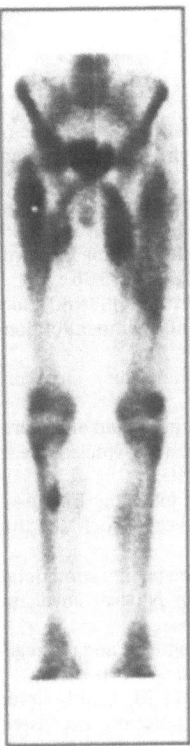

Fig. 10.14. Scintigraph of the lower extremities of an ultramarathon runner who completed 62 miles of a 100-mile race. This anterior view shows markedly increased radionuclide concentration in several muscle groups, indicating rhabdomyolysis in these muscles. The skeletal abnormality in the right tibia was present prior to the race and is shown in Fig. 10.1.

illustration of a rather extreme example of muscle injury in the thigh and calf muscles of a runner who completed 62 miles of the 100 mile race before having to withdraw because of severe leg pain.

We have learned that the amount of radionuclide concentration in the muscle is generally proportional to the creatinine kinase elevation and, in general, to the degree of pain experienced by the athlete. This, of course, is subjective because of the varying pain tolerance in individuals. Follow-up studies showed that the muscle injury is no longer detectable by bone scan by approximately 1 week after the muscle injury. This is essentially the same time course found when studying patients who have had acute myocardial infarcts.

The explanation of why the bone-imaging agents detect muscle necrosis probably begins with an influx of calcium ions into acutely necrotic muscle. The phosphate bone-imaging agents follow the calcium and become concentrated in the acutely necrotic muscle cells, where they may be imaged with any standard nuclear medicine camera. The scintigraphs are usually abnormal within a few hours of the injury. The most intense abnormality on the bone scan appears to be within 24–48 h of injury, with a gradual decrease in the intensity of the abnormality until the region of muscle injury is no longer detected.

The individual muscles involved can usually be well delineated. The use of emission tomographic imaging has helped in the analysis of which individual muscles are involved. This information can be of considerable use when attempting to correct the gait of a runner who demonstrates muscle injury only to isolated muscle groups. Of course, overuse is the most typical cause for the rhabdomyolysis associated with extreme exercise. The only treatment required, in our experience, is rest of the muscles until the pain experienced by running has subsided. This technique has also been useful in studying acute muscle injuries experienced by other athletes such as hurdlers, football players, weight lifters etc.

Figure 10.15 is an example of a runner who experienced pain in his thighs following a 100-mile foot race. The bone scan was performed approximately 24 h after the race, with a repeat study

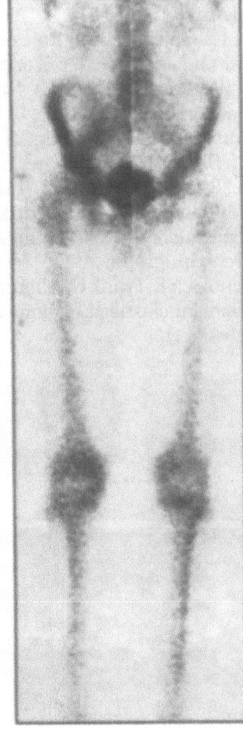

a   b

Fig. 10.15. a Demonstrates increased muscle concentration in an ultramarathon runner who completed the entire 100-mile ultramarathon race. The abnormalities are present in several muscle groups but are less intense than those demonstrated in Fig. 10.14. b Follow-up study performed 5 days after the original study. Note that the abnormalities in his muscles have completely disappeared.

approximately 5 days following the initial examination. The initial study shows significantly increased muscle uptake in the quadriceps and hamstring muscles. The follow-up study, performed approximately 6 days after the race, was completely normal.

An interesting sequel to these findings is that the incorrect diagnosis of myocardial infarction may have been applied to some older runners who collapsed during strenuous long-distance running events. It is possible that these patients were admitted to the hospital where an electrocardiogram was performed and found to be abnormal (perhaps as a result of the exertion alone) and subsequent blood samples showed significant elevation of the creatinine kinase MB isoenzyme. We now know that the isoenzyme can be elevated as a result of skeletal muscle necrosis alone and that the only way to diagnose a myocardial infarct would probably be to image the patient's myocardium with scintillation camera. The same injection of radiopharmaceutical used to detect the skeletal muscle necrosis can also be used to detect any myocardial injury, if present.

The ability to detect skeletal muscle abnormalities as well as skeletal and connective tissue disorders helps us to diagnose specifically the various types of lesions which might be associated with pain in the lower extremities or elsewhere in an athlete. If performed within a few days of the onset of pain, nuclear medicine studies utilising the bone-seeking radiopharmaceuticals can be used to differentiate between acute muscle injury, true shin splints, skeletal injury (periosteal reaction or stress fracture) or an abnormality which is entirely associated with a joint or connective tissues. The resulting management of the patient with the injury can be directed in a much more specific and scientific manner.

References

Abdel-Dayem HM, Barodawala Y, Papademetriou T (1981) Scintigraphic arthrography: a new imaging procedure. Clin Nucl Med 6: 246–248

Brill DR (1981) Radionuclide imaging of non-neoplastic soft tissue disorders. Semin Nucl Med 11: 277–288

Brill DR (1983) Sports nuclear medicine. Bone imaging for lower extremity pain in athletes. Clin Nucl Med 8: 101–106

Desai A, Alavi A, Dalinka M, Brighton C, Esterhai J (1980) Role of bone scintigraphy in the evaluation and treatment of non-united fractures. J Nucl Med 21: 931–934

Gartland JJ (1979) Fundamentals of orthopaedics, 3rd edn. Saunders, Philadelphia

Holder LE, Matthews LS (1984) The nuclear physician and sports medicine. In: Freeman LM, Weissmann HS (eds) Nuclear medicine annual. Raven, New York, pp. 81–140

Matin P (1979) Appearance of bone scans following fractures: including immediate and long-term studies. J Nucl Med 20: 1227–1231

Matin P (1982) Bone scanning of trauma and benign conditions. In: Freeman LM, Weissmann HS (eds) Nuclear medicine annual. Raven, New York, pp 81–118

Matin P (1983) Bone scintigraphy in the diagnosis and management of traumatic injury. Semin Nucl Med 13: 104–122

Matin P, Lang G, Carretta RF, Simon G (1983) Scintigraphic evaluation of muscle damage following extreme exercise. J Nucl Med 24: 308–311

Meurman KA, Elfving S (1980) Stress fractures in soldiers: multifocal bone disorders; comparative radiologic and scintigraphic studies. Radiology 134: 483–487

Norfray JF, Schlachter L, Kernahan WT, Arenson DJ, Smith SD, Roth IE, Schlefman BS (1980) Early confirmation of stress fractures in joggers. JAMA 243: 1647–1649

Prather JL, Nusynowitz ML, Snowdy HA, Hughes AD, McCartney WH (1977) Scintigraphic findings in stress fractures. J Bone Joint Surg [Am] 59: 869–874

Rosenthall L, Lisbona R (1980) Role of radionuclide imaging in benign bone and joint diseases of orthopedic interest. In: Freeman LM, Weissmann HS (eds) Nuclear medicine annual. Raven, New York, pp 267–301

Roub LW, Gumerman LW, Hanley EN Jr, Clark MW, Goodman M, Herbert DL (1979) Bone stress: a radionuclide imaging perspective. Radiology 132: 431–438

Werner JA, Botvinick EH, Shames DM, Parmley WW (1977) Clinical application of technetium-99m stannous pyrophosphate infarct scintigraphy. West J Med 127: 464–478

Zwas ST, Elkanovich R, Frank G, Aharonson Z (1985) Stress fracture development classified by bone scintigraphy. J Nucl Med 26: P77 (abstract)

11 · The Bone Scan in Arthritis

L. Rosenthall

Introduction

The aetiology of many of the arthritides is unknown, and a satisfactory scientific classification based on causation is yet to be developed. For purposes of radionuclide imaging they can be grouped into primarily inflammatory and non-inflammatory types, although the latter may be associated with an element of synovitis, and bone erosion may occur later in the former. Included in the inflammatory joint diseases are rheumatoid arthritis, psoriatic arthritis, Reiter's syndrome, ankylosing spondylitis, systemic lupus erythematosus, infection and other less frequently encountered entities. The most frequent non-inflammatory condition is osteoarthritis, but this category also includes trauma, neuroarthropathy, reflex sympathetic dystrophy, mechanical abnormalities etc.

Radionuclide methods are capable of disclosing synovitis, subchondral bone destruction, or both, but do not specify the cause. Historically, test agents such as ^{131}I albumin, ^{131}I globulin, [131]NaI, [24]Na and ^{133}Xe saline were injected into the joint cavity and their rate of disappearance was found to vary directly with the degree of synovial inflammation (Ahlstrom et al. 1956; Dick et al. 1970). Although useful as a quantitative research tool, it was not practical for screening a large population, nor patients with multiarticular involvement. The introduction of intravenously administered ^{131}I-labelled albumin to depict the expanded blood pool of the inflamed synovium made it possible to study many joints in the same patient with a single injection (Weiss et al. 1965). Other radiopharmaceuticals were later suggested. These can be divided into three groups:

1. The vascular compartment markers, viz. [131]I albumin, ^{131}I iodipamide (Maxfield et al. 1968), radiopertechnetate (Hays and Green 1972), ^{99m}Tc albumin (Cohen and Lorber 1971), [113m]In (Martinez-Villesenor and Katon 1968) and ^{99m}Tc-DTPA (Maxfield et al. 1972)

2. Bone seekers, viz. [85]Sr (Holopainen and Rekonen 1966), [87]Sr, [18]F (Jeremy et al. 1969) and ^{99m}Tc phosphate complexes (Desaulnier et al. 1974)

3. Inflammatory site markers, viz. [67]Ga citrate (Colman et al. 1982; Tannenbaum et al. 1984) and ^{111}In leucocytes

The vascular compartment markers make visible the enlarged synovial blood pool and synovial interstitial extravasation, whereas the bone seekers demonstrate increased periarticular bone concentration because the hyperaemia of synovitis induces an increased blood flow to adjacent bone through anastomotic vascular channels. When there is subchondral bone damage the augmented focal uptake is a manifestation of the normal bone response to the insult. [67]Ga has a propensity to concentrate in septic and non-septic inflammatory sites and thereby visualises the inflamed synovium directly. ^{111}In-labelled leucocytes accumulate at sites of leucocyte migration and should therefore be specific for septic synovitis. However, there is a relatively small and variable leucocyte accumulation in rheumatoid arthritis which may render visible ^{111}In leucocyte uptake in the joint region.

Synovitis

The synovial membrane is highly vascular with an extensive capillary network. There are also anastomoses with the juxtaepiphyseal and epiphyseal vessels of adjacent bone, so that changes in synovial blood flow are reflected in periarticular bone flow. Inflammation triggers increases in blood flow, blood pool volume and vascular permeability. These changes occur primarily in the terminal arterioles, capillaries and venules. In the acute phase there is a cellular response consisting of an accumulation of polymorphonuclear leucocytes, located predominantly in the joint fluid. The chronic inflammatory response, which is longer in duration in the course of events, is characterised by an infiltration of lymphocytes, macrophages and plasma cells in the interstitium, while polymorphonuclear cells are still present in the joint fluid.

In light of these histological changes in active inflammatory disease, it is understandable that a perfusion study with a ^{99m}Tc label will demonstrate increased transit on first pass, increased concentration in the static image immediately after perfusion, and increased periarticular bone concentration in the delayed ^{99m}Tc phosphate images (Figs. 11.1, 11.2). It also explains the observed concentration of ^{67}Ga citrate and the potential for low-grade ^{111}In leucocyte deposition.

The normal synovium cannot be distinguished from adjacent structures by blood compartment markers (Fig. 11.2). When the synovium is inflamed most of the radiopertechnetate of ^{99m}Tc albumin is found in the membrane. A small amount is present in the synovial fluid, but it does not contribute significantly to the overall count rate (Hays and Green 1972). The distribution of radiopertechnetate and ^{99m}Tc pyrophosphate were studied in a rabbit model of arthritis induced by the intra-articular injection of ovalbumin into sensitised animals. Radiopertechnetate was found to be in bone and soft tissue like radiophosphate, but with radiopertechnetate the maximum uptake was in the synovium while the maximum uptake with radiophosphate was in bone (Rosenspire et al. 1981). A similar animal study utilising ^{67}Ga and a zymosan-induced knee arthritis showed a predominant uptake in the synovium; however, increases were also registered in the fat pad, patella, meniscus and adjacent tendons, but not periarticular bone (Tannenbaum et al. 1984). There is a report showing a correlation between the synovial fluid white cell concentration and ^{67}Ga knee/femur count ratio in patients with active rheumatoid arthritis, implying that these ratios are a reflection of the degree of synovial inflammation (McCall et al. 1983).

A blood compartment tracer is the preferable agent to use in screening patients with arthralgia, because it visualises the inflamed synovium directly and the concentration is a reflection of the degree of inflammation. There are few false-positive scan results and these are caused mainly by overlying oedema and cellulitis. Osteoarthritic joints are usually normal, unless complicated by a synovitis (Dick et al. 1972). In contrast, radiophosphate uptakes

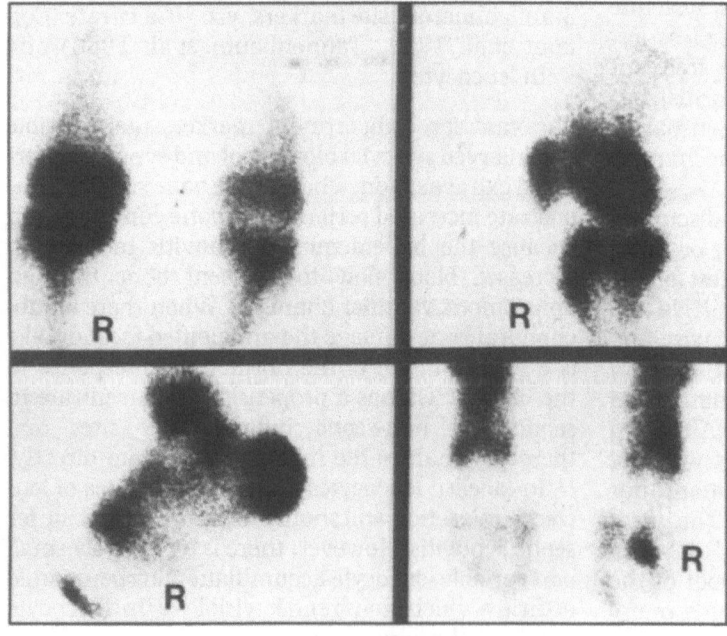

Fig. 11.1. Reiter's disease. Twenty-year-old male demonstrating increased periarticular uptake of radiophosphate about the right knee, right second metatarsophalangeal joint, and both ankles and tarsal bones, but it is particularly intense in the right calcaneus, so-called lover's heel.

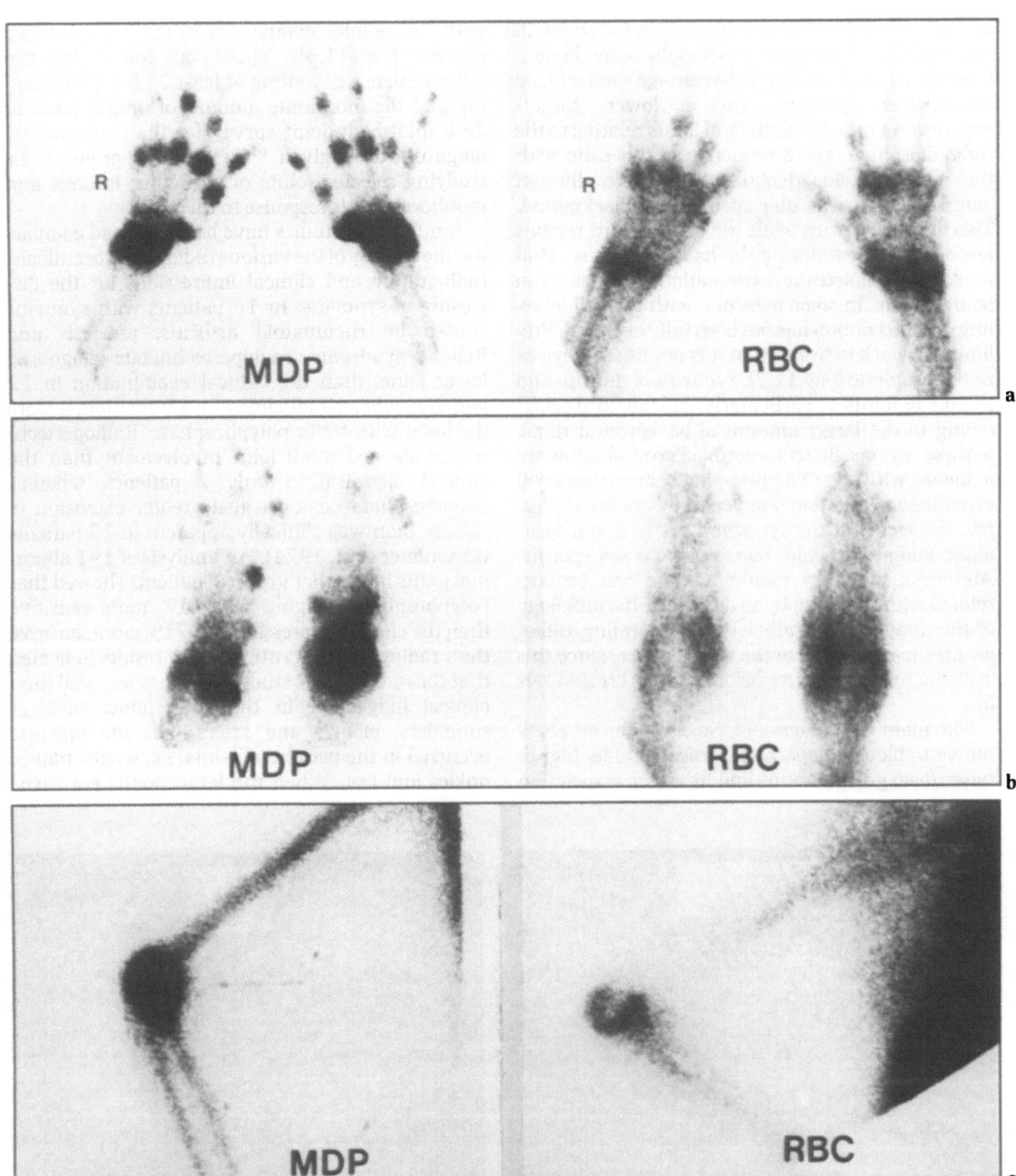

Fig. 11.2a–c. Comparison of radiophosphate (*MDP*) and ⁹⁹ᵐTc-labelled red blood cells (*RBC*) in a patient with active rheumatoid arthritis. **a** The ⁹⁹ᵐTc-MDP images of the hands show intense uptake in both wrists, most of the metacarpophalangeal joints and several proximal interphalangeal joints of both hands. Corresponding images with labelled red blood cells exhibit the expanded blood pool of the inflamed wrists and metacarpophalangeal joints, but the target/background ratio is lower than those of radiophosphate. The abnormal proximal interphalangeal joints of the left hand involving the third and fifth digits are not seen with the blood compartment marker. **b** ⁹⁹ᵐTc-MDP depicts intense uptake in the involved ankles and lower relative concentrations in several metatarsophalangeal joints and toes. The inflamed synovium of the ankles are well demonstrated with labelled red cells, but the synovial concentrations in the other affected joints are either absent or too subtle to be of diagnostic value. **c** Intense uptake of the inflamed elbow is registered with radiophosphate. The labelled red cells also show an intense uptake, but in the distribution of the synovium.

are not exclusive to synovitis, but may occur in osteoarthritis, bone injury, metabolic bone disease, blood dyscrasias etc. The disadvantages of the blood compartment tracers are a lower target/background ratio for peripheral joints relative to the radiophosphate, and a reduction of this ratio with time as the radiopertechnetate or ^{99m}Tc albumin enters the extravascular space of the backgound. This drift takes place while the various joint regions are being imaged during the half-hour, or so, that it takes to complete the investigation. Perhaps it can be overcome, in some measure, with red cell labelling, but this notion has not been fully explored. Preliminary work indicates that it is not as sensitive as radiophosphate (Fig. 11.2). Synovitis of the hips and sacroiliac joints is particularly difficult to disclose owing to the larger amount of background tissue in these regions. Better target/background ratios are achieved with the ^{99m}Tc phosphate complexes at all articulations and they are generally preferred, despite the fact that the synovium per se is not visualised and periarticular bone uptake is not specific. Abnormal joints by radiophosphate can be correlated with radiography to determine the aetiology of the abnormality, rather than performing radiographic joint surveys in the first instance, since this is distinctly less sensitive before pannus erosion sets in.

The main advantages of ^{67}Ga citrate as an alternative to blood compartment tracers are its higher target/background ratios and its closer association with the cellular component of the inflammatory process (Fig. 11.3). These are offset by the inconvenience of waiting at least 24 h before imaging and the inordinate amount of time it takes to do a total body joint survey for the conventional diagnostic doses given. ^{67}Ga is more appropriate for studying selected joints of particular interest and monitoring their response to therapy.

A number of studies have been reported comparing the efficacy of the various radiopharmaceuticals, radiography and clinical impressions for the disclosure of synovitis. In 16 patients with synovitis caused by rheumatoid arthritis, psoriasis and Reiter's syndrome, radiopertechnetate diagnosed fewer joints than the clinical examination in 12 patients, whereas all clinically affected joints were disclosed with ^{99m}Tc polyphosphate. Radiopertechnetate showed more joint involvement than the clinical appraisal in only 2 patients, whereas polyphosphate demonstrated greater extension of disease than was clinically apparent in 15 patients (Desaulnier et al. 1974). An analysis of 191 abnormal joints in another group of patients showed that polyphosphate imaging was 11% more sensitive than the clinical impression and 72% more sensitive than radiography. Scrutiny of the results indicated that the radionuclide study performed less well than clinical judgement in the large joints such as shoulders, elbows and knees, but the opposite occurred in the peripheral joints, i.e. wrists, hands, ankles and feet. When the larger joints portrayed

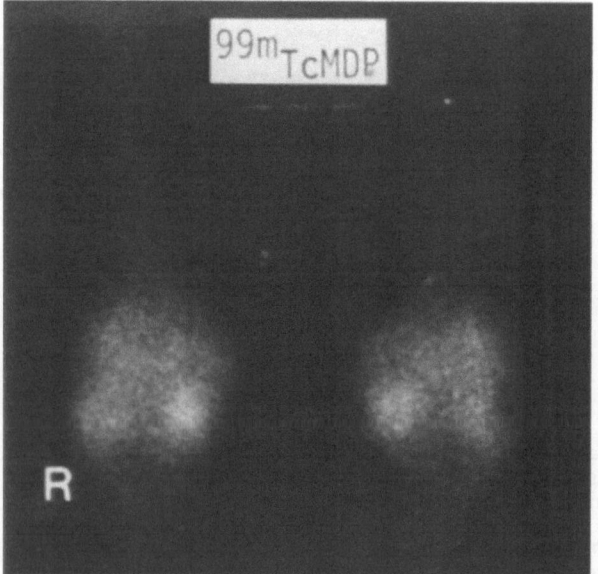
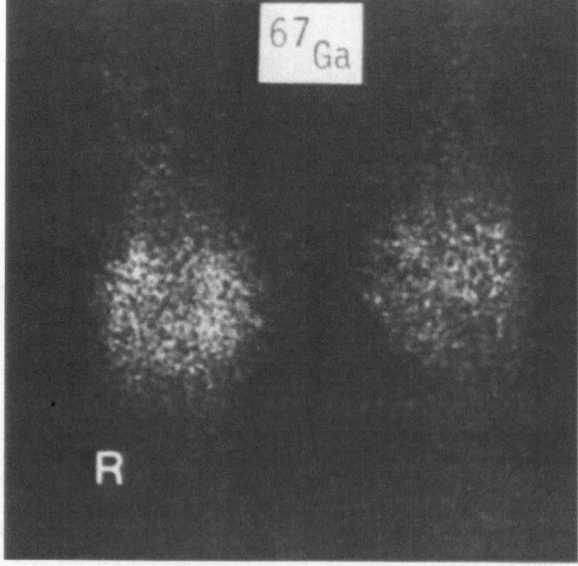

Fig. 11.3. Active rheumatoid arthritis of the knees. The ^{99m}Tc-MDP images show bilateral diffuse periarticular bone uptake characteristic of synovitis. Corresponding ^{67}Ga citrate images also demonstrate an elevated uptake in the region, but most of it is in the inflamed synovia, although this cannot be appreciated from the frontal images presented.

asymmetrical increases in uptake there was no difficulty in making the diagnosis, but small to moderate symmetrical increases were difficult to distinguish from the normally higher concentrations of radiophosphate that accumulate at these articulations. Some help may accrue from the use of blood pool markers at these sites (Greyson 1980). Similar results were published by another group of investigators who found that ^{99m}Tc pyrophosphate imaging was better than radiographic and clinical appraisal of the peripheral joints, but interpretative difficulties arose at the larger joints (Weisberg et al. 1978). Radiophosphate disclosed 172 abnormal joints compared with 105 by radiopertechnetate for a 64% improvement in an analysis limited to the hands of adult patients with rheumatoid arthritis and reflex sympathetic dystrophy. In this set of patients fine detailed radiography detected 7% more joints than radiopertechnetate, but radiophosphate disclosed 32% more than radiography (Beckerman et al. 1976).

It has been reported that radiopertechnetate is 96% sensitive in disclosing polymyalgia rheumatica, whereas radiophosphate is usually normal (O'Duffy et al. 1976). Synovitis in polymyalgia rheumatica features a non-specific chronic inflammation with infiltrations of lymphocytes and plasma cells that extend beyond the synovium to include the joint capsule and adjacent tissues, unlike the acute proliferative synovitis of rheumatoid arthritis. It can be postulated that there may not be sufficient increase in blood flow to produce a visibly discernible increase in radiophosphate uptake, but the vascular blood pool is large enough relative to adjacent tissue to be seen with radiopertechnetate, or some other blood compartment marker.

The proximal joints, shoulders and hips, are usually involved in polymyalgia rheumatica, and symmetrical incremental increase in radiophosphate uptake, if it occurs, can be difficult to appreciate, just as it is in the more proliferative inflammatory conditions. Synovitis associated with lupus erythematosus is also of the non-proliferative type, and the detection of peripheral joint disease with radiophosphate is variable and very often falsely negative. A definitive crossover study comparing a blood pool marker and radiophosphate in polymyalgia rheumatica and lupus erythematosus has yet to be done.

Juvenile Rheumatoid Arthritis

The diagnosis of synovitis in the presence of unfused epiphyses is difficult when using radiophosphate, because the high uptake in the growth plates obscures the periarticular increases caused by the hyperaemia. This is particularly troublesome in the small peripheral joints. When there is asymmetry, or some of the small joints are not involved and act as reference points, the diagnosis of synovitis may be less difficult. An exception is the knee, because increased accretion in the patella, resulting from its vascular anastomosis with the synovial network, can be seen in the lateral projection free of the growth plate. [67]Ga citrate may be successful where radiophosphate fails, but this approach has not been fully explored for juvenile rheumatoid arthritis. The synovitis of rheumatic fever can show avid radiophosphate and ^{67}Ga uptakes (Fig. 11.4).

Response to Treatment

Successful clinical treatment with steroidal or nonsteroidal anti-inflammatory drugs implies a relief of pain, increased range of joint movement, subsidence of joint swelling, improved grip strength etc. Underlying this is a defervescence of the inflammatory reaction in the synovium, and this should be reflected in a decreasing concentration of blood compart-

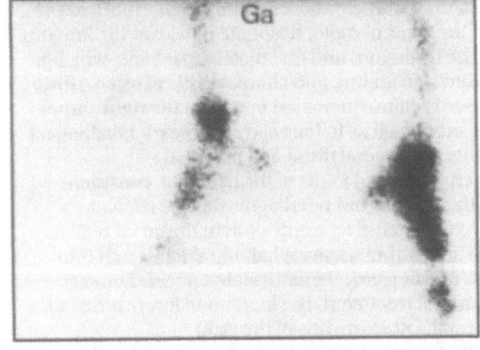

Fig. 11.4a,b. Rheumatic fever. Synovitis of the ankle and tarsal bones demonstrates a regional diffuse increase in radiophosphate uptake (a) and an increase in radiogallium localised to the synovium (b).

ment markers, radiophosphates and ^{67}Ga citrate (Fig. 11.5). Generally this is true, but there are caveats to keep in mind. Persistent high accretion of radiophosphate in the face of clinical remission could be due either to subclinical synovitis or histological remission with reactive bone repair of the pannus erosion. These erosions may even elude fine detailed radiography. A blood compartment marker may help in the differential diagnosis.

Radiopertechnetate measurements before and after corticosteroid treatment proved to be more sensitive to the efficacious effects of the drug than either grip strength or joint circumference (Collins et al. 1971). In another study consisting of 11 patients with knee pain, but no definite indication of warmth, swelling or both, there was increased uptake of radiopertechnetate only when synovial biopsy showed histological evidence of hyperaemia. It was concluded that the radiopertechnetate uptake was a more sensitive parameter of synovitis than clinical impressions of warmth and joint swelling (Boerbooms and Buys 1978).

Radionuclide remission may lag behind clinical remission. There can be a stage in treatment when the symptoms have abated, but the hyperaemia continues at a subclinical level and the radionuclide

uptake persists. This requires continued anti-inflammatory therapy to quash completely (Tannenbaum et al. 1986).

Radionuclide monitoring of arthritis treatment is not clinically important, because the thrust of medication is to relieve symptoms and not to improve the appearance of the joint images. Its main attribute lies in pharmacological testing and comparison of anti-inflammatory drugs.

Quantitative Joint Imaging

Various methods of joint uptake quantitation have been tried in order to obviate the subjective nature of image interpretation. The usual approach is to obtain a ratio of the uptakes over individual affected joints to adjacent normal bone or soft tissue at a fixed time interval after administration of the test agent. Some have used joint uptakes compared with an outside standard source. One suggestion consisted of measuring radioactivity over groups of small joints in the hands and comparing it with the uptake of an internal reference source (Park et al. 1977).

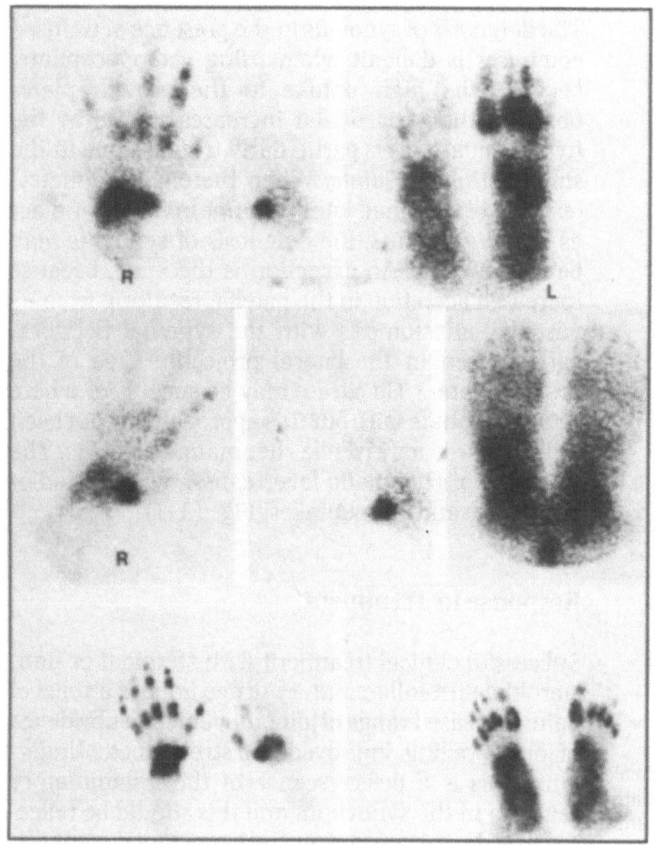

Fig. 11.5. Psoriasis under treatment. *Upper panel:* Prior to treatment the left hand was normal except for the focus of radiophosphate uptake at the juncture of the trapezium and first metacarpal bone, which is a common finding and characteristic of osteoarthritis. There is diffuse increased uptake in the right carpal region as well as in four of the metacarpophalangeal joints and several distal and proximal interphalangeal joints of the left hand, consistent with synovitis but not diagnostic. The left foot exhibits intense concentration in the tarsal region, the first four metatarsophalangeal joints and third toe. *Middle panel:* 9 months later, after an intense course of treatment, the hands and feet reverted to normal. Osteoarthritis of the right trapeziometacarpophalangeal joint, previously obscured by the synovitis, is now apparent. *Lower panel:* 1 year after the last study the patient returned with a recrudescence of the psoriatic arthritis. It affected both feet and right hand predominantly.

An exhaustive study compared four parameters, utilising ^{99m}Tc pyrophosphate as the test agent: ratio of joint to non-joint bone using count rate per unit area; ratio of joint to non-joint bone total uptake using count rate only; absolute uptake per unit area normalised for body weight and dose; and absolute total uptake normalised for body weight and dose. The mid-radius and mid-ulna were the non-joint reference bones when normal and inflamed articulations of the hand were measured, and the mid-femur was the non-joint reference for the knee assessments. These parameters were evaluated in controls and in patients afflicted with rheumatoid arthritis. The best separation was obtained with the absolute uptake per unit area, i.e. without reference to a non-joint bone. However, the overlap between abnormals and normals was large and this undermined its value as a screening procedure to disclose synovitis. The least discriminating parameter was the ratio of joint uptake to non-joint uptake (Rosenspire et al. 1980a).

Most studies utilising the joint/non-joint ratio have assumed that the reference bone is unaffected by the inflammation. There is growing evidence that this is not so. It was found, for instance, that the mid-third of the radius and ulna in patients with active rheumatoid arthritis of the hand on the same side was about 35% higher than controls (Rosenspire et al. 1980b). The lumbar spine/soft tissue ratio was enhanced by 28% in patients with rheumatoid arthritis compared with an age- and sex-matched control group. Rheumatoid arthritis usually does not involve the lumbar spine, nor was there clinical evidence of it in this group of patients (Helfgott et al. 1982). The 24-h whole-body retention (WBR) measurements of ^{99m}Tc-MDP by two different methods demonstrated increases of 45% and 33%, respectively, in rheumatoid patients. Although these increases could be attributed to the periarticular uptake rather than the non-joint bone, nevertheless there was no correlation of the 24-h WBR values with the number and size of abnormal joints (Lansbury index), sedimentation rate, functional class or rheumatoid factor titre. From this it can be inferred that the results of the lumbar spine/soft tissue ratio and 24-h WBR support the hypothesis of a generalised bone reaction superimposed on a local articular process. Increased 24-h WBR in rheumatoid arthritis was found by another group of investigators. Inpatients had higher retentions than outpatients, and those on steroids registered the highest retentions (Steven et al. 1982). This lack of neutral reference bone can explain the failure of the joint/non-joint ratios to clearly distinguish actively inflamed rheumatoid from control joints. There is no acceptable quantitative parameter at this time that can be used as a screening procedure. There is some merit in these parameters for monitoring numerically the response to treatment, as ratios in the normal range have been shown to decrease in response to inflammatory suppression. Whichever parameter is adopted, the ultimate confirmation of its meaning and value will be its correlation with synovial biopsy, not with clinical or radiographic impressions.

Normal paired joints do not necessarily exhibit symmetrical periarticular accretions of radiophosphate. Some of the discrepancy can be explained by the person's dominant side or handedness. A numerical analysis in non-pathological joint pairs showed a significantly higher accretion on the right side in 37%, the left side in 21%, and no difference in 42% of the joint pairs. The highest incidence of disparity occurred in the shoulder joints (Norbjerg et al. 1980).

Value of a Negative Joint Scan Result

It is well appreciated that a positive radiophosphate joint scan result is not specific for synovitis, and the findings must be interpreted within the clinical context. In fact, the number of false-positive results is unknown and of some editorial concern (Green 1979). More important, perhaps, is the significance of a negative joint study result in a patient with polyarthralgia. Polyarthralgia is a frequent complaint, but a causal synovitis is less common. A normal radiophosphate bone scan is purportedly significant for an absence of synovitis, but documentation by long-term clinical follow-up has been reported in only one small series of patients (Shearman et al. 1982). This was a retrospective study of two groups of patients. Group A consisted of 22 patients with polyarthralgia of at least 3 months' duration, normal radiophosphate joint scans, or non-inflammatory joint scans typical of osteoarthritis (i.e. they did not demonstrate diffuse periarticular concentrations, but rather focal uptake limited to one compartment of a knee joint or focal uptake within a wrist). Group B contained the same number of patients, who were age and sex matched with Group A but had abnormal inflammatory joint scans featuring diffuse juxta-articular bone uptake in one or more joints. The patients in group A were recalled for clinical examination 3.6 ± 0.9 years later, and none of the 22 patients with previous normal joint scans had evidence of inflammatory disease. Group B patients were re-examined 4.0 ± 1.0 years later, and 21 of the 22 patients had clinically active synovitis. There were 12 cases of rheumatoid arthritis, 5 of psoriasis, and 1 each of

Reiter's syndrome, ankylosing spondylitis, mixed connective tissue disease and undifferentiated connective tissue disease. The single patient who was free of inflammatory disease on recall had documented juvenile rheumatoid arthritis but was in complete remission. Three patients in group A were originally thought to have clinical synovitis, but these were later diagnosed as two with polymyalgia rheumatica and one with lupus erythematosus—entities known to yield normal radiophosphate scans. The conclusion derived from this isolated study is that a normal radiophosphate joint survey in a patient with polyarthralgia makes it unlikely for an inflammatory polyarthritis to develop if a thorough rheumatological evaluation fails to demonstrate evidence of inflammatory joint disease.

Sacroiliitis

Sacroiliitis is characterised by an enhanced accretion of radiophosphate at the sacroiliac joint. This can be difficult to appreciate visually, because there is normally a high concentration in the area and mild to moderate symmetrical increases may escape

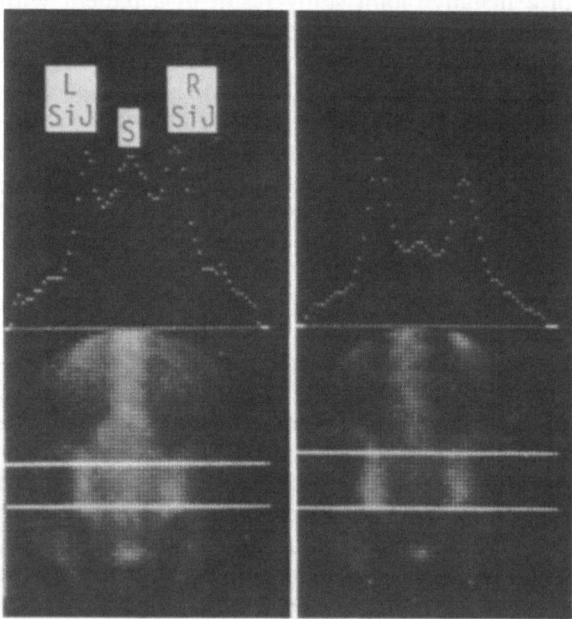

Fig. 11.6. Analysis of sacroiliac joints (*SiJ*). A profile slice through the full length of the joint and sacrum (*S*) is obtained. The parameter for measuring joint activity is a ratio of peak SiJ to peak S counts. *Left:* Normal patient. SiJ/S = 1.03. *Right:* Enteropathic sacroiliitis. SiJ/S = 1.84 (normal less than 1.35 for this laboratory using ^{99m}Tc-MDP).

detection. Various quantitative techniques have been proposed to obviate the subjective interpretation. A ratio of the peak sacroiliac joint count rate to the peak sacral count rate was originally introduced (Fig. 11.6). Early results indicated clear separation of the controls from an experimental group of ankylosing spondylitis (Russell et al. 1975). A modification was proposed in which background corrected sacroiliac joint/sacrum ratios were obtained in the upper, middle and lower thirds of the joint, instead of the full length of the joint as originally proposed (Fig. 11.7). This manoeuvre was allegedly more sensitive in disclosing inflammatory disease which was limited to the lower half of the joint—the location of the synovium (Namey et al. 1977). It has also been suggested that the ratio of the peak joint count rate to the minimum count rate in a profile slice through the joints and sacrum favours better separation between normal and diseased joints (Ayres et al. 1981).

If the radionuclide procedure is to have clinical utility it must possess a high sensitivity at a stage of the disease when the radiographic stigmata are inapparent or dubious, i.e. radiographic grades 0 and 1. Otherwise, there is no need for nucleography. It is imperative that the study be performed when the patient is not receiving anti-inflammatory drugs and that a standardised procedure be used. Specifically, the same radiophosphate test agent must be used in all cases in order to avoid varying pharmacokinetics. The time of imaging should be fixed between 4 and 5 h, a time when the rate of accumulation of radioactivity has levelled off; 24 h after injection is probably better, but this can be impractical. The patient should also be rested for the examination, as physical exertion induces a hyperaemia that may affect the ratio. A prospective study has been reported in which these variables were rigidly controlled and which used ^{99m}Tc-MDP and the full length of the joint. It showed a significant difference between controls and ankylosing spondylitis with radiographic grades 0–1, 2, 3 and 4 respectively. There was a substantial overlap of the patients with radiographic grades 0–1 disease and the normal 2 standard deviation range, despite the statistically significant group difference. The absence of a sharp separation weighs heavily against the technique as a modality for population screening (Esdaile et al. 1980). The technique does have merit in monitoring treatment, however, because there was a group of patients in this series with false-negative ratios that decreased with successful anti-inflammatory therapy.

An unpublished study investigating the value of the triple profile slice, i.e. upper, middle and lower thirds of the sacroiliac joint, in 26 patients with

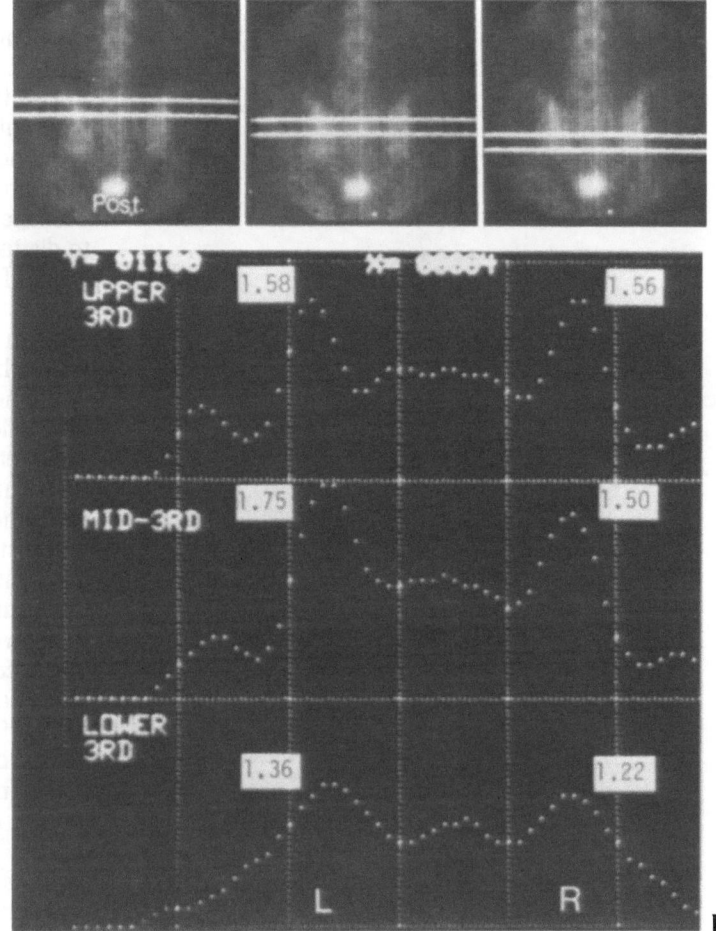

Fig. 11.7a,b. Fractionated analysis of sacroiliac joints in a patient with ankylosing spondylitis. **a** Location of the three profile slices. **b** Histograms of the upper, middle and lower third profile slices. *Inset numbers* represent the sacroiliac joint/sacrum ratios for the left and right sacroiliac joints at the different levels.

ankylosing spondylitis demonstrated no material improvement over the single full-length profile slice. There were ten more abnormalities detected with this fractionation compared with the unfractionated analysis, but nine of these were in radiographic grades 3 and 4; only one was in grade 0.

It is apparent that quantitative sacroiliac scintigraphy offers a substantial improvement over subjective interpretation, but there is no absolute separation of diseased and normal groups, and the reported degree of overlap varies from acceptable to unacceptable for clinical utility (Berghs et al. 1978; Dequeker et al. 1978; Goldberg et al. 1978; Spencer et al. 1979; Domeij-Nyberg et al. 1980). There is also a lack of specificity, because high ratios can be obtained in osteoarthritis and metabolic bone disease. Age, sex and laterality may also influence the ratios. One communication states that the normal ratio is on average higher on the right side than the left in all ages (both male and female), the right joint ratios are higher in males than females, and that there is no variation of the ratio with age in either sex (Vyas et al. 1981). In contrast, another report related a decrease in the normal ratio values with increasing age in both sexes (Dodig et al. 1984). To confuse matters more, it also claimed that the normal ratios decreased with advancing years in females, but not males (Ayres et al. 1981).

An assumption in all these ratio stratagems is that the sacrum, the reference bone, does not participate in the inflammatory process. There is growing evidence that the sacrum is not immune. Significantly higher uptakes of radiophosphate in the sacrum of patients suffering from ankylosing spondylitis and Reiter's disease than those of controls have been found. Additionally, sacral uptake in degenerative disc disease and diffuse idiopathic skeletal hyperostosis were normal (Paquin et al. 1983). The implication of these findings is that the ratios in sacroiliitis are not just a function of the numerator, the sacroiliac joint count rate, but also of the denominator, the sacral count rate. This tends to lower the ratio and probably contributes to the loss of sensitivity.

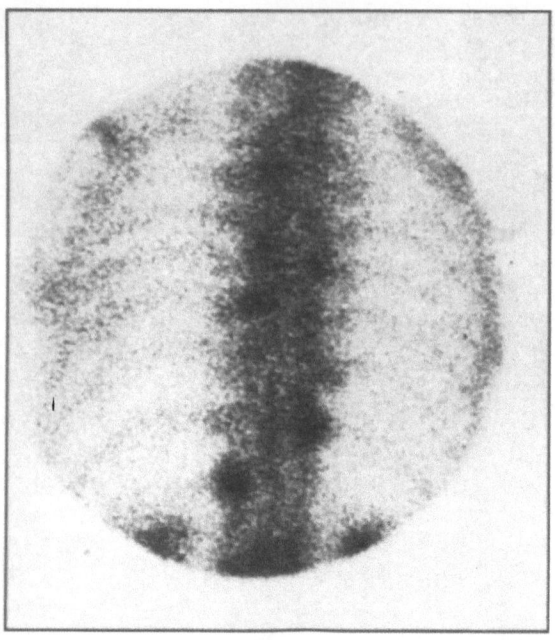

Fig. 11.8. Apophysitis in ankylosing spondylitis. The radiophosphate scan demonstrates focal concentrations at scattered apophyseal joints in the thoracolumbar spine.

Ankylosing Spondylitis

Lesions other than sacroiliitis can be detected with radiophosphate in ankylosing spondylitis. Features such as spinal apophyseal, sternoclavicular, manubriosternal and sternocostal joint involvement have been detected as foci of elevated radiophosphate uptake (Lentle et al. 1977; Lin et al. 1980). The ankylosed spine is rigid and osteoporotic, and therefore susceptible to fractures which may not be symptomatic, endure continued movement for long periods and result in pseudoarthrosis. Adjacent bone proliferation and ankylosis tend to obscure the fracture lines in conventional radiography, but they are readily revealed by radiophosphate imaging (Resnick et al. 1981; Figs. 11.8, 11.9).

Osteoarthritis

Osteoarthritis is a common disease of the diarthrodial and, to some degree, amphiarthrodial joints. It is characterised by a non-inflammatory deterioration of the articular cartilage and reactive new bone formation at joint surfaces and margins, but there is still a debate as to whether it originates in the cartilage or in the subchondral bone. There is fibrotic thickening of the joint capsule and, at times, a mild synovitis.

The induced radiophosphate response can vary from subtle to pronounced, depending on the metabolic activity of the lesions. Blood compartment markers are usually normal in osteoarthritis, because the synovitis is not flagrant. It is impossible to distinguish osteoarthritis of the peripheral small joints of the hands and feet from a synovitis, because the resolution of the imaging equipment is not fine enough. In large joint areas, such as the wrists, knees, hips and shoulders, the focal nature of the radiophosphate uptake can be better appreciated in distinction to the diffuse juxta-articular concentration seen in synovitis (Figs. 11.10, 11.11, 11.12).

In a multiple crossover study comparing clinical assessment, conventional radiography, double-contrast arthrography, arthroscopy, surgical observations and radiophosphate bone imaging it was found that radionuclide imaging was superior to arthrography and radiography in disclosing the presence and degree of osteoarthritis of the medial, lateral and patellofemoral compartments (Thomas et al. 1975). These findings were important considerations in planning remedial knee surgery.

Degenerative changes in the spinal column may induce low-grade radiophosphate accretions that can be troublesome in assigning an aetiology in patients with known malignancy. In a small group of patients with diffuse idiopathic skeletal hyperostosis, the vertebral column did not exhibit remarkable focal uptakes of radiophosphate. The lumbar spine/soft tissue and sacrum/soft tissue quotients in this set were, on the average, higher than controls, but not significant to a 0.05 probability level. These indices for degenerative disc disease were indistinguishable from normal (Paquin et al. 1983). In another study of ten patients with proved herniation of the lumbar discs, there was no evidence of an associated abnormal radiophosphate uptake (Johansen et al. 1980).

Radiophosphate imaging can be used to differentiate degenerative disease of the temporomandibular joints from myofacial disorders without pathological joint involvement. Planar scintigraphy correlated completely with microscopy in eight patients with osteoarthritis and in one without bone changes. In the same group of patients radiography missed four of the osteoarthritis joints (Goldstein and Bloom 1980). Single photon emission computed tomography (SPECT) has been applied to the screening of temporomandibular disorders and it seems to improve the sensitivity, because of greater contrast and better localisation (Collier et al. 1983; Fig. 11.13). In one series of patients SPECT with

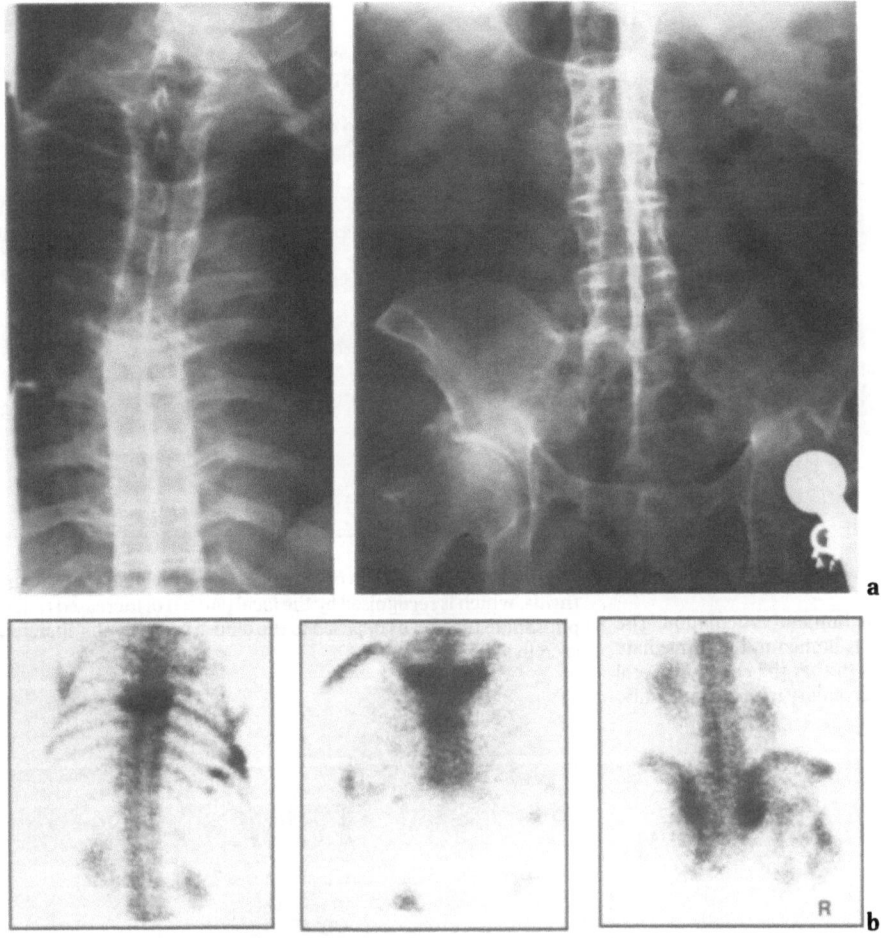

Fig. 11.9a,b. Ankylosing spondylitis. This 57-year-old male with advanced ankylosing spondylitis sustained a minor fall which resulted in a fracture of the thoracic spine and several ribs because of the rigidity of the axial skeleton. **a** Conventional radiograph of the thoracic spine shows the features of spinal fusion with no definite evidence of fracture. **b** Radiograph of the lumbar spine and pelvis demonstrates fusion of the sacroiliac joints and lumbar vertebra. **c** Radiophosphate images depict an intense uptake in the T-4 to T-5 region and in some of the ribs on the right. There is also an augmented uptake at the manubrioclavicular and manubriosternal junctions, which are features of ankylosing spondylitis. Although the radiographs showed fusion of the sacroiliac joints, the scan depicted some residual activity in the right sacroiliac joint. When fusion is metabolically complete radiophosphate uptake is normal.

radiophosphate gave positive results in 6 of 11 patients with internal derangement, 9 of 10 patients with degenerative joint disease, and negative results in 4 patients with myofacial disorders.

There is a high incidence of enhanced accretion of radiophosphate in the patella, often without corresponding radiographic abnormalities. A retrospective review of 100 consecutive adult patients found that it occurred bilaterally in 15%, and unilaterally in 5%. Osteoarthritis was seen in the radiographs in 7 out of 20 patients, and other confirmed lesions included fractures, osteomyelitis, bursitis and Paget's disease. However, a number of abnormally radioactive patellae remained undocumented and these were presumed to be secondary to chondromalacia and osteoarthritis which eluded

radiographic detection (Kipper et al. 1982). In 130 patients ranging in age from 4 to 83 years, increased patellar radioactivity with normal radiographic findings occurred with a 44% frequency, whereas the incidence of increased patellar radioactivity associated with radiographic evidence of patellar degeneration occurred in only 33% (Lin et al. 1981). The medial and lateral knee compartments were also studied in this series of patients, and increased radiophosphate concentration was found in the presence of normal radiographic knees in 33%. Moreover, 100% of radiographically abnormal knees also had corresponding abnormal radiophosphate uptakes. The authors postulated that the increased patellar radioactivity not accompanied by increased knee radioactivity or radiographically

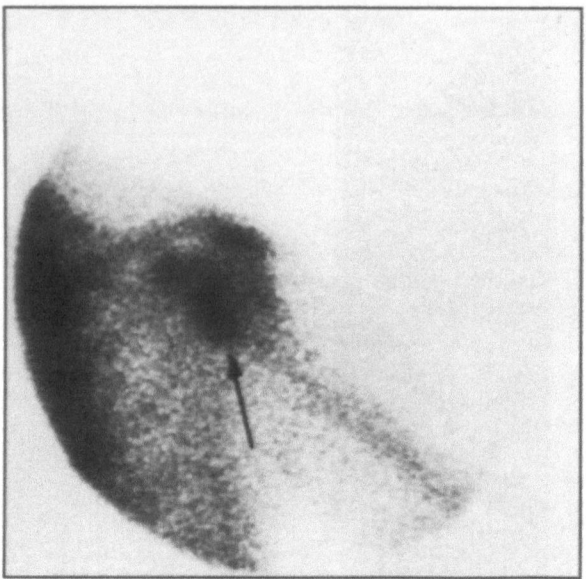

Fig. 11.10. Osteoarthritis of the glenohumeral articulation. The increased uptake of radiophosphate is limited to the immediate joint area (*arrow*). A synovitis differs in that the entire humeral head would show increased uptake secondary to the hyperaemia.

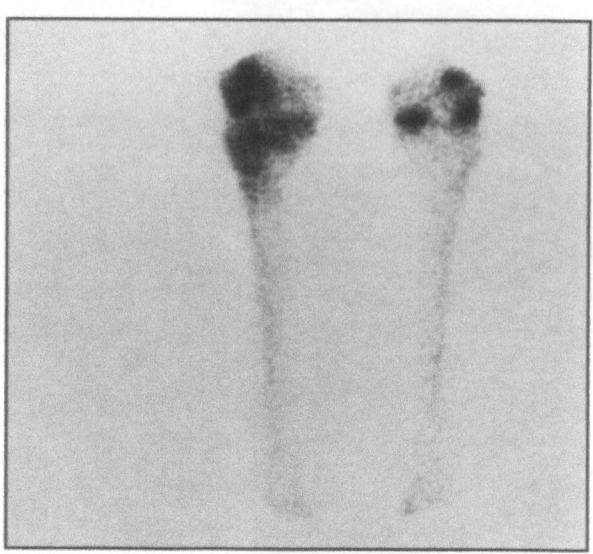

Fig. 11.12. Osteoarthritis of the knees. There is bilateral osteoarthritis, which is recognised by the focal pattern of increased radiophosphate uptake, as opposed to the diffuse periarticular increase seen in synovitis.

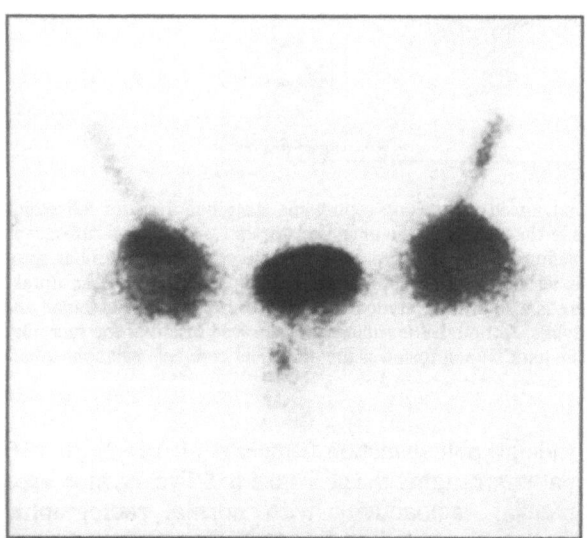

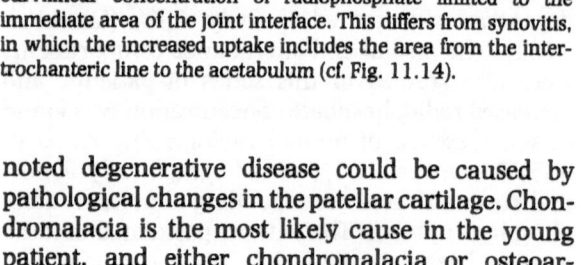

Fig. 11.11. Bilateral osteoarthritis of the hips. There is an intense curvilinear concentration of radiophosphate limited to the immediate area of the joint interface. This differs from synovitis, in which the increased uptake includes the area from the intertrochanteric line to the acetabulum (cf. Fig. 11.14).

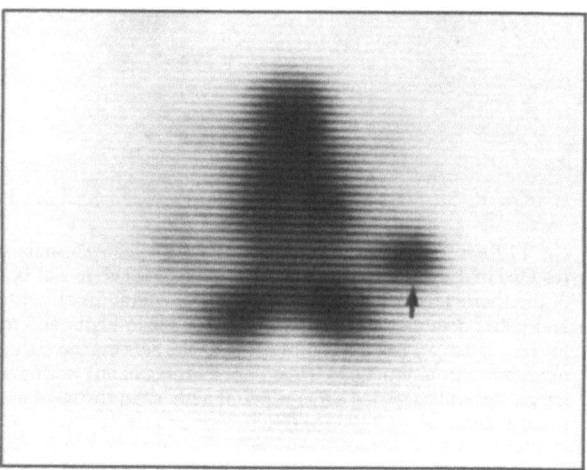

Fig. 11.13. Osteoarthritis of the right temperomandibular joint (*arrow*). Transverse slice from a SPECT study using radiophosphate.

Transient (Toxic) Synovitis of the Hip

noted degenerative disease could be caused by pathological changes in the patellar cartilage. Chondromalacia is the most likely cause in the young patient, and either chondromalacia or osteoarthritis, or both, in the older patient (Lin et al. 1981).

Transient synovitis is an ailment that generally occurs in children under 10 years of age. The cause is not known. It may be due to occult trauma, but an association between the synovitis and a preceding viral infection of the upper respiratory tract has

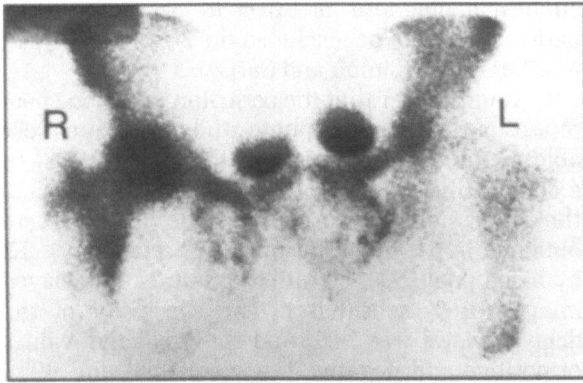

Fig. 11.14. Transient synovitis in a 24-year-old male who complained of right hip pain after a football game. The joint aspirate was clear and showed no evidence of sepsis by cytological examination and culture. Treatment consisted of bed rest. Note the increased periarticular bone uptake in the right hip, beginning abruptly in the intertrochanteric region and extending to include the femoral neck, epiphysis and acetabulum—the extent of the hyperaemia.

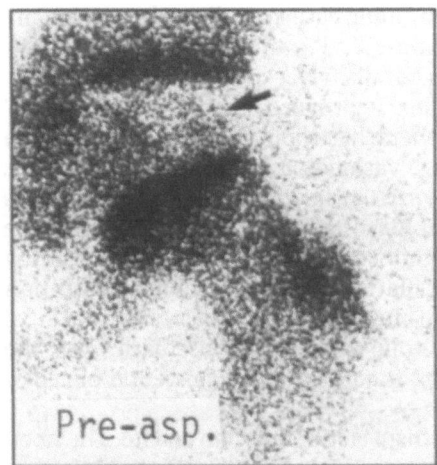

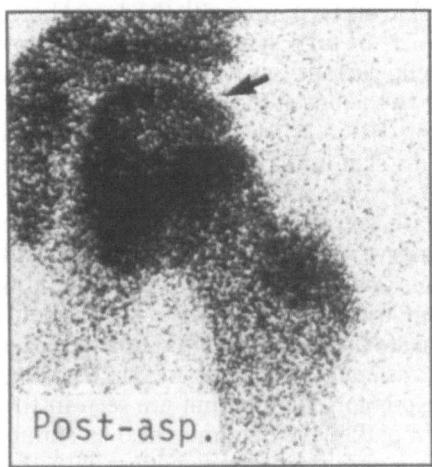

Fig. 11.15. Transient synovitis in the left hip of a 7-year-old child. The blood pool images were normal, but the delayed image showed a decrease in the radiophosphate concentration in the left femoral epiphysis (*arrow*). The blood supply was normal in the study obtained 2 days after aspiration.

been noted. It can produce signs of mild inflammation and must be distinguished from bacterial infection. Some authors claim that as many as 10% of these patients may develop Legg–Perthes disease as a complication. Transient synovitis is usually self limiting and treated with bed rest.

Transient synovitis has been investigated by all three phases of radiophosphate nucleography, i.e. perfusion, blood pool and delayed images. The anatomical disposition of the vascular supply is such that vessels which supply the femoral capital epiphysis pass through the joint capsule, and a sufficient rise in intracapsular pressure by the effusion can impair the blood supply and delivery of radiophosphate to the epiphysis. This can result in a variable radionuclide portrayal (Fig. 11.14).

In one series of 13 patients, the periarticular uptake of radiophosphate in the delayed images was normal in 9, increased in 3 and decreased in 3 (Heyman et al. 1980). Similar variations were reported by other authors (Murray 1980; Sutherland et al. 1980). In a well-documented study of 19 cases of transient synovitis, there were 6 that demonstrated normal blood pool and delayed images. One patient showed increased radioactivity in the blood pool image, and ten showed it on the delayed images, but not in the blood pool phase. Eight patients exhibited photon deficiency in the blood pool phase. Six of these eight patients had a reduced, but not absent, epiphyseal uptake in the delayed views. All six patients reverted to normal after joint aspiration (Kloiber et al. 1983; Fig. 11.15). It would appear that transient synovitis can demonstrate reduced,

normal or increased concentrations of radiophosphate in the blood pool and delayed images, and the direction of change in both phases is not necessarily the same in a given patient.

Reflex Sympathetic Dystrophy Syndrome

The reflex sympathetic dystrophy syndrome (RSDS) is not well understood, and this is reflected in the many appellations applied to the symptoms, such as "causalgia", "acute atrophy of bone", "Sudeck's atrophy", "peripheral acute trophoneurosis", "traumatic angiospasm", "post-traumatic osteoporosis", "traumatic vasospasm", "reflex dystrophy of the extremities", " minor causalgia", "post-infarction sclerodactyly", "shoulder-hand syndrome", "reflex neurovascular dystrophy" and " reflex sympathetic dystrophy". It is associated with pain, swelling, vasomotor disturbances with signs of increased vascular flow, trophic dermal changes and radiographic osteoporosis. Histologically, the synovium demonstrates proliferation of the lining cells and capillaries and perivascular infiltration with chronic inflammatory cells. The lack of sympathetic tone and hypervascularity of the synovium abet the periarticular accretion of radiophosphate.

The mechanism is still subject to debate. The nociceptive (pain) nerve system carries afferent information from the skin and synapses with the dorsal horn neurones, which in turn synapse with the motor and sympathetic efferents, as well as the ascending tracts leading to the brain. Partial peripheral nerve injury and soft tissue crush induce a number of responses. With skin injury there is a local release of bradykinin, prostaglandin, seratonin and Substance P (a neurotransmitter). These affect the sympathetic nerve ends and skin capillaries and excite and sensitise the skin nociceptors. It is also postulated that with nerve injury the sympathetic nerves may excite the nociceptors and influence the release of the various algesic substances in the skin, and cause vasomotor changes that are seen in the RSDS. The sympathetic system may also be stimulated through a short-circuit connection with the excited and sensitised nociceptor afferent nerves.

The most frequent varieties of the syndrome are Sudeck's atrophy and shoulder-hand syndrome. Shoulder-hand syndrome is bilateral in about 30% of cases and is associated with myocardial infarction, trauma, spinal disc disease, neoplasia, cerebrovascular accident and drugs. However, a specific precipitant cannot be found in 35% of cases.

Triple-phase radiophosphate imaging has been applied to the investigation of patients with RSDS. In one study consisting of 39 patients with definite, probably or possible RSDS, 69% demonstrated radiographic osteopenia. The radionuclide abnormalities, i.e. increased perfusion and diffuse enhanced periarticular uptake in the affected area, occurred in 60%. It was also found that patients with an abnormal radionuclide study were considerably more responsive to steroid control than those with normal images. From this it was concluded that the degree of radiophosphate uptake is a reflection of the activity and potential reversibility of the disordered blood flow, and thus a valuable prognosticator of the response to systemic steroid therapy (Kozin et al. 1976, 1981). Radiophosphate scans

enabled a diagnosis of RSDS to be made in 13 patients and to be excluded in 5, according to another report (Simon and Carlson 1980).

It would appear that the perfusion and blood pool phases of the radiophosphate study are not as reliable as the delayed images in disclosing RSDS. In a clinical investigation of 23 patients with RSDS of the hands and forearms, positive results were obtained in 10 by perfusion (45% sensitivity), 12 by blood pool (52% sensitivity), but 22 by delayed images (96% sensitivity). The specificity of the delayed views was 98% and the predictive values of positive and negative test were 88% and 99%, respectively (Mackinnon and Holder 1984).

A group of 85 patients with cerebrovascular accidents were investigated by the three-phase radiophosphate study. There were 21 patients with increased uptake in the delayed views, of which 13 (62%) had increased blood flow and 8 (38%) had decreased blood flow, and these results were consistent with the clinical suspicion of RSDS. Abnormal delayed views antedated clinical symptoms in two patients. Of the cerebrovascular accident patients without RSDS 55 (65%) portrayed decreased blood flow and blood pool images of the hands and wrists on the affected side, but all had normal delayed radiophosphate images. This was attributed to the paralysis, disuse, or both. The remaining nine patients were normal in all three phases. It was postulated that the decreased blood flow and blood pool radioactivity which occurred in 38% of the patients with RSDS was caused by the reduced nutrient demands for blood by the paralysed or immobilised limb, while the increased blood flow to bone remained unaffected. Since the main contribution to blood flow and pool radioactivity is from soft tissue, the resultant portrayal is decreased perfusion and blood pool concentrations and enhanced periarticular accretions in delayed views (Greyson and Tepperman 1984; Fig. 11.16).

Regional Migratory Osteoporosis

Regional migratory osteoporosis is a syndrome of acute periarticular painful soft tissue swelling, usually involving the lower extremities, which migrates from joint to joint. If the patient is not followed for long enough, the migratory nature of the disease may be missed. However, there are variants of this affliction which seem to be limited to one joint. The variable course and lack of known cause has

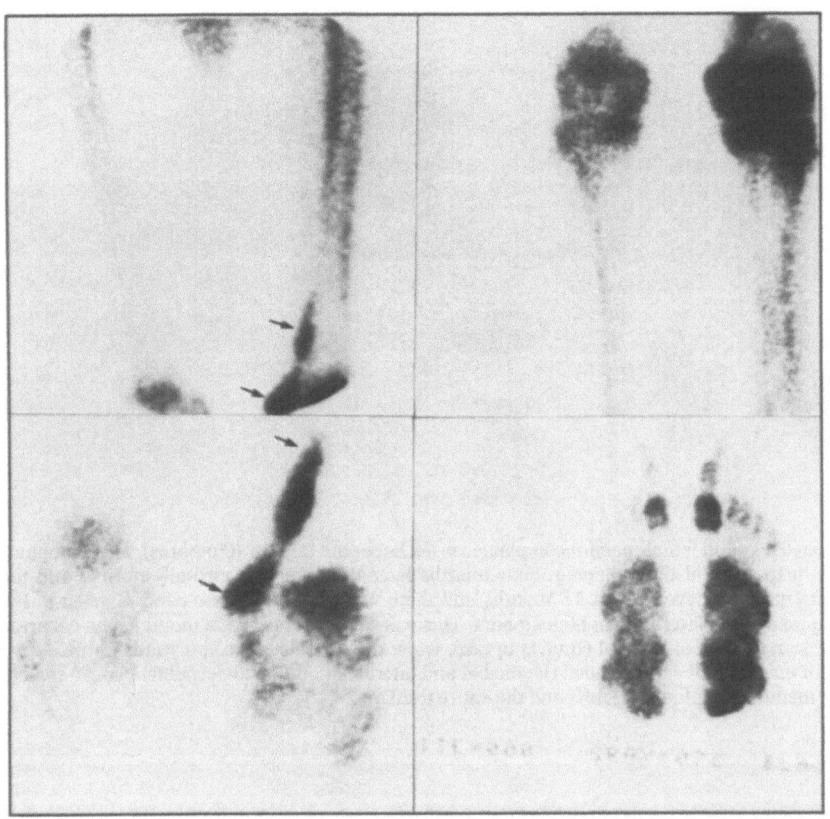

Fig. 11.16. RSDS. This male patient attempted suicide by shooting himself in the abdomen with buckshot. This caused considerable visceral and bone damage. About a month after this episode he developed signs and symptoms suggesting RSDS in the entire left lower extremity. A radiophosphate perfusion and blood pool study of the feet demonstrated relative increases in the left foot, but a greater disparity was shown in the delayed images. There was increased uptake in the long bones with emphasis at the periarticular zones. Additionally, there was the development of heterotopic bone (myositis ossificans) along the medial aspect of the distal femur (*arrows*), a rare complication. The radiophosphate manifestation of heterotopic bone antedated the radiographic appearance.

resulted in a variety of terms, such as "transient osteoporosis", "migratory osteolysis", "algodystrophy" and "partial algodystrophy". Occurrence of the disease is usually spontaneous in otherwise healthy middle-aged adults, without any known precipitating cause. Males outnumber females by a factor of three. About half the reported female cases presented in the last trimester of pregnancy or shortly after giving birth. Episodes of regional migratory osteoporosis last about a year or less and resolve spontaneously without specific therapy. The most frequent site of initial involvement is the hip, but the disease may start in the knees, ankles or feet. Once remission occurs in a given joint it is not likely to be affected again. The interval of time between migration from one joint to the next can be a few months to many years.

Bone biopsy shows increased vascularity, vascular dilatation, fibrillosis of fatty marrow and bone remodelling with formation of lamellar and woven bone (Strashun and Chayes 1979; Lagier

1983). This histological picture is similar to that found in Sudeck's atrophy. The synovial membranes can be normal or show chronic hyperplastic changes.

The radiophosphate presentation is that of a high, non-specific uptake on one or both sides of a joint, involving the full or partial width of the bone. Radionuclide findings antedate the radiographic changes; the latter show subchondral demineralisation without loss of cartilage space (O'Mara and Pinals 1970; Gaucher et al. 1979; Tannenbaum et al. 1980; Rozenbaum et al. 1984; Fig. 11.17).

Trochanteric Bursitis

Trochanteric bursitis tends to occur in middle-aged and elderly patients and it consists of a non-

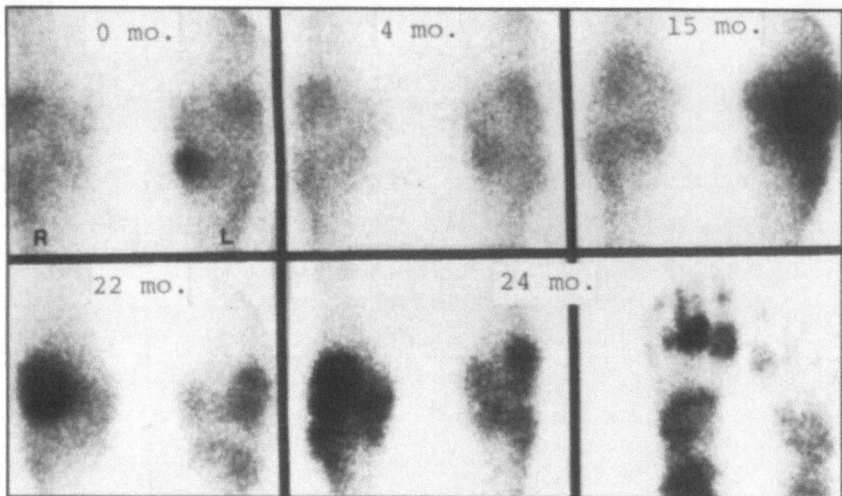

Fig. 11.17. Regional migratory osteoporosis. This adult female patient complained of left knee pain initially (0 months). The radiophosphate scan demonstrated a focal uptake in the medial tibial plateau. Four months later the scan was virtually normal and the patient was asymptomatic. Recurrent left knee pain developed at 15 months and there was now an intense concentration in the left lateral femoral condyle and a lesser uptake in the lateral tibial plateau area. This pain receded, but at 22 months pain occurred in the right knee, which showed an intense right lateral femoral condyle uptake, while the left side receded towards normal. Two months later (24 months) the involvement on the right side included the medial and lateral femoral condyles, tibial plateau region, the right ankle, tarsal bones, the first four metatarsophalangeal joints and the entire third toe.

infectious inflammation of one or more bursa about the gluteus medius insertion on the femoral trochanter. It causes pain on external rotation of the hip and is recognised by exquisite tenderness over the trochanteric area. Radiophosphate imaging may show an increased accretion in the greater trochanter underlying the bursa (Fig. 11.18).

Plantar Fasciitis (Calcaneal Periostitis)

Chronic plantar fasciitis is one cause of the painful heel syndrome, wherein pain and tenderness are concentrated at the site of attachment of the long plantar tendon into the base of the calcaneus. The radiophosphate portrayal is that of a focal high accretion in the calcaneus at the point of insertion of the tendon. Radiography may be normal when the radionuclide study is abnormal, or it may manifest marginal erosions, spurs and periosteal new bone formation at the base of the calcaneus (Sewell et al. 1980). [67]Ga may demonstrate enhanced uptake in the fascia over its entire length.

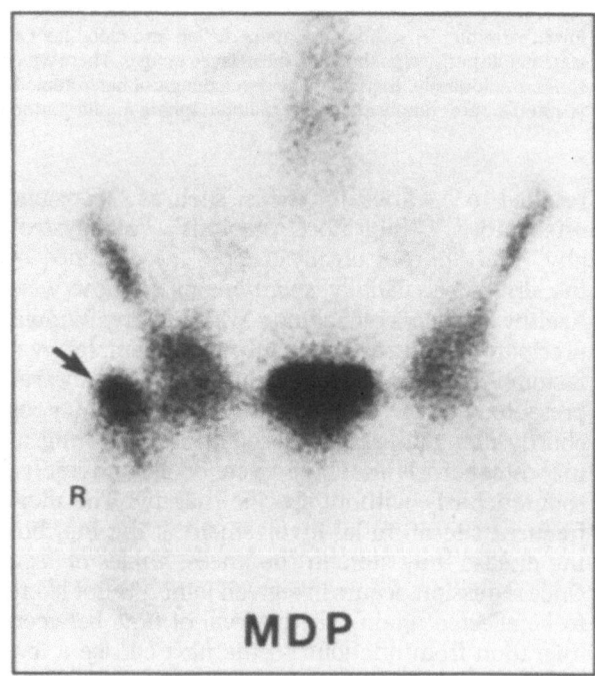

Fig. 11.18. Tronchanteric bursitis. This patient had exquisite point tenderness over the right greater trochanter which was clinically diagnosed as bursitis. There was an intense focus of radiophosphate uptake in the right greater trochanter (*arrow*).

References

Ahlstrom S, Gedda PO, Hedberg H (1956) Disappearance of radioactive serum albumin from joints in rheumatoid arthritis. Acta Rheum Scand 2: 129–135

Ayres J, Hilson JW, Maisey MN, Laurent R, Panayi GS, Saunders AJ (1981) An improved method for sacroiliac joint imaging: a study of normal subjects, patients with sacroiliitis and patients with low back pain. Clin Radiol 32: 441–445

Beckerman C, Genant HK, Hoffer PB, Kozin F, Ginsberg M (1976) Radionuclide imaging of the bone and joints of the hand. Radiology 118: 653–659

Berghs H, Remans J, Dreiskens L, Keiboom S, Polderman J (1978) Diagnostic value of SI joint scintigraphy with Tc-99m-pyrophosphate in sacroiliitis. Ann Rheum Dis 37: 190–194

Boerbooms AM, Buys WC (1978) Rapid assessment of Tc-99m-pertechnetate uptake of the knee joint as a parameter of inflammatory activity. Arthritis Rheum 21: 348–352

Cohen MB, Lorber A (1971) Avoiding false positive joint scans by the use of labelled albumins. Arthritis Rheum 14: 32–40

Coleman RE, Samuelson CO, Baim S, Christian PE, Ward JR (1982) Imaging with Tc-99m-MDP and GA-67-citrate in patients with rheumatoid arthritis and suspected septic arthritis. J Nucl Med 23: 479–482

Collier BD, Carrera GF, Messer EJ, Ryan DE, Gingrass D, Angell D, Palmer DW, Isitman AT, Hellman RS (1983) Internal derangement of the temporomandibular joint: detection of single-photon emission computed tomography. Radiology 149: 557–561

Collins KE, Deodhar S, Naki G, Whaley K, Buchanan WW, Dick WC (1971) Radioisotope study of small joint inflammation in rheumatoid arthritis. Ann Rheum Dis 30: 401–405

Desaulnier M, Rosenthall L, Fuks A, Lacourciere Y, Hawkins D (1974) Radiotechnetium polyphosphate joint imaging. J Nucl Med 15: 417–423

Dequeker J, Goddeeris T, Walravens M, DeRoc M (1978) Evaluation of sacroiliitis: camparison of radiological and radionuclide techniques. Radiology 128: 687–689

Dick C, Whaley K, St Onge RA, Downie RA, Boyle JA, Nuki G, Gillespie FC, Buchanan WW (1970) Clinical studies on inflammation in human knee joints: xenon (Xe-133) clearances correlated with clinical assessment in various arthritides and studies on the effect of intra-articularly administered hydrocortisone in rheumatoid arthritis. Clin Sci 38: 123–130

Dick WC, Collins KE, Buchanan W (1972) Clinical studies on inflammation in small diarthrodial joints. Clin Sci 42: 383–393

Dodig D, Popovic S, Domljan Z (1984) Influence of age on quantitative sacroiliac joint imaging. Eur J Nucl Med 9: 177–179

Domeij-Nyberg B, Kjallman M, Nylen O, Pettersson NO (1980) The reliability of quantitative bone scanning in sacroiliitis. Scand J Rheumatol 9: 77–79

Esdaile JM, Rosenthall L, Terkeltaub R, Kloiber R (1980) Prospective evaluation of sacroiliac scintigraphy in chronic inflammatory back pain. Arthritis Rheum 23: 998–1003

Gaucher A, Colomb JN, Naoun A, Faure G, Netter P (1979) The diagnostic value of Tc-99m diphosphonate bone imaging in transient osteoporosis of the hip. J Rheumatol 6: 574–583

Goldberg RP, Genant HK, Shimchak D, Shames D (1978) Applications and limitations of quantitative sacroiliac joint scintigraphy. Radiology 128: 683–686

Goldstein HA, Bloom CY (1980) Detection of degenerative disease of the temporomandibular joint by bone scintigraphy. J Nucl Med 21: 928–930

Green FA (1979) Joint scintiscans: present status. J Rheumatol 6: 370–376

Greyson ND (1980) Radionuclide bone and joint imaging in rheumatology. Bull Rheum 30: 1034–1049

Greyson ND, Tepperman PS (1984) Three-phase bone scans in hemiplegia with reflex sympathetic dystrophy and the effect of disuse. J Nucl Med 25: 423–429

Hays MT, Green FA (1972) The pertechnetate joint scan: timing. Ann Rheum Dis 31: 272–281

Helfgott S, Rosenthall L, Esdaile J, Tannenbaum H (1982) Generalised skeletal response to Tc-99m-MDP in rheumatoid arthritis. J Rheumatol 9: 939–941

Heyman S, Goldstein HA, Crowley W, Treves S (1980) The scintigraphic evaluation of hip pain in children. Clin Nucl Med 5: 109–115

Holder LE, Mackinnon SE (1984) Reflex sympathetic dystrophy in the hands. Clinical and scintigraphic criteria. Radiology 152: 517–522

Holopainen T, Rekonen A (1966) Uptake of radioactive strontium (Sr-85) in joints damaged by rheumatoid arthritis disease. Acta Rheum Scand 12: 102–108

Jeremy R, Cato J, Scott BW (1969) Investigation of bone and joint disease using 18-fluorine. Med J Aust 1: 492–499

Johansen JP, Fossgreen J, Hansen HH (1980) Bone scanning in lumbar disc herniation. Acta Orthop Scand 51: 617–620

Kipper MS, Alazraki NP, Feiglin DH (1982) The "hot" patella. Clin Nucl Med 7: 28–30

Kloiber R, Parlosky N, Portner O, Gartke K (1983) Bone scintigraphy of hip joint effusions in children. AJR 140: 995–999

Kozin F, McCarty D, Sims J, Genant H (1976) The reflex sympathetic dystrophy syndrome. Am J Med 60: 321–331

Kozin F, Soin JS, Ryan LM, Carrera GF, Wortmann RL (1981) Bone scintigraphy in the reflex sympathetic dystrophy syndrome. Radiology 138: 437–443

Lagier R (1983) partial algodystrophy of the knee. J Rheumatol 10: 255–260

Lentle BC, Russell AS, Percy JS, Jackson FI (1977) Scintigraphic findings in ankylosing spondylitis. J Nucl Med 18: 524–528

Lin D, Alavi A, Dalinka M (1981) Bone scan evaluation of patellar activity. Int J Nucl Med Biol 8: 105–109

Lin MS, Fawcett HD, Goodwin DA (1980) Bone scintigraphy demonstrating arthropathy of central joints in ankylosing spondylitis. Clin Nucl Med 5: 364–366

Mackinnon SE, Holder LE (1984) The use of three-phase radionuclide bone scanning in the diagnosis of reflex sympathetic dystrophy. J Hand Surg 9: 556–563

Martinez-Villasenor D, Katona G (1968) Scintigraphy by means of radioisotopes of short half-life for diagnosing diseases of the joints. In: Medical radioisotope scintigraphy, vol 2. International Atomic Energy Agency, Vienna, pp 295–305

Maxfield WS, Weiss TE, Tutton RH, Hidalgo JU (1968) Detection of arthritis by joint scanning. In: Medical radioisoptope scintigraphy, vol 2. International Atomic Energy Agency, Vienna, pp 307–323

Maxfield WS, Weiss TE, Schuler SE (1972) Synovial membrane scanning in arthritic disease. Semin Nucl Med 2: 50–70

McCall IW, Sheppard H, Haddaway M, Park WM, Ward DJ (1983) Gallium-67 scanning in rheumatoid arthritis. Br J Radiol 56: 241–243

Murray IP (1980) Bone scanning in the child and young adult. Skeletal Radiol 5: 65–76

Namey TC, McIntyre J, Buse M, LeRoy EC (1977) Nucleographic studies of axial spondylarthritides. Quantitative sacroiliac scintigraphy in early HLA-B27 associated sacroiliitis. Arthritis Rheum 20: 1058–1064

Norbjerg M, Heerfordt J, Dissing I, Jensen M, Moller J, Sneppen O (1980) Numerical assessment of asymmetry at scintigraphy of normal joints pairs. Acta Radiol [Diagn] (Stockh) 21: 235–238

O'Duffy JD, Wahner HW, Hunder GG (1976) Joint imaging in

polymyalgia rheumatica. Mayo Clin Proc 51 : 519–524

O'Mara RE, Pinals RS (1970) Bone scanning in regional migratory osteoporosis. Radiology 97 : 579–581

Paquin J, Rosenthall L, Esdaile J, Warshawski R, Damtew B (1983) Elevated uptake of Tc-99m methylene diphosphonate in the axial skeleton in ankylosing spondylitis and Reiter's disease: implications for quantitative sacroiliac scintigraphy. Arthritis Rheum 26 : 217–220

Park H, Terman SA, Ridolfo AS, Wellman HN (1977) A quantitative evaluation of rheumatic activity with Tc-99m-EHDP. J Nucl Med 18 : 973–976

Resnick D, Williamson S, Alazraki NP (1981) Focal spinal abnormalities on bone scans in ankylosing spondylitis: a clue to the presence of fracture or pseudoarthrosis. Clin Nucl Med 6 : 213–217

Rosenspire KC, Kennedy AC, Russomano L, Steinbach J, Blau M, Green FA (1980a) Comparison of four methods of analysis of TC-99m pyrophosphate uptake in rheumatoid arthritic joints. J Rheumatol 7 : 461–468

Rosenspire KC, Kennedy AC, Steinbeck J, Blau M, Green FA (1980b) Investigation of the metabolic activity of bone in rheumatoid arthritis. J Rheumatol 7 : 469–473

Rosenspire KC, Blau M, Kennedy AC, Green FA (1981) Assessment and interpretation of radiopharmaceutical joint imaging in an animal model of arthritis. Arthritis Rheum 24 : 711–716

Rozenbaum M, Zenman C, Nagler A, Pollack S (1984) Transient osteoporosis of the hip joint with liver cirrhosis. J Rheumatol 11 : 241–243

Russell, AS, Lentle BC, Percy JS (1975) Investigation of sacroiliac disease: comparative evaluation of radiological and radionuclide techniques. J Rheumatol 2 : 45–51

Sewell JR, Black CN, Chapman AH, Statham AH, Hughes GRV, Lavender JP (1980) Quantitative scintigraphy in diagnosis and management of plantar fasciitis. J Nucl Med 21 : 633–636

Shearman J, Esdaile J, Rosenthall L, Hawkins D (1982) Predictive value of radionuclide joint scans. Arthritis Rheum 25 : 83–86

Simon H, Carlson DH (1980) The use of bone scanning in the diagnosis of reflex sympathetic dystrophy. Clin Nucl Med 5 : 116–121

Spencer DG, Adams FG, Horton PW, Buchanan WW (1979) Scintiscanning in ankylosing spondylitis: a clinical radiological and quantitative study. J Rheumatol 6 : 426–431

Steven MM, Sturrock RD, Fogelman I, Smith ML (1982) Whole body retention of diphosphonate in rheumatoid arthritis. J Rheumatol 9 : 873–877

Strashun A, Chayes Z (1979) Migratory osteolysis. J Nucl Med 20 : 129–132

Sutherland AD, Savage JP, Patterson DC, Foster BK (1980) The nuclide bone scan in the diagnosis and management of Perthes' disease. J Bone Joint Surg [Br] 62 : 300–306

Tannenbaum H, Esdaile J, Rosenthall L (1980) Joint imaging in regional migratory osteoporosis. J Rheumatol 7 : 237–244

Tannenbaum H, Rosenthall L, Greenspoon M, Ramelson H (1984) Quantitative joint imaging using gallium-67 citrate in a rabbit model of zymosan induced arthritis. J Rheumatol 11 : 687–691

Tannenbaum H, Rosenthall L, Arzoumanian A (1986) Quantitative scintigraphy in patients with rheumatoid arthritis. J Rheumatol (in press)

Thomas RH, Resnick D, Alazraki NP, Daniel D, Greenfield R (1975) Compartmental evaluation of osteoarthritis of the knee. Radiology 16 : 585–592

Vyas K, Eklem M, Seto H, Bobba VR, Brown P, Haines J, Krishnamurthy GT (1981) Quantitative scintigraphy of sacroiliac joints: effect of age, gender and laterality. AJR 136 : 589–592

Weisberg DL, Resnick D, Taylor A, Becker M, Alazraki N (1978) RA and its variants: analysis of scintiphotographic, radiologic and clinical examinations. Am J Roentgenol Radium Ther Nucl Med 131 : 655–673

Weiss TE, Maxfield WS, Murison PJ, Tutton RH, Hidalgo RH (1965) Iodinated human serum albumin (I-131) localization studies of rheumatoid arthritis joints by scintillation scanning. Arthritis Rheum 8 : 976–987

12 · The Bone Scan in Avascular Necrosis

L. Rosenthall

Introduction

The histological features of osteonecrosis are death of the osteocyte and the cellular elements in the adjacent marrow. Most investigators concede that the stage immediately preceding cellular demise is the interruption of the blood supply. The debate centres around the evolution of events that lead to the end stages of ischaemia and necrosis. The list of conditions associated with ischaemic osteonecrosis is long and the aetiological connections are frequently tenuous. The list has been divided into definite and probable association (Ficat and Arlet 1980). Definite aetiological associations include major trauma, caisson disease, sickle cell disease, post-irradiation necrosis, necrosis of arterial origin, Gaucher's disease, frostbite and electrical injury. In these conditions the effect follows the cause, and their linkage and mechanism of bone death are not too controversial. More doubt surrounds the probable causes: minor trauma, exogenous corticosteroids, cancer chemotherapy, gout and hyperuricaemia, venous disease, bone dysplasia (particularly in the hip), lipid disturbances (including alcohol abuse), connective tissue disease (e.g. rheumatoid arthritis and systemic lupus erythematosus not treated with steroids), osteoporosis and osteomalacia. The nexus between osteonecrosis and probable cause is the higher incidence of necrosis in these conditions, but the mechanism of bone death production, as in corticosteroid therapy and alcohol abuse, is not settled. Idiopathic osteonecrosis of the capital femoral epiphysis (Legg–Perthes disease), head of the second or third metatarsal (Freiberg's disease), lunate (Kienbock's disease), medial end of the clavicle (Friedrich's disease), and many other locations are well recognised, but the causative factors are unknown.

Steroid-induced Osteonecrosis

Several hypotheses on the pathogenesis of steroid-induced osteonecrosis have been advanced, but all are disputed. One theory states that there is a continual process of microfracture and repair in normal bone. The suppression of osteoblastic activity by exogenous steroids retards the lamellar bone repair process, and, as the number of unhealed fractures increase, the bony structure weakens and finally collapses (McFarland and Frost 1961). Further support for this thesis was obtained from an exhaustive investigation of iliac crest bone histology in 77 adult patients with aseptic osteonecrosis of various bone sites and normal renal function. Nine patients, four of whom were alcoholics, had osteomalacia. The remaining 68 patients consisted of 15 who were treated with steroids, 29 alcoholics and 24 with no identifiable associated disorder other than primary osteoporosis; all of them depicted a common histomorphometric profile. There was a reduction in trabecular bone volume and in the thickness of osteoid seams, and dynamically in the calcification rate and in total labelled surfaces determined with tetracycline. This implied a reduction in osteoblastic appositional rate and in bone formation rate at the cell and tissue level, which could impair the healing of microfractures (Arlot et al. 1983). This has been criticised by reports that the microfractures have not always been found in osteonecrotic femoral heads, but the discrepancy may be due to the histological technique employed (Fisher 1978; Glimcher and Kenzora 1979). Routine histological techniques visualise the microcallus as evidence of microfracture, but special methods are required to visualise the microfracture directly, and these are seen to be more numerous in patients with osteonecrosis than in controls (Frost 1964).

A variation of this theory has been advanced to account for the high incidence of osteonecrosis in renal transplants. It is claimed that the persistent secondary hyperparathyroidism after homotransplantation, particularly in the presence of hypercalcaemia, causes trabecular erosion. Aggravated by steroid-induced osteoporosis and loss of pain sensitivity, the bone becomes susceptible to frac-

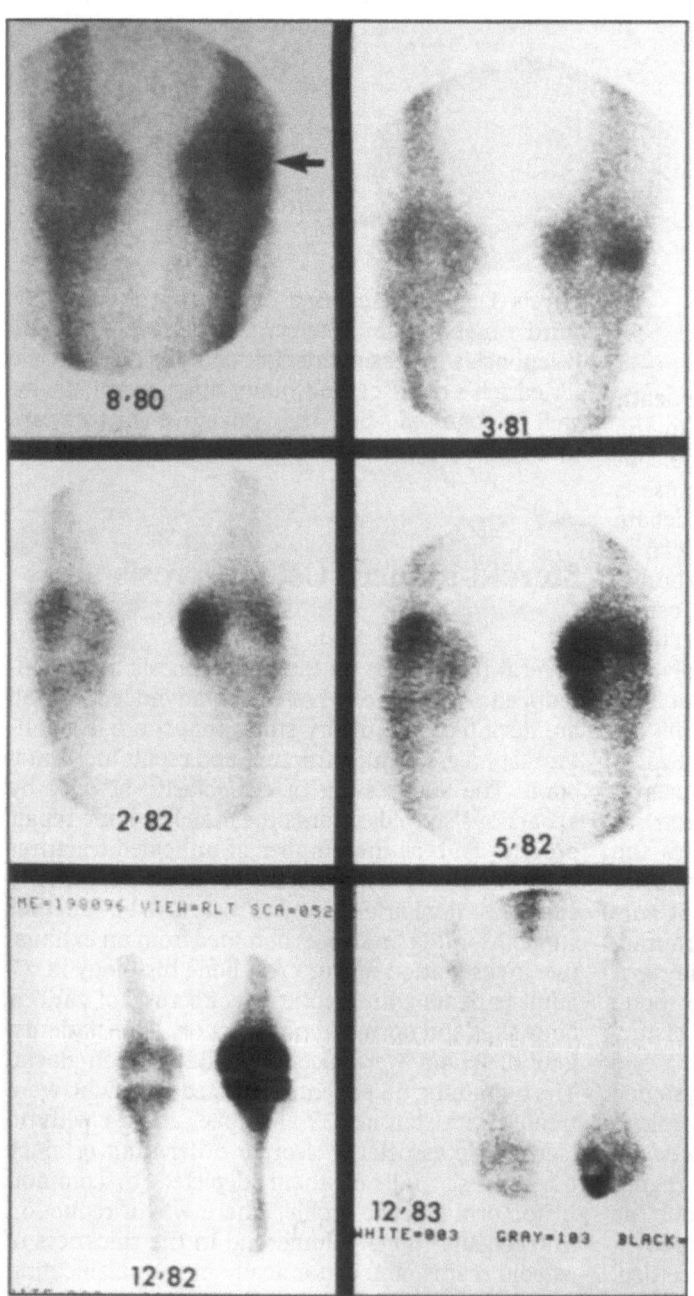

Fig. 12.1. Multiple areas of steroid-induced osteonecrosis in a renal transplant recipient. In August 1980 the patient presented with left knee pain. Radiophosphate demonstrated increased concentration in the left lateral femoral condyle (*arrow*). In March 1981 the intensity in the lateral condyle decreased, but the medial condyle exhibited enhanced uptake for the first time. Further intensification developed in the medial condyle in February 1982. In May 1982 the left medial tibial plateau exhibited evidence of osteonecrosis. Seven months later both femoral condyles and the entire tibial plateau showed hyperconcentration of radiophosphate. Soon afterwards a prosthesis was implanted in the medial compartment of the knee joint and a bone biopsy taken at the time confirmed the presence of necrosis. In December 1983 the left knee area was normal, except for persistent augmented accretion in the medial tibial plateau.

ture and necrosis at weight-bearing sites (Ibels et al. 1978). The hyperparathyroid aspect of the theory was invoked, because osteonecrosis occurs earlier in renal transplants than in patients receiving steroids for collagen-vascular diseases, and therefore could not be caused by steroids alone. Osteonecrosis is rare in primary hyperparathyroidism, and this implies that a synergism exists between hyperparathyroidism and exogenous steroids to promote the occurrence of osteonecrosis (Fig. 12.1). The microfracture theory is somewhat at odds with the hypothesis of ischaemia as the last stage before cell death. However, it is possible that the lesion that surrounds the fracture can obliterate the lumina of the adjacent vessels.

Several investigators claim to have found intravascular fat emboli in human bone involved with ischaemic necrosis (Cruess et al. 1968; Jones 1971). It is postulated that steroids produce fatty metamorphosis of the liver which release fat globules the size of emboli into the general circulation. Repeated showers of these fat emboli to the subchondral end-arteries are followed by intravascular coagulation, fibrin thrombus propagation, focal marrow necrosis, osteon anoxia and osteocytic death. Alcohol abuse also induces hepatic fatty metamorphosis and it is postulated to cause osteonecrosis by the same mechanism as steroids. This theory is still being argued. It is difficult to tell whether the observed intravascular fat caused the necrosis, or is the result of it, i.e. the bone collapse caused the extrusion of intramedullary fat into the Haversian canals (Solomon 1973).

It has been alleged that steroids can cause blood sludging, thrombosis or haemorrhage, and thereby produce bone death (Cosgriff 1951; Boettcher et al. 1970). Arterial occlusion secondary to a steroid-induced vasculitis has also been implicated (Kemper et al. 1957; Cruess et al. 1968). Neither notion has withstood histological scrutiny.

In an attempt to produce femoral head necrosis, growing and adult rabbits were subjected to large doses of cortisone over a 5-month interval. There was an increase in serum cholesterol and fatty metamorphosis of the liver, and fat emboli were seen to be partially obliterating the microcirculation of the subchondral vessels of the femoral head. The average diameter of the marrow fat cells was also increased, and this resulted in displacement of the myeloid tissue. This intramedullary lipocyte hypertrophy within a closed volume is postulated to cause compression of the vascular sinusoids, venous stasis, arterial insufficiency, ischaemia of dependent tissue, fat necrosis and finally bone necrosis, in that order; therefore it is an important primary pathogenetic mechanism in steroid-

associated osteonecrosis (Wang et al. 1977). Similar histological findings were seen in patients receiving large doses of corticosteroids, where the lipocyte increased 68% in area at the expense of the other myeloid elements (Solomon 1981). The early stages of fatty congestion, venous stasis and marrow necrosis may be unsymptomatic and depict normal radiographic images. Measurements of intramedullary pressure at this stage are either elevated, show an abnormally high pressure increase in response to an intramedullary saline infusion, or both. A decompression procedure has been advocated which involves the removal of a 10-cm core of bone from the femoral head and neck in order to relieve the vascular congestion and preclude necrosis. This bone forage technique is most effective in the preclinical or early radiographic stages of the disease before femoral head deformity sets in (Hungerford and Zizic 1980; Zizic et al. 1980).

The first definite radiographic sign of femoral head steroid-induced osteonecrosis is a thin linear subchondral lucency (crescent sign), and it represents fracture through dead bone (Fig. 12.2). Patchy increase in density reflects reactive new bone formation and is a late manifestation of the disease, sometimes occurring several years after bone death (Glimcher and Kenzora 1978).

Disclosure of the early pathological changes is necessary in order to preclude the development of femoral head deformity and articular complications. Intraosseous venography will show a decreased washout and reflux along the shaft when contrast agent is injected into a diseased site, if the intramedullary pressure is elevated. The intraosseous saline infusion stress test will also be abnormal under these circumstances. Both modalities are invasive and not practical for routine study, even in high-risk patients. Radiocolloid imaging is theoretically attractive, because the test agent concentrates in the reticuloendothelial system, and in the course of events the decrease in myeloid elements antedates intramedullary hypertension, ischaemia and bone death. However, it can only be utilised when the area of interest contains myeloid, such as the proximal femur, but not the femoral condyles. There is also a variation in normal uptake of radiocolloid in the femoral heads. In 200 patients with no predisposing factor to osteonecrosis, the femoral heads were visualised bilaterally with ^{99m}Tc sulphur colloid in only 70% (Webber and Wagner 1973). Another study related that half the femoral head-pairs were not visualised (Spencer et al. 1982). This evidence weighs heavily against the usefulness of radiocolloid to disclose potential or impending bone death. When there is gross asymmetry between the femoral heads, then the diagnostic con-

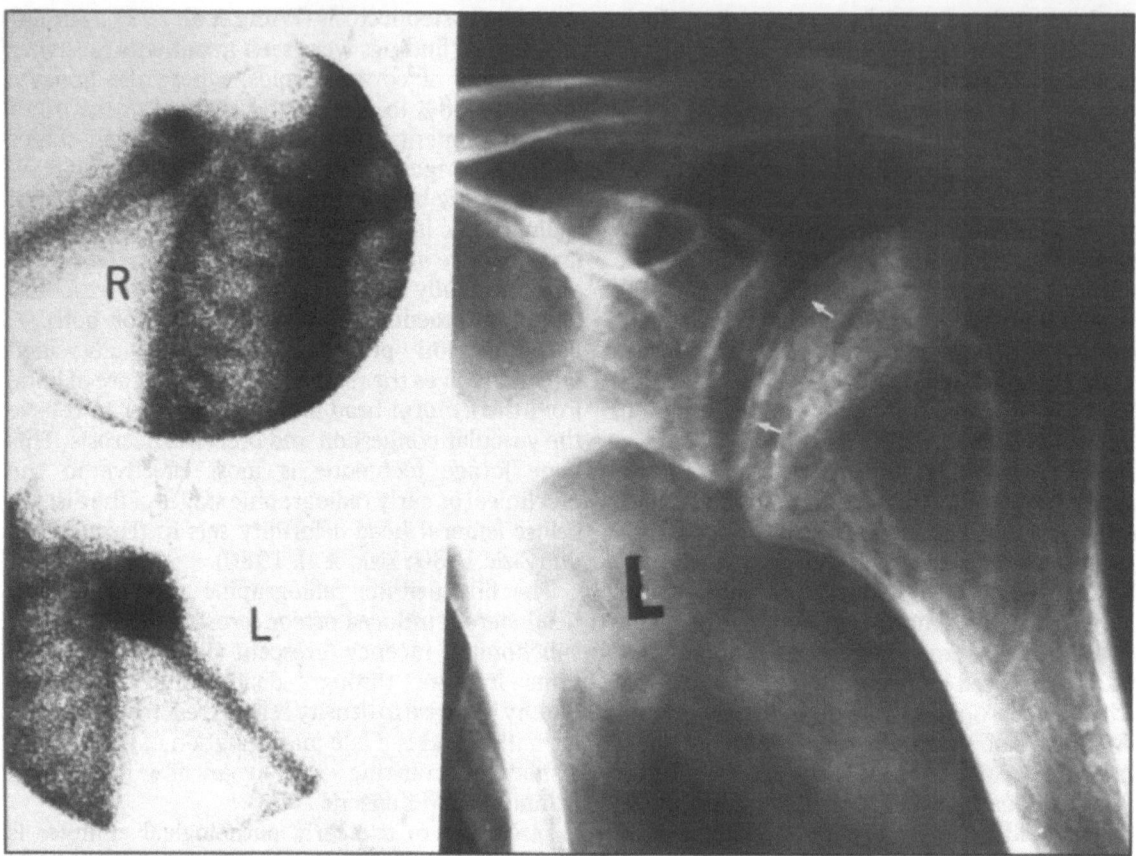

Fig. 12.2. Steroid-induced osteonecrosis of the left humeral head. The radiophosphate uptake in the area is increased and the radiograph shows the late features of necrosis, viz. flattening of the contour, sclerosis and a linear subchondral fracture (*arrows*).

fidence level for unilateral disease is high. Better candidates for radiocolloid imaging are children, who normally have more abundant myeloid tissue in the proximal femurs, and adults with blood dyscrasias and peripheral expansion of the red marrow. The use of a smaller particle size may improve the visualisation of the femoral heads in adults, because it has been shown that colloids one-tenth the size of sulphur colloid have a threefold greater concentration in the marrow (Kloiber et al. 1981).

Radiophosphate imaging is generally used to disclose steroid-induced osteonecrosis. Avascular bone is seen as a photon-deficient zone, and the repair process as hyperconcentration. These portrayals may antedate radiographic stigmata of osteonecrosis by several months. The photon-deficient phase is not often seen in practice, unless high-risk patients are scanned routinely before they are symptomatic. One such study on renal transplant recipients showed that photon-deficient femoral heads were not uncommon before the onset of symptoms (Hull et al. 1979). Two cases were described of photon-deficiency in the femoral condyle

and tibial plateau which progressed to hyperconcentration. One of the patients complained of knee pain during the photon-deficient phase, whereas the other did not (Burt and Mathews 1982). With high-quality images combined increased and decreased concentrations can be resolved in the intermediate phases of osteonecrosis repair (Fig. 12.3). If the osteonecrosis consists of a thin subchondral band, then the photon deficiency will probably escape detection with radiophosphate and only the reactive hyperconcentration will be seen.

Drug-induced Osteonecrosis

Drugs other than steroids have been implicated in the causation of osteonecrosis. There is an alleged association between malignant lymphoma (preponderantly Hodgkin's disease) and bone

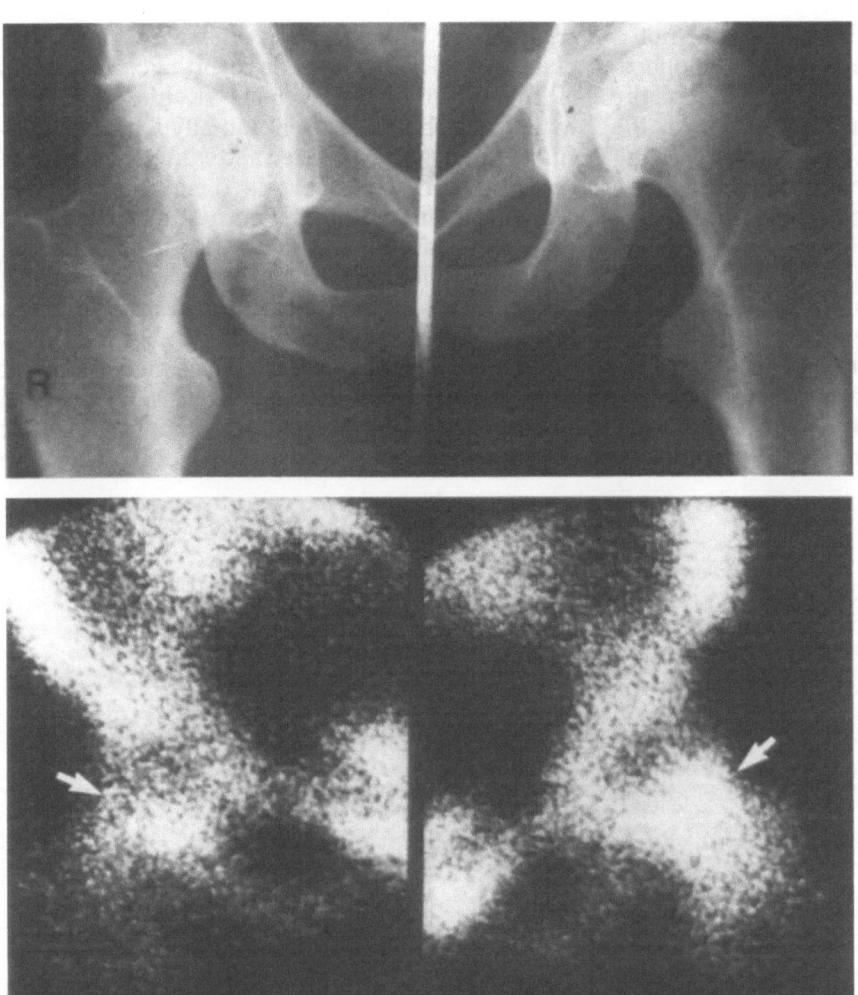

Fig. 12.3. Bilateral steroid-induced osteonecrosis of the femoral heads. This patient had been on steroids for treatment of lupus erythematosus. She complained of bilateral hip pain, but the radiographs of the hips were normal (*above*). Corresponding radiophosphate scans (*below*) demonstrated increased concentration in the femoral necks (*arrows*). She later required bilateral total hip arthroplasties. The increased concentration represents the healing response. There is probably photon deficiency in part of the femoral heads, but this is obscured by the encompassing acetabuli.

necrosis, but no definite evidence exists to prove that the lymphoma itself predisposes to the condition (Thorne et al. 1981; Editorial 1982; Harper et al. 1984). The avascular femoral heads that were removed were not infiltrated with lymphoma, but all patients had courses of steroids and other chemotherapeutic agents such as vincristine, alkylating agents and procarbazine. The steroid doses were not high, and perhaps the other drugs catalysed the propensity of the steroid to induce osteonecrosis. However, osteonecrosis has been reported with bleomycin, cyclophosphamide, methotrexate and 5-fluorouracil in the absence of steroids. The rare case of osteonecrosis developing during pregnancy has been reported (McGuigan and Fleming 1983). The radiophosphate manifestation is that of increased uptake in the affected region of bone.

Idiopathic Osteonecrosis

Idiopathic epiphyseal/metaphyseal bone necrosis has been described in about 30 different sites. Some of these were later shown to be developmental or congenital defects or normal variants and not a result of ischaemia and necrosis. The radiophosphate images are variable and are contingent on the size of the lesion, time of imaging relative to the onset of the disease, and probably the underlying pathogenesis, e.g. microfracture and secondary necrosis, or ischaemia secondary to elevated intramedullary pressure. The early stages of Legg–Perthes disease is readily seen as a photon-deficient zone. Osteochondritis dissecans invariably presents as a focus of increased uptake which represents the reactive process, while the button of separated dead bone is too small to be resolved as a photon-deficient focus. Osteonecrosis of the heads of the second or third metatarsals (Freiberg's disease) have all been reported as demonstrating increased radiophosphate only. There is a single report of osteonecrosis of the tarsal navicular bone (Kohler's disease), which was photon deficient initially while the concurrent radiograph depicted flattening, sclerosis and fragmentation. On follow-up 6 months later the concentration returned to normal and there was some reconstitution of the bone on the radiograph (McCauley and Kahn 1977). Necrosis of the medial end of the clavicle (Friedrich's disease) exhibits increased uptake of radiophosphate (Fig. 12.4).

Spontaneous osteonecrosis of the medial femoral condyle and medial tibial plateau are well-defined clinical and pathological entities (Houpt et al. 1982; Greyson 1982; Aglietti et al. 1983). They are

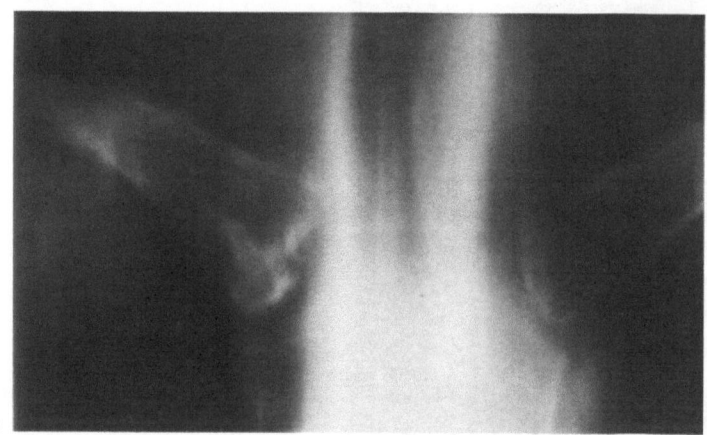

a

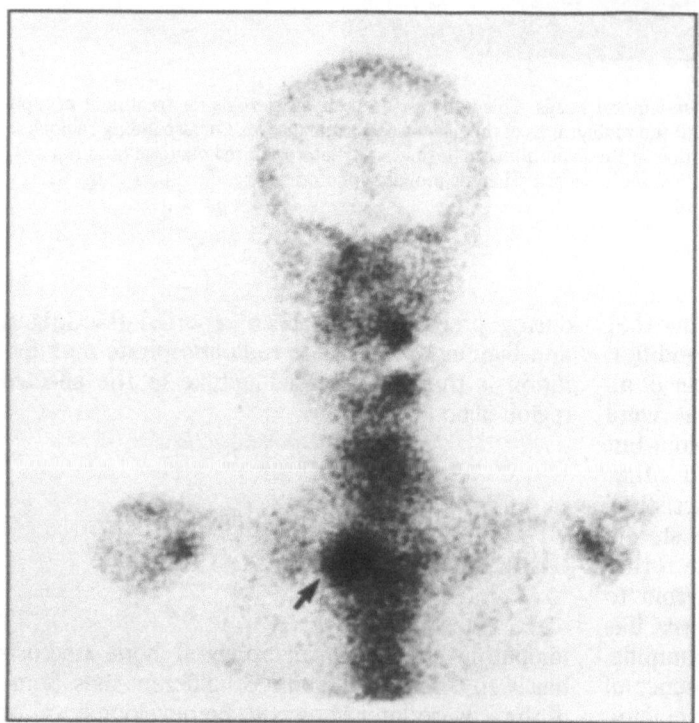

b

Fig. 12.4a,b. Osteonecrosis of the medial end of the right clavicle (Friedrich's disease) in a 75-year-old woman. She complained of sternoclavicular pain, and there was a mild swelling in the region. a The radiograph demonstrated sclerosis and irregularity of the medial cortex. b An intense focus of radiophosphate concentration appeared in the region, which by itself is non-specific (arrow). An open biopsy of the region showed fibrosis of the marrow and absence of osteocytes, i.e. necrosis.

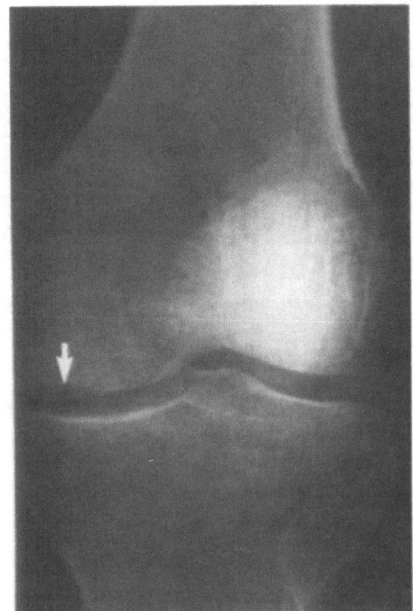
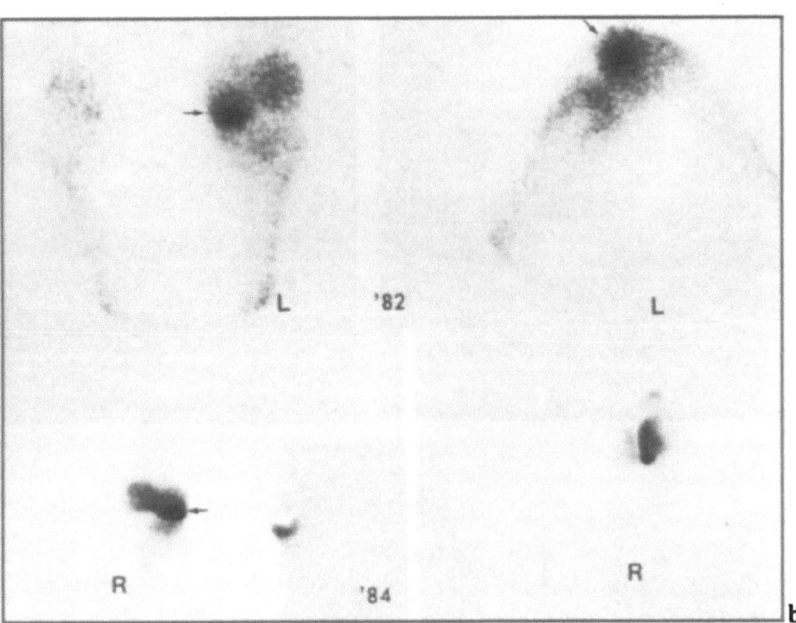

a   b

Fig. 12.5a,b. Spontaneous osteonecrosis of the medial femoral condyles 2 years apart in a 71-year-old woman. **a** The radiograph shows a cortical depression (*arrow*). The initial radiograph was normal at the time the radiophosphate scan was abnormal (3 months earlier). **b** Anterior and lateral radiophosphate scans. The initial episode in 1982 depicted intense concentration of tracer in the left medial femoral condyle (*arrows*). A knee prosthesis was implanted. Two years later, in 1984, spontaneous onset of pain occurred in the right medial femoral condyle and the radiophosphate scan was abnormal.

characterised by a sudden onset of knee pain and a later development of radiographic articular changes, similar to osteochondritis dissecans, on the weight-bearing surface. Unlike the latter, which occurs in a younger athletic age group, spontaneous osteonecrosis is an affliction of older people with a mean age of 65 years, with women outnumbering men by a factor of two to three. It also differs from steroid necrosis, which is not age and sex dependent, and occurs in either the medial or lateral knee compartments. Spontaneous osteonecrosis of the lateral compartment is an infrequent event. In the acute phase the radiophosphate perfusion, blood pool and delayed images are all abnormally high and remain so while healing is in progress. Later in the process, as the revascularisation subsides and remodelling sets in, the perfusion and blood pool phases tend towards normal, while the delayed views remain abnormal. The end result is complete radionuclide resolution or a picture simulating osteoarthritis, particularly if there are radiographic changes at the articular surface. Nucleographic abnormalities may antedate the radiographic changes by several months (Fig. 12.5). In fact, the process may resolve without ever producing radiographic changes (Lotke et al. 1977). The three-phase bone study is most useful in distinguishing spontaneous osteonecrosis from osteoarthritis; the latter demonstrates abnormal delayed views only. Regional

hyperaemia may cause enhanced uptake beyond the focus of necrosis on the same or both sides of the joint, but the intensity is maximal at the focus. The aetiology is not known.

Osteonecrosis Following Trauma

The femoral head is very susceptible to necrosis following femoral neck fractures. Displaced fractures run a greater risk of femoral head necrosis than do undisplaced fractures. In one report 40% of healed displaced fractures resulted in osteonecrosis when followed for at least 2 years, compared with 14% for healed undisplaced fractures. The incidence of absent blood flow to the femoral head immediately following fracture varies from 66% to 84%, which implies that about 50% of them revascularise without sequelae (Catto 1965). Posterior hip dislocations may also be complicated by ischaemia and necrosis. Radiography is not helpful in diagnosing avascular necrosis at its onset, because the telltale signs may be delayed by several months after an intracapsular fracture (Bayliss and Davidson 1977). There is a significant correlation between the degree of displacement of the femoral head and ischaemia,

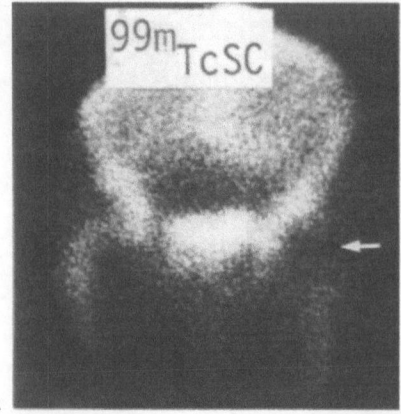
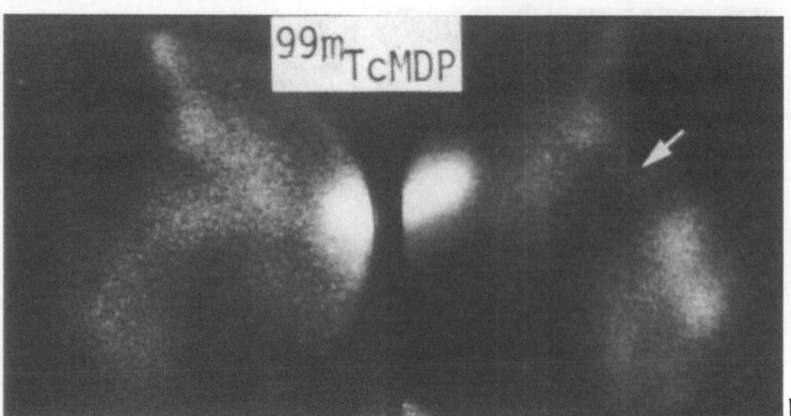

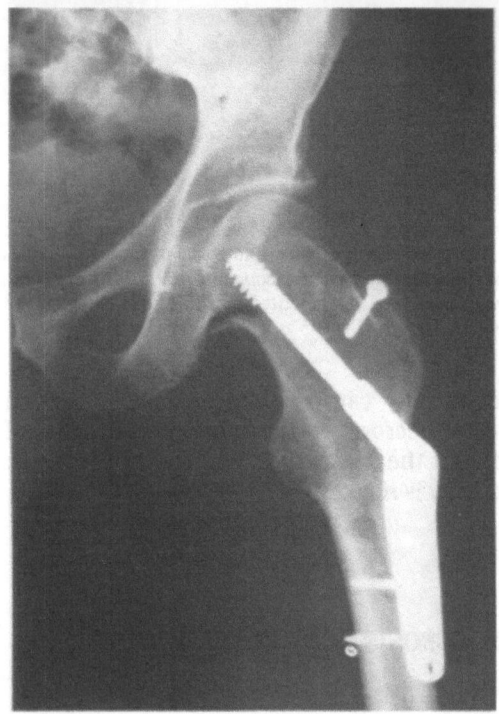

Fig. 12.6a–c. Avascular necrosis of the left femoral head treated by compression screw and side plate, and a posterior pedicle bone graft. a Preoperative 99mTc sulphur colloid scan depicting photon deficiency of the left femoral head (*arrow*). b Two days postoperatively the radiophosphate study showed photon deficiency of the femoral head and proximal portion of the femoral neck. The increased concentration in the greater trochanter was caused by excision of bone for grafting. c Postoperative radiograph showing the fixation and bone graft.

but it is of limited predictive value in the individual patient (Calandrucco and Anderson 1980). Earlier radionuclide methods for diagnosing ischaemia consisted of intravenous administration of ^{32}P followed by intraosseous measurement of its concentration, or intraosseous deposition of ^{133}Xe, ^{131}I albumin, ^{131}I antipyrine or ^{24}Na, followed by external monitoring of their washout. None of these gained favour because they proved to be less simple and efficacious than anticipated.

Bone- and marrow-seeking radiopharmaceuticals are potentially more valuable, because they do not entail operative intervention. ^{18}F was shown to have the same distribution as tetracycline in both vascular and avascular heads (Stadalnik et al. 1975). Radiophosphate deposition is primarily a

function of the integrity of the local microvasculature, as is the uptake of radiocolloid by the reticuloendothelial cells of the marrow. High-resolution external imaging with these tracers provides information on the vascular status of the femoral heads (Figs. 12.6, 12.7).

^{32}P autoradiography in a series of 113 femoral head specimens from subcapital fractures of less than 2 weeks' duration showed that 47% were segmentally, not uniformly, ischaemic. Potentially, this group could depict various degrees of reduced, but not absent, uptake, unless the photon-deficient focus is resolvable by the equipment. Numerical ratios of the radiophosphate uptake in the involved femoral head to the normal contralateral side have been advocated as an improvement over visual

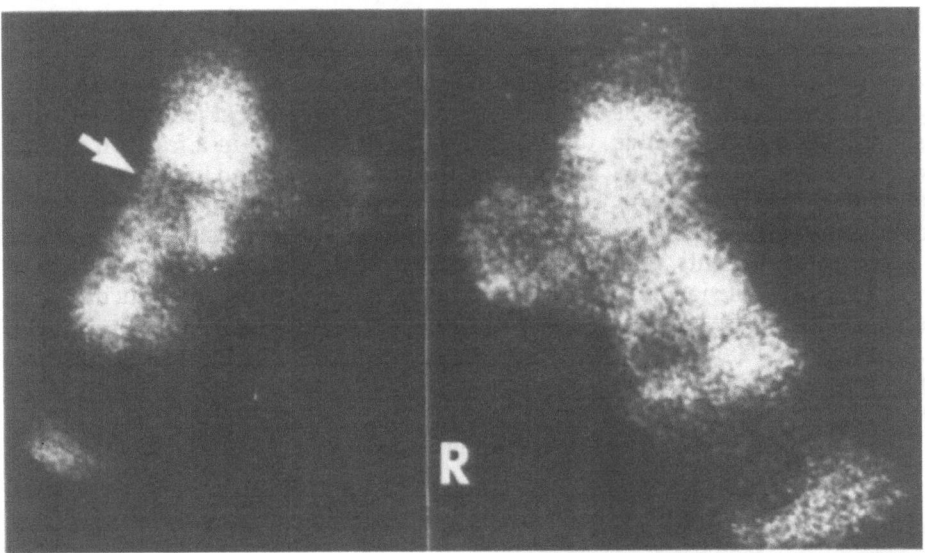

Fig. 12.7. Osteonecrosis of the left talus. This teenager sustained a talar neck fracture as a result of a fall. The radiophosphate scan demonstrated photon deficiency (*arrow*).

assessment and as a means of monitoring progress of repair (Bauer et al. 1980; Stromqvist et al. 1984). Less than half the activity monitored over a normal femoral head has been shown to be emitted from the head itself; most of the radiation emanates from the soft tissues anterior and posterior to the head. Trauma induces a regional hyperaemia which includes the soft tissues. During the first 48 h the elevated soft tissue background of radiophosphate may obfuscate the femoral head ischaemia, particularly if it is segmental, and thereby cause a falsely negative interpretation.

Radiocolloid imaging for viability of the femoral head has been claimed to be superior to radiophosphate within the first 24 h of the fracture. This is based on the observation that the death of the myeloid elements precedes osteocytic death by up to several days (Catto 1965). A rabbit model consisting of subcapital osteotomy and division of the ligamentum teres demonstrated absent uptake of 99mTc antimony colloid in all animals within 24 h, whereas a small subset which also received radiophosphate showed no reduction in uptake. In a patient study the accuracy of 99mTc sulphur colloid imaging was reported to be 95% as confirmed by histological findings and clinical course (Meyers et al. 1977). Using 99mTc antimony colloid, the presence or absence of femoral head uptake preoperatively predicted normal healing or subsequent osteonecrosis, respectively, in 28 out of 30 (93%) patients who were followed for a maximum of 2 years (Turner 1983). This implies that a preoperative finding of absent femoral head uptake

indicates no chance of healing normally—an arguable deduction. One of the factors governing the radiophosphate uptake in bone is blood flow; however, even though the osteocyte is known to survive for a time after ischaemia, this should not override the lack of normal delivery to the area and present a falsely positive indication of bone viability. Perhaps there is a radiophosphate photon deficiency of the femoral head that is being obscured by the traumatic soft tissue hyperaemia in the immediate area during the initial 24–48 h. Conversely, it has been shown in an experimental bone graft revascularisation study that radiophosphate uptake corresponded spatially to the neovasculature and that it could take place in the absence of live osteocytes; it was strictly a chemical adsorption process onto the apatite crystal (Bos 1979). In other words, it was flow limited. Good correlations between external radiophosphate femoral head count ratios, bone biopsy assay of radiophosphate and intravital bone staining with tetracycline in fresh subcapital fractures in patients has been reported (Stromqvist et al. 1984). Many authors are sceptical about the validity of radiocolloid imaging, because of the variation in the number of reticuloendothelial cells in the femoral head, particularly in the older age group. While it is true that three to four times more marrow uptake is achieved with small colloid sizes, such as antimony colloid, which is a factor of 10 to 20 smaller than sulphur colloid, the dearth of reticuloendothelial cells is a limiting factor. A definitive crossover study between the two radiopharmaceuticals is yet to be done.

It has been shown that femoral heads that are visualised as vascular by radiophosphate preoperatively may become avascular after reduction and nailing, implicating the surgical procedure as the cause. This is a reason to obtain postoperative images for a more realistic assessment of the status of the femoral head. Radiocolloid is at a disadvantage here, because the orthopaedic nail replaces part of the marrow. In one series of 15 patients with ischaemic femoral heads, normal perfusion and blood pool images were obtained in 3 in the immediate perioperative period, whereas the delayed views were all abnormal. This was attributed to the regional traumatic soft tissue hyperaemia (Bauer et al. 1980).

The controversy over the relative merits of radiocolloid and radiophosphate, or whether these studies are indicated, rests largely on the philosophy of management of transcervical femoral fractures. If the disclosure of ischaemia in a fracture dictates removal of the femoral head and implantation of an endoprosthesis as opposed to reduction and fixation, then selection of the most sensitive test is mandatory. On the other hand, if the tendency is to reduce and fix all fractures, particularly in the younger age group, then nucleography is redundant, except perhaps sometimes in the postoperative period to document the vascularity of the femoral head. If the degree of displacement is a determining factor, radiography is all that is needed.

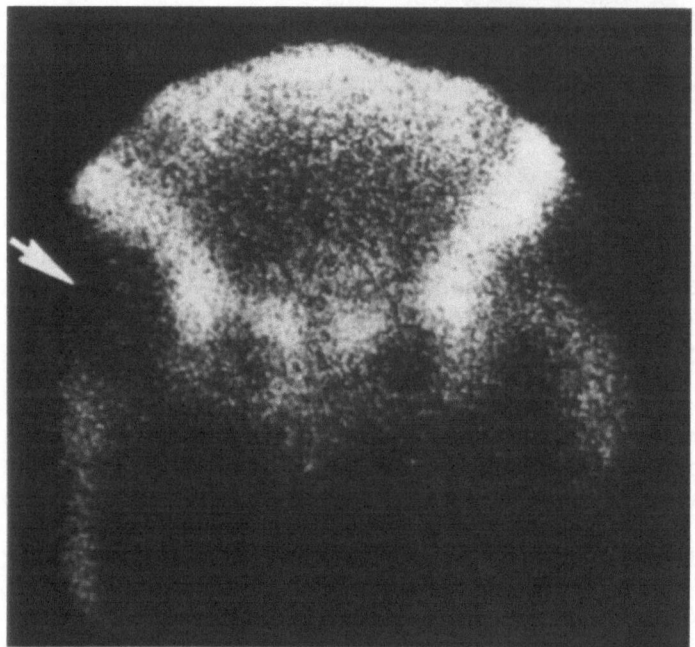

a

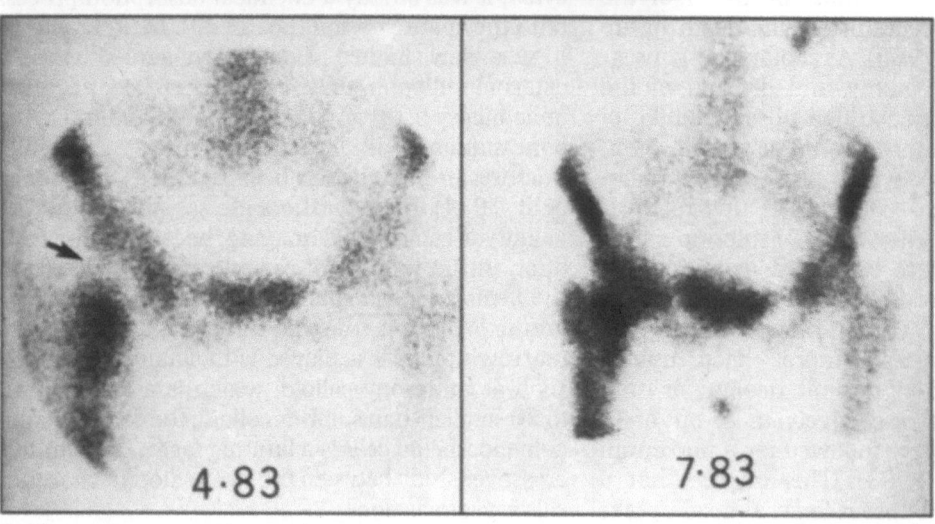

b

Fig. 12.8a,b. Osteonecrosis and revascularisation of a femoral head. This elderly woman fell and suffered a left femoral neck fracture. It was reduced and fixed with pins. a Preoperative ^{99m}Tc sulphur colloid scan demonstrates the avascular left femoral head (*arrow*). b Preoperative radiophosphate scan (April 1983) also shows photon deficiency in the left femoral head (*arrow*). Three months later (July 1983) the head has revascularised. There is increased intensity at the fracture line, which is undergoing remodelling.

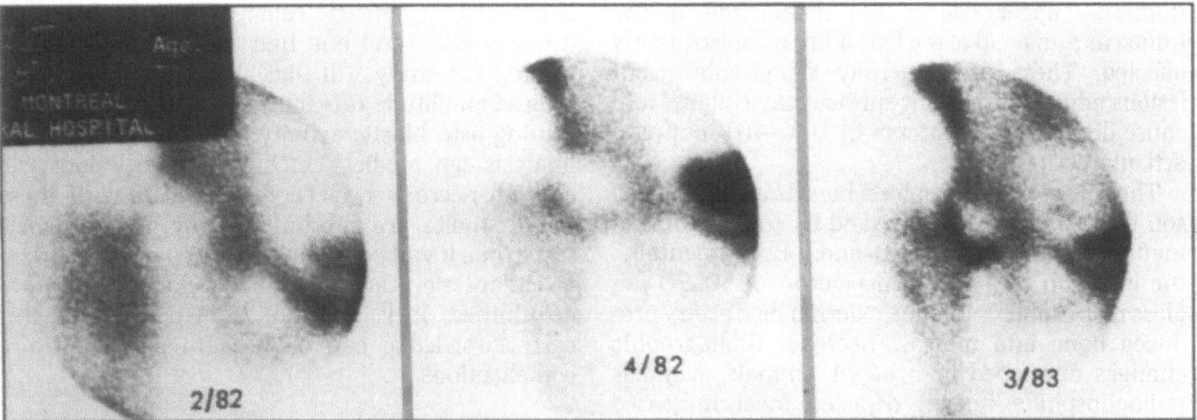

Fig. 12.9. Aborted revascularisation of the femoral head following a transcervical fracture. In February 1982 the patient sustained a fracture, and the radiophosphate scan the following day demonstrated an avascular head. This was reduced and fixed with five Knowles pins. Two months later (April 1982) there was no appreciable revascularisation. In March 1983 only a small curvilinear segment of the femoral head depicted creeping substitution. The head was removed and replaced with an endoprosthesis. Histologically the head was dead, and a barrier of fibrocartilage separated it from the femoral neck.

Arthroplasty has its complications and the long-term results are poor, although it can always be used if healing is complicated by necrosis after reduction and fixation. A survey showed a 20% 6-month mortality in elderly patients and an incidence of good results in only 28% of those treated by primary prosthetic arthroplasty (Hunter 1980). There is also some debate about the value of supplementing reduction and fixation with a posterior pedicle bone graft. a more lengthy operative procedure. Allegedly, it reduces the incidence of osteonecrosis following ischaemia in displaced fractures, but this has to be confirmed. The preoperative role of radionuclide imaging is yet to be defined and it will vary with the institution.

Revascularisation of an ischaemic head is seen as a progressive inroad of radiophosphate deposition, commencing at the fracture line. In an uncomplicated course revascularisation and disappearance of the photon-deficient zone are completed in about 3 months (Fig. 12.8). This can be frustrated by the development of a fibrocartilagenous barrier which halts the healing process and encourages collapse and deformation of the articular surface of the femoral head. It provides a mixed picture of persistent photon deficiency and adjacent hyper-concentration of radiophosphate (Fig. 12.9).

Caisson Disease

The commonly held theory of causation of caisson disease, viz. bone necrosis caused by infarction from gas bubbles appearing during decompression and interfering with the blood supply to bone, is being questioned (McCallum 1984). Large areas of bone are often infarcted, which implies that a large vessel or several medium-sized vessels are occluded by gas bubbles of considerable size. Also, infarctions in other parts of the body, e.g. liver, spleen and kidney, do not occur. This restriction to bone suggests a mechanism that must be rationalised in terms of the peculiarities of the osseous anatomy. It has been reported that there is a decrease in blood flow in the bones of animals during exposure to compressed air. Exposing fat cells to similar conditions increased their size, presumably as a result of oxygen toxicity. The mechanism propounded is somewhat similar to that of steroid-induced osteonecrosis; an increase in fat cell size within the rigid intraosseous extra-vascular compartment, venous compression and congestion, reduction in blood flow and inhibition of the clearance of gas from the marrow during decompression, which somehow contributes to the onset of necrosis (Pooley and Walder 1980; Gregg et al. 1980). Other proffered mechanisms include fat embolism, intravascular erythrocyte agglutination, platelet thrombi and the osmotic effect of gas dissolved in the tissues. None have gained acceptance.

The radiographic incidence of bone necrosis in divers, in one or more sites, is 4%. In descending order, the lower end of the femur, head of the humerus, upper end of the tibia, shaft of the humerus and head of the femur are most frequently affected. These are generally symptomless, but lesions adjacent to a joint surface may collapse and cause disability. This occurs in 10%–40% of juxta-articular lesions.

The role of radiophosphate bone imaging in caisson disease is under study, and its contribution to management is not fully defined. Experimentally, the injection of a saline suspension of 50–70 μm glass microspheres into the external iliac artery produced bone and marrow necrosis. Radiographic changes developed in 2 of 14 animals, whereas radiophosphate images depicted focal increased uptake in 12 of the 14 animals 3 weeks after vascular blockage. The increased uptake persisted for 3 months. No mention was made of the radiophosphate portrayal soon after the vascular occlusion, so that it is not known whether the hyperconcentration was preceded by photon deficiency (Gregg and Walder 1980). Biopsy of the areas exhibiting focal accretion showed the typical picture of bone and marrow necrosis. It was concluded that bone scintigraphy was more sensitive than radiography.

Radiophosphate bone scans in divers were found to be abnormal as early as a few days after decompression. About 18% of the lesions progressed to produce visible changes on the radiograph, and those that did were usually smaller in area on the radiograph than on the scan. The radiographic appearance is most often of sclerosis, but a mixed pattern of sclerosis and lucency can also occur. In a study of 12 men who ceased working in a hyperbaric environment for at least 10 years it was found that the radiographic lesions changed very little with time. Ten men had 18 sites of increased focal accretion by radiophosphate imaging, and some of these were not detected by radiography. It can be inferred that the healing process may continue for many years after the insult, whereas those lesions which appear radiographically sclerotic but normal on the radiophosphate bone scan are quiescent (Gregg and Walder 1981).

In a small series of eight divers it was found that parametric or functional radiophosphate imaging may be helpful in predicting which lesions will develop radiographic changes, or true unrevascularised osteonecrosis. Using a gamma camera and a computer program to image two rate constants, accretion and amplitude, functional images were produced. The amplitude images reflect osteoblastic activity and the accretion images relate the status of the microvasculature. Three patients had accretion rate images which depicted little or no increased intensity, i.e. a dearth of perfusion; two

eventually produced radiographic evidence of osteonecrosis; and one had these changes at the time of the study. All had abnormal delayed and intense amplitude rate images consistent with continuing osteoblastic activity. The claim is that this analysis can predict which bone scan lesions will develop necrosis (MacLeod et al. 1982). If these initial studies are substantiated by further experience then it will be possible to forecast which juxta-articular lesions are at risk of developing structural deformities. It is still not known whether this early knowledge can be used to prevent future complications.

Legg–Perthes Disease

The pathological evidence of Legg–Perthes disease is an osteonecrosis of the capital femoral epiphysis that may extend to the epiphyseal plate and metaphysis with secondary changes in contours of the acetabulum in a growing child. The aetiology is still obscure. It is believed to be vascular in origin, perhaps from multiple infarcts (Sanchis et al. 1973). Alterations in blood coagulability and a relatively insufficient blood supply to a growing epiphysis have also been suggested mechanisms. Transient synovitis is considered by some investigators to be a predisposing cause through a process of intracapsular tamponade and secondary ischaemia. In an experimental animal model in which the synovial cavity was filled with fluid under pressure it was shown that about 4 h of this intracapsular tamponade induced marrow cell death, whereas more than 6 h caused osteocyte and osteoblast death as well, although the vessels appeared histologically normal and their lumina remained patent (Kemp 1973). It is for this reason that immediate aspiration and decompression is advised for transient synovitis in order to reduce the duration of ischaemia, if it exists, and thereby forestall the onset of bone necrosis. Transient synovitis occurs equally in both sexes, but osteonecrosis is five times more prevalent in boys. The reason for this disparity is unknown.

Radiocolloid and radiophosphate are both capable of disclosing the ischaemia. High-resolution images with a pin-hole or convergent collimator, or electronic magnification are necessary for a detailed assessment of the distribution pattern. The entire femoral head is not always ischaemic; some may show quadrant involvement only (LaMont et al. 1981). The reparative process is visualised earlier

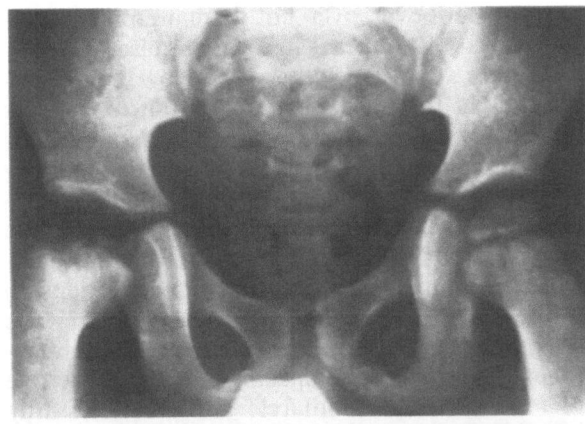

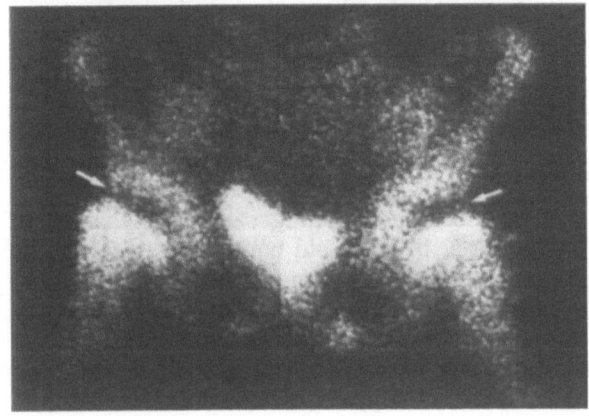

Fig. 12.10a,b. Bilateral Legg–Perthes disease. a The radiograph showed fragmentation and resorption of the left capital femoral epiphysis. An intact femoral epiphysis was seen on the left. b Bilateral avascular femoral epiphyses were depicted with the radiophosphate images (*arrows*).

with radiophosphate, because osteal repair antedates marrow repopulation.

Before revascularisation takes place the radiophosphate portrayal is that of photon deficiency involving all or part of the femoral head (Fig. 12.10). The manifestation of healing is hyperconcentration, and it begins at the periphery of the photopaenic zone, and progressively surrounds and invaginates the necrotic area. With complete uncomplicated repair, the femoral head uptake of radiophosphate returns to normal. The spatial deposition of radiophosphate reflects the areas of neovasculature penetration and creeping substitution.

The diagnostic sensitivity and specificity of radiophosphate imaging for Legg–Perthes disease are 0.98 and 0.95, respectively, compared with radiography, in which they are 0.92 and 0.78, respectively. An analysis of 147 patients with osteonecrosis demonstrated an association between the size of the radiophosphate zone of photopaenia and the sub-

sequent degree of radiographic deformity, i.e. epiphyseal flattening and fragmentation. In this series, the signs of radiophosphate healing preceded those of radiography by 3–6 months (Fisher et al. 1980). Radiophosphate scintigraphy was performed in 24 patients within 4 months of the onset of symptoms. In 18 patients out of 24 patients 20 hips developed Legg-Perthes disease, and all showed photon deficiency with radiophosphate, whereas 2 had normal radiographs at the initial examination. The remaining six patients had normal imaging studies throughout the follow-up period and were presumed to have had transient synovitis (Fasting et al. 1978). A true-positive frequency of 100% has also been reported in 59 patients with documented Legg–Perthes disease by utilising radiophosphate and a pin-hole collimator (Danigelis 1976).

Slipped Capital Femoral Epiphysis

Epiphyseal slippage is classified into three types: minimal slip, marked slip without osteonecrosis and marked slip with osteonecrosis. The cause of this disorder is conjectural, and it may be manifold. Severe trauma can doubtless produce a fracture through the growth plate and slipping of the epiphysis, but the usual history obtained is that of minimal or moderate trauma. Other predisposing conditions have been suggested and these include mechanical stress (Chung et al. 1976), biochemical disorders (Eisenstein and Rothschild 1976), hormonal abberrations (Harris 1950), inflammation (Howarth 1966), genetic abnormalities (Rennie 1967) and radiation therapy (Libshitz and Edeiken 1981). The site of fissure and slipping is the zone of hypertrophic chondrocytes of the growth plate; 40% of the patients present with bilateral involvement (Fig. 12.11). Both radiophosphate and radiocolloid can be used to determine the vascular integrity of the femoral head in this age group.

Sickle Cell Disease

The proposed pathogenic mechanism for infarction is occlusion of small vessels in marrow and bone by sickled cells. While any bone may be involved, weight-bearing areas of long bones adjacent to articular surfaces are most frequently affected. In 81 patients, it was found that the sites most often afflic-

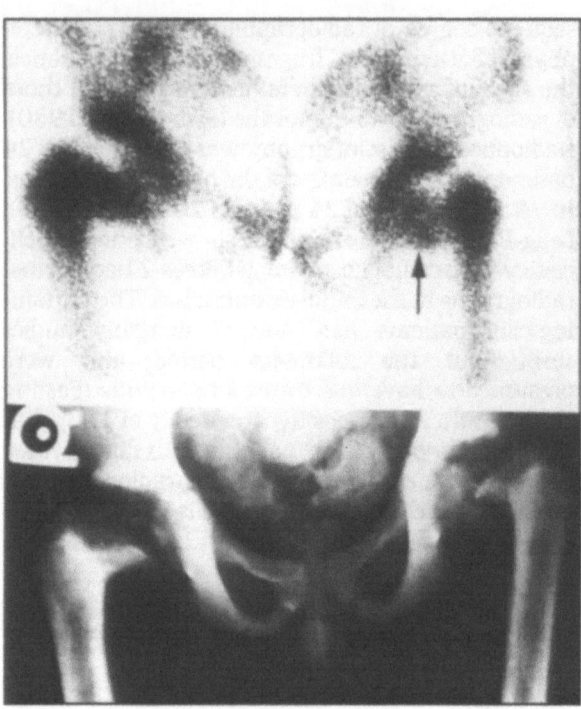

Fig. 12.11. Slipped epiphyses in a 5-year-old girl with hypophosphatasia and rickets. Radiograph (*below*) showed fragmentation and resorption of the right capital femoral epiphysis and marked slipping of the left epiphysis. Corresponding radiophosphate images (*above*) portrayed an absence of uptake in the right epiphysis, but there was concentration in the slipped left epiphysis, indicating viability (*arrow*).

ted, in descending order, were the femur, tibia, humerus, fibula, radius and ulna; 24% of the group had symmetrical infarcts (Bohrer 1970). Radiographic signs of ischaemic necrosis are either late in developing or may never appear at all and are therefore not helpful when the patient is in an acute crisis (Lutzker and Alavi 1976). The clinical presentation of sickle cell infarction is that of fever, acute localised bone pain and swelling of overlying soft tissues if periosteal bone is involved (Lukens 1981). These signs and symptoms are not dissimilar to those of osteomyelitis, and since an opportunistic osteomyelitis may complicate infarcted marrow and bone, an early differentiation of the two entities is required. To sort this out three radiopharmaceuticals have been utilised: radiocolloid to visualise the reticuloendothelial cells of the marrow, radiophosphate to identify the bone, and ^{67}Ga to delineate the septic tissue. ^{67}Ga is not ideal, because it has a normal propensity to concentrate in marrow and bone, but it has been used successfully when the relative uptakes in different parts of the bone are being considered. Indium-labelled white cells might be an

improvement over ^{67}Ga, but there are no substantive reports of its efficacy in sickle cell disease.

There is expansion of the red marrow into the distal ends of the appendicular skeleton in patients afflicted with sickle cell disease, and this broadens the application of radiocolloid imaging. A marrow infarct is seen as a photon-deficient zone in a radiocolloid image. In time an infarct may repopulate completely, partially or not at all. Therefore, disclosure of photon deficiency bears no relationship to the time of the event, unless there are previous studies for comparison, in which case an enlargement of the area of photopaenia is highly suggestive of a recent infarct. Infarcts are not necessarily accompanied by local symptoms; silent infarcts are known to occur. It is estimated that about 50% of patients imaged with ^{99m}Tc sulphur colloid during the asymptomatic period will manifest focal areas of decreased or absent radioactivity, probably representing fibrosis of previous infarctions (Alavi et al. 1974).

Radiophosphate imaging can identify a recent bone infarct, because old bone infarcts caused by sickle cell disease heal. Immediately after the onset of ischaemia there is a zone of photon deficiency (Fig. 12.12). This is followed by a repair process at the periphery which is reflected on the scan as a ring of hyperconcentration surrounding the photopaenic zone. With further progress the photopaenia disappears and the area exhibits a hyperconcentration which can be mistaken for osteomyelitis at this point of healing. At the end stage of repair the radiophosphate concentration is normal (Greyson and Kassel 1976).

The area of marrow infarction is usually larger than the bone component. Bone has a dual blood supply, endosteal and periosteal, and the presence of the latter probably minimises the extent of necrosis and hastens its repair. In a set of nine patients with uncomplicated bone infarctions, the ^{67}Ga portrayal was that of absent or decreased uptake within the first week of the insult, but the older ones were normal (Fig. 12.13). This normal uptake occurred even when the corresponding radiophosphate scans demonstrated hyperconcentration (Armas and Goldsmith 1984).

Osteomyelitis is an uncommon complication and it may occur as the primary event in sickle cell disease, or more likely develop as an opportunistic infection in an infarcted area. In either case it must be distinguished from a sickle cell crisis, because the treatment is different. There are no large radionuclide studies recorded from which to draw statistical conclusions, but from anecdotal reports there emerge several diagnostic portrayals using combinations of radiotracers. If the contentious area

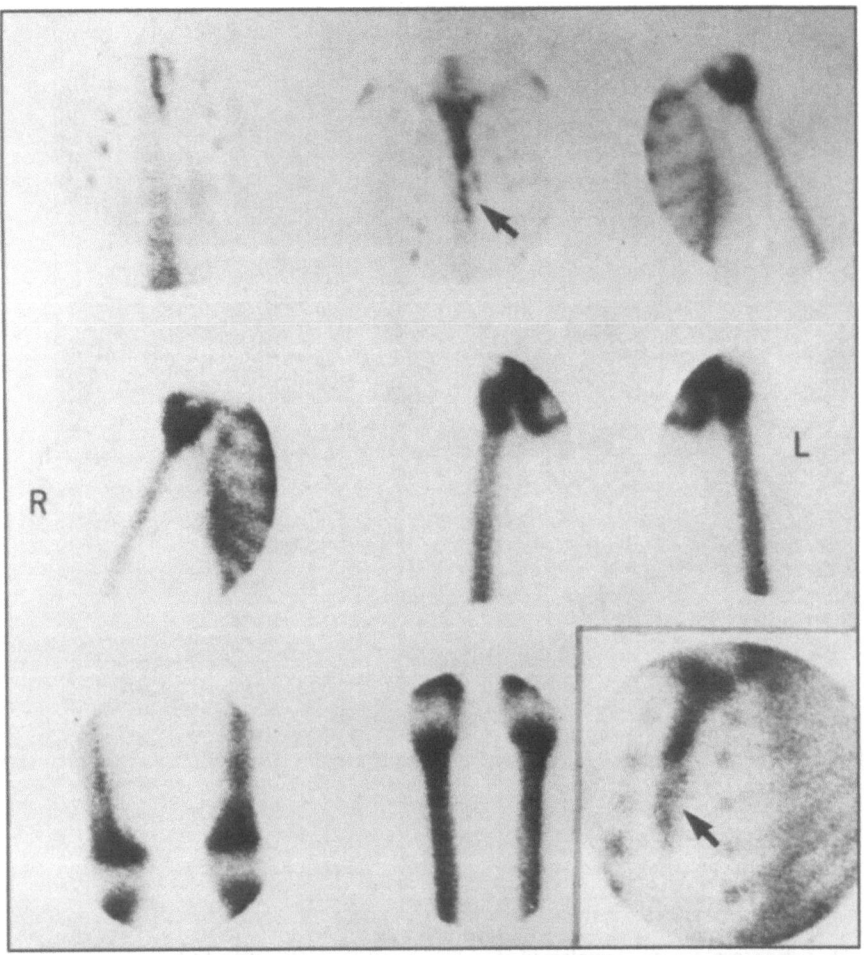

Fig. 12.12. Sickle cell crisis. The radiophosphate whole-body survey demonstrated photopaenia in the lower half of the body of the sternum (*arrow*), indicative of a recent infarct. Both tibiae exhibited diffusely high uptake consistent with ongoing repair of previous infarctions. Lower grades of concentration were observed in the distal femoral shafts which could represent either a subsiding repair process or a reaction to a very cellular marrow.

shows intense uptake of radiophosphate, but no radiocolloid photon deficiency, then osteomyelitis is highly probable. If this area also shows an intense ^{67}Ga uptake, then the diagnosis is even more certain. Absent radiocolloid deposition and a surrounding rim of radiophosphate strongly favours osteonecrosis, but if there is also an intense ^{67}Ga concentration then osteomyelitis is more likely.

Gaucher's Disease

Gaucher's disease features an abnormal accumulation of cerebroglycosides in the reticuloendothelial cells. Within the rigid confines of bone, this encroaches upon the lumina of the marrow capil-

laries and reduces intramedullary circulation. This can ultimately lead to ischaemia and osteonecrosis. The clinical presentation may mimic osteomyelitis in that there can be fever and local pain. Photopaenia with radiocolloid, radiophosphate and ^{67}Ga is characteristic of an acute infarction, whereas osteomyelitis depicts an intense ^{67}Ga uptake. The criteria are the same as for sickle cell infarction. Packing of the marrow with these Gaucher cells can cause bone resorption and fracture.

Radiation Osteonecrosis

Originally it was thought that the primary effect of radiation was on the bone cells, i.e. osteocytes,

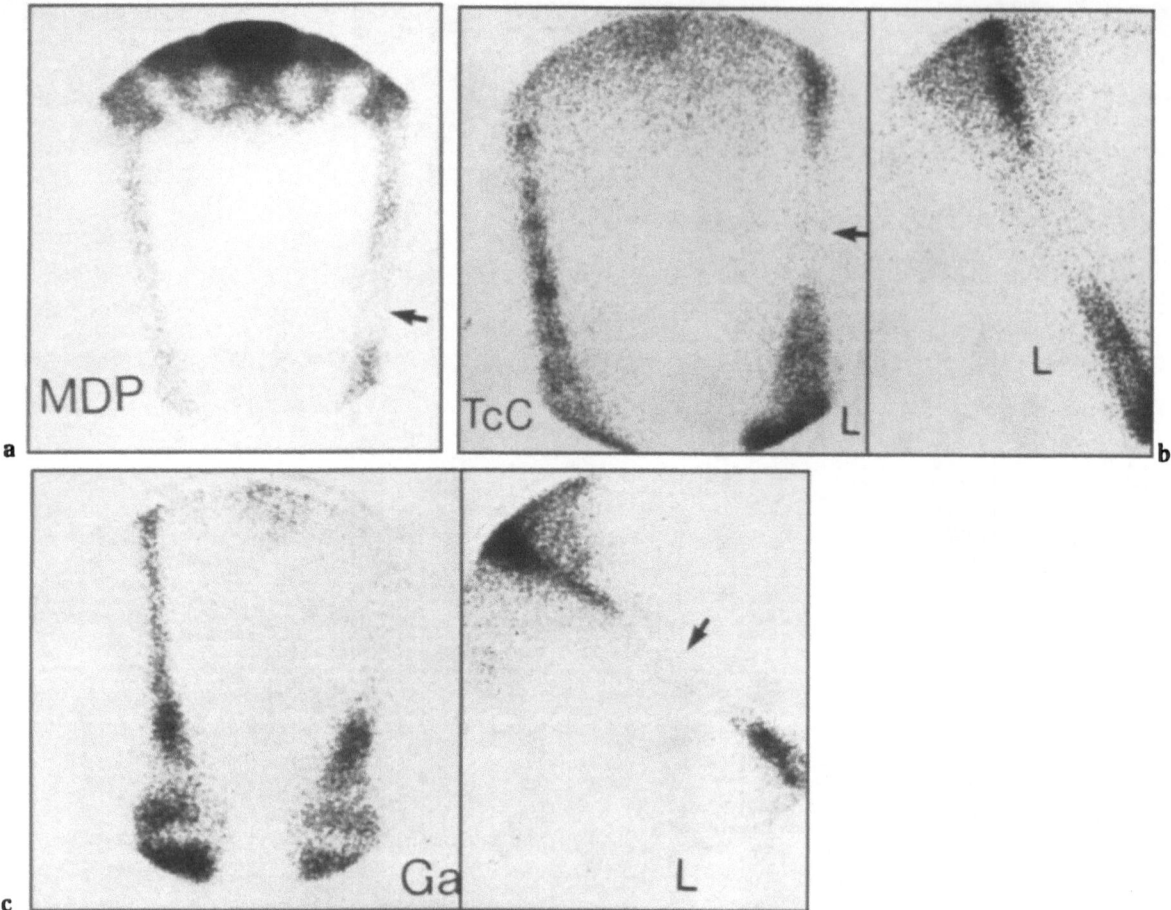

Fig. 12.13a–c. Bone infarction in sickle cell disease. Patient complained of sudden onset of thigh pain which was accompanied by local tenderness and warmth, and pyrexia. Osteomyelitis was considered in the differential diagnosis. **a** Radiophosphate scan demonstrated an area of photon deficiency in the left femoral diaphysis (*arrow*). **b** The ⁹⁹ᵐTc sulphur colloid scan showed a larger, more clearly defined area of photopaenia (*arrow*). **c** Anterior and lateral ⁶⁷Ga images also depicted a large photopaenic zone, similar to the radiocolloid (*arrow*). This effectively excluded osteomyelitis.

osteoblasts and osteoclasts. The bulk of evidence currently supports the concept that radiation damage is mediated through alterations in the microvasculature, which becomes partially or completely occluded (King et al. 1979). The direct affect on bone cells constitutes a minor contribution to the radiation sequelae, and their demise is primarily a result of ischaemia. Shortly after radiation there may be an increase in radiophosphate uptake secondary to an inflammatory hyperaemia. In time this recedes, and the radiophosphate uptake may be less than normal, depending on the patency of the microvasculature, which in turn is a function of the dose administered. Doses of about 30 Gy (3000 rads) in 3 weeks induce a depression in marrow and bone uptake of radiocolloid and radiophosphate, respectively, and this is strictly limited to the outlines of the treatment field (Bell et al. 1969; Cox 1974). Marrow depression is greater than bone for the same dose. The likelihood of irreversible osteonecrosis is increased with absorbed doses in the neighbourhood of 60 Gy (6000 rads) in 6 weeks. Loss of bone viability makes the bone susceptible to injury and infection, and the expected response of hyperconcentration of radiophosphate to these complications may be frustrated (Fig. 12.14). Sarcomatous degeneration is also an uncommon complication (Fig. 12.15).

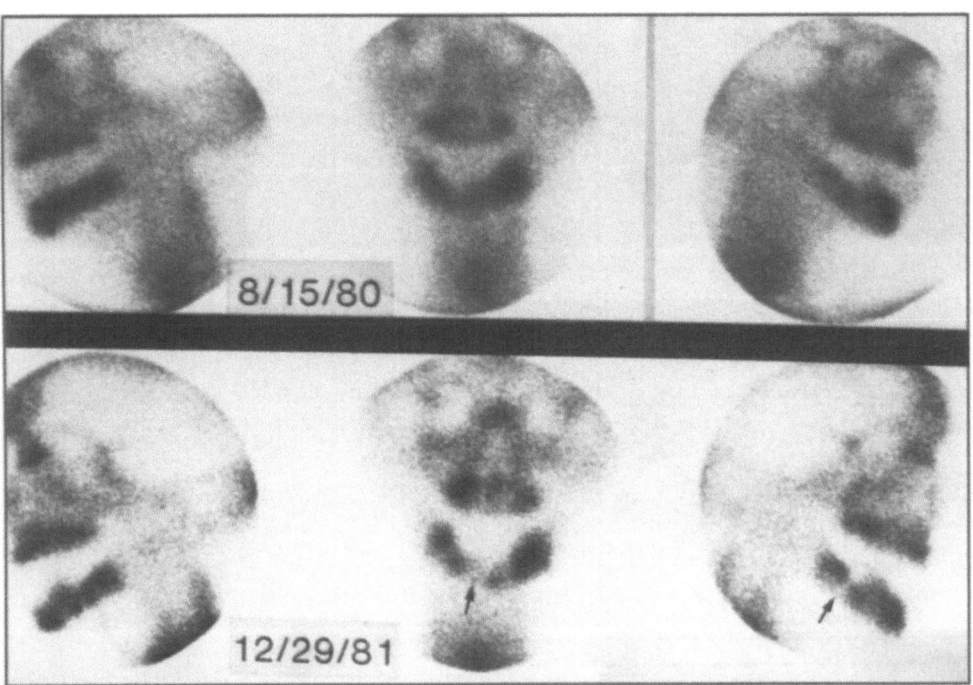

Fig. 12.14. Radiation osteonecrosis. This patient received 60 Gy (6000 rads) to the mandible through parallel opposing fields as treatment for a submandibular tumour 15 years previously. A smouldering, chronic osteomyelitis with acute flare-ups developed in a bed of revitalised bone and soft tissue. A sinus tract extended to the floor of the mouth anteriorly and spicules of sequestered bone were removed periodically. There was no focal reactive radiophosphate uptake to the osteomyelitis (nor ^{67}Ga; not shown) on 15 August 1980. On 29 December 1981 the radiophosphate images of the mandible exhibited two avascular areas (*arrows*). The segment of bone at the mentum had separated from the mandible.

Frostbite

Frostbite injuries of bone can result from microvascular occlusion and bone cell disruption. There is evidence of crystal formation directly causing bone cell damage, but the major cause of osteonecrosis is felt to be due to trauma of the endothelial lining of the microvasculature. This leads to increased vessel wall permeability, plasma transudation, erythrocyte stasis and sludging, and arteriovenous shunting of the nutritive blood flow proximal to the injured area. Injury to the overlying soft tissue usually exceeds the incidence and extent of bone necrosis, because of the existing thermal gradient between the superficial and deep tissues in cold injury. Plain film radiography of the affected part soon after the bone insult demonstrates normal density and architecture and gives no indication of osteonecrosis. The presence of subcutaneous gas at this time, when it occurs, is a bad prognostic sign (Tishler 1972).

Radiophosphate is eminently suited for defining the area of necrosis, which presents as absent uptake (Fig. 12.16; Lisbona and Rosenthall 1976). Invariably, there is an adjacent increased concentration as a result of reactive hyperaemia. Muscle injury may, on occasion, concentrate radiophosphate, but this lasts about a week—a course similar to the concentration in myocardial infarcts (Rosenthall et al. 1981).

Electrical Burns

High-tension electrical burns cause soft tissue and bone necrosis. The deep muscles often show greater involvement than the skin. Osteonecrosis manifests as absent uptake of radiophosphate, which may not necessarily involve the full thickness of bone, and there may be an adjacent reactive hyperconcentration (Fig. 12.17). Between 24 h and 6 days after the insult, there is radiophosphate deposition in the damaged muscle, and this has clinical utility in the selection of sites for debridement (Hunt et al. 1979).

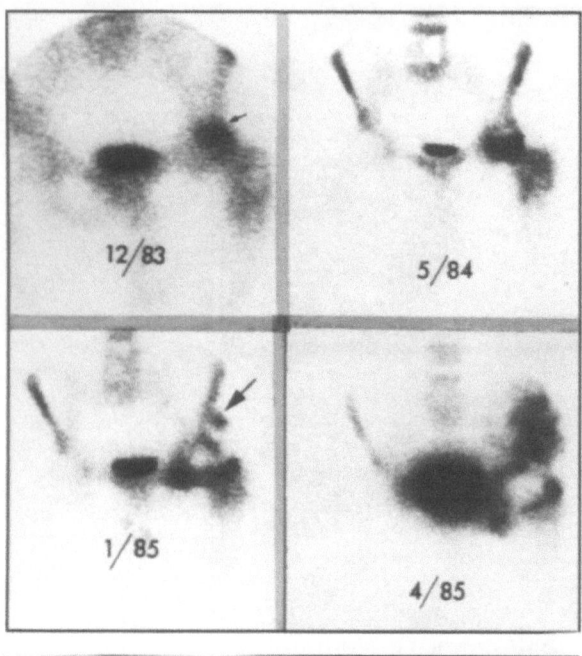

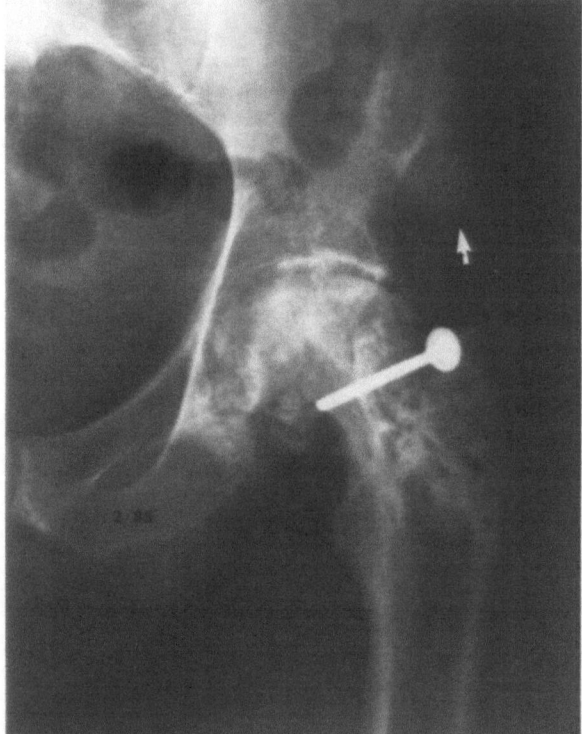

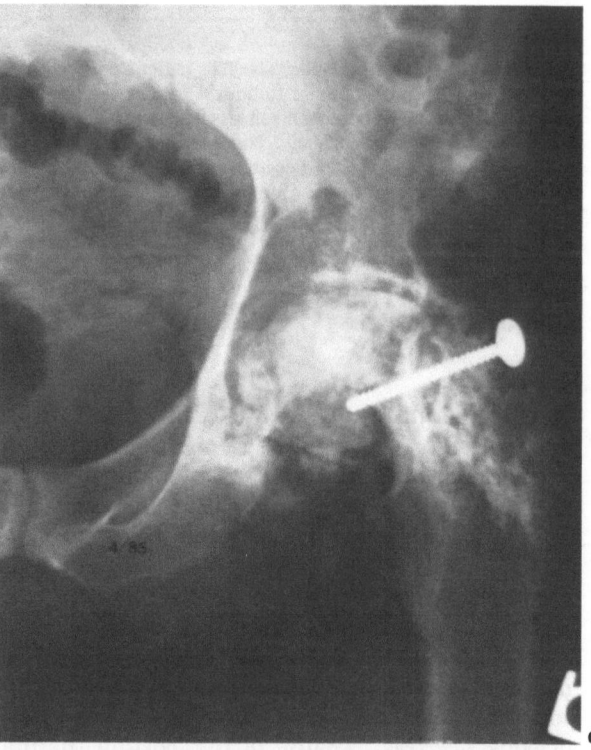

Fig. 12.15a,b. Radiation necrosis and radiation-induced osteosarcoma. At 23 years of age (1962) this man was given 62 Gy (6200 rads) in 58 days to the left hip for treatment of a giant cell tumour in the intertrochanteric region. This was delivered through parallel opposed treatment portals measuring 15 × 15 cm. **a** Twenty-one years after treatment (December 1983) he developed left hip pain secondary to avascular necrosis. The radiophosphate scan showed a focus of increased concentration (*arrow*). A gluteus medius vascular pedicle graft was applied, and the radiophosphate bone scan 3 months later (May 1984) demonstrated increased activity which represented the bone graft and perhaps partial revascularisation of the head. In January 1985 a femoral neck fracture occurred and the head lost its blood supply. More serious was the development of a focus of increased radiophosphate uptake just superior to the left acetabulum and extending into the soft tissues (*arrow*). This was an osteosarcoma arising at the edge of the treatment fields applied 23 years previously. The scan taken in April 1985 showed rapid enlargement of the osteosarcoma over a 3-month interval. **b** Radiograph of the left hip taken in February 1985 showed the osteosarcoma (*arrow*) and the femoral neck fracture. **c** Radiograph taken 2 months later (April 1985) showed further enlargement of the osteosarcoma.

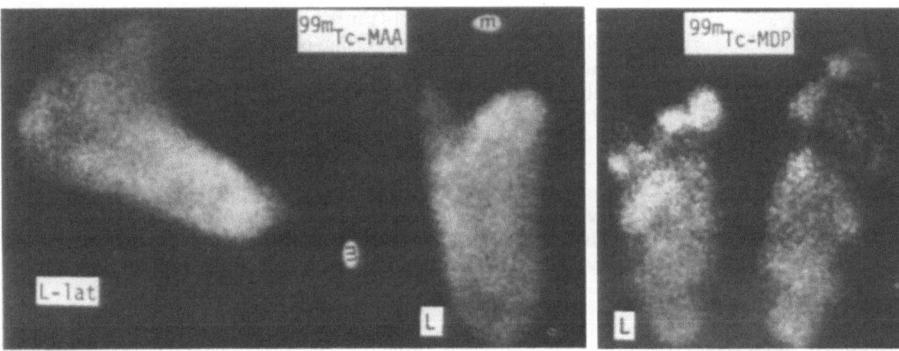

Fig. 12.16. Frostbite of the left foot. The radiophosphate images ($^{99m}Tc\text{-}MDP$) portrayed absent uptake in the bones of the first, second, third and fourth phalanges, and head of the third metatarsal of the left foot. Normal right foot. ^{99m}Tc macroaggregates of albumin ($^{99m}Tc\text{-}MAA$) were injected into the left femoral artery to delineate the status of the microcirculation. (*m*, a radioactive marker at the distal tip of the foot.) The extent of soft tissue and bone necrosis is the same as shown in the radiophosphate images.

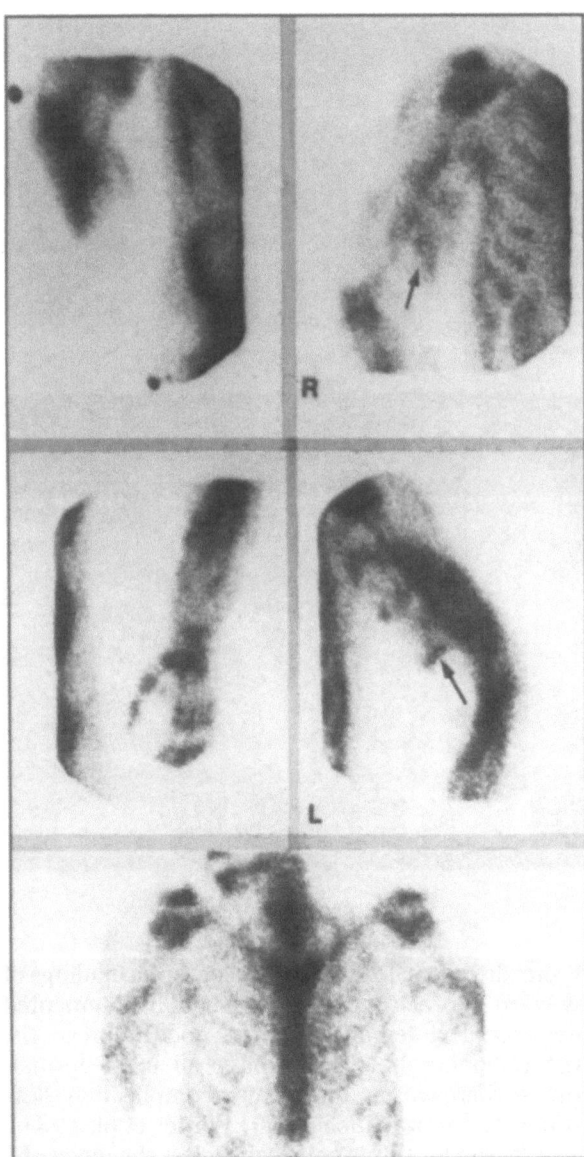

Fig. 12.17. Electrical burn causing bone and muscle necrosis. A 12 000 V current entered the right hand and exited at the left elbow. There is complete death of the flesh and bone just distal to the right elbow, as seen by the complete absence of radiophosphate concentration. The right humerus depicts irregular uptake throughout the shaft, consistent with irregular necrosis. A reactive hyperaemia is present in the humeral head. Radiophosphate deposition in the soft tissue represents muscle necrosis (*arrows*). The left upper extremity shows extensive soft tissue deposition of the test agent from the proximal arm to the proximal forearm, obscuring the status of the underlying bones. Hyperaemia of the left hand is noted. (Courtesy of Dr. R. Lisbona)

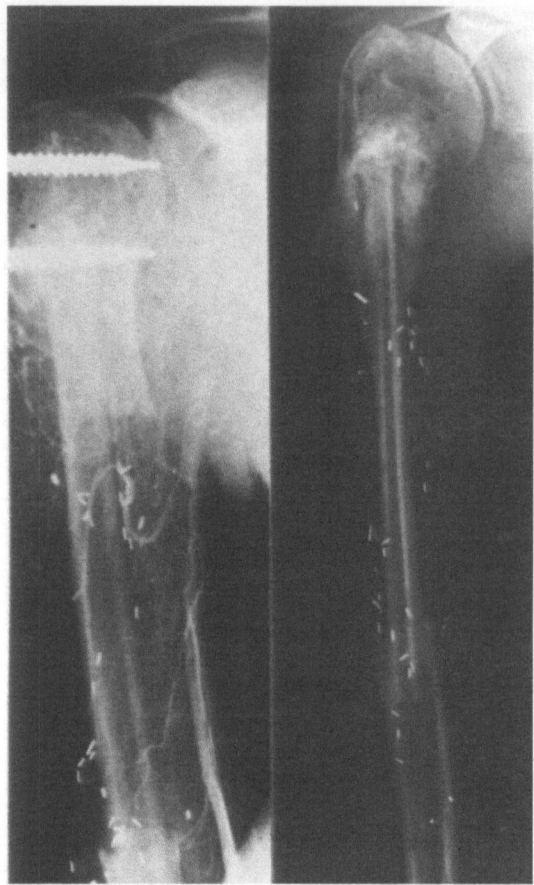

Fig. 12.18a,b. Successful microvascular bone graft. This 17-year-old boy had an en bloc resection of a recurrent cyst in the right humerus, and the gap was spanned with a microvascularised fibular transplant graft. a *Left*: Arteriogram 6 weeks postoperatively demonstrates a patent vascular supply. *Right*: Incorporation of the graft edges at 5 months. b Periodic follow-up radiophosphate bone images. At 2 days (*2d po*) the fibular graft depicts concentration indicating viability of the vascular microanastomosis (*arrows*). One week later (*1w po*) there is a higher concentration in the graft, and this is probably due to a remission of an initial vasospasm and oedema. At 5 months (*5m po*) the graft is still thriving.

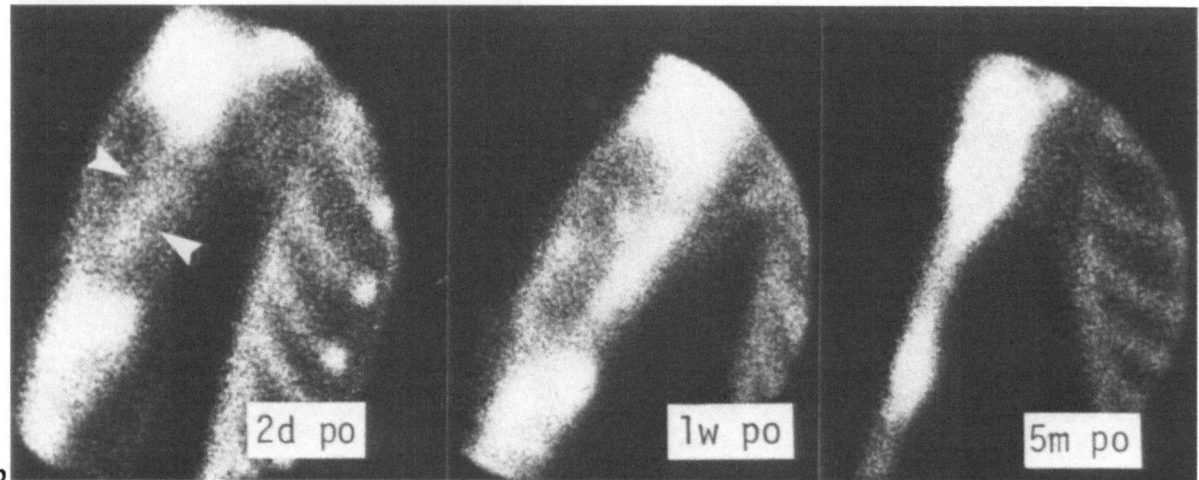

Juvenile Kyphosis

Juvenile kyphosis is also known as Scheuermann's disease, and its aetiology has been attributed to osteonecrosis of the vertebral end-plates, disc herniation, mechanical stress and endocrine or nutri-tional disorders. Despite the radiographic findings of wedged thoracic vertebrae, irregular fragmented epiphyseal plates and Schmorl node impressions, the radiophosphate scans have all been normal, unless there was an intervening complication (Kettunen and Karjalainen 1969; Winter et al. 1981). The reason for this is not clear, unless the metabolic reaction to the disorder subsides long before the radiographic changes become apparent, or the reaction is too low grade to be resolved by external imaging

Bone Graft Revascularisation

Bone graft revascularisation and viability can be studied by radiography, tetracycline labelling and tissue biopsy, but these methods are either insensitive, subjective or inherently destructive. Radiophosphate bone imaging provides an innocuous method of monitoring the progress of bone graft healing, and it has been shown to provide information on the status of the graft earlier than radiogra-

phy (Stevenson et al. 1974). Four types of bone graft have been used: bone without inherent vascular supply; bone graft vascularised via intact pedicles of nutrient blood vessels, skin, muscle and omentum; bone graft transferred with its nutrient vessel(s) and microanastomosed to the vessels in the recipient bed; bone graft transferred with an artery, vein or vascular bundle implanted into a hole drilled in the graft.

In a conventional bone graft, where there is no inherent vascular supply, revascularisation takes place by vessel ingrowth from the points of contact with the host-bone via the old circulatory cavities. It is estimated that the neovasculature penetrates the cancellous bone at a rate of 0.2–0.4 mm/day and the cortical bone at 0.15–0.3 mm/day (Albrektson 1980). New bone is deposited on necrotic bone in the cancellous part, thereby provoking increased density on the radiograph. The process differs in cor-

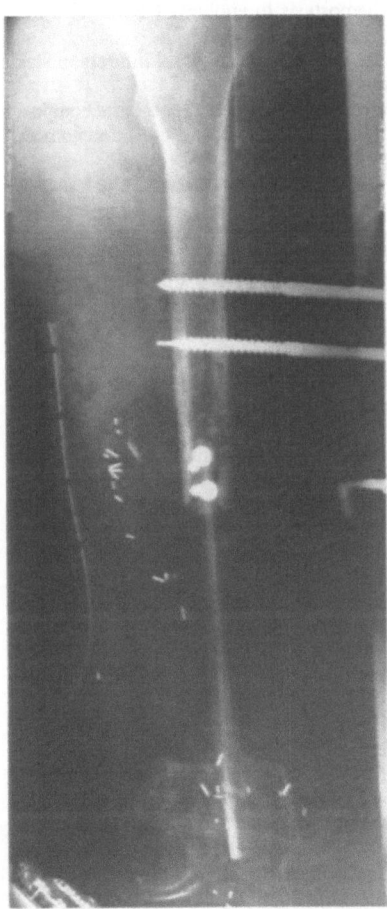
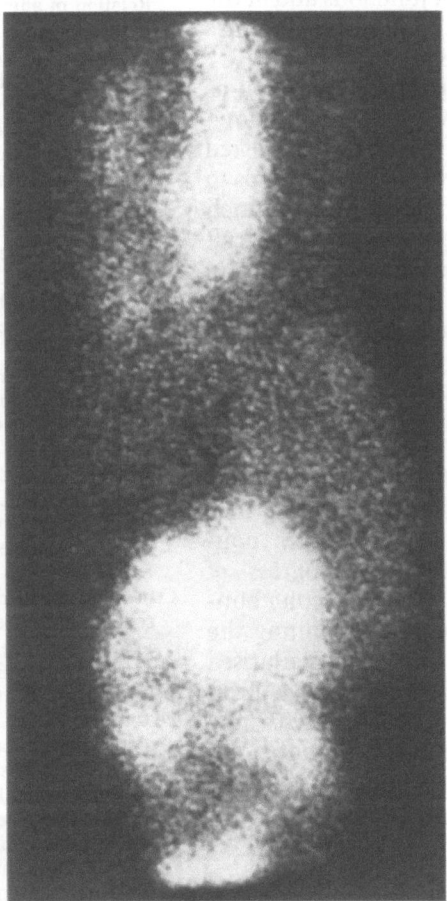

a   b

Fig. 12.19a,b. Failed microvascular bone graft. **a** Postoperative radiograph following block resection of a primary sarcoma of the left femur and the transplant of a microvascular fibular graft. **b** Radiophosphate study 3 days postoperatively shows no deposition in the graft, an indication of occlusion of the micro-anastomosed vessels. Surgical muscle injury and host–bone reaction account for the enhanced uptakes in the scan.

tical bone wherein there is an initial resorption of bone along the old osteons with neovascular penetration, making the graft weaker and more radiolucent. There is appositional new bone formation following the resorption, but it takes some time for normal bone strength to be restored. In man, the incidence of fatigue fractures in long-bone autografts caused by resorption weakness is greatest between 6 and 18 months after grafting. The radiophosphate portrayal is that of increased uptakes at the host–graft junctions, which will extend towards each other and coalesce with successful revascularisation. A failed graft does not concentrate radiophosphate.

Microvascularised and functioning pedicle bone grafts have their blood supply intact from the beginning and these show normal or increased radiophosphate concentration. The increased uptake is probably a manifestation of hyperaemia secondary to opening of normally dormant vascular channels. Vascular bundle implanted grafts exhibit enhanced concentration at the host–graft junctions and at the point of vascular implantation. The three sites fuse with successful revascularisation.

A microvascular transplant can still function as a conventional graft if its blood supply fails. However, the sleeve of soft tissue which is transferred with the bone undergoes necrosis, and this tends to frustrate conventional bone graft healing, in much the same way as the incidence of conventional graft success is reduced when applied in a bed of devitalised tissue (Bos 1979). Necrotic soft tissue is known to concentrate radiophosphate, and this can be a potential source of error in judging bone graft viability. A recent experimental study utilising dog rib grafts has shown this to be an insignificant factor and not a source of interpretative error (Papanastasiou et al. 1983; Figs. 12.18, 12.19).

Mounting evidence supports the contention that radiophosphate imaging is an accurate, non-invasive method of assessing the progress of revascularisation of conventional and vascular bundle implanted bone grafts, and in determining the integrity of the blood supply in microvascularised bone grafts. The radiophosphate uptake has been shown to have a spatial congruence with the neomicrovasculature penetration (Lisbona et al. 1980; Berggren et al. 1982; Lalonde et al. 1984).

References

Aglietti P, Insall JN, Buzzi R, Deschamps G (1983) Idiopathic osteonecrosis of the knee. J Bone Joint Surg [Br] 65: 588–597

Alavi A, Bond JP, Kul DE (1974) Scan detection of bone marrow infarcts in sickle cell disorders. J Nucl Med 15: 1003–1006

Albrektsson T (1980) Repair of bone grafts. Scand J Plast Reconstr Surg 14: 1–9

Arlot ME, Bonjean M, Chavassieux PM, Meunier PJ (1983) Bone histology in adults with aseptic necrosis. J Bone Jt Surg [Am]: 1319–1327

Armas RR, Goldsmith SJ (1984) Gallium scintigraphy in bone infarction with bone imaging. Clin Nucl Med 9: 1–3

Bauer G, Weber DA, Ceder L, Darte L, Egund N, Hanson I, Stromqvist B (1980) Dynamics of technetium-99m methylenediphosphonate imaging of the femoral head after hip fracture. Clin Orthop 152: 85–92

Baylis AP, Davidson JK (1977) Osteonecrosis of the femoral head following intracapsular fracture: incidence and earliest radiological features. Clin Radiol 28: 407–414

Bell EG, McAfee JG, Constable WV (1969) Localized radiation damage to bone and marrow demonstrated by radioisotope imaging. Radiology 92: 1083–1088

Berggren A, Weiland AJ, Ostrup LT (1982) Bone scintigraphy in evaluation viability of composite bone grafts revascularized by microvascular anastomoses, conventional autogenous bone grafts and free nonrevascularized periosteal grafts. J Bone Joint Surg [Am] 64: 799–809

Boettcher WG, Bonfiglio M, Hamilton HH, Sheets RF, Smith K (1970) Non-traumatic necrosis of the femoral head. Part 1. Relation of altered hemostasis to etiology. J Bone Joint Surg [Am] 52: 312–321

Bohrer SP (1970) Acute long bone diaphyseal infarcts in sickle cell disease. Br J Radiol 43: 685–697

Bos KE (1979) Bone scintigraphy of experimental and composite bone grafts revascularized by microvascular anastomoses. Plast Reconstr Surg 64: 353–360

Burt RW, Mathews TJ (1982) Aseptic necrosis of the knee. AJR 138: 571–573

Calandrucco RA, Anderson WE (1980) Postfracture avascular necrosis of the femoral head: correlation of experimental and clinical studies. Clin Orthop 152: 49–84

Catto M (1965) A histological study of avascular necrosis of the femoral head after transcervical fracture. J Bone Joint Surg [Br] 47: 749–776

Chung SMK, Batterman SC, Brighton CT (1976) Shear strength of the human femoral capital epiphyseal plate. J Bone Joint Surg [Am] 58: 94–103

Cosgriff SW (1951) Thromboembolic complications associated with ACTH and cortisone therapy. JAMA 147: 924–926

Cox PH (1974) Abnormalities in skeletal uptake of Tc-99m polyphosphate in areas of bone associated with tissues which have been subjected to radiation therapy. Br J Radiol 47: 851–856

Cruess RL, Blennerhassett J, MacDonald FR, MacLeod LD, Dosseter J (1968) Aseptic necrosis following renal transplantation. J Bone Joint Surg [Am] 59: 1577–1590

Danigelis JA (1976) Pinhole imaging in Legg-Perthes disease. Semin Nucl Med 6: 69–82

Editorial (1982) Osteonecrosis caused by combination chemotherapy. Lancet I: 433–434

Eisenstein A, Rothschild S (1976) Biochemical abnormalities in patients with slipped capital femoral epiphysis and chondrolysis. J Bone Joint Surg [Am] 58: 459–467

Fasting OJ, Langeland N, Bjerkreim I, Hertzenberg L, Nakken K (1978) Bone scintigraphy in early diagnosis of Perthes disease. Acta Orthop Scand 49: 169–174

Ficat RP, Arlet J (1980) Ischemia and bone necrosis. Williams and Wilkins, Baltimore

Fisher DE (1978) The role of fat embolism in the etiology of corticosteroid-induced avascular necrosis. Clin Orthop 130: 68–80

Fisher RL, Roderique JW, Brown DC, Danigelis JA, Ozonoff MB, Sziklas JJ (1980) The relationship of isotopic bone image findings to prognosis in Legg-Perthes disease. Clin Orthop 150: 23–29

Frost HM (1964) The etiodynamics of aseptic necrosis of the femoral head. In Proceedings of the conference on aseptic necrosis of the femoral head, St. Louis, Missouri, 1964, pp 393–413

Glimcher MJ, Kenzora JE (1978) The biology of osteonecrosis of the human femoral head and its clinical implications. Clin Orthop 130: 47–50

Glimcher MJ, Kenzora JE (1979) The biology of osteonecrosis of the human femoral head and its clinical implications. Clin Orthop 140: 273–312

Gregg PJ, Walder DN (1980) Scintigraphy versus radiography in the early diagnosis of experimental bone necrosis. J Bone Joint Surg (Br): 214–221

Gregg PJ, Walder DN (1981) A study of old lesions of caisson disease of bone by radiography and bone scintigraphy. J Bone Joint Surg [Br] 63: 132–137

Gregg PJ, Walder DN, Rannie I (1980) Caisson disease of bone: a study of the Gottingen mini-pig as an animal model. Br J Exp Pathol 16: 39–53

Greyson ND, Kassel EF (1976) Serial bone scan changes in recurrent bone infarction. J Nucl Med 17: 184–186

Greyson ND, Lotem MM, Gross AE, Houpt JB (1982) Radionuclide evaluation of spontaneous femoral osteonecrosis. Radiology 142: 729–735

Harper PG, Trask C, Souhami RL (1984) Avascular necrosis of bone caused by combination chemotherapy without corticosteroids. Br Med J 288: 267–268

Harris WR (1950) The endocrine basis for slipping of the upper femoral epiphysis. An experimental study. J Bone Joint Surg [Br] 32: 5–16

Houpt JB, Alpert B, Lotem M, Greyson ND, Pritzker KPH, Langer F, Gross AE (1982) Spontaneous osteonecrosis of the medial tibial plateau. J Rheumatol 9: 81–90

Howarth B (1966) Pathology. Slipping of the capital femoral epiphysis. Clin Orthop 48: 33–45

Hull A, Hattner R, Vincente F (1979) Prospective scintigraphic evaluation of avascular necrosis of the femoral head in renal transplant recipients. J Nucl Med 20: 20 (abstract)

Hungerford DS, Zizic TM (1980) The treatment of ischemic necrosis of bone in systemic lupus erythematosus. Medicine 59: 143–148

Hunt J, Lewis S, Parkey R, Baxter C (1979) The use of technetium-99m stannous pyrophosphate scintigraphy to identify muscle damage in acute electrical burns. J Trauma 19: 409–413

Hunter GA (1980) Should we abandon primary prosthetic replacement for freshly displaced fractures of the neck of the femur. Clin Orthop 152: 158–161

Ibels LS, Alfrey AC, Huffer WE, Weil R (1978) Aseptic necrosis of bone following renal transplantation: experience in 194 transplant recipients and review of the literature. Medicine 57: 25–42

Jones JP (1971) Alcoholism, hypercortisonism, fat emboli and osseous avascular necrosis. In: Zinn WM (ed) Idiopathic ischemic necrosis of the femoral head in adults. Thieme, Stuttgart, pp 112–132

Kemp HBS (1973) Perthes disease: an experimental and clinical study. Ann R Coll Surg Engl 52: 18–35

Kemper JW, Baggenstoss AH, Slocumb CH (1957) The relationship of therapy with cortisone to the incidence of vascular lesions in rheumatoid arthritis. Ann Intern Med 46: 831–834

Kettunen K, Karjalainen P (1969) External counting of radiostrontium in the differential diagnosis of juvenile osteochondrosis of the spine. Ann Chir Gynaecol 58: 9–16

King M, Cassarett GW, Weber DA (1979) A study of irradiated bone: histopathic and physiologic changes. J Nucl Med 20: 1142–1149

Kloiber R, Damtew B, Rosenthall L (1981) A crossover study comparing the effect of particle size on the distribution of radiocolloid in patients. Clin Nucl Med 6: 204–206

Lalonde DH, Williams HB, Rosenthall L, Viloria JB (1984) Circulation, bone scans and tetracycline labeling in microvascularized and vascular bundle implanted rib grafts. Ann Plast Surg 13: 366–374

LaMont RL, Muz J, Heilbronner D, Bouwhuis JA (1981) Quantitative assessment of femoral head involvement in Legg–Calve–Perthes disease. J Bone Joint Surg [Am] 63: 746–752

Libshitz HI, Edeiken BS (1981) Radiotherapy changes of the pediatric hip. AJR 137: 585–588

Lisbona R, Rosenthall L (1976) Assessment of bone viability by scintiscanning in frostbite injuries. J Trauma 16: 986–992

Lisbona A, Rennie WRJ, Daniel RK (1980) Radionuclide evaluation of free vascularized bone graft viability. AJR 134: 387–388

Lotke PA, Ecker ML, Alavi A (1977) Painful knees in older patients: radionuclide diagnosis of possible osteonecrosis with spontaneous resolution. J Bone Joint Surg [Am] 59: 617–621

Lukens JN (1981) Sickle cell disease. Disease-a-Month 27: 16

Lutzker LG, Alavi A (1976) Bone and marrow imaging in sickle cell disease. Diagnosis of infarction. Semin Nucl Med 6: 83–93

MacLeod MA, McEwan AJB, Pearson RR, Houston AS (1982) Functional imaging in the early diagnosis of dysbaric osteonecrosis. Br J Radiol 55: 497–500

McCallum RI (1984) Bone necrosis due to decompression. Philos Trans R Soc Lond 304: 185–191

McCauley RGK, Kahn PC (1977) Osteochondritis of the tarsal navicular. Radioisotope appearances. Radiology 123: 705–706

McFarland PH, Frost HM (1961) A possible new cause for aseptic necrosis of the femoral head. Henry Ford Hosp Med Bull 9: 115–122

McGuigan L, Fleming A (1983) Osteonecrosis of the humerus related to pregnancy. Ann Rheum Dis 42: 597–599

Meyers MH, Telfer N, Moore TM (1977) Determination of the vascularity of the femoral head with technetium-99m sulfur colloid. J Bone Joint Surg [Am] 59: 658–664

Mould JJ, Adam NM (1983) The problem of avascular necrosis of bone in patients treated for Hodgkin's disease. Clin Radiol 34: 231–236

Papanastasiou VW, Lalonde DH, Williams HB, Rosenthall L (1983) Role of bone scintigraphy in the postoperative evaluation of microvascularized rib grafts. Surg Forum 34: 613–615

Pooley J, Walder DN (1980) Reduction in bone marrow blood flow during simulated dives: investigation of the mechanism. J Bone Joint Surg [Br] 62: 635 (abstract)

Rennie AM (1967) Familial slipping of the upper femoral epiphysis. J Bone Joint Surg [Br] 49: 534–541

Rosenthall L, Kloiber R, Gagnon R, Damtew B (1981) Frostbite with rhabdomyolysis and renal failure. AJR 137: 387–390

Sanchis M, Zakir A, Freeman MAR (1973) The experimental stimulation of Perthes disease by consecutive interruptions of the blood supply to the capital femoral epiphysis in the puppy. J Bone Joint Surg [Am] 55: 335–342

Solomon L (1973) Drug-induced arthropathy and necrosis of the femoral head. J Bone Joint Surg [Br] 55: 246–261

Solomon L (1981) Idiopathic necrosis of the femoral head: pathogenesis and treatment. Can J Surg 24: 573–578

Spencer RP, Lee YSC, Sziklas JJ (1982) Radiocolloid imaging of the femoral heads: a possible interpretative fallacy. J Nucl Med 23: 29 (abstract)

Stadalnik RC, Riggins RL, D'Ambrosia R, De Nardo GL (1975) Vascularity of the femoral head: 18-fluorine scintigraphy validated with tetracycline labeling. Radiology 114: 663–666

Stevenson JS, Bright RW, Dunson GL, Nelson FR (1974) Technetium-99m phosphate bone imaging: a method for assessing bone graft healing. Radiology 110: 391–394

Stromqvist B, Brismar J, Hansson LI, Thorngren KG (1984) External and biopsy determination of Tc-99m-MDP femoral-head labeling in fracture neck. J Nucl Med 25: 854–858

Thorne JC, Evans WK, Alison RE, Fournasier V (1981) Avascular necrosis of bone complicating treatment of malignant lymphoma. Am J Med 71: 751–758

Tishler JM (1972) The soft tissue and bone changes in frostbite injuries. Radiology 102: 511–513

Turner JH (1983) Post-traumatic avascular necrosis of the femoral head predicted by preoperative technetium-99m antimony-colloid scan. J Bone Joint Surg [Am] 65: 786–797

Wang GJ, Sweet DE, Reger SI (1977) Fat-cell changes as a mechanism of avascular necrosis of the femoral head in cortisone-treated rabbits. J Bone Joint Surg [Am] 59: 729–735

Webber M, Wagner J (1973) Demonstration of vascularity of the femoral head using technetium-99m. J Bone Joint Surg [Am] 55: 1315

Winter WA, Veraat BEEMJ, Verdegaal WP (1981) Bone scintigraphy in patients with juvenile kyphosis. Diagn Imaging 50: 186–199

Zizic TM, Hungerford DS, Stevens MB (1980) Ischemic bone necrosis in systemic erythematosus. The early diagnosis of ischemic necrosis of bone. Medicine 59: 134–142

13 · Orthopaedic Applications of Single Photon Emission Computed Tomographic Bone Scanning

B. D. Collier

Introduction

When compared with planar bone scanning, single photon emission computed tomography (SPECT) has technical advantages of potential diagnostic significance. Planar imaging often superimposes substantial underlying or overlying activity on the bony structures of medical interest. SPECT, however, can be used to remove such unwanted activity. For example, in the hip the acetabulum extends downwards behind the femoral head. Therefore, when using planar bone scanning techniques, the photon-deficient defect typical of avascular necrosis (AVN) of the femoral head may be obscured by activity originating in the underlying acetabulum. By using SPECT, underlying and overlying distributions of activity can be separated into sequential tomographic planes. For this reason SPECT facilitates the detection of AVN of the femoral head (Collier et al. 1984a, 1985b).

When referring a patient without a history of malignancy for bone scanning, the orthopaedic surgeon usually has a specific clinical question involving a limited portion of the skeleton. Orthopaedic surgeons at our institution commonly use bone scanning to clarify the cause of back, hip or knee pain; to determine with a physiological test the significance of radiographic findings; and to establish the extent of disease at symptomatic skeletal sites such as the three compartments of the knee. In instances such as these, when clinical concern is limited to a specific anatomical region, a bone scan procedure that includes SPECT imaging of only a portion of the skeleton is appropriate. To date, SPECT of the skeletal system has most frequently been used to evaluate patients with pain in the larger joints and bony structures such as the lumbar spine, hips, knees, or temporomandibular joints (TMJ).

Principles

In comparison with planar imaging, SPECT bone scanning increases image contrast by removing from the diagnostic image the activity (noise) from in front and behind the plane in which activity of medical interest (signal) is distributed. As is shown in Fig. 13.1, removal of activity from underlying

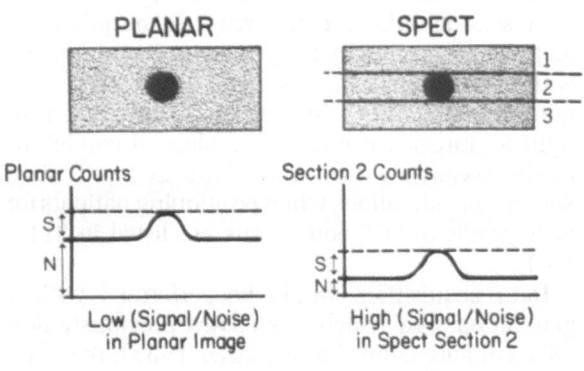

Fig. 13.1 Improved signal/noise ratio with SPECT.

and overlying planes improves the SPECT signal/ noise ratio. This improvement in signal/noise ratio increases image contrast and facilitates detection of skeletal lesions. An added benefit of SPECT bone scanning is improved positional information which allows the observer to distinguish between bony structures that overlap on planar images.

It is important to recognise that the spatial resolution of SPECT bone scanning is inferior to that which can be obtained using planar techniques. Therefore, when examining the hands, feet or other relatively small bony structures there is a trade-off between spatial resolution and image contrast which usually favours high-resolution planar imaging.

Techniques

SPECT supplements but does not replace planar bone scanning. In addition, many patients complaining of back, hip or knee pain may benefit from a radionuclide flow study and blood pool imaging procedure. At our institution, the imaging sequence for such patients is as follows:

1. Flow study (5 s/frame)
2. Blood pool image (500 000 counts)
3. Planar bone scanning
4. SPECT bone scanning

For some adult patients the diagnostic quality of SPECT may be count limited. Therefore, an adult dose of 25 mCi (925 MBq) of ^{99m}Tc medronate is used.

Positioning for SPECT bone scanning at our institution requires that the patient lies supine and immobile on the imaging table for 21 min while a gamma camera rotates through 360° to complete data acquisition. The importance of bilaterally symmetrical skeletal positioning for an optimal SPECT bone scan should be emphasised. Bilaterally symmetrical positioning of bony structures, e.g. having both knees equally extended and in a neutral position, results in SPECT images for which any left-to-right asymmetry is due to pathological conditions in the skeleton rather than flaws in positioning. Special considerations when positioning patients for orthopaedic SPECT bone scans are listed in Table 13.1.

Data acquisition should be performed with a gamma camera which has passed previously described quality control tests (Eisner 1985). Based on an acceptable trade-off between sensitivity and

Table 13.1. Patient positioning for orthopaedic SPECT bone scanning

Bony structures	Special positioning	Pitfalls
1. Knees	5- to 7-cm (2- to 3-in) pad between knees. Secure knees with straps to prevent motion. Secure feet in neutral position to prevent rotation	For obese patients both knees may not fit in field of view
2. Hips and pelvis	Empty bladder before examination. Position hips symmetrically and secure knees and/ or feet to prevent motion	Bladder filling during examination creates artefacts
3. Lumbar spine	Keep arms out of field of view. A pillow under the knees may relieve back pain	Patients with back pain often move during the examination

resolution, a low-energy general-purpose collimator is recommended for SPECT bone scanning. For the circular gamma cameras with 400 mm field of view[1] used at our institution for over 2000 orthopaedic SPECT bone scans, data acquired using a standard protocol (64 × 64 matrix, 64 projections over 360° of circular rotation, 20 s per projection) has routinely produced SPECT images of good technical and diagnostic quality (Collier et al. 1985c). In clinical practice, no artefacts caused by incomplete angular sampling, gamma camera nonuniformity, variations in centre of rotation, or gantry instability have occurred in this series.

Data processing begins with a 9-point spatial smooth on each of the 64 projections. After this "preprocessing" of the 64 projections, one slice thick transaxial, coronal and sagittal tomograms (approximately 6 mm thick tomograms for our gamma camera system) are reconstructed using filtered backprojection with a straight ramp (Hanning filter with cut-off frequency of at least 10 cycles per pixel). Attenuation correction is not used. For most orthopaedic SPECT bone scans, a linear map is used when photographing SPECT images onto transparencies. However, in searching for a photondeficient defect in the femoral head at risk for AVN, a log map is usually preferred. Review and interpretation of orthopaedic SPECT bone scans by nuclear medicine physicians requires that all three orthogonal sets of SPECT images as well as planar views

---

[1] General Electric Medical Systems Group, Milwaukee, Wisconsin 53201 USA.

be simultaneously available. In addition to viewing transparencies, physicians seeking to assure themselves that optimal image enhancement has been used may need to review SPECT images at the computer terminal.

Clinical Applications

Many of the bony structures suitable for SPECT imaging have not been studied in detail, and the potential of SPECT bone scanning for oncological imaging has not been thoroughly investigated. However, experience to date has shown a role for SPECT in examining orthopaedic patients with low back, hip, knee, or TMJ pain.

Lumbar Spine

When interpreted without radiographic correlation, SPECT bone scanning can rarely identify a specific cause of low back pain (LBP) in adult patients without a history of malignancy. Trauma, infection, osteoarthritis, spondylolysis and numerous other causes for LBP may all produce an increase in scintigraphic activity in the lumbar spine. Therefore, in evaluating the case of an adult patient with LBP, SPECT complements rather than replaces radiography. The optimal diagnostic strategy is to interpret the two examinations together, thereby correlating anatomy and function so as to arrive at a more reliable diagnosis of the cause for LBP. To date, this complementary role of bone scintigraphy is best established for evaluating spondylolysis or spondylolisthesis as the aetiology for LBP.

Plain film radiography or transmission computed tomography detects most anatomical defects of the bony neural arch (Wiltse et al. 1975; Rhea et al. 1980; Grogan et al. 1982; Libson et al. 1982). However, it is not possible with radiography alone to determine whether spondylolysis or spondylolisthesis is the cause of LBP or is in fact an incidental finding of no clinical significance. The prevalence of spondylolysis in populations undergoing radiographic examination is reported to be between 3% and 10% with a lower prevalence for spondylolisthesis (Bailey 1947; Roche and Rowe 1952; Splithoff 1953; Wiltse and Hutchinson 1964; Torgerson and Dotter 1976; Eisenstein 1978; Libson et al. 1982). However, spondylolysis is almost as common among symptomatic as among asymptomatic populations (Bailey 1947; Torgerson and Dotter

1976; Libson et al. 1982). In only one series (Magora and Schwartz 1980) was LBP universal among patients with radiographic evidence of spondylolisthesis (Meyerding 1941; Bailey 1947; Splithoff 1953; Torgerson and Dotter 1976; Libson et al. 1982). Furthermore, the clinical presentation of LBP caused by spondylolysis or spondylolisthesis may mimic the signs and symptoms of herniation of the nucleus pulposus with nerve root compression and may be confused with bone metastases, osteomyelitis, disc space infections, spinal stenosis, osteoarthritis, or muscular strain. Therefore, correlation of clinical findings with the results of X-ray imaging frequently does not yield a specific diagnosis.

The role of planar bone scanning in conjunction with radiographic examination of the bony posterior neural arch has been frequently limited by the inability to distinguish between lumbar vertebral body and posterior neural arch. For example, by altering the alignment of vertebral bodies, high-grade spondylolisthesis often leads to osteoarthritic changes in vertebral body end-plates. This may be associated with increased scintigraphic activity at both the bilateral pars interarticularis defects and at the sites of osteoarthritis over the vertebral body end-plates. When using planar imaging techniques, such vertebral body and posterior neural arch activity are superimposed on straight posterior views and are often difficult to localise on posterior oblique views. However, with the recent availability of SPECT, more accurate scintigraphic localisation is now possible.

To determine the usefulness of SPECT in this clinical setting, 19 adult patients with radiographic evidence of spondylolysis and/or spondylolisthesis were studied (Collier et al. 1985a). This group of patients included individuals with and without symptoms of LBP. Planar and SPECT scans were interpreted independently. Planar scintigraphy was credited with identification of a pars interarticularis defect when increased scintigraphic activity was correctly localised to either the left or right of midline at the appropriate lumbar vertebral level. SPECT was credited with correct localisation only if increased scintigraphic activity was seen over the appropriate portion of the posterior neural arch (Fig. 13.2). SPECT was more sensitive than planar scanning when used to identify 31 sites of pars interarticularis defects in 13 patients with "painful" spondylolysis or spondylolisthesis (Table 13.2). A group of five adults without any history of LBP, undergoing bone scintigraphy for other purposes, had been studied previously to establish the normal SPECT appearance of the adult lumbar spine. For these normal adults both sides of the posterior

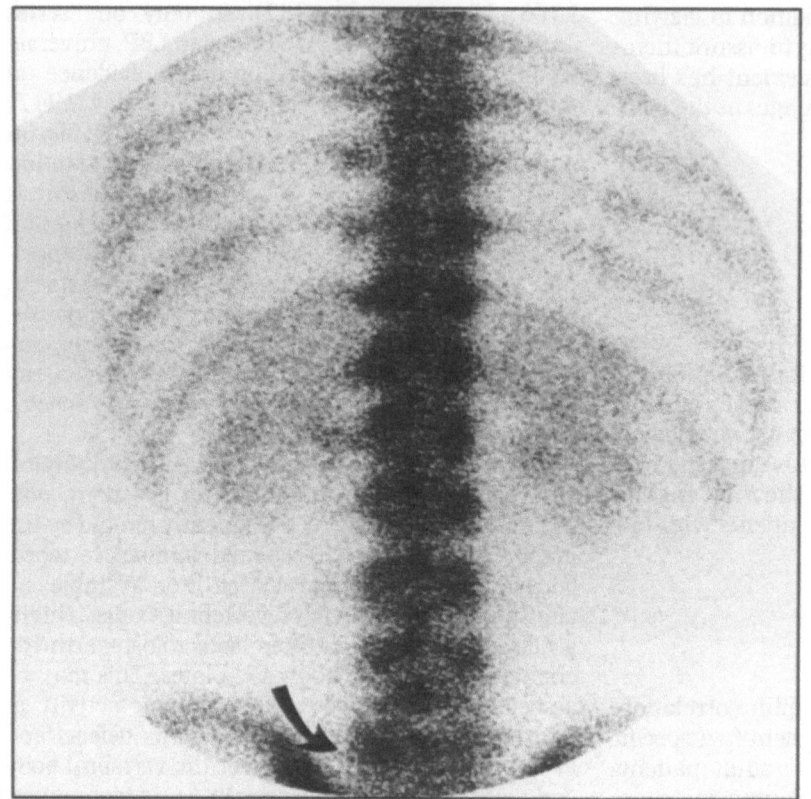

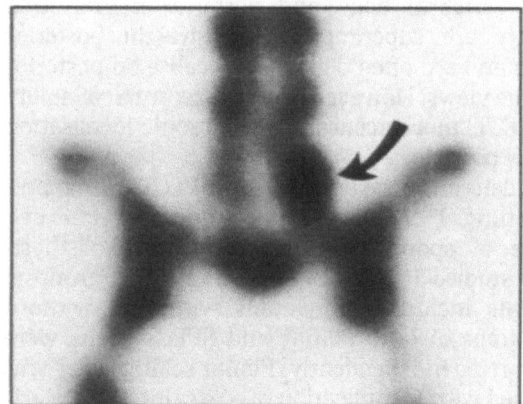

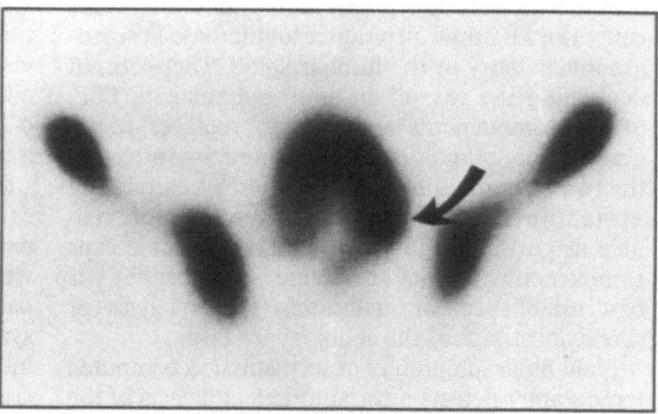

Fig. 13.2a–c. A 22-year-old man with a 9-month history of severe LBP and radiographs showing spondylolysis of L-5 on the left. Posterior planar bone scan (a) shows minimal increased activity over the left side of L-5 (*arrow*). Coronal (b) and transaxial (c) SPECT bone scans demonstrate that the increased activity is located in the left side of the L-5 neural arch (*arrows*). Spinal fusion relieved the pain. (Collier et al. 1985a)

Table 13.2. Sensitivity of SPECT and planar bone scanning for detecting "painful" spondylolysis or spondylolisthesis

	SPECT	Planar
Patients ($n = 13$)	0.85	0.62
Pars interticularis defects ($n = 31$)	0.68	0.42

neural arch along with the spinous process were visualised at all levels in the lumbar spine. There was no left-to-right asymmetry in the posterior neural arch, and activity in the posterior neural arch was less intense than activity in the vertebral bodies. Among the patients with symptomatic spondylolysis or spondylolisthesis, there were eight involved lumbar vertebral levels at which SPECT

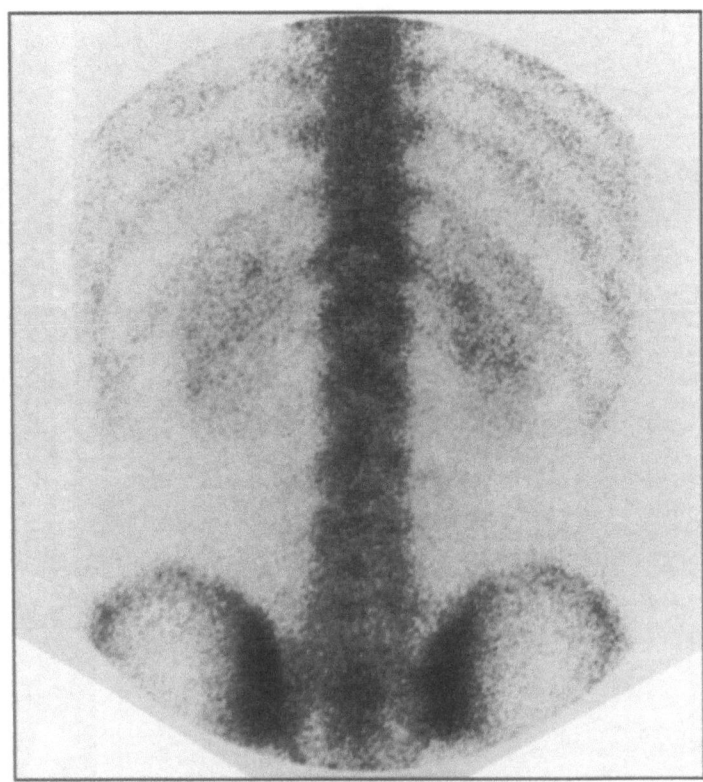

a

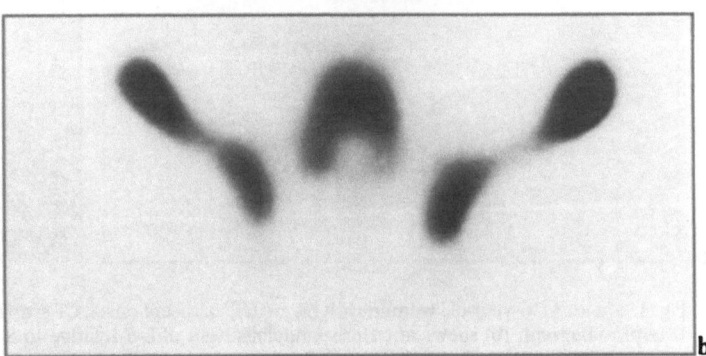

b

Fig. 13.3a,b. An 18-year-old-man with a 1-year history of severe LBP and radiographs showing a defect of the pars interarticularis on the right side of L-5. Posterior planar bone scintigram (a) is normal. Transaxial SPECT bone scan (b) shows increased activity over the right side of the L-5 neural arch corresponding to the site of the pars defect. (Collier et al. 1985a)

identified sites of increased posterior neural arch activity judged to be normal on the planar images (Fig. 13.3). Included in the analysis are three patients whose LBP was eventually attributed to causes other than spondylolysis or spondylolisthesis after SPECT of the posterior neural arch was deemed normal (Fig. 13.4). Based on these results it was concluded that when spondylolysis or spondylolisthesis is the cause of LBP, pars interarticularis defects are frequently associated with increased scintigraphic activity that is best detected and localised by SPECT. These preliminary results suggest that pars interarticularis defects are not responsible for LBP when SPECT and planar bone scintigraphy are normal. Studies of a much larger

number of patients are necessary in order to confirm this hypothesis.

Other promising orthopaedic applications of SPECT bone scanning in the diagnosis of LBP include the detection of symptomatic osteoarthritis of the articular facets, occult fractures, sacroiliitis, pseudoarthrosis following spinal fusion, infection and bone metastases.

Hips

Many investigators using ^{99m}Tc diphosphonates and planar imaging techniques report that AVN of the

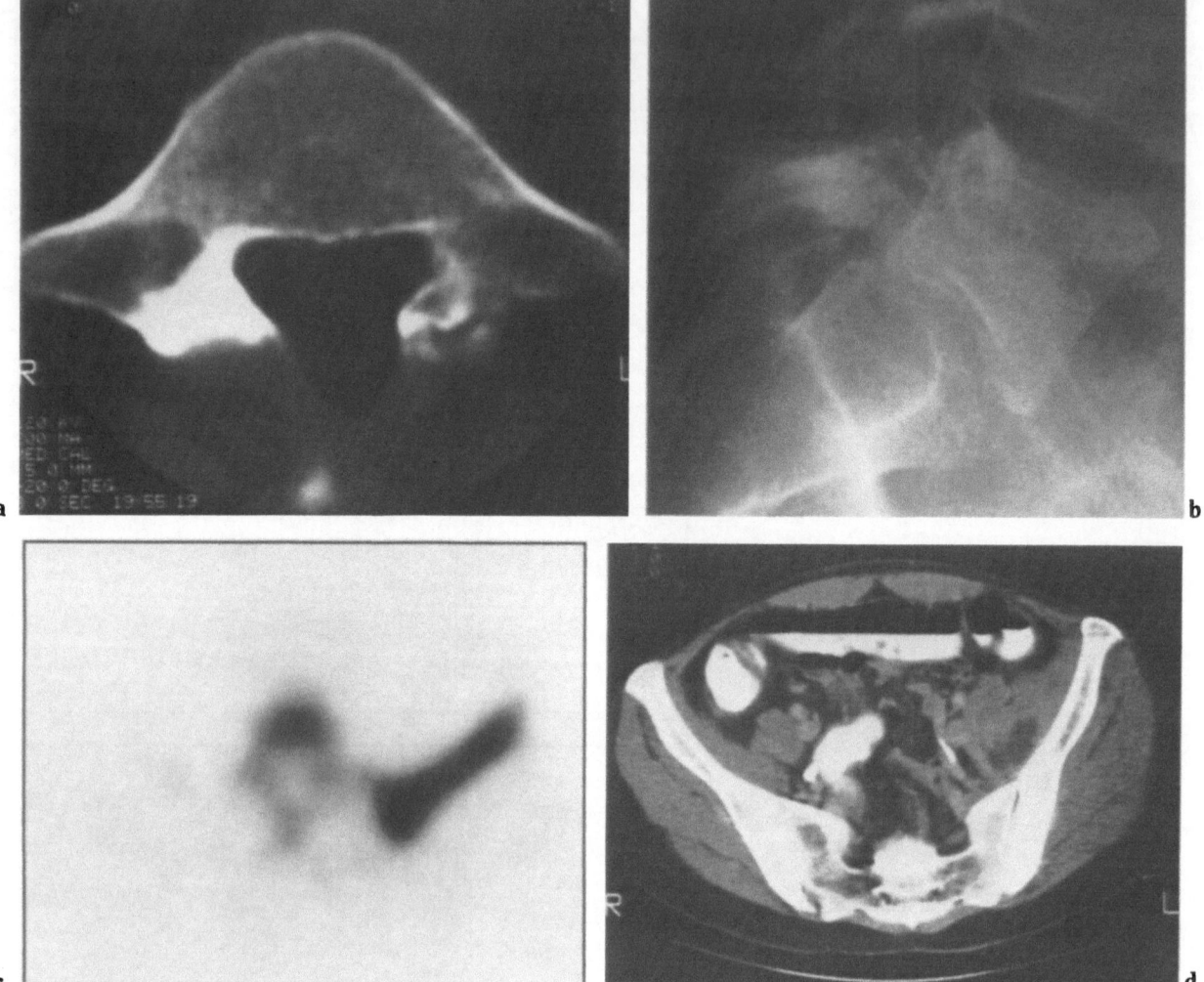

Fig. 13.4a–d. A 26-year-old woman with severe LBP of recent onset. CT scan (a) shows bilateral L-5 spondylolysis with bony sclerosis. Lateral radiograph (b) shows anterior spondylolisthesis of L-5 relative to S-1. Transaxial SPECT bone scan (c) is normal over the L-5 posterior neural arch but shows increased activity in the left iliac wing. CT scan (d) of the pelvis shows a left iliopsoas abscess. (Collier 1985a)

adult femoral head initially appears as a photon-deficient defect (Greyson and Kassel 1976; D'Ambrosia et al. 1978; Hull et al. 1979; Bauer et al. 1980; Greiff 1980; Grieff et al. 1980; Rosenthall and Lisbona 1980; Bassett et al. 1981; Kirchner and Simon 1981; Lucie et al. 1981; Matin 1982; Conklin et al. 1983; Lull et al. 1983; Stromqvist et al. 1984). On planar anterior views of the pelvis, increased scintigraphic activity over the acetabulum and the proximal femoral metaphysis may be present at the time of initial scintigraphy or may develop over the course of weeks to months (D'Ambrosia et al. 1978; Hull et al. 1979; Matin 1982). Subsequently, the photon-deficient defect is often lost on planar bone scans amidst the ingrowth

of osteoblasts upwards into the adult femoral head and the increasingly severe osteoarthritic change in the joint (D'Ambrosia et al. 1978; Hull et al. 1979; Bassett et al. 1981; Matin 1982; Lull et al. 1983; Stromqvist et al. 1984). Osteoarthritic change in the posterior rim of the acetabulum may in part obscure a persistent photon-deficient defect within the femoral head. Furthermore, a rim of increased activity in the subchondral bone over the articular surfaces of the hip often develops in response to AVN-induced bony collapse. This may obscure an underlying photon-deficient defect at the centre of the femoral head. Stromqvist's published data suggests that for planar bone scanning of the normal hip "less than half of the emission ascribed to the

femoral head is derived from the femoral head itself"
(Stromqvist et al. 1984). Late in the course of AVN,
increased uptake adjacent to the avascular femoral.
head undoubtedly reduces the target/background
ratio even further. However, by removing overlying
and underlying activity from the tomographic plane
containing the femoral head, SPECT bone scintigraphy improves image contrast and thereby
facilitates detection of any photon-deficient defects.

Twenty-one adult patients with the clinical
diagnosis of femoral head AVN were examined by
planar and SPECT bone scanning (Collier et al.
1984a, 1985b). SPECT bone scans of the hips
obtained using the techniques described above were
compared with planar 500 000-count images from
a gamma camera with a large field of view and
equipped with a high-resolution collimator. A final
diagnosis of AVN was established for 15 symptomatic patients who had a total of 20 involved hips.
SPECT and planar bone scanning were considered
positively diagnostic of AVN only if a photon-
deficient defect could be identified. Using SPECT, 17
of the 20 involved hips were correctly identified,
whereas with planar imaging only 11 of 20 involved
hips were detected. There were no false-positive
diagnoses of AVN for either SPECT or planar bone
scans when independently interpreted. Included in
this series were patients who had photopaenic
defects detected only with SPECT (Fig. 13.5). One
case of bilateral femoral head AVN with late,
symptomatic involvement in the left hip and early,
asymptomatic disease in the right hip was encountered (Fig. 13.6). For the 20 hips with AVN, 13
had radiographic abnormalities at the time of the
initial SPECT bone scan. However, a subchondral
fracture—the most specific radiographic finding of
early femoral head AVN—was present in only six
instances. The other seven radiographically abnormal hips showed either osteoarthritic changes and/
or flattening of the femoral head—signs generally
not considered to be specific for AVN. The conclusions from this study would indicate that when a
photon-deficient defect is used as the criterion for
early AVN, SPECT bone scanning is more sensitive
than either planar imaging or radiography.

Knees

With recent improvements in arthroscopic technique, direct visual inspection of the knee is now
commonly used to provide highly specific diagnostic
information. However, the general availability of
such a highly specific, invasive and relatively expensive test creates the need for a non-invasive screening examination. If bone scanning could be

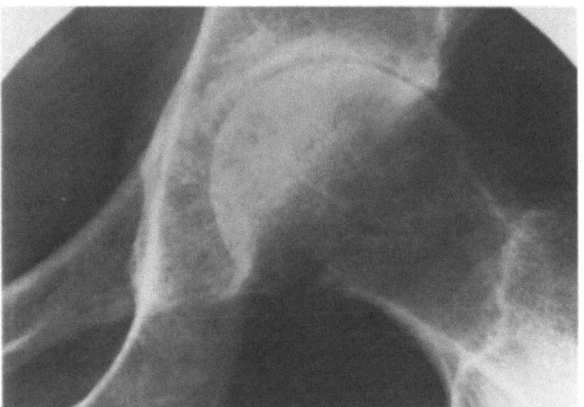
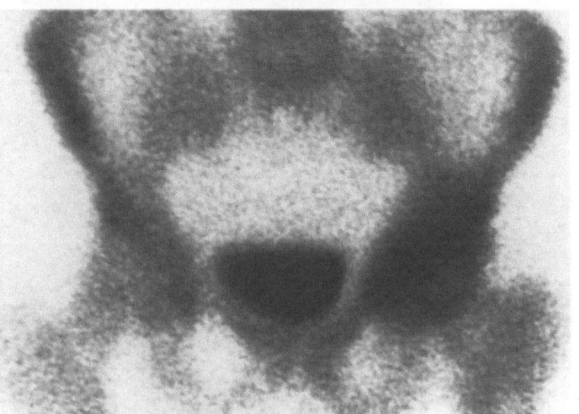
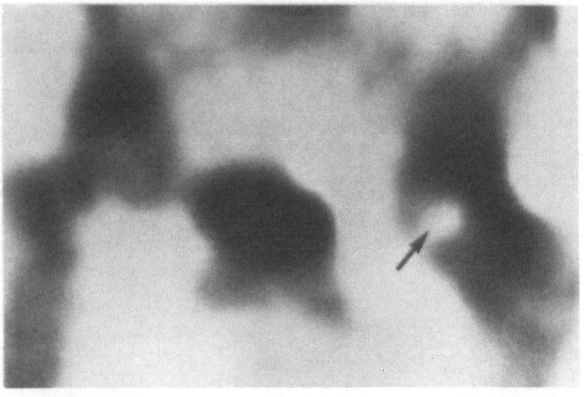

Fig. 13.5a–c. A 57-year-old man with onset of severe left hip pain
3 months previously. Left hip radiograph (a) shows sclerosis, joint
space narrowing and osteophyte formation. Planar bone scintigram (b) shows increased scintigraphic activity over the left
femoral head and left acetabulum with no photon-deficient defect
within the femoral head. Coronal SPECT image (c) shows a
photon-deficient defect in the left femoral head (arrow). (Collier
et al. 1985b)

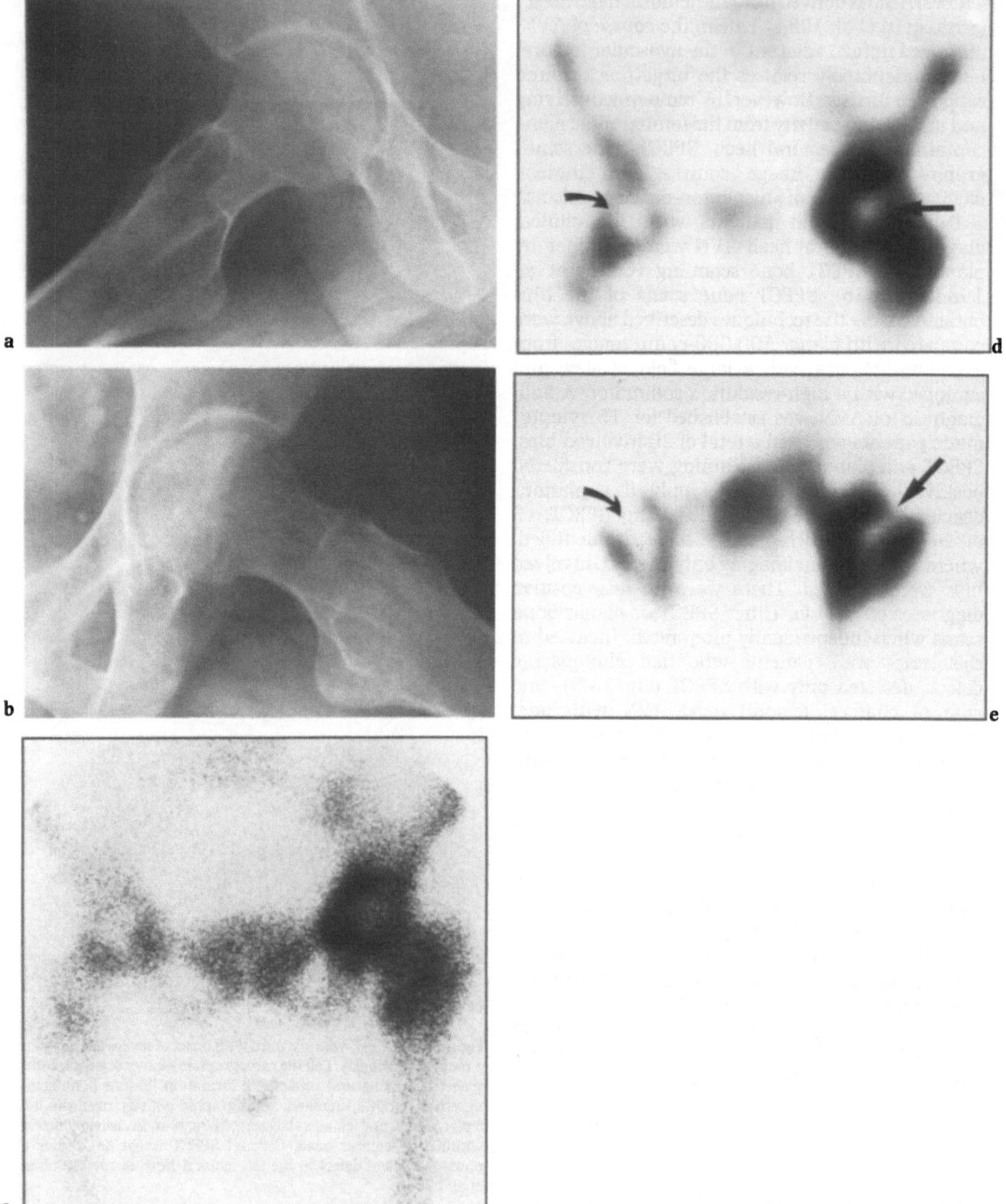

Fig. 13.6a–e. A 52-year-old woman treated with prednisone for chronic active hepatitis had experienced left hip pain for 4 months. Normal right hip radiograph (**a**). Left hip radiograph (**b**) shows sclerosis and flattening of the femoral head. Anterior view planar bone scan (**c**) shows increased activity over the acetabulum and proximal left femur without convincing evidence of a photon-deficient defect in the left femoral head. Coronal (**d**) and transaxial (**e**) SPECT bone scintigrams through both hips clearly demonstrate a central photon-deficient defect surrounded by increased activity within the left femoral head (*straight arrow*). In addition, a photon-deficient defect is seen within the asymptomatic right femoral head (*curved arrow*). (Collier et al. 1985b)

developed as a highly sensitive, albeit non-specific, screening examination for degenerative cartilage damage, meniscus tears and other internal derangements of the knee, then orthopaedists could use bone scanning to select patients more appropriately for invasive diagnosis and treatment. Furthermore, by using the bone scan as a "roadmap" to guide subsequent intra-articular visual inspection, the orthopaedist would be free to concentrate on sites of potentially significant abnormality.

Planar bone scanning has been shown to be more sensitive than history and physical examination, conventional radiography, or double-contrast arthrography for evaluating the extent of osteoarthritis of the knee (Thomas et al. 1975). More recently, planar bone scanning has been used to detect torn menisci (Marymont et al. 1983). When compared with direct visual inspection at the time of arthroscopy or arthrotomy, planar bone scanning frequently identified involved medial and lateral

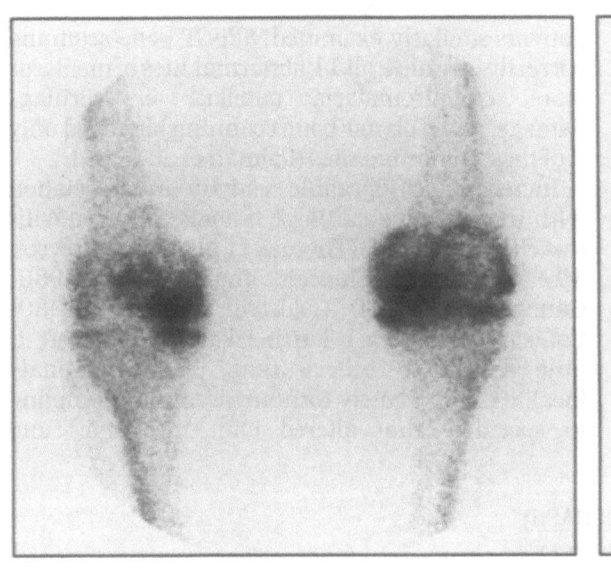
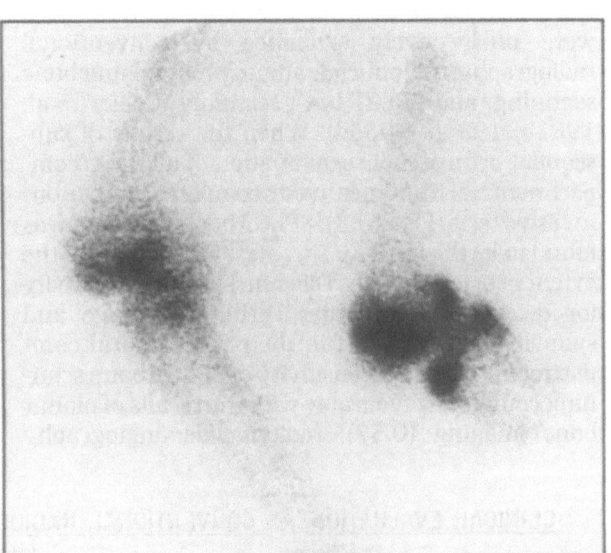
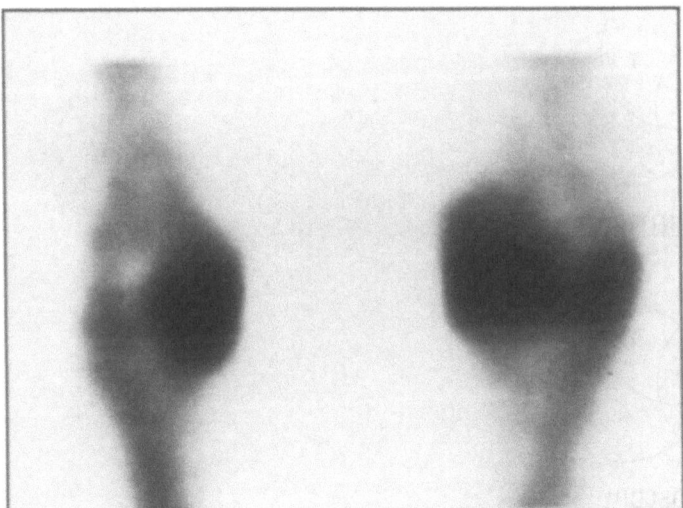
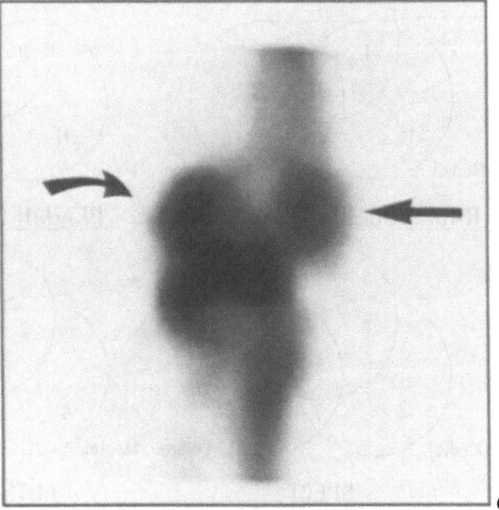

Fig. 13.7a–d. A 30-year-old woman with a 3-year history of left knee pain. Radiographs show varus angulation of the left knee with osteophytes involving the medial and lateral compartments along with joint space narrowing over the medial compartment. Anterior (a) and lateral (b) planar bone scans show convincing evidence of increased activity over the medial and lateral compartments of the left knee with the patella and patellofemoral articulation remaining obscured. Coronal SPECT bone scan (c) through the weight-bearing surfaces of the medial and lateral compartments confirm the increased bony repair at the level of the joint space, which is more pronounced medially. Sagittal SPECT bone scan (d) shows increased activity at the site of articulation of the patella with the interchondral notch (*straight arrow*), which is separate from increased activity along the dorsal surface of the distal end of the femoral condyle (*curved arrow*).

compartments in which osteoarthritis went undetected on other examinations (Thomas et al. 1975). However, when used to detect patellofemoral osteoarthritis, planar bone scintigraphy reportedly has a relatively low sensitivity (Thomas et al. 1975) and a poor specificity (Kipper et al. 1982; Fogelman et al. 1983). Such patellofemoral involvement is more frequently detected by SPECT bone scanning, which separates activity about the patellofemoral articulation from otherwise superimposed activity originating in the medial and lateral femoral condyles (Fig. 13.7).

Twenty-seven patients with chronic knee pain were prospectively examined by conventional radiography, radionuclide angiography, planar bone scanning, and SPECT bone scanning (Collier et al. 1983b, 1984b, 1985d). When the results of subsequent arthroscopic examination of all three compartments of the knee were compared with non-invasive tests (Fig. 13.8), SPECT bone scanning was found to be the most sensitive test for evaluating the extent of osteoarthritis. Differences in the sensitivity for detection of articular cartilage damage and synovitis were greatest in the patellofemoral compartment. The 0.91 sensitivity of SPECT bone scanning compared favourably with the results of planar bone imaging (0.57), radionuclide angiography

(0.39), conventional radiography (0.22), and clinical examination (0.17). Of the 27 patients in this series 14 had the pre-arthroscopic diagnosis of a torn medial and/or lateral meniscus. Arthroscopic examination of 15 knees in this group of 14 patients revealed 7 knees with intact menisci: 3 knees were totally normal, while in the other 4 knees synovitis (2), cartilage damage (1) or chondromalacia patellae (1) were present. SPECT showed increased scintigraphic activity in all compartments where torn menisci (Fig. 13.9) were found but had a specificity of only 0.68 when used to exclude a torn medial or lateral meniscus. For a separate series of 12 patients similarly examined, SPECT bone scanning correctly identified all 11 abnormal sites of meniscus tears, chondromalacia patellae, or cartilage damage, while planar bone scanning identified only 9 of these abnormal sites (Fajman et al. 1985).

Increased scintigraphic activity in association with degenerative cartilage damage and synovitis is well documented (Thomas et al. 1975; Greyson 1979–1980; Christensen and Arnoldi 1980; Gaucher et al. 1980; Goldstein and Bloom 1980; Collier et al. 1983a). Furthermore, while there is little reason to believe that ^{99m}Tc medronate localises in an acutely torn meniscus, it is tempting to speculate that altered joint mechanics and

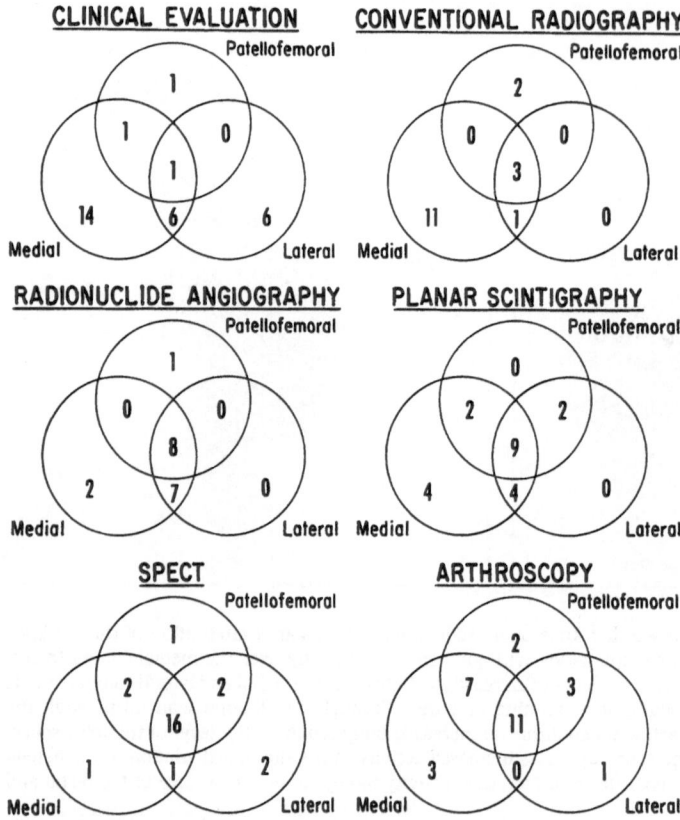

Fig. 13.8. Distribution of abnormal findings for non-invasive compartmental examinations of the knee compared with the distribution of cartilage damage and/or synovitis detected by arthroscopy.

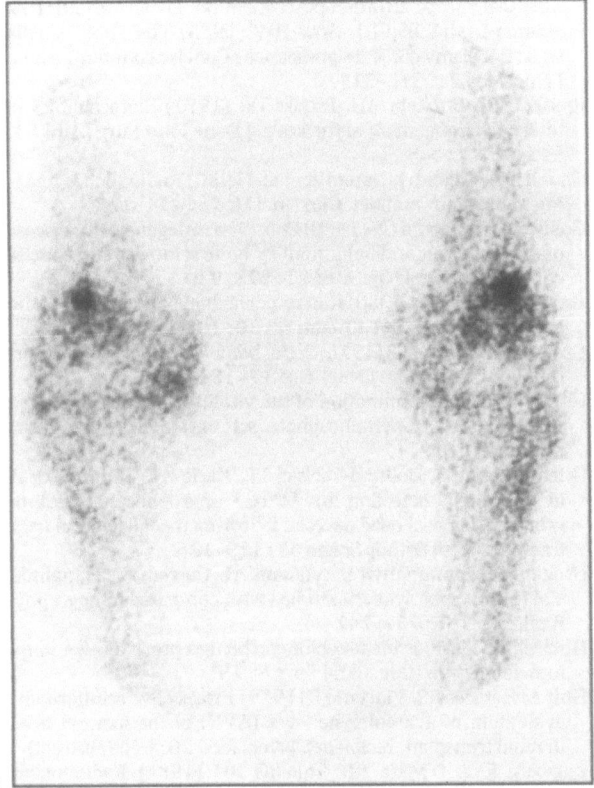

a

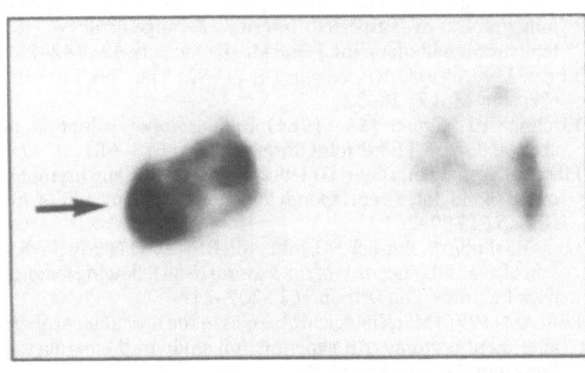

b

Fig. 13.9a,b. A 63-year-old man with 2 months of right knee pain and locking. Radiographs showed only small patellar osteophytes bilaterally. Anterior view planar bone scan (**a**) shows moderately intense increased activity over both patellae with no major scintigraphic abnormalities in the medial or lateral compartments of the painful right knee. Transaxial SPECT image (**b**) at the level of the joint space shows a crescent-shaped band of increased activity in the lateral compartment of the right knee (*arrow*) corresponding closely to the location of a longitudinal lateral meniscus tear identified at the time of subsequent arthroscopy.

degenerative changes secondary to a long-standing meniscus tear eventually predispose to increase scintigraphic activity in the adjacent subchondral bone (Huckell 1965; Frankel et al. 1971; Dandy and Jackson 1975; Lufti 1975; Walker and Erkman 1975; Noble and Erat 1980; Sonne-Holm et al.

1980). Testing of a larger and more varied group of patients with clinical suspicion of internal derangement of the knee is needed to evaluate fully the diagnostic efficacy of this technique. None the less, for patients with chronic knee pain and clinical suspicion of a meniscus tear or other significant degenerative internal derangement, SPECT bone scanning appears to be a highly sensitive screening test worthy of additional investigation. Further research will probably show that increased scintigraphic activity in the medial or lateral compartments of the knee cannot be used to distinguish a meniscus tear from cartilage damage, synovitis, intra-articular loose bodies or most other morbid conditions associated with chronic knee pain. However, it is the ability to detect and localise such lesions of bone and cartilage—not the ability to make a specific diagnosis—which argues for the use of SPECT bone scanning as a pre-arthroscopic screening examination.

Temporomandibular Joints

Oral surgeons seeking to confirm the diagnosis of internal derangement of the TMJ have found SPECT to be a valuable screening test. When used to examine 36 oral surgery patients undergoing preoperative evaluation, the sensitivity of SPECT (0.94) was comparable with arthrography (0.96) and significantly better than planar bone scanning (0.76) or conventional radiography (0.04) (Collier et al. 1983a). While data from a larger asymptomatic control population are needed, preliminary results give SPECT a diagnostic specificity of 0.70 for internal derangement of the TMJ requiring surgical correction. Lower sensitivities but comparable specificities for SPECT have been reported in series using arthrography rather than surgery to confirm the status of the TMJ (O'Mara et al. 1983; Katzberg et al. 1984).

Summary and Conclusions

During the day-to-day operation of a busy nuclear medicine laboratory, the addition of SPECT imaging to an orthopaedic bone scanning procedure requires an extra 5 min for setup and patient positioning, 21 min for data acquisition, and 15 min for processing and filming. However, when examining patients with knee, hip and low back pain, SPECT bone scanning frequently gives images of greater clarity and in many instances provides unique diagnostic information. Specific advantages of SPECT in identifying and localising skeletal pathology have already been established, and further diagnostic applications both for skeletal oncology and for the study of LBP are anticipated.

References

Bailey W (1947) Observations on the etiology and frequency of spondylolisthesis and its precursors. Radiology 48: 108–112

Bassett LW, Gold RH, Webber MM (1981) Radionuclide bone imaging. Radiol Clin North Am 19: 675–702

Bauer G, Weber DA, Ceder L et al. (1980) Dynamics of technetium-99m methylenediphosphonate imaging of the femoral head after hip fracture. Clin Orthop 152: 85–92

Christensen SB, Arnoldi CC (1980) Distribution of Tc-99m-phosphate compounds in osteoarthritic femoral heads. J Bone Joint Surg [Am] 62: 90–96

Collier BD, Carrera GF, Messer EJ et al. (1983a) Internal derangement of the temporomandibular joint: detection by single photon emission computed tomography. Radiology 149: 557–561

Collier BD, Johnson RP, Carrera GF, Palmer DW, Isitman AT, Hellman RS (1983b) Single photon emission computed tomography in suspected internal derangements of the knee. J Nucl Med 24: P41

Collier BD, Johnson RP, Carrera GF, Isitman AT, Hellman RS, Zielonka JS (1984a) Detection of avascular necrosis in adults by single photon emission computed tomography. J Nucl Med 25: P25

Collier BD, Johnson RP, Carrera GF et al. (1984b) Use of bone scintigraphy as a screening examination for torn menisci in patients with chronic knee pain. Radiology 153: P212

Collier BD, Johnson RP, Carrera GF et al. (1985a) Painful spondylolysis or spondylolisthesis studied by radiology and single-photon emission computed tomography. Radiology 154: 207–211

Collier BD, Carrera GF, Johnson RP et al. (1985b) Detection of femoral head avascular necrosis in adults by SPECT. J Nucl Med 26: 979–987

Collier BD, Dellis CJ, Peck DC, Krohn L (1985c) Bone SPECT. J Nucl Med Tech 13: 230–236

Collier BD, Johnson RP, Carrera GF et al. (1985d) Chronic knee pain assessed by SPECT: comparison with other modalities. Radiology 157: 795–802

Conklin JJ, Alderson PO, Zizic TM et al. (1983) Comparison of bone scan and radiograph sensitivity in the detection of steroid-induced ischemic necrosis of bone. Radiology 147: 221–226

D'Ambrosia RD, Shoji H, Riggins RS, Stadalnik RC, DeNardo GL (1978) Scintigraphy in the diagnosis of osteonecrosis. Clin Orthop 13: 139–143

Dandy DJ, Jackson RW (1975) Meniscectomy and chondromalacia of the femoral condyle. J Bone Joint Surg [Am] 57: 1116

Eisenstein S (1978) Spondylolysis. A skeletal investigation of two population groups. J Bone Joint Surg [Br] 60: 488–494

Eisner RL (1985) Principles of instrumentation in SPECT. J Nucl Med Tech 13: 23–31

Fajman WA, Diehl M, Dunaway E et al. (1985) Tomographic and planar radionuclide imaging in patients with suspected meniscal injury: arthroscopic correlation. J Nucl Med 26: P77

Fogelman I, McKillop JH, Gray HW (1983) The "hot" patella sign: is it of any clinical significance? Concise communication. J Nucl Med 24: 312–315

Frankel VH, Burstein AH, Brooks DB (1971) Biomechanics of internal derangement of the knee. J Bone Joint Surg [Am] 53: 945–962

Gaucher A, Colomb J, Naoun A et al. (1980) Radionuclide imaging in hip abnormalities. Clin Nucl Med 5: 214–226

Goldstein HA, Bloom CY (1980) Detection of degenerative disease of the temporomandibular joint by bone scintigraphy: concise communication. J Nucl Med 21: 928–930

Greyson ND (1979–1980) Radionuclide bone and joint imaging in rheumatology. Bull Rheum Dis 30: 1032–1039

Greyson ND, Kassel EE (1976) Serial bone-scan changes in recurrent bone infarction. J Nucl Med 17: 184–186

Grieff J (1980) Determination of the vitality of the femoral head with Tc-99m-Sn-pyrophosphate scintigraphy. Acta Orthop Scand 51: 109–117

Grieff J, Lanng S, Hoilund-Carlsen PF, Karle AK, Uhrenholdt A (1980) Early detection by ^{99m}Tc-Sn-pyrophosphate scintigraphy of femoral head necrosis following medial femoral neck fractures. Acta Orthop Scand 51: 119–125

Grogan JP, Hemminghytt S, Williams AL, Carrera GF, Haughton VM (1982) Spondylolysis studied with computed tomography. Radiology 145: 737–742

Huckell JR (1965) Is meniscectomy a benign procedure? A long-term follow-up study. Can J Surg 8: 254

Hull A, Hattner RS, Vincente F (1979) Prospective scintigraphic evaluation of avascular necrosis (AVN) of the femoral head in renal transplant recipients. J Nucl Med 20: 646 (abstract)

Katzberg RW, O'Mara RE, Tallents RH (1984) Radionuclide skeletal imaging and single photon emission computed tomography in suspected internal derangements of the temporomandibular joint. J Oral Maxillofac Surg 42: 782–787

Kipper MS, Alazraki NP, Feiglin DH (1982) The "hot" patella. Clin Nucl Med 7: 28–32

Kirchner PT, Simon MA (1981) Radioisotope evaluation of skeletal disease. J Bone Joint Surg [Am] 63: 673–681

Libson E, Bloom RA, Dinari G (1982) Symptomatic and asymptomatic spondylolysis and spondylolisthesis in young adults. Int Orthop 6: 259–261

Lucie RS, Fuller S, Burdick DC, Johnston RM (1981) Early prediction of avascular necrosis of the femoral head following femoral neck fractures. Clin Orthop 161: 207–214

Lufti AM (1975) Morphological changes in the articular cartilage after meniscectomy. An experimental study in the monkey. J Bone Joint Surg [Br] 57: 525

Lull RJ, Utz JA, Jackson JH et al. (1983) Radionuclide evaluation of joint disease. In: Freeman LM, Weissman HS (eds) Nuclear medicine annual. Raven, New York, pp 281–328

Magora A, Schwartz A (1980) Relation between low back pain and x-ray changes. 4. Lysis and olisthesis. Scand J Rehabil Med 12: 47–52

Marymont JV, Lynch MA, Henning CE (1983) Evaluation of meniscus tears of the knee by radionuclide imaging. Am J Sports Med 11: 432–435

Matin P (1982) Bone scanning of trauma and benign conditions. In: Freeman LM, Weissman HS (eds) Nuclear medicine annual. Raven, New York, pp 81–118

Meyerding HW (1941) Low backache and sciatic pain associated with spondylolisthesis and protruded intervertebral disc: incidence, significance, and treatment. J Bone Joint Surg 23: 461–470

Noble J, Erat K (1980) In defence of the meniscus. J Bone Joint Surg [Br] 62: 7–11

O'Mara RE, Katzberg RW, Weber DA, Wilson GA, Tallents RH (1983) Skeletal imaging and SPECT in temporomandibular joint disease. Radiology 149: P101

Rhea JT, DeLuca SA, Llewellyn JH, Boyd RJ (1980) The oblique view: an unnecessary component of the initial adult lumbar spine examination. Radiology 134: 45–47

Roche MB, Rowe GG (1952) The incidence of separate neural arch and coincident bone variations. A summary. J Bone Joint Surg [Am] 34: 491–494

Rosenthall L, Lisbona R (1980) Role of radionuclide imaging in benign and joint diseases of orthopedic interest. In: Freeman LM, Weissman HS (eds) Nuclear medicine annual. Raven, New York, pp 267–302

Sonne-Holm S, Fledelius I, Ahn N (1980) Results after meniscectomy in 147 athletes. Acta Orthop Scand 51: 303–309

Splithoff CA (1953) Lumbosacral junction. Roentgenographic comparisons of patients with and without backaches. JAMA 152: 1610–1613

Stromqvist B, Brismar J, Hansson LI, Palmer J (1984) Technetium-99m-methylenediphosphonate scintigraphy after femoral neck fracture. Clin Orthop 182: 177–189

Thomas RH, Resnick D, Alazraki NP, Daniel D, Greenfield R (1975) Compartmental evaluation of osteoarthritis of the knee. Radiology 116: 585–594

Torgerson WR, Dotter WE (1976) Comparative roentgenographic study of the asymptomatic and symptomatic lumbar spine. J Bone Joint Surg [Am] 58: 850–853

Walker PS, Erkman MJ (1975) The role of the menisci in force transmission across the knee. Clin Orthop 109: 184

Wiltse LL, Hutchinson RH (1964) Surgical treatment of spondylolisthesis. Clin Orthop 35: 116–135

Wiltse LL, Widell EH Jr, Jackson DW (1975) Fatigue fracture; the basic lesion in isthmic spondylolisthesis. J Bone Joint Surg [Am] 57: 17–22

14 · The Bone Scan in Paediatrics

I. Gordon and A. M. Peters

Introduction

In 1984, a survey carried out in 21 countries in Europe showed that bone scintigraphy comprised 16% of all paediatric radioisotope scans. Although the value of bone scans in paediatrics is potentially great, their quality varies greatly, and poor-quality images are giving this valuable technique a bad reputation (Harcke 1978).

The handling of children requires a sensitive staff and the provision of a few simple inexpensive items of distraction. Attempting simply to scan a child between two adult patients in a busy general department is a recipe for an unhappy, uncooperative child with the probable result of poor images. The intravenous injection of isotope should be given adjacent to the gamma camera room, unless dynamic scans are required, so that the child does not associate the camera with the injection. This injection is best carried out by someone competent in paediatric venipunture; the entire procedure should be explained to the child and parent, who should remain with the child throughout. It is naive to think that silence makes for a cooperative child (Carty 1984).

Following the intravenous injection the child should be encouraged to drink as much as possible. This is of great assistance in ensuring the bladder is free of radioactivity when the later images are obtained. Simple sand bags at the side of the child, coupled with wide Velcro straps, help the child to keep still. All images should be obtained with the patient lying on top of the camera so that at no time does the child feel sandwiched between camera and table top. This is obviously not possible for pin-hole images, which should therefore be done last.

Books for children of different ages, a few cuddly toys and a musical box frequently convert the atmosphere in the gamma camera room to a pleasant welcoming one. These facilities, together with a dedicated technician sensitive to children, result in the high-quality images so essential to paediatric nuclear medicine.

Radioisotopes

The sensitivity of bone-seeking radioisotope tracers and the marked improvement in gamma camera resolution has allowed bone scanning to become an integrated technique in the assessment of children suspected of suffering from pathological bone conditions. The tracer most commonly used for routine bone scanning is ^{99m}Tc diphosphonate (MDP); other isotopes used include ^{99m}Tc colloid for bone marrow scans and ^{67}Ga citrate and ^{111}In white blood cells (^{111}In WBC) for investigation of inflammatory/infective lesions.

^{99m}Tc-MDP

Following intravenous injection ^{99m}Tc-MDP is absorbed onto the hydroxyapatite of the bone. Images 1 min after the intravenous injection reflect

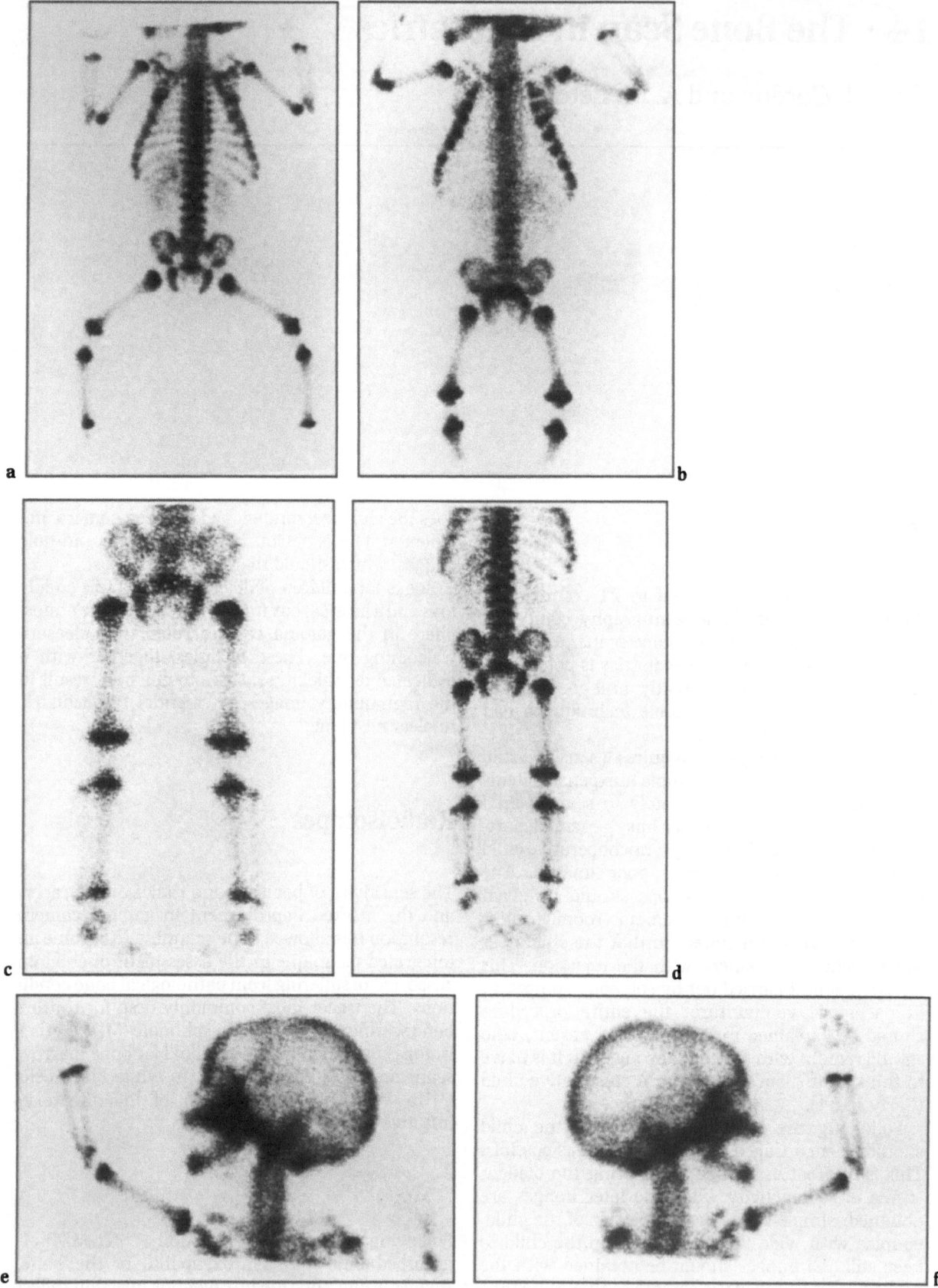

◀ **Fig. 14.1a–f.** Normal bone scan in a neonate. **a,b** Posterior and anterior non-magnified views; **c** posterior magnified view of lower limbs; **d** posterior non-magnified view of spine, pelvis and lower limbs; **e** left lateral view of skull and left arm; **f** right lateral view of skull and right arm.

Note high uptake of tracer in sites of active bone growth, such as the epiphyseal plates of the long bones and the sutures of skull. A high-resolution collimator and attention to technical detail were essential for these high-quality images. Note separate visualisation of the tibia and fibula in the lower limbs and radius and ulna in the upper limbs, and note also that the bladder is empty. The proximal epiphyses of the tibia and distal epiphysis of the femora are visible, but the ossification centres for the femoral heads have not appeared. The patient had neuroblastoma. Although the skeleton is normal, abnormal soft tissue uptake by the primary can be seen in the left suprarenal region (**a,b**).

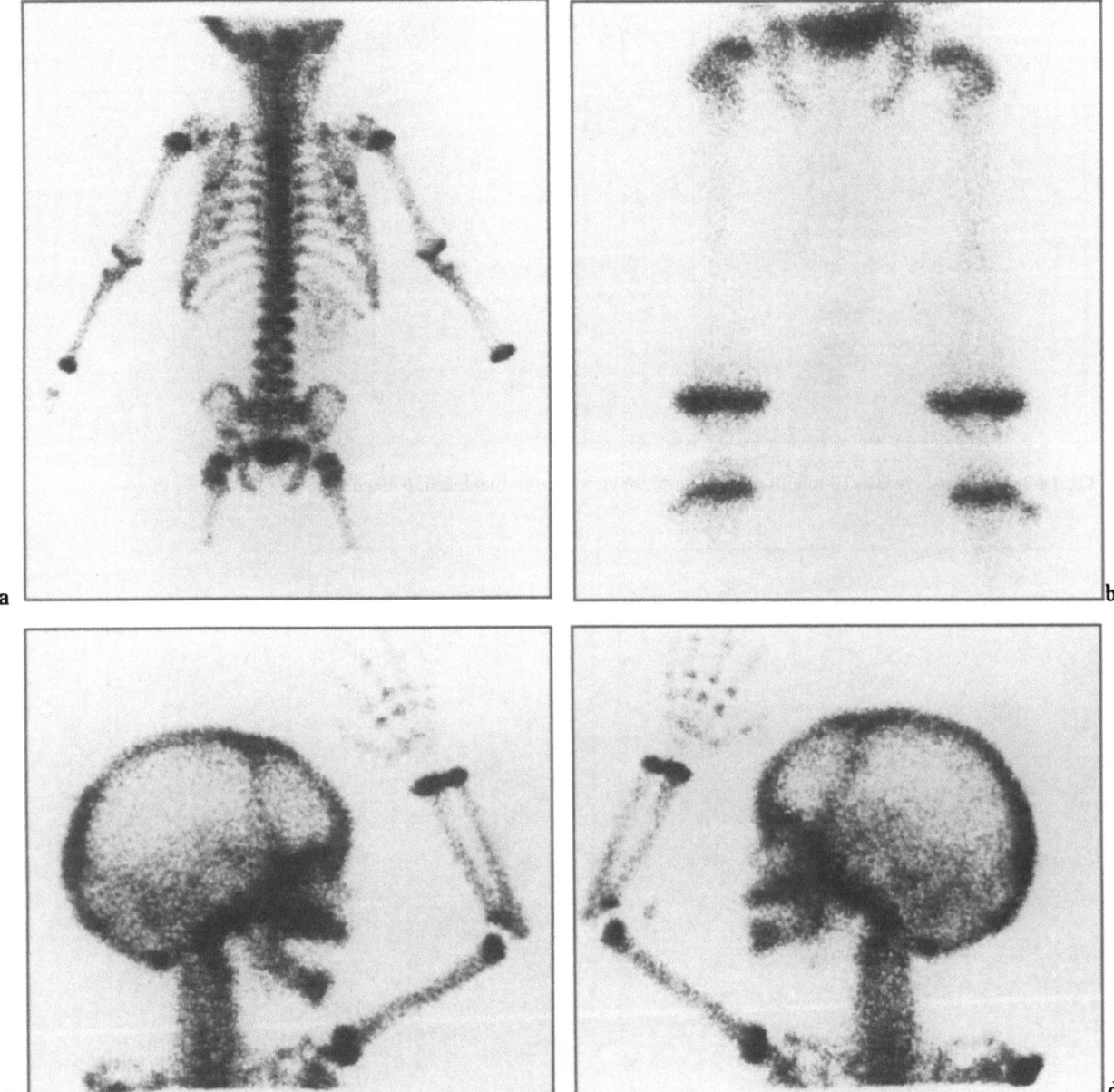

Fig. 14.2a–d. The same infant as in Fig. 14.1 re-scanned at age 18 months. The skeleton remains normal. **a** Posterior non-magnified view. Note "shine through" in chest from the anterior ends of the ribs, giving impressions of "hot spots" in posterior ribs. **b** Posterior magnified views of lower limbs. The growth plates can be seen very clearly and the epiphyses around the knee are more obvious than in the previous scan. The femoral heads are also now visible. **c,d** Lateral skull views with upper limbs.

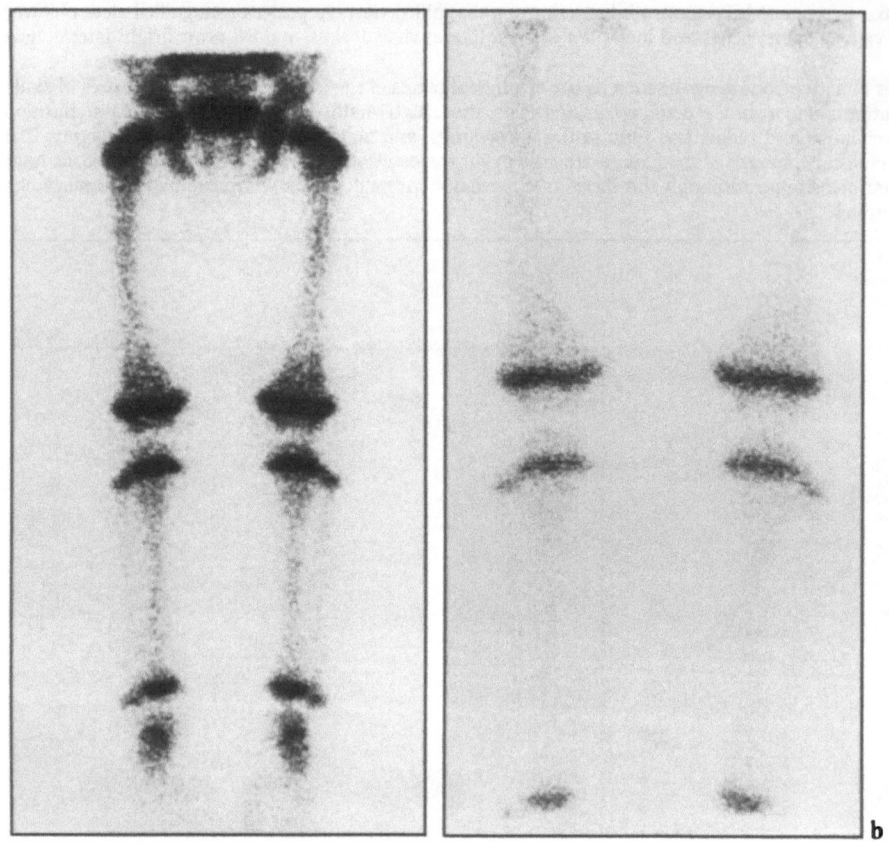

Fig. 14.3a,b. Normal knees in 18-month-old boy. Posterior views: a non-magnified; b magnified.

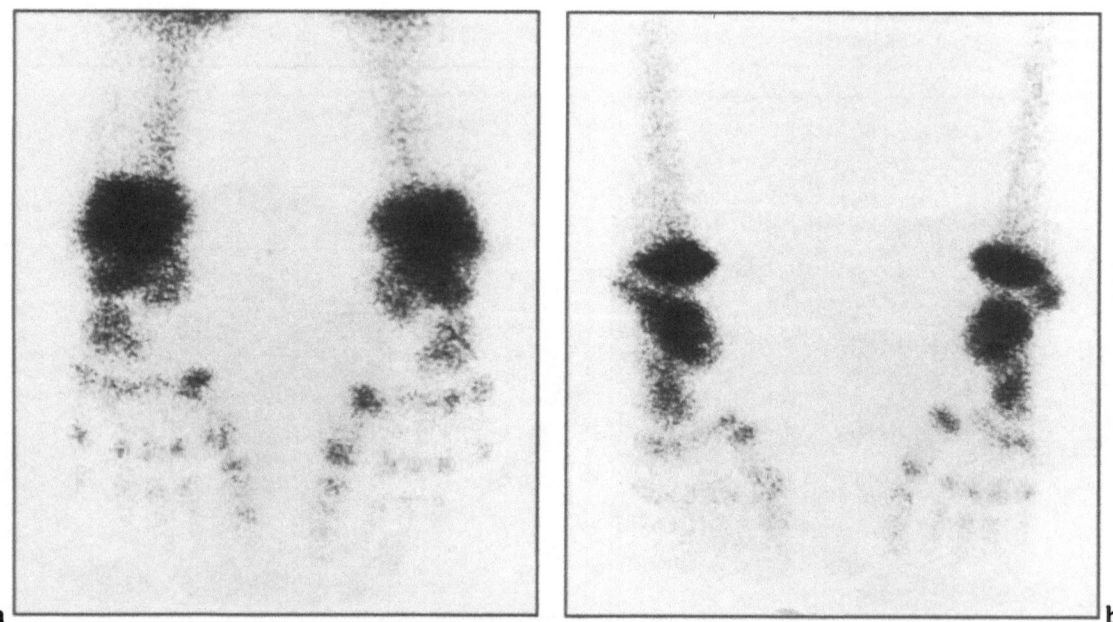

Fig. 14.4a,b. Normal foot in an 18-month-old child. a Plantar view; b dorsal view. The distal epiphyses of the fibula and tibia are separately visible in the dorsal view but are seen as one in the plantar view. Ossification centres have appeared in the talus, calcaneum, cuboid and lateral cuneiform, but not in the navicular and medial and intermediate cuneiforms. The growth plates of the metatarsals and phalanges are clearly visible

blood flow to the bone, while the images at 2–4 h reflect the bone turnover. The dose of isotope to be injected is calculated on a body surface area basis. An adult dose of 13.5 mCi (500 MBq) for 1.73 m² is used and scaled down. However, in infants under 5 kg a minimum dose of 1.08 mCi (40 MBq) is given. The radiation dose to the whole body is acceptable for a diagnostic procedure (Treves and Kirkpatrick 1985).

The ^{99m}Tc-MDP scan shows increased uptake of isotope even when minimal bone abnormality is present, but this is non-specific. For this reason a good-quality radiograph of the abnormal areas on the ^{99m}Tc-MDP bone scan is recommended in order to give the test a high sensitivity and specificity. Examples of normal bone scans are given in Figs. 14.1–14.9.

An adequate ^{99m}Tc-MDP bone scan requires high-quality images upon which the full value of the scan is dependent (see Fig. 14.4). When the lower limbs are imaged the tibia and fibula must be clearly distinguishable (see Fig. 14.6), as must the radius and ulna in the upper limb (see Figs. 14.1, 14.2, 14.5). When the lumbar spine and pelvis are the centre of attention, an empty bladder is important so that urinary activity does not obscure true pathological conditions. In suspected hip abnormality, the acetabular roof must be clearly seen apart from the capital epiphysis and the femoral head (see Fig. 14.7). When an infiltrative disorder, e.g. neuroblastoma, is suspected, then images of the knees in the centre of the field of view, with clear distinction of the tibia from the head of the fibula, are essential (see Figs. 14.3, 14.5). Good positioning is very important and there is no substitute for a dedicated radiographer/technician. In certain circumstances, e.g. Perthes disease (see Figs. 14.11, 14.12), discitis and back pain, a whole-body scan is not essential (see Figs. 14.8, 14.9).

The major indications for bone imaging include osteomyelitis, Perthes disease (see p. 198), longstanding pain of skeletal and/or joint origin and malignancy. Bone scans are more sensitive than radiographs in detecting secondary deposits in malignancy and also in osteomyelitis. The one area where caution must be exercised is in the neonate, since rampant osteomyelitis may not be revealed on bone scintigraphy (Ash and Gilday 1980). High-quality hip views with an empty bladder are essential if Perthes disease is not to be overlooked.

^{99m}Tc Colloid

The radioisotope is attached to a very small sized particle +/− 100 ng, which is avidly taken up by the reticuloendothelial system. This scan is reserved for certain haematological disorders for the monitoring of bone marrow recovery, and also in determining distribution of disease in certain cases of marrow aplasia. The marrow scan also gives good images of the liver and spleen, but this has the disadvantage of obscuring the marrow in the lower dorsal and upper lumbar spine. (Siddiqui et al. 1979).

^{111}In WBC

The removal, labelling and reinjection of blood involved in performing the ^{111}In WBC scan means that this scan is somewhat more complex than other scans. Coupled with the relatively high radiation dose (Gordon and Vivian 1984) this scan should be reserved for certain difficult problems. It is a second-line investigation but does have a place in the ill neonate with suspected osteomyelitis, and also possibly in chronic multifocal osteomyelitis. Following osteomyelitis in the older infant and child, the bone scan may remain "hot" for a varying period and there may be no other way of determining whether this increased uptake of isotope is due to ongoing infection or simple remodelling following infection. In this setting, the ^{111}In WBC scan may be useful or, if it is unavailable, then the ^{67}Ga scan may be used.

^{67}Ga Citrate

The isotope ^{67}Ga was routinely used for bone scans in the 1960s but it is not ideal for the gamma camera because it has three energy peaks. It is also excreted via the biliary and gastrointestinal tract and is not an ideal agent for bone scanning. However, this isotope does accumulate in infective/inflammatory sites and also in certain malignant tumours. Its clinical use is similar to that of ^{111}In WBC. It has been used with good results in suspected early acute osteomyelitis when the ^{99m}Tc-MDP bone scan may well be normal (Handmaker and Giammona, 1984). Its use in osteomyelitis is in distinguishing between infection and simple new bone formation.

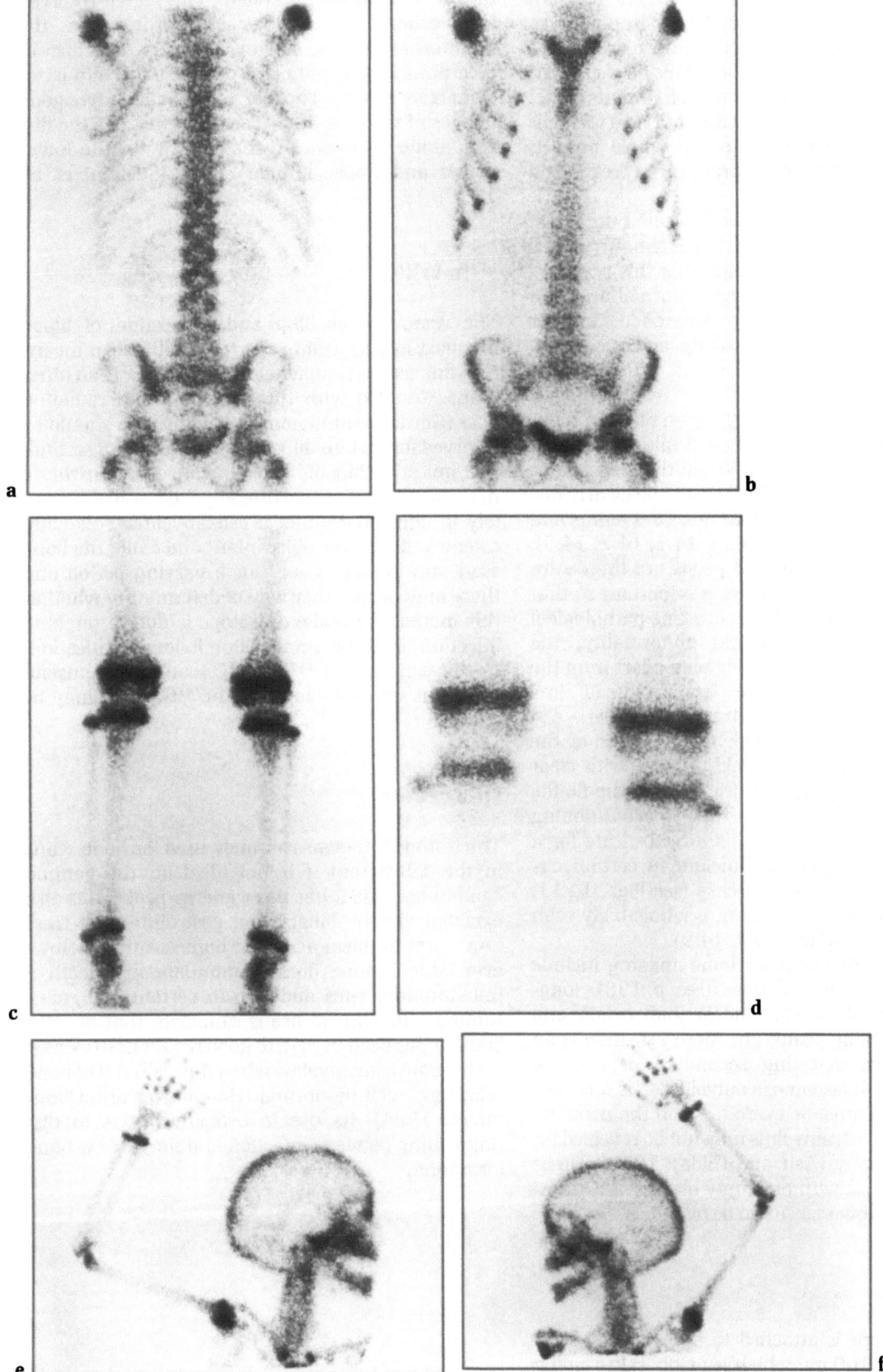

◀ Fig. 14.5a–f. Normal skeleton in a 5-year-old girl. a Posterior spine and pelvis; b anterior spine and pelvis; c posterior knees and ankles (non-magnified); d posterior knees (magnified); e,f lateral skulls and upper limbs. Note that the ossification centre for the greater trochanter is visible at this age.

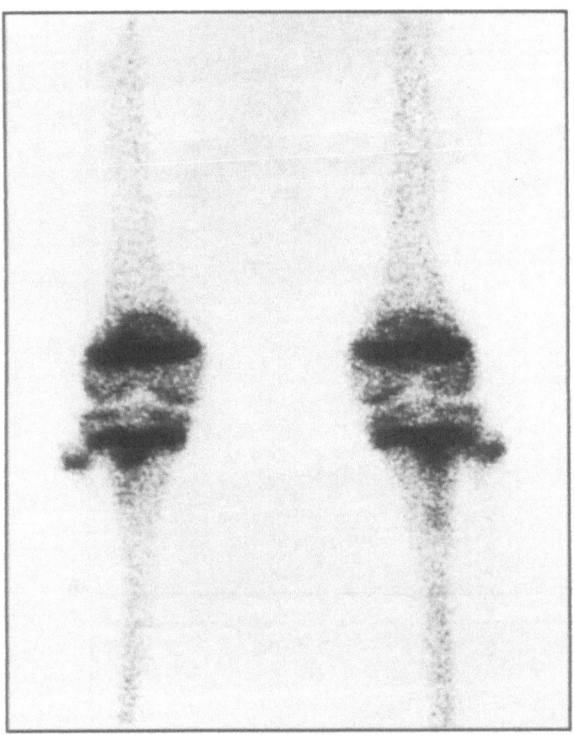

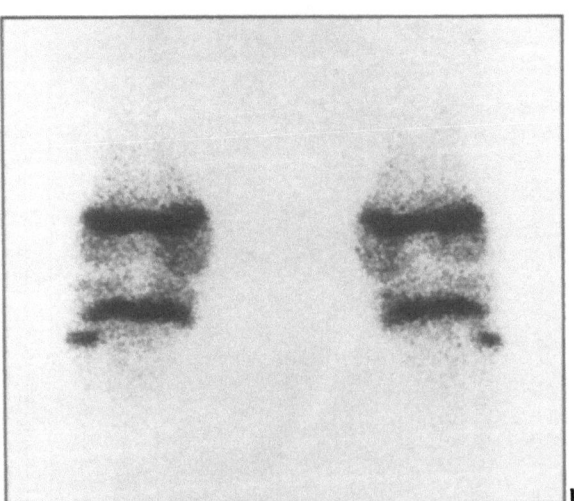

▲
Fig. 14.6a,b. Normal knees in the older boy (age 14 years). a Anterior view; b posterior view. The patella and tibial tuberosities are clearly visible on the anterior view.

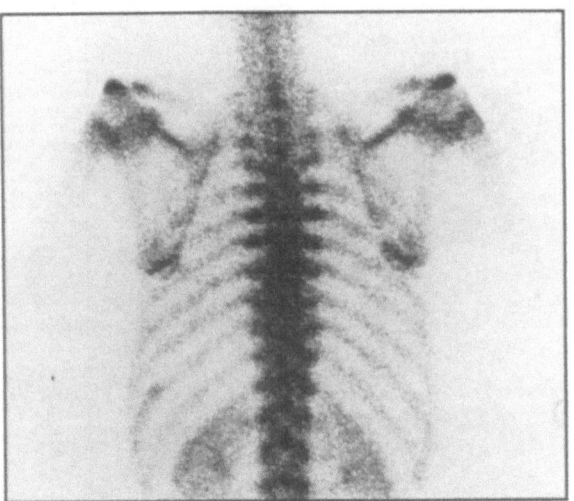

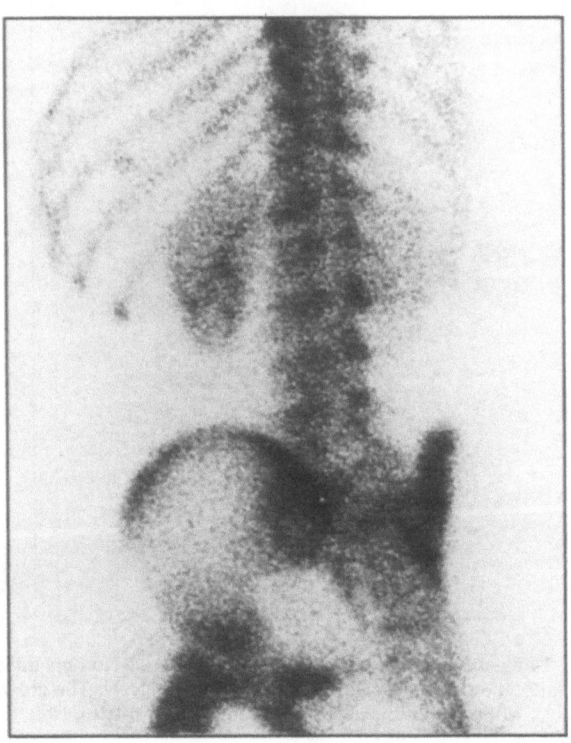

▲
Fig. 14.7a,b. Normal spine and pelvis in a 14-year-old boy. The value of the oblique spinal view (a) is demonstrated in that the apparent rib lesions on the posterior view (b) are seen to lie between the 10th and 11th left ribs on the oblique view.

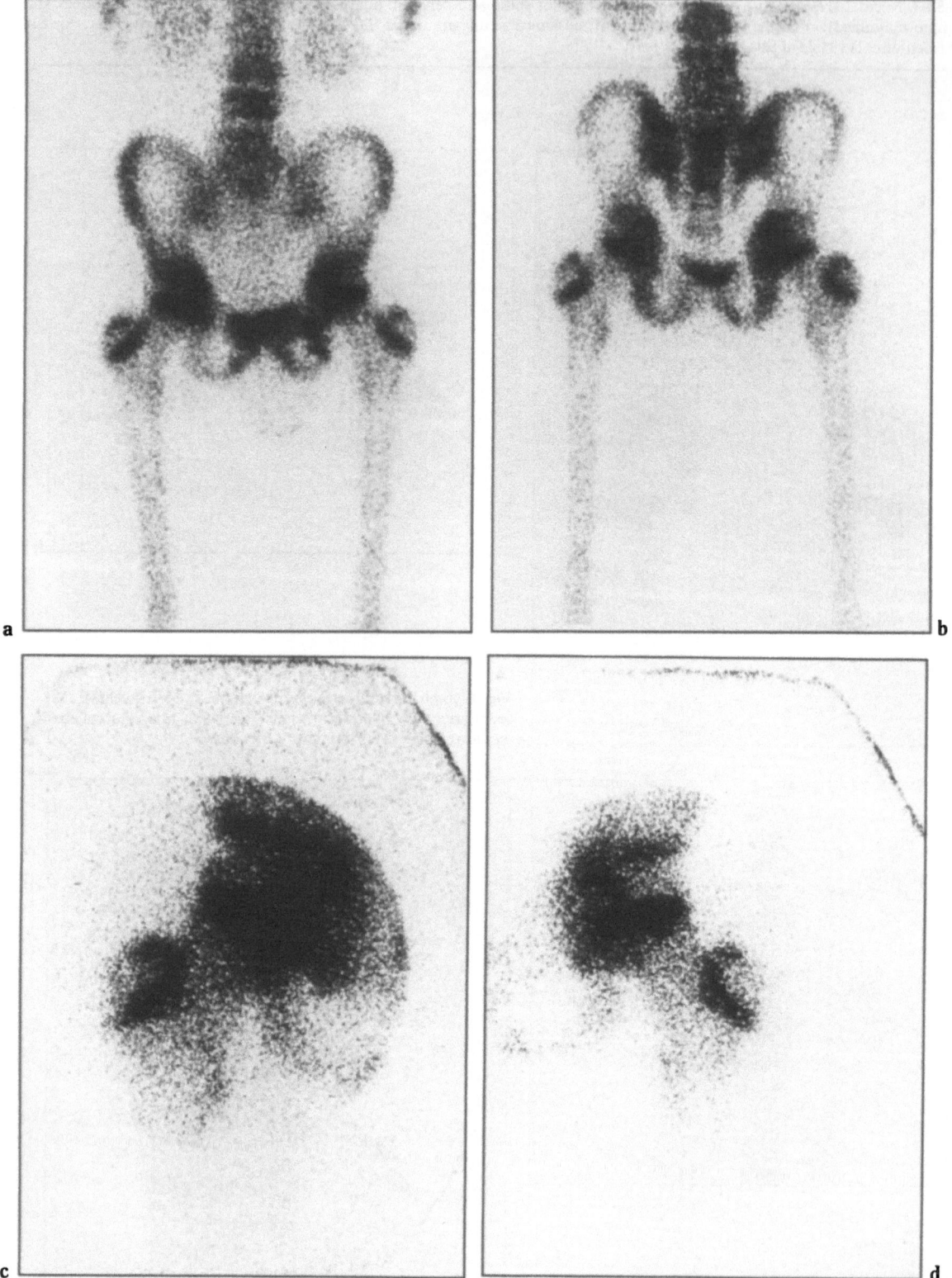

Fig. 14.8a–d. Normal hips in a 12-year-old child. **a,b** Non-magnified views, anterior and posterior respectively. **c,d** Anterior pin-hole magnification views of right and left hips respectively. The growth plates of the femoral head and greater trochanter are clearly visible, while that of the lesser trochanter is only just so. Note that the lateral part of the femoral head has less activity than the medial part.

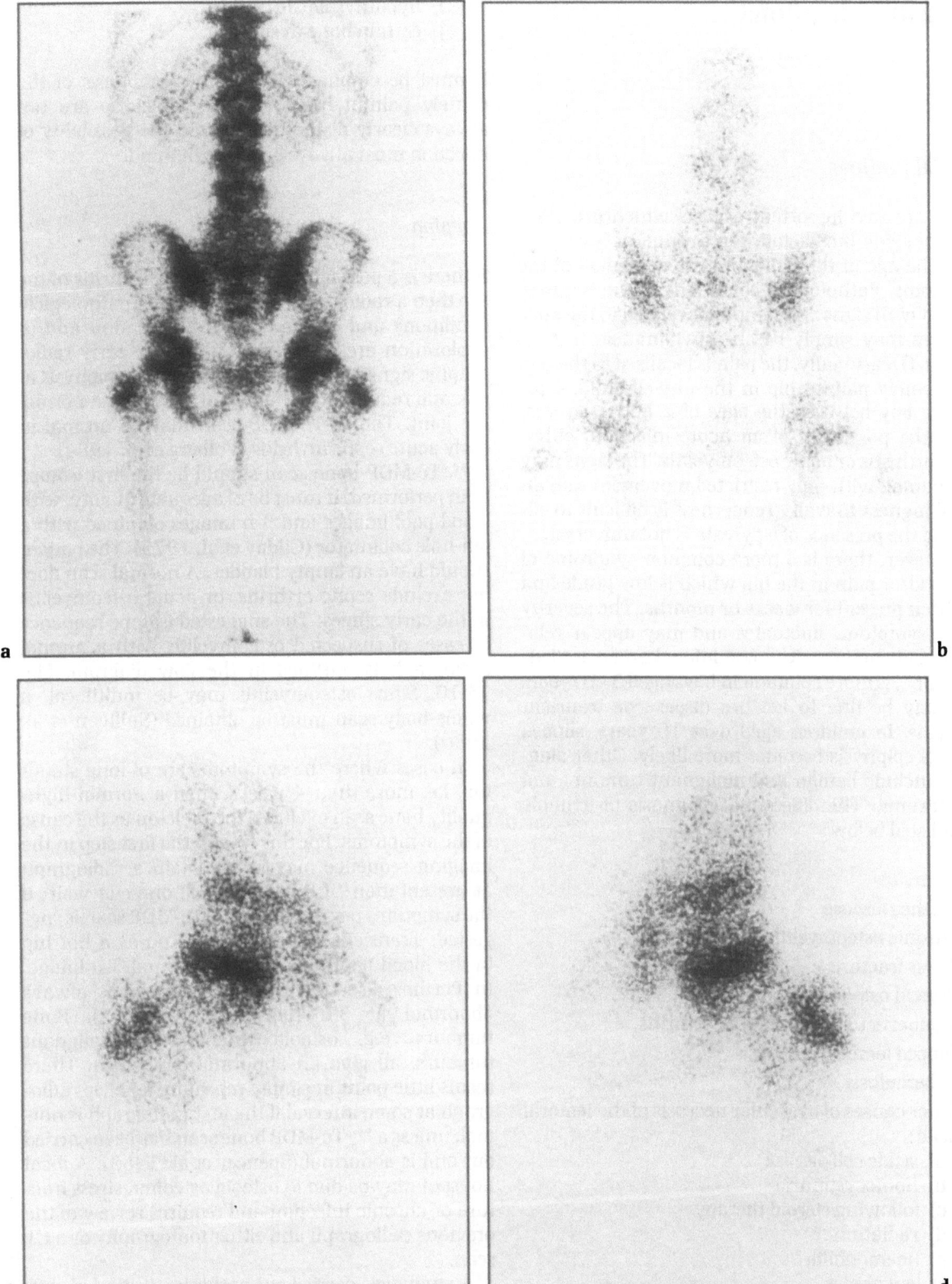

Fig. 14.9a–d. Normal hips in a 6-year-old girl. **a,b** Posterior views, non-magnified and magnified respectively. **c,d** Anterior pin-hole magnification views, right and left respectively. The growth plates of the femoral head and greater trochanter are visible. The lesser trochanter is just visible. Note that the lateral point of the femoral head is less active than the medial part.

Clinical Indications

Hip

Clinical Features

There are two important aspects which are clinically obvious but dictate the avenue of investigation: the age of the child and the acuteness of the symptoms. Pathological conditions in the hip may present with signs and symptoms related to the knee or there may simply be an unwillingness to bear weight. Occasionally, the pain is localised to the hip. The acutely painful hip in the unwell child, especially a boy between the ages of 2 and 10 years, raises the possibility of an acute infection, either septic arthritis or acute osteomyelitis. The signs may be minimal, with only restricted movement and an unwillingness to walk. Tenderness is difficult to elicit, and the presence of a pyrexia is not universal.

However, there is a more common syndrome of limp and/or pain in the hip which is low grade and has been present for weeks or months. The severity of the symptoms fluctuates and may appear relatively acute at times. This condition, known as "irritable hip", is more common in boys aged 3–10 years and may be due to Perthes disease or transient synovitis. In children aged over 10 years, slipped femoral epiphysis becomes more likely. Other diagnoses include benign and malignant tumours and also trauma. The differential diagnosis of irritable hip is listed below:

1. Synovitis
2. Perthes disease
3. Chronic osteomyelitis
4. Stress fracture
5. Osteoid osteoma
6. Monoarticular rheumatoid arthritis
7. Slipped femoral epiphysis
8. Tuberculosis
9. Other causes of avascular necrosis of the femoral head:
    a) sickle cell disease
    b) homocystinuria
    c) following steroid therapy
    d) radiation
    e) haemophilia
    f) leukaemia
    g) trauma, including surgical manipulation in congenitally dislocated hips
    h) Gaucher's disease

i) hypothyroidism
j) certain bone dysplasias

It must be emphasised that the symptoms of the acutely painful hip and of irritable hip are not always clearly distinguished, and the possibility of infection must always be borne in mind.

Imaging

If there is a possibility of acute septic arthritis of the hip then a radiograph to exclude other pathological conditions and an urgent joint aspiration and/or exploration are essential. Waiting for early radiographic signs places the femoral capital epiphysis at risk and reduces the chances of salvaging a normal hip joint. The ^{99m}Tc-MDP scan may be normal in early acute septic arthritis (Volberg et al. 1984).

^{99m}Tc-MDP bone scan should be the first isotope scan performed. It must be of adequate quality, with blood pool images and 3-h images obtained with a pin-hole collimator (Gilday et al. 1975). The patient should have an empty bladder. A normal scan does not exclude septic arthritis, or acute osteomyelitis in the early stages. The suggested isotope sequence in cases of suspected osteomyelitis with a normal radiograph is outlined in the flow diagram, Fig. 14.10. Since osteomyelitis may be multifocal, a whole-body scan must be obtained (Sullivan et al. 1980).

In cases where the symptoms are of long standing, i.e. more than 4 weeks, then a normal high-quality bone scan excludes the skeleton as the cause of the symptoms. For this reason the first step in the imaging sequence may be to obtain a radiograph at presentation; if this is normal, one can wait; if the symptoms persist, then a ^{99m}Tc-MDP scan is suggested. Transient synovitis shows up as a hot hip in the blood pool phase with a normal 3-h image. In Perthes disease, however, the scan is always abnormal at 3 h (Figs. 14.11, 14.12). Bone tumours, e.g. osteoid osteoma or malignant tumours, all give an abnormal bone scan. There seems little point in simply repeating a pelvic radiograph at some interval if the first radiograph is normal, unless a ^{99m}Tc-MDP bone scan has been carried out and is abnormal (Spencer et al. 1983). A focal hot spot may be due to osteoid osteoma, stress fracture or chronic infection and requires review of the previous radiograph and either tomography or a CT scan.

A study was carried out at this institution of children with long-standing symptoms (i.e. lasting over 4 weeks) related to the hip. All the children had a normal radiograph at presentation and underwent

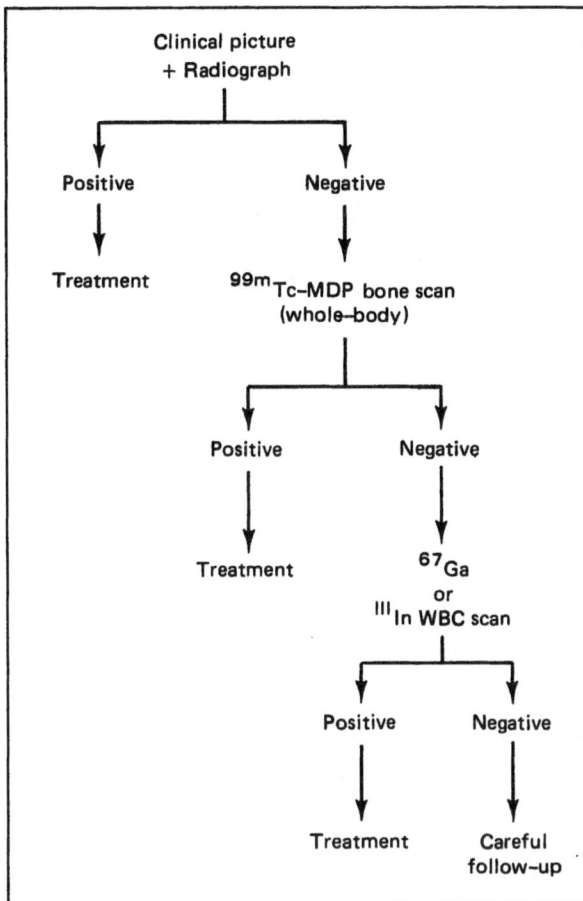

Fig. 14.10. Flow diagram of suggested isotope sequence in cases of suspected acute osteomyelitis.

a ^{99m}Tc-MDP bone scan. All those children with a normal scan failed to demonstrate any significant pathological findings on follow-up. This study strongly suggests that a normal ^{99m}Tc-MDP bone scan in the presence of long-standing hip symptoms excludes the pelvis and hips as the cause for the symptoms.

Conclusion

When there is clinical evidence of acute septic arthritis a normal radiograph or ^{99m}Tc-MDP bone scan does not exclude the diagnosis. Aspiration and exploration may be the only diagnostic avenue.

In children with long-standing symptoms a plain radiograph and ^{99m}Tc-MDP bone scan will detect all significant pathological conditions of bone. If both these examination results are normal then transient synovitis/irritable hip may be present; however, this disease runs a benign course.

Symptoms in Other Joints

Clinical Features

Frequently the child is suffering from a known chronic disorder and the skeleton is imaged not so much in the search for a diagnosis, but in order to assess complications of the underlying disease. The most common general diseases in this category are blood dyscrasia—usually sickle cell disease—or a connective tissue disorder—usually juvenile chronic arthritis. Only 8% of children with this latter disease have the adult seropositive rheumatoid arthritis. Localised long-standing disease may be present, e.g. old septic arthritis or traumatic arthritis. In these various disorders, joint symptoms wax and wane. In the majority of cases the clinical picture and physical examination allow an accurate diagnosis to be made, and the role of imaging is secondary. Occasionally, trauma or infection may result in damage to a part of the epiphyseal plate, causing premature fusion of that part of the growth plate only and without directly damaging the articular surface itself. With subsequent growth the unaffected part of the metaphysis continues to increase in length, resulting in distortion of the adjacent joint and premature osteoarthritis.

Less commonly, a child may present with pain localised to a single joint. The pain may be low grade, and if a weight-bearing joint is involved there may be a limp. Systemic signs may be totally absent.

Osteochondritis is an avascular necrosis of a developing epiphysis or apophysis of unknown aetiology and is usually seen in the first decade. Certain epiphyses are more susceptible, and sometimes there may be a history of stress or trauma. The changes are usually unilateral, but when bilateral they are asynchronous. The capital femoral epiphysis is most commonly affected—Perthes disease. Although almost any epiphysis may be involved, some are more commonly affected and have acquired eponyms. It is in this context that a high-quality radiograph is helpful. Clinically there may be a pointer to the diagnosis, but there is a differential diagnosis:

1. Infection
   a) viral
   b) bacterial
   c) tuberculosis
2. Trauma—chronic repetitive trauma (exercise)
3. Monoarticular juvenile arthritis
4. Arthritis in inflammatory bowel disease
5. Osteochondritis

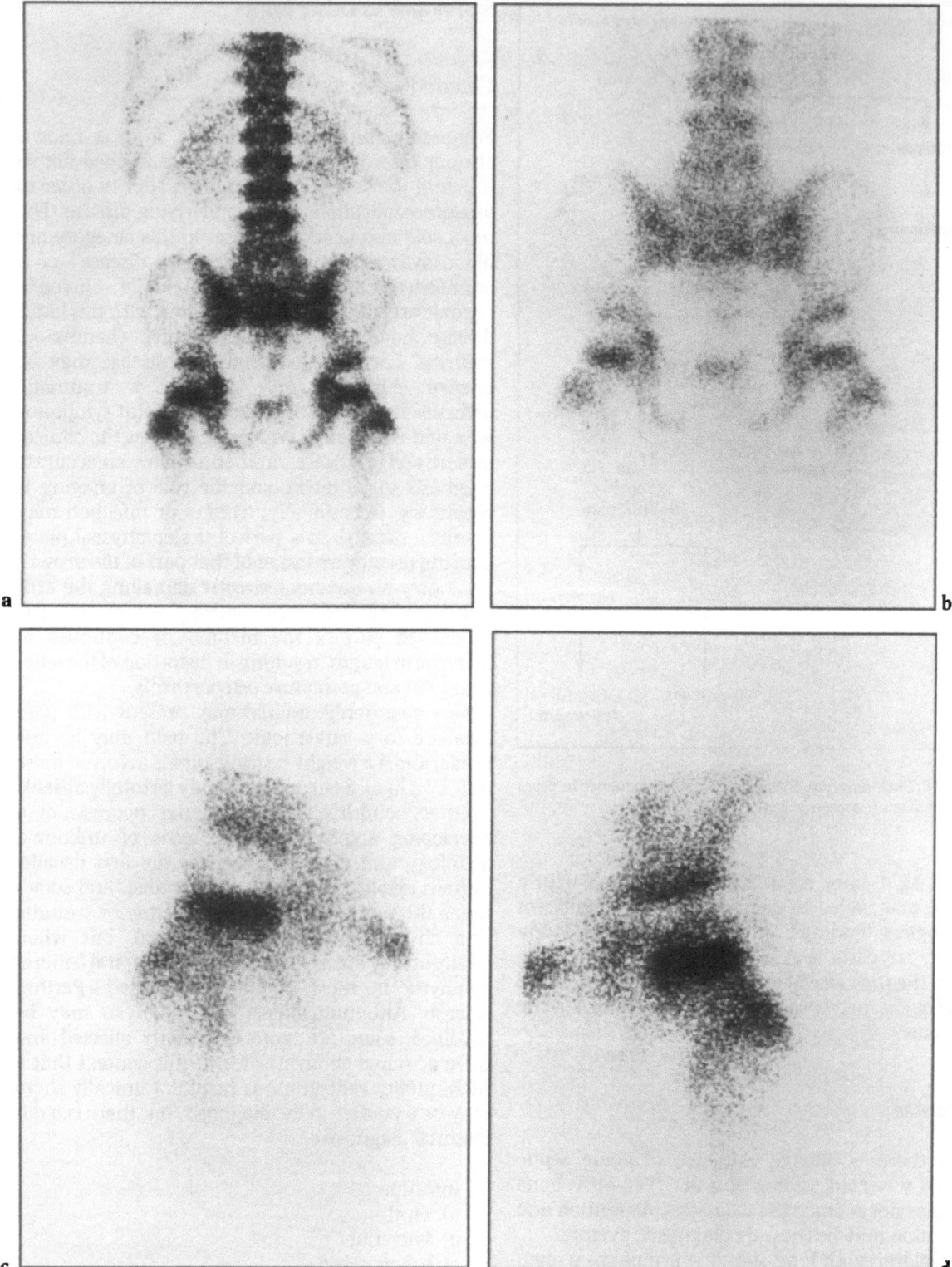

Fig. 14.11a–d. Perthes disease in a boy of 7 years. **a** Non-magnified posterior view, showing loss of activity in the right head of femur. **b** Magnified posterior image. The loss of uptake is seen to involve virtually the whole of the femoral head. **c,d** Anterior pin-hole magnified views of right (**c**) and left (**d**) hips. A column of normal uptake can be seen in the femoral head laterally. This indicates that revascularisation has commenced. The left femoral head has slightly decreased uptake and is flattened, suggesting bilateral Perthes disease.

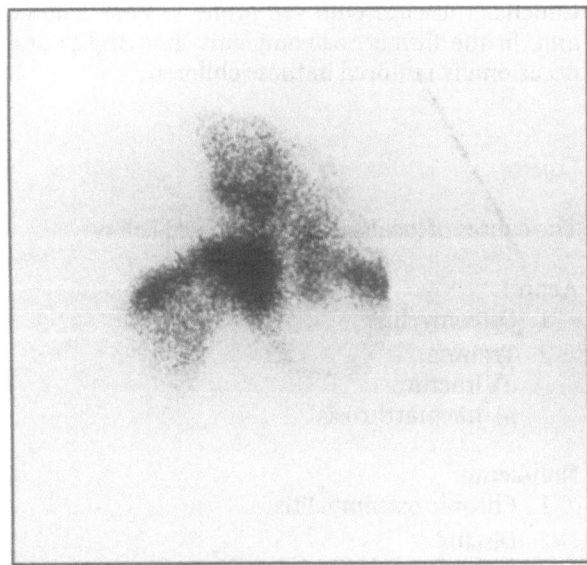

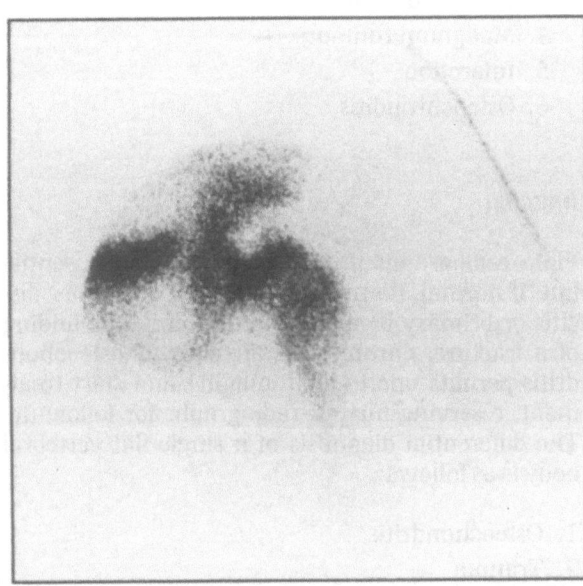

Fig. 14.12a,b. Bilateral Perthes disease. Anterior pin-hole magnified views of right (a) and left (b) hips. The left hip (b) shows the classic appearance of a cold lesion in the lateral two-thirds of the femoral head, the result of avascular necrosis. Revascularisation has commenced, however, as shown by the activity just visible in the femoral head above the lateral margin of the epiphyseal plate. The right hip (a) is also abnormal, with increased uptake in the somewhat flattened femoral head. These are the appearances of revascularisation of a stage more advanced than that of the left hip.

Imaging

In children with known underlying disease, radio-isotopes offer little help. In the child with acute septic arthritis the bone scan may be normal, in which case ^{67}Ga or ^{111}In WBC may be useful. Both are time consuming and not universally available; therefore this diagnosis should be excluded by a joint aspiration/exploration in the majority of cases.

In the child with long-standing, grumbling symptoms and a normal radiograph then a ^{99m}Tc-MDP bone scan is indicated. In monoarticular juvenile arthritis the joint is usually diffusely hotter than the opposite joint. A focal abnormality may be seen, suggesting either an osteoid osteoma or a Brodie's abscess. Such a finding demands review of the radiographs and then either tomography or computed tomography (CT) if the pathological condition cannot be accurately determined.

Conclusion

When there is a known underlying disease, imaging should be as infrequent as is compatible with high-quality care, investigations being requested only to answer specific pertinent clinical questions. When the symptoms are of long standing one should proceed from a radiograph to a ^{99m}Tc-MDP bone scan. This combination will allow accurate diagnosis of most conditions, but occasionally a synovial biopsy may still be required to establish a diagnosis. The history of juvenile arthritis varies from a non-specific synovitis to the typical changes. Unusual infections have been diagnosed from synovial culture.

Localised Bone Pain

Introduction

Children may have difficulty in verbalising their complaint. This section deals with the child considered by the clinician to have localised pain of probable skeletal origin as a major feature. A full examination and a radiograph go a long way towards resolving this problem in many children.

Clinical Features

It is useful to subdivide these children into those with acute symptoms and those with long-standing or flitting symptoms.

Acute pain in a child, with or without other signs or symptoms, raises the possibility of a fracture or infection. Acute osteomyelitis results generally in an unwell child with systemic signs. Most benign tumours do not present with acute pain; many are incidental findings (non-ossifying fibroma, enchondroma) and others are localised bony deformities—exostoses. Occasionally, these benign tumours may present as acute pain resulting from a pathological fracture. This is usually through an area of cortical thinning, as, for example, in simple bone cysts. More usually, however, the pain is of longer duration, as in osteoid osteoma, osteoblastoma and eosinophilic granuloma. Acute backache is fortunately very rare.

When the symptoms are of long standing and/or flitting there may be no systemic upset. However, these two groups are not quite so well separated, and children may present with severe pain of some weeks' or months' duration who are off their food and generally miserable. Included in this group is a significant number of children with backache. There may be time lost from school—a useful indicator of "significant symptoms". Intermittent pain, occurring mainly at night, which is relieved by salicylates, may be due to an osteoid osteoma. This benign bone tumour has within it a high vascular nidus, which may calcify. Although found in any part of the skeleton, it occurs most commonly in the upper femur and upper tibia and the pain may be referred to the adjacent joints. Radiographically the changes may be diagnostic (Omojola et al. 1981). Localised bone pain is usually the presenting feature in primary malignant bone tumours. Children with backache are worthy of special mention, since it is in this group that it may prove most difficult to discover a cause. If there are any neurological signs then a intraspinal lesion must be considered. In the absence of neurological or other signs doubt always exists as to whether "true organic pathology" exists. However, disease such as discitis, osteochondritis or a primary benign bone tumour may be the cause of the symptoms, even in the presence of a normal radiograph.

There is a small but significant number of children, usually girls between the ages of 10 and 13 years, who present with pain around the knee. Frequently the pain seems to be localised to the region of the patella. These girls have repeated radiographs which invariably are normal. To date, the role of ^{99m}Tc-MDP scans in this condition has not been evaluated. These girls should probably be examined by high-quality radiographs of the knees, which, if normal, should be followed by a ^{99m}Tc-MDP bone scan, including lateral views of both knees. If no abnormality is seen, then no further imaging need be carried out.

In children with a known systemic disease, acute bone pain may demand repeated medical attention but not necessarily repeated imaging. This includes children with sickle cell disease (Fig. 14.13) or Gaucher's disease who are prone to bone infarcts and, in the former, osteomyelitis. Imaging is only occasionally required in these children.

Causes

The causes of localised pain are listed below:

Acute:
1. Osteomyelitis
2. Trauma
    a) fracture
    b) haemarthrosis

Non-acute:
1. Chronic osteomyelitis
2. Discitis
3. Benign tumours
4. Malignant tumours
5. Infarction
6. Osteochrondeitis

Imaging

Plain radiographs in two projections are essential but, if normal, do not exclude acute infection, discitis or primary benign bone tumours. The finding of a fracture, chronic osteomyelitis or osteochondritis permits one to stop imaging and start treatment, reserving further radiographs for follow-up. The differential diagnosis of a single flat vertebral body is as follows:

1. Osteochondritis
2. Trauma
3. Histiocytosis X
4. Leukaemia

If the symptoms are considered to be skeletal in origin and the plain radiographs are normal, then a ^{99m}Tc-MDP bone scan is indicated. In the presence of acute symptoms the imaging sequence set out in Fig. 14.10 is suggested. With long-standing symptoms a normal ^{99m}Tc-MDP bone scan excludes the possibility of a benign bone tumour as well as discitis. It is highly likely that if both the radiograph and isotope bone scan are normal then the non-acute symptoms are not skeletal in origin (Fig. 14.14). If a focal abnormality is shown on the bone scan it requires accurate anatomical localisation, either with simple radiography, fluoroscopy, tomography or CT scanning.

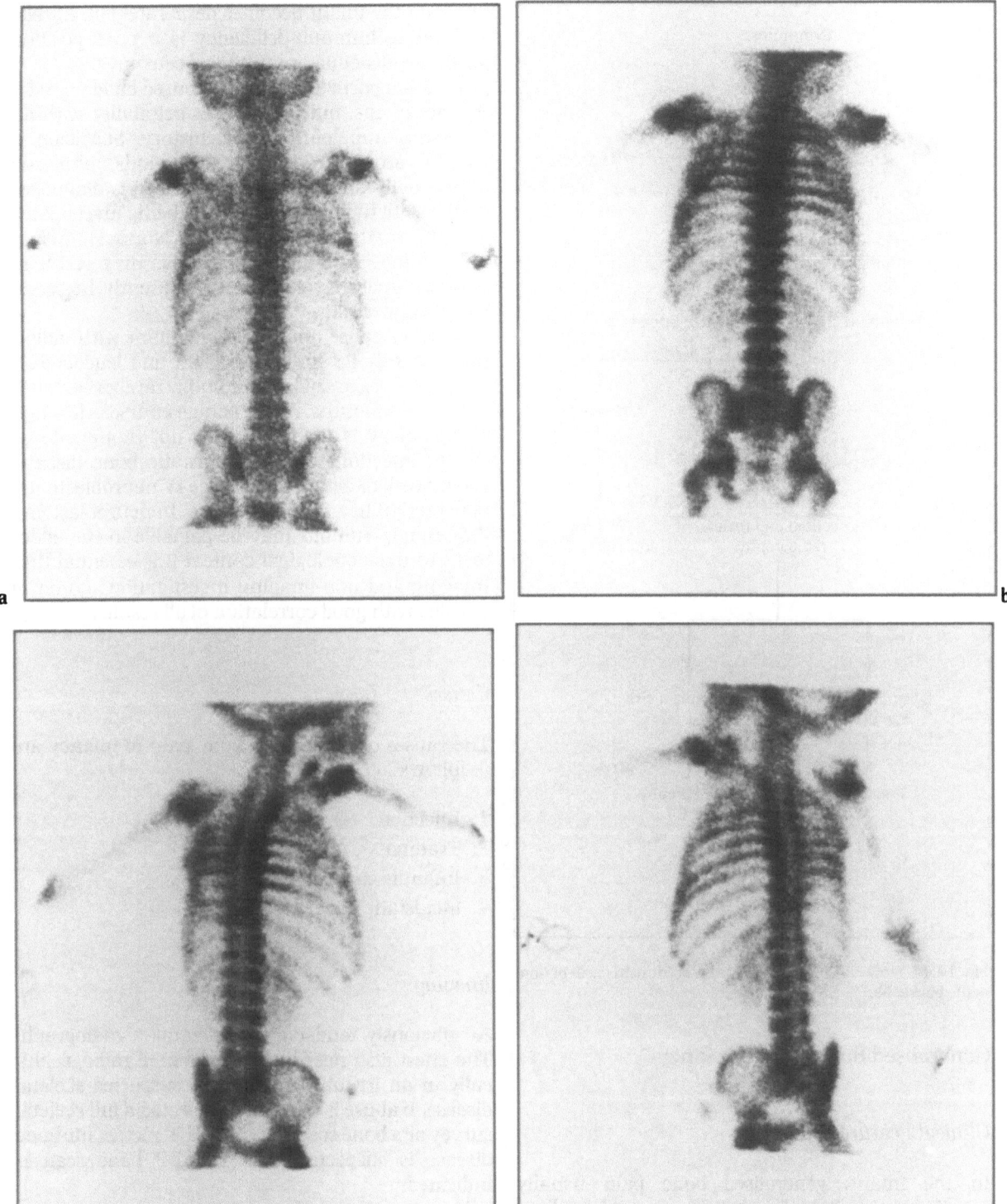

Fig. 14.13a–d. Sickle cell disease in a child of 4 years. **a** This poor-quality image of the posterior spine shows only a diffusely increased count density in both upper hemithoraces, more on the left. **b** Better image clearly shows increased uptake in almost all of the upper ribs on both sides. On the left, the 7th, 8th and 10th ribs, and probably the 11th rib, are also involved, and this is well shown on the left posterior oblique view (**d**). The right posterior oblique view is also shown (**c**). In addition to the rib lesions, there is a focus of increased uptake in the mid-shaft of the right humerus. These appearances are compatible with either bone infarcts or complicating osteomyelitis. In some cases of sickle cell disease the spleen shows prominent uptake of MDP, but this was not apparent in this case.

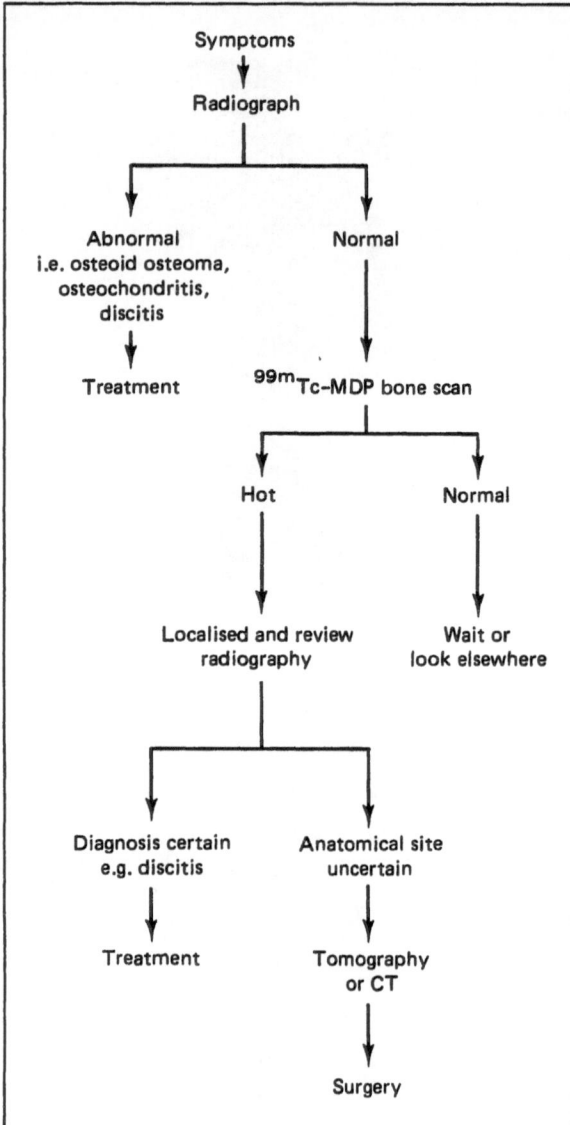

Fig. 14.14. Flow diagram of suggested procedure in cases of non-acute backache.

Generalised Bone Pain in Infancy

Clinical Features

In the infant, generalised bone pain usually manifests as irritability, particularly on handling. The associated clinical features may lead to an accurate diagnosis. Systemic signs of an infection, especially evidence of septicaemia, suggest multifocal osteomyelitis, which may be a complication or cause of the septicaemia. Vomiting, together with poor feeding, may be a prominent feature. The clinical picture may begin in an apparently benign manner,

but soon the infant becomes desperately ill. Rarely, underlying immuno-deficiency is a predisposition for the septicaemia or multifocal osteomyelitis.

Trauma, particularly in the abused child of under 3 years of age, may present as irritability with an otherwise unhelpful clinical history. Suspicion is usually aroused on clinical grounds, although occasionally an unsuspected fracture is diagnosed on the skull radiograph in a child being investigated for failure to thrive and irritability. Normal handling of an infant with abnormal bones may result in multiple fractures, seen most frequently in osteogenesis imperfecta.

Another cause of an irritable infant with pallor, pseudoparalysis, an elevated ESR and leucocytosis is Caffey's disease. This condition, rarely seen after the age of 6 months, runs a benign course. Although the aetiology is unknown, it is not thought to be due to infection. Diffuse metastatic bone disease, caused by leukaemia or by Stage IV neuroblastoma, may present in a similar manner. In neuroblastoma the primary tumour may be palpable in the abdomen. In this aetiological context it is essential that imaging and non-imaging investigations go on in parallel with good correlation of all results.

Causes

The causes of generalised bone pain in infancy are as follows:

1. Infection
2. Trauma
3. Infantile cortical hyperostosis
4. Metastatic bone disease

Imaging

An obviously tender area warrants a radiograph. The chest also needs to be examined radiographically in an irritable infant with suspected skeletal disease. If abuse is clinically suspected a full skeletal survey or a bone scan is indicated. If metastatic bone disease is suspected a ^{99m}Tc-MDP bone scan is indicated.

However, if the diagnosis is uncertain and the infant is being investigated for irritability and other non-specific signs like vomiting and/or failure to thrive but without focal signs, then a ^{99m}Tc-MDP bone scan is warranted, with radiographs obtained of any area which is abnormal on bone scan. This approach is only valid for the infant over 1–2 months of age (see p. 207).

A ^{99m}Tc-MDP bone scan with its high sensitivity makes it a useful screening procedure when multiple abnormal bony areas may be present. It is non-specific; therefore a radiograph of each abnormal area must be obtained. The main drawback in cases of child abuse is the difficulty in estimating the ages of any hot areas. Skull fractures may also fail to show up on the bone scan. Negative scans are well reported in unifocal osteomyelitis but not multifocal osteomyelitis. The bone scan may remain abnormal for a prolonged period and cannot be used to judge when to stop antibiotic therapy. In this context ^{111}In WBC or ^{67}Ga have been suggested. If either of these scans changes from abnormal to normal then it can be confidently concluded that infection has resolved. If a new abnormal site is seen on the ^{99m}Tc-MDP or ^{111}In WBC or ^{67}Ga scan then a new pathological site is suggested. If there is no change it cannot be assumed that infection is still active, since an inflammatory response following infection may still give an abnormal scan.

Generalised Bone Pain in Childhood, Including Malignancy

Clinical Features

There is no clear-cut distinction between infancy and childhood, although certain pathological states are more common in certain age groups. When there is a known underlying disease such as malignancy, sickle cell disease or chronic renal failure, imaging may be important in follow-up. However, a child may present with generalised aches and pains, irritability, tiredness and weight loss with no previous illness, in which case the initial radiograph may suggest the diagnosis of acute leukaemia. It is rare for a child with histiocytosis X to present with this picture, but it is seen.

Causes

The causes of generalised bone pain in childhood are given in Table 14.1.

Imaging

Bone scanning has a very small role to play in establishing the diagnosis of malignancy but is very helpful in defining the extent of the disease. ^{99m}Tc-MDP scans should be undertaken in all children

Table 14.1. Causes of generalised bone pain in childhood

A. *Known underlying disease*
  1. a) neuroblastoma
     b) leukaemia
     c) hepatoblastoma
     d) histiocytosis X
  2. Sickle cell disease
  3. Bone dysplasia:
     a) osteogenesis imperfecta
     b) osteopetrosis
     c) diaphyseal dysplasia
     d) melorrheostosis
     e) pachydermoperiostosis
     f) fibrous dysplasia
     g) homocystinuria
  4. Chronic renal failure
B. *De novo:*
  1. Malignancy:
     a) neuroblastoma
     b) leukaemia
  2. Metabolic—idiopathic juvenile osteoporosis
  3. Trauma, including child abuse

with a primary malignant bone tumour at diagnosis in order to detect a skip lesion close to the primary tumour and also to see if the remainder of the skeleton is free of disease. Follow-up bone scans are important and should be routinely done at 3-monthly or 6-monthly intervals for up to 2 years and then at 6-monthly or yearly intervals for up to 5 years (Nair 1985).

In neuroblastoma a ^{99m}Tc-MDP scan (Figs. 14.15, 14.16, 14.17), a ^{99m}Tc colloid marrow scan and a ^{123}I-MIBG scan should be performed at the time of diagnosis. Scans should also be obtained near the completion of chemotherapy (Fig. 14.18), but scans between these two points have no value.

In 8 children with known malignancy at this institution all had an abnormal ^{99m}Tc-MDP scan with an associated abnormal radiograph at the time of diagnosis. The ^{99m}Tc-MDP scan remained abnormal when the children were in clinical remission and not receiving chemotherapy. Bone biopsies were obtained in all these children and no malignancies were seen. The clinical course subsequently confirmed that these abnormal sites on ^{99m}Tc-MDP scan were not due to malignancy. This has led to the feeling that follow-up bone scans in children with known malignancy must be carefully evaluated. If an abnormal area remains abnormal then caution should be exercised before calling it malignant. If a new abnormal area develops on follow-up bone scan then there should be a high index of suspicion of recurrence of the malignancy. In the so-called bone-metastasising Wilms' tumour ^{99m}Tc-MDP bone scan is suggested at 6-monthly or yearly intervals.

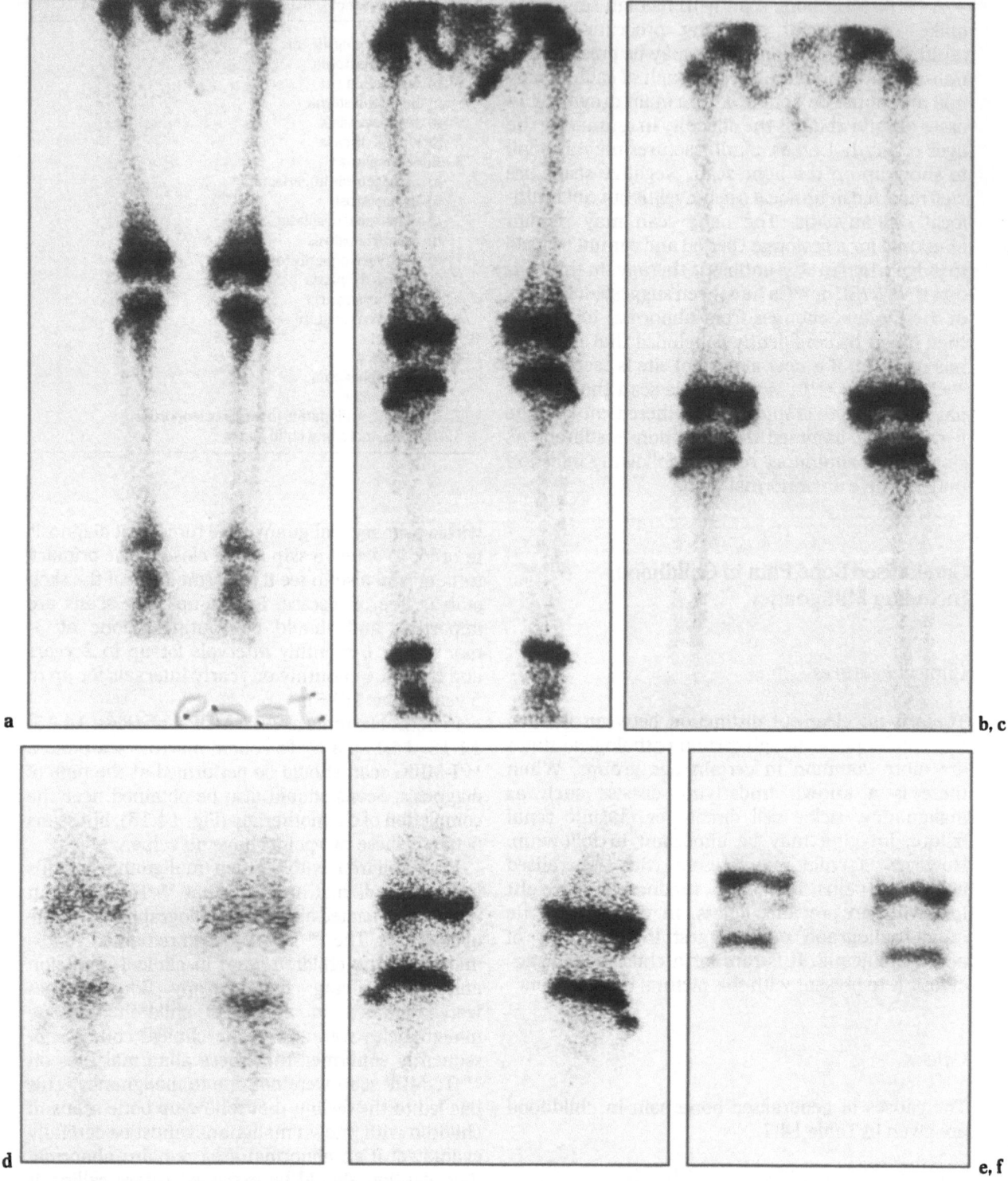

Fig. 14.15a–f. The knees in metastatic neuroblastoma. Three pairs of images (non-magnified, *top row*; magnified, *bottom row*) taken on three successive occasions in a girl with Stage IV neuroblastoma. **a,d** Prior to treatment (age 3 years 6 months) the knees are grossly abnormal with almost complete loss of the sharp boundary between the metaphysis and growth plates in both distal femora and proximal tibiae. This is the result of an increase in metaphyseal uptake giving a count rate comparable with that in the growth plate. The ankles are also abnormal. This is the typical appearance of long bone metastases in this condition. **b,e** Three months later, following treatment, there has been a considerable improvement. **c,f** A further 15 months later, the child is disease free and the knees look quite normal.

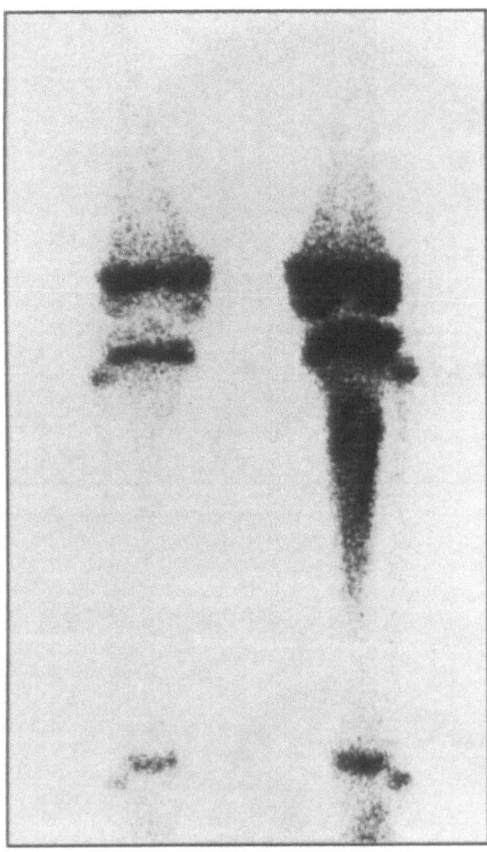

Fig. 14.16. Recurrent neuroblastoma in a child aged 5 years 3 months. This image shows an obvious focus of increased uptake in the upper half of the shaft of the tibia. The whole of the remainder of the abnormal limb shows increased activity compared with the contralateral limbs as a result of hyperaemia. This is a less common appearance of metastatic neuroblastoma, the commoner picture being a more diffuse uptake in the metaphysis, as in Fig. 14.15.

In histiocytosis X there is controversy about the value of bone scans. In the experience of most authors, ourselves included, the bone scan does not detect all the lesions and therefore a radiographic skeletal survey is more sensitive and specific; however, other authors do not hold to this view (Parker et al. 1980).

At present the bone scan is of little use in metabolic disorders, but new developments may change this (Fogelman and Carr 1980).

The Neonate/Infant

The response to acute disease processes in the neonatal skeleton differs significantly from those in the older child (see Fig. 14.1).

Clinical Features

The signs of bone abnormality may be minimal or absent. One may simply be faced with an irritable neonate who is failing to thrive or whose only symptom is dehydration caused by reduced fluid intake. Pyrexia may not be a feature, even in the presence of severe osteomyelitis. The diagnosis of skeletal disease may be incidental when a radiograph is carried out for another reason.

Imaging

Osteomyelitis/Septic Arthritis. Well-established osteomyelitis may show up radiographically as a highly destructive lesion. A normal radiograph of a bone or joint does not, however, rule out significant pathological features. In acute osteomyelitis the ^{99m}Tc-MDP bone scan has been particularly disappointing in the neonate. The bone scan may remain normal even 4–8 weeks after the beginning of osteomyelitis. In septic arthritis the bone scan may also be normal (Ash and Gilday 1980).

Since a bacteriological diagnosis is also required the only certain proof of infection is aspiration and/or exploration. The timing of radiography is difficult in the absence of focal signs. It is preferable to do a ^{99m}Tc-MDP bone scan as the initial screening test since if this gives a positive result it indicates where to look for bacteria. If the bone scan result is negative then a skeletal survey may be undertaken. In this context the use of ^{111}In WBC or ^{67}Ga may be useful. ^{111}In WBC has been reported as giving a positive result in a 4-week-old infant with osteomyelitis (Gordon and Vivian 1984).

Bone Infarction. In neonates and infants a specific finding of bone infarction may be that of a dactylitis, with multifocal extensive diaphyseal destruction of phalanges and metacarpals associated with florid periosteal new bone formation. This appearance is usually seen in sickle cell disease. The radiographic changes may be identical to tuberculous dactylitis at the same age. More commonly, the bone infarcts of sickle cell disease are seen at an older age, with symmetrical changes of avascular necrosis of the epiphyses, usually affecting the capital femoral epiphyses and the humeral heads but also the central portions of the vertebral end-plates.

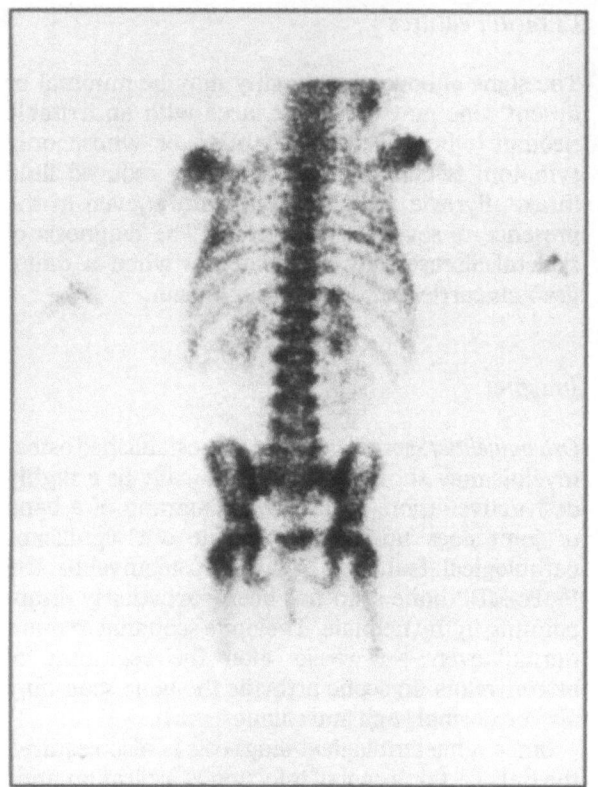

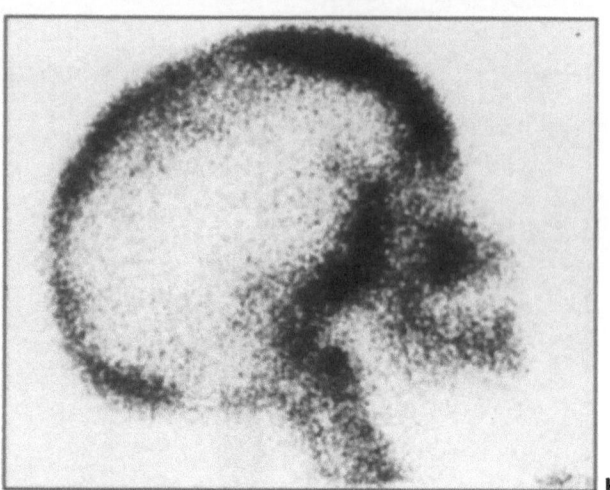

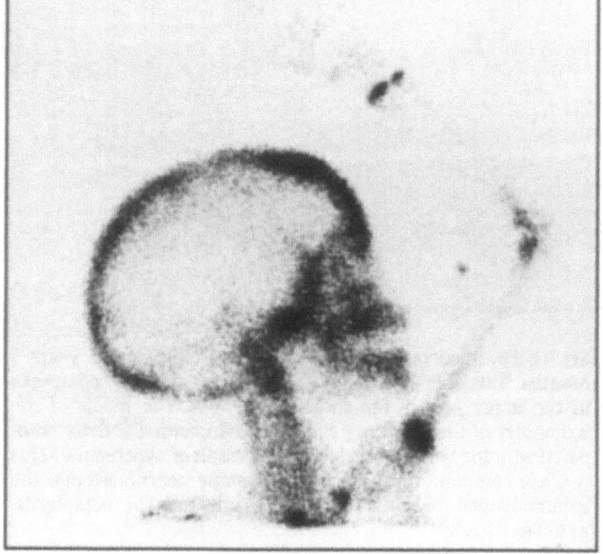

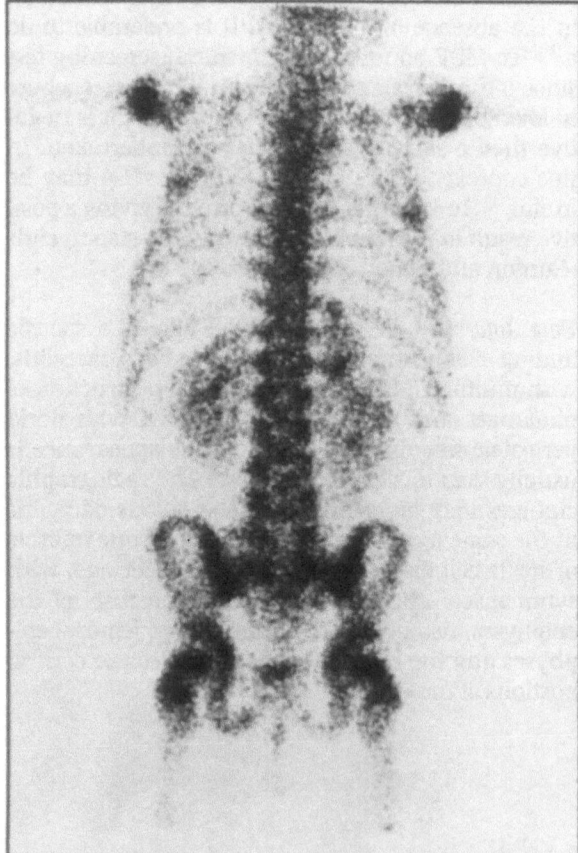

Fig. 14.17a–d. Stage IV neuroblastoma in a girl aged 4 years 6 months. a,b Posterior spine, right lateral skull prior to treatment. The skull vault, which is clearly abnormal, is a common site for neuroblastoma deposits. The right 7th rib is also abnormal and the left 7th and 8th ribs provoke suspicion. The primary is avidly concentrating activity and pushing the right kidney laterally and inferiorly. c,d Corresponding images obtained 2½ months following treatment. The skull vault, although still abnormal, has improved. The ribs now look normal, while the primary is taking up less activity than previously.

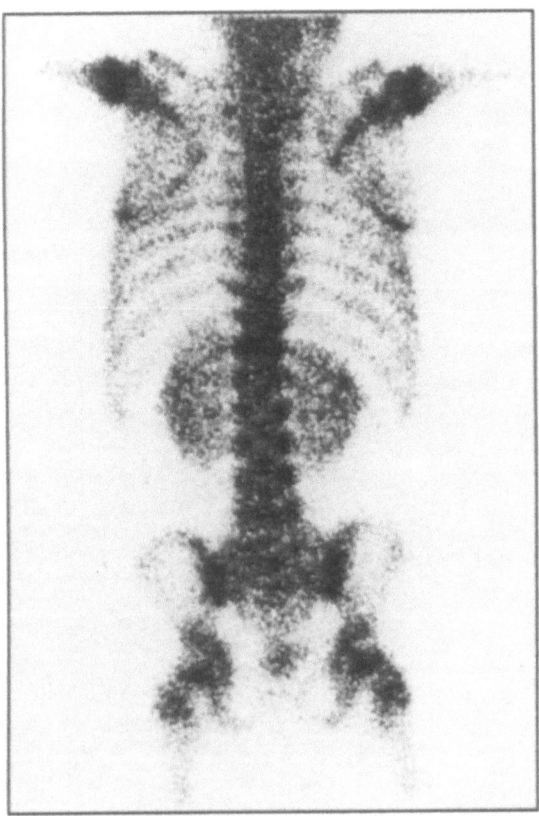

Fig. 14.18. Increased renal uptake following chemotherapy. This 2½-year-old girl had been treated for rhabdomyosarcoma which had metastasised to bone. Here the skeleton is within normal limits.

Omojola MF, Cockshott WP, Beatty EG (1981) Osteoid osteoma. An evaluation of diagnostic modalities. Clin Radiol 32: 199–204

Parker BR, Pinckney L, Etcubonas E (1980) Relative efficacy of radiographic and radionuclide bone surveys in the detection of skeletal lesions of histiocytosis X. Radiology. 134: 377–380

Siddiqui AR, Oseas RS, Wellman HN, Doerr DR, Bachner RL (1979) Evaluation of bone marrow scanning with Tc99m sulphur colloid in paediatric oncology. J Nucl Med 21: 379–386

Spencer RP, Lee YS, Sycklas JJ, Rosenberg RJ, Karimeddini MK (1983) Failure of uptake of radiocolloid by the femoral heads. A diagnostic problem: concise communication. J Nucl Med 24: 116–118

Sullivan DC, Rosenfield NS, Ogden J, Ghottschalk A (1980) Problems in the scintigraphic detection of osteomyelitis in children. Radiology 135: 731–736

Treves ST, Kirkpatrick JA (1985) Bone. In: Treves ST (ed) Paediatric nuclear medicine. Springer, Berlin Heidelberg New York, pp 1–48

Volberg FM, Summer TE, Abramsom JS, Winchester PH (1984) Unreliability of radiographic diagnosis of septic hip in children. Pediatrics 74: 118–120

References

Ash JM, Gilday DL (1980) The futility of bone scanning in neonatal osteomyelitis: concise communication. J Nucl Med 21: 417–420

Carty H (1984) Successful imaging in paediatrics. Nucl Med Comm 5: 775–779

Fogelman I, Carr D (1980) A comparison of bone scanning and radiology in the evaluation of patients with metabolic bone disease. Clin Radiol 31: 321–326

Gilday DL, Eng B, Paul DJ (1975) Diagnosis of osteomyelitis in children by combined blood pool and bone imaging. Radiology 117: 331–335

Gordon I, Vivian G (1984) Radiolabelled leucocytes. A new inflammatory diagnosis tool in occult infection. Arch Dis Child 59: 62–66

Handmaker H, Giammona ST (1984) Improved early diagnosis of acute inflammatory skeletal articular disease in children. A two radiopharmaceutical approach. Pediatrics 73: 661–669

Harcke HT (1978) Bone imaging in infants and children. A review. J Nucl Med 19: 325–329

Nair N (1985) Bone scanning in Ewing's sarcoma. J Nucl Med 26: 349–352

15 · Soft Tissue Uptake of Bone Agents

H. W. Gray

Introduction

This volume, and others, attest to the wide-ranging application of bone-seeking radiopharmaceuticals to diagnostic problems in clinical practice. There was early recognition that valuable information on the kidney and urinary tract could be obtained incidentally (Park et al. 1973) by virtue of the prompt renal excretion of these agents. Other soft tissues were thought to take up the ^{99m}Tc phosphates because of macro- or microscopic tissue calcification (Silberstein et al. 1975). The last 10 years, however, have witnessed a plethora of case reports showing accumulation of bone-seeking agents in both neoplastic and non-neoplastic soft tissue. Our simplistic concept of a uniform mechanism for soft tissue deposition has therefore become untenable, and despite considerable research effort our overall understanding of the process is still in its infancy.

The often non-specific and occasionally artefactual nature of soft tissue uptake provides the unwary or inexperienced observer with a source of uncertainty and error. Conversely, awareness of specific conditions with soft tissue uptake of tracer greatly enhances the diagnostic value of the study. The purpose of this chapter is to review the wide range of disease processes where recognition of non-skeletal soft tissue uptake of ^{99m}Tc phosphates is of value in clinical practice. No attempt has been made to produce a gamut for uptake of bone tracer by soft tissue. (For this purpose readers are directed to the many excellent articles and texts available: Chew et al. 1981; Brill 1981; Silberstein 1984; Neely et al. 1984; Rosenthall 1984; McAfee and Silberstein 1984.) Instead, emphasis has been placed firstly upon the diagnosis which can be made by chance from the bone scan and secondly on the use of bone imaging for specific detection of conditions known to cause accumulation of bone agents in soft tissues. Artefactual uptake in soft tissue is also briefly discussed. No distinction has been made between the different ^{99m}Tc-labelled phosphate complexes because of the evidence that they behave qualitatively in a similar manner (Charkes 1979).

Pathophysiology

The mechanism for uptake of bone-seeking agents in soft tissue remains uncertain, except for heterotopic new bone formation (e.g. myositis ossificans) where it is similar to that for the skeleton (Francis et al. 1969; King et al. 1971; Rossier et al. 1973; Charkes 1979).

Several theories to account for soft tissue uptake of ^{99m}Tc phosphates have been proposed. Increased blood flow through an organ or tissue would allow more tissue contact with tracer, and certainly the effect can be recognised in the syndrome of reflex sympathetic dystrophy (Carlson et al. 1977). However, Chew et al. (1981) found no evidence of hypervascularity in soft tissue sarcomas which accumulated bone tracer, while Siddiqui et al. (1982) reported that tracer uptake in neuroblastoma was a later rather than an early phenomonen. There is no evidence as yet to substantiate this particular theory.

It has been suggested that alteration of capillary permeability might increase the concentration of bone tracer bathing tumour cells, thereby increasing their uptake. What little evidence is available suggests that this is an unimportant consideration (McCartney et al. 1976).

Soft tissue calcification has been recognised as an important causal factor in the uptake of ^{99m}Tc phosphates since Francis et al. (1969) showed strong chemiadsorption of diphosphonates onto hydroxyapatite crystals, and Silberstein et al. (1975) confirmed in patients that ^{99m}Tc phosphate uptake in tissue is proportional to its calcium content. This mechanism is thought to be operative in dystrophic calcification from whatever cause since most tissue calcium is in the form of hydroxyapatite (Gatter and McCartney 1967). Absence of ^{99m}Tc phosphate uptake in some tumours, despite recognisable calcification on the radiograph cannot be explained (Garcia et al. 1977; Martin-Simmerman et al. 1984).

Metastatic calcification occurs in the presence of renal failure when the solubility product for calcium and phosphate is exceeded and hydroxyapatite crystals precipitate in the soft tissue extracellular space (Richards 1975). McLaughlin (1975) and Rosenthal et al. (1977) confirmed the affinity of ^{99m}Tc phosphate for calcium precipitates by correlating diffuse lung uptake of tracer in hypercalcaemic patients with the pathological identification of calcium deposition in the alveolar septa. Watson et al. (1977) showed resolution of the lung uptake upon correction of the hypercalcaemia. Conger and Alfrey (1976) demonstrated in vitro that ^{99m}Tc phosphates form a strong chemical bond to hydroxyapatite crystals and a weak bond to the amorphous salt (Whitlockite) found in the lungs of uraemic patients (Conger et al. 1975). This may explain the lack of sensitivity of bone tracers in detecting metastatic lung calcification in dialysis patients (Alfrey et al. 1976).

The abnormal intracellular flux of ionic calcium induced by ischaemic or other damage to cell membrane integrity has been clearly shown to be a preliminary factor in the increased uptake of ^{99m}Tc phosphates by ischaemic or dying cells (Wahner and Dewanjee 1981). The intracellular solubility product for calcium and phosphate may be exceeded with precipitation of calcium salts around mitochondria which have nucleating properties (Shen and Jennings 1972a, b). ^{99m}Tc pyrophosphate localises to intracellular calcium as amorphous calcium phosphate and crystalline hydroxyapatite but

also to calcium complexed to myofibrils and other macromolecules in the myoplasm (Dewanjee and Kahn 1976; Buja et al. 1977). It is conceivable that release of colloidal calcium phosphate from damaged mitochondria into the myoplasm could provide a mechanism by which continuous production of hydroxyapatite crystals is initiated in the presence of extracellular fluid (Russell and Kanis 1984).

There is evidence that transchelation of ^{99m}Tc may occur where there is a high local tissue concentration of calcium or iron to facilitate dissociation of ^{99m}Tc from the phosphate ligand and lead to its deposition at the reaction site (McRae et al. 1976). This mechanism would be operative for uptake in infarction or in tissues with a high iron content like iron injection sites (Van Antwerp et al. 1975a; Byun et al. 1976) or the spleen in haemolysis (Nisbet and Maisey 1982). McRae also suggested that ionic iron may catalyse the formation of a new ^{99m}Tc ligand with a tissue distribution different from ^{99m}Tc phosphate. This could explain the high renal uptake of ^{99m}Tc when bone imaging is performed in systemic iron overload (Choy et al. 1981).

Binding of ^{99m}Tc phosphate to receptor sites on tissue enzymes such as acid phosphatase has been suggested to account for breast uptake in normal or cancer patients (Schmitt et al. 1974; Zimmer et al. 1975). Little hard evidence is available to substantiate this theory.

Collagen can nucleate the growth of hydroxyapatite crystals (Glimcher and Krane 1968), and Rosenthall and Kaye (1975) have argued that ^{99m}Tc phosphates may have a greater affinity for immature collagen than for the crystal surface of bone. Their theory is supported by the localisation of bone-seeking agents in healing surgical scars (Poulose et al. 1975) and in fibrothorax (Ravin et al. 1977).

Finally, Richman et al. (1975) suggested that local tissue anoxia with increased lactate production and pH reduction might lead to increased tissue affinity for the ^{99m}Tc phosphate or, alternatively, an increase in release of reduced ^{99m}Tc from the phosphate ligand. Again, little evidence is available to support this theory.

Bone Scan Appearances

Incidental Findings

As a bone scan is invariably obtained to assess skeletal abnormalities, the detection of soft tissue abnormalities is usually an unexpected bonus. Most relevant information thus obtained relates to the kidney and urinary tract because of the high photon density achieved within this organ system during radiopharmaceutical excretion. Less commonly, new information is gained which delineates unsuspected benign or malignant tumours, areas of unsuspected infarction or unforeseen effects or complications from known disease processes. The prevalence of renal abnormalities on unselected bone scans is approximately 15% (Park et al. 1973; Maher 1975; Sty et al. 1979a; Adams et al. 1980). No equivalent figures are available for other soft tissue abnormalities.

Kidney and Urinary Tract

In the early days of bone imaging with ^{99m}Tc phosphates, the high renal excretion of up to 70% of dose in 6 h (Citrin et al. 1975) provided renal images of excellent quality for detection of most sizeable abnormalities. As the skeletal uptake of more up-to-date bone agents has risen, however, so the renal excretion has fallen, reducing the quality of incidental renal images at 4 h. Since our institution changed to ^{99m}Tc-MDP, we have had to contrast the digitised lumbar views to obtain renal images of diagnostic quality (Gray and McKillop 1985, unpublished work). It is our view that those using the analogue mode would have to overexpose the lumbar view and "burn out" the spine to obtain acceptable kidney images. Other workers have routinely imaged kidneys at 5-min after injection to ensure adequate high-count-density views (Chayes and Strashun 1980), but it is not clear whether this extra time and effort is worthwhile. Occasionally, the diagnostic value may be enhanced by extra views in the lateral or oblique position for kidney or squat position (Fig. 15.1) for bladder.

The most specific signs of renal disease on bone scans can be classified as renal asymmetry, mass lesions, urinary or renal tract dilatation or abnormalities of uptake, size or displacement. Less valuable signs are bilateral decreased renal uptake and focal areas of increased uptake.

Renal Asymmetry. Renal asymmetry is a sensitive and specific sign of renal abnormality (Vieras and Boyd 1975; Sty et al. 1979a) and may be noted in up to 10% of routine bone scans (Hattner et al. 1975). Specificity is poor when the asymmetry is minor, and the abnormal kidney may be difficult to pinpoint. Anterior, oblique or lateral views may confirm the abnormality in such cases or show horizontal orientation of one kidney (Neely et al. 1984).

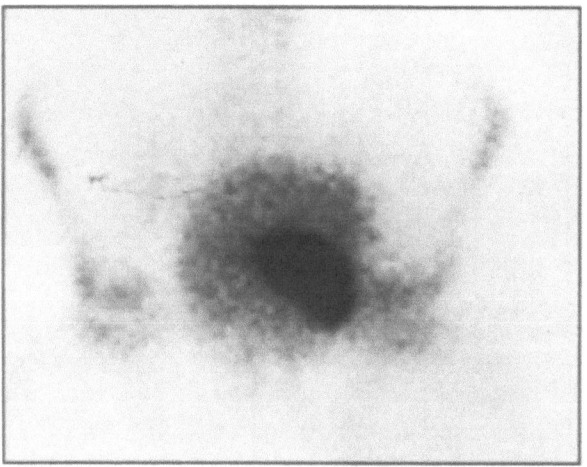

▲ Anterior   Caudal ▼

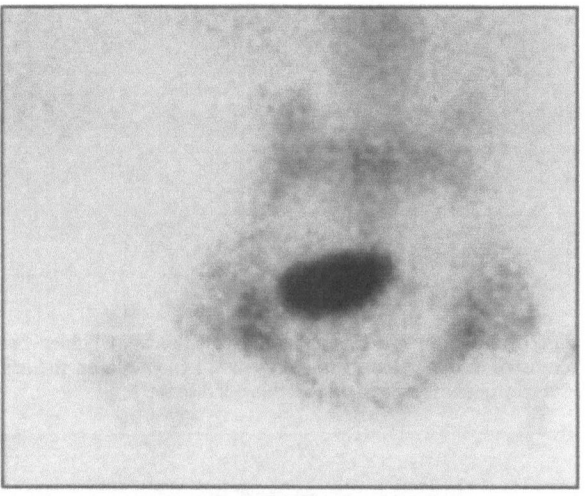

Fig. 15.1a,b. A bladder diverticulum can be confused with urine contamination. The caudal view (b) clearly shows that the abnormal activity seen on the anterior view (a) represents a bladder diverticulum and not abdominal wall contamination.

In the first pattern, a unilateral non-functioning kidney is accompanied by a normal or hypertrophied contralateral kidney (Fig. 15.2). This may occur in congenital absence, chronic pyelonephritis, following nephrectomy or in idiopathic nonfunction (Maher 1975; Vieras and Boyd 1975; Adams et al. 1980). In the second pattern, a unilateral small kidney may result from chronic pyelonephritis (Fig. 15.3), radiation nephritis (Sty et al. 1979a), idiopathic small kidney, chronic hydronephrosis without urinary stasis (Vieras and Boyd 1975; Adams et al. 1980), or renal artery stenosis (Neely et al. 1984). A unilateral small kidney may be simulated by the presence of a renal mass at either pole which is not directly visualised (Biello et al. 1976). The third pattern of unilateral

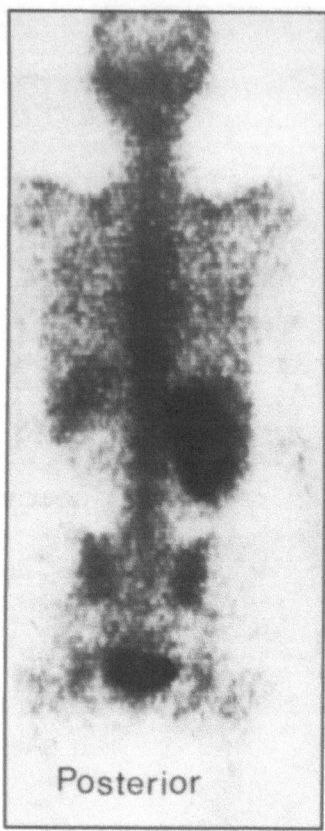

Fig. 15.2. Compensatory enlargement of the right kidney has occurred in this patient with congenital hypoplasia on the left. Splenic uptake is secondary to sickle cell disease.

enlargement with a normal contralateral kidney has been reported in hydronephrosis (Vieras and Boyd 1975) and in the presence of renal cell carcinoma (Neely et al. 1984) or Wilms' tumour (Edeling 1983). Sty et al. (1979a) suggested that this pattern might also be seen in acute events such as renal vein thrombosis (Lamki and Wyatt 1983), acute renal infarction and pyelonephritis. Lantieri et al. (1980) reported that high uptake of bone agent can occur in the kidney with renal artery stenosis and cited ischaemia and urinary hyperconcentration as mechanisms. Excessive uptake in a neuroblastoma (Fig. 15.4) can mimic a large kidney, as can increased uptake in stomach.

Mass Lesions. The mass lesion represented by a focal area of reduced or absent tracer accumulation is an uncommon but reliable indicator of renal disease. In paediatrics, Sty et al. (1979a) reported that Wilms' tumour was the most common neoplasm while lymphoma and sarcoma were rare. Solitary cysts, polycystic disease and renal abscess were uncommon in their experience. In an adult population, primary renal cell carcinoma (Fig. 15.5) and single or multiple renal cysts are equally common, while metastatic disease (Fig. 15.6) and renal abscess are less common (Maher 1975; Vieras and Boyd 1979; Adams et al. 1980).

It seems likely that many small lesions will be missed despite the acquisition of good-quality images.

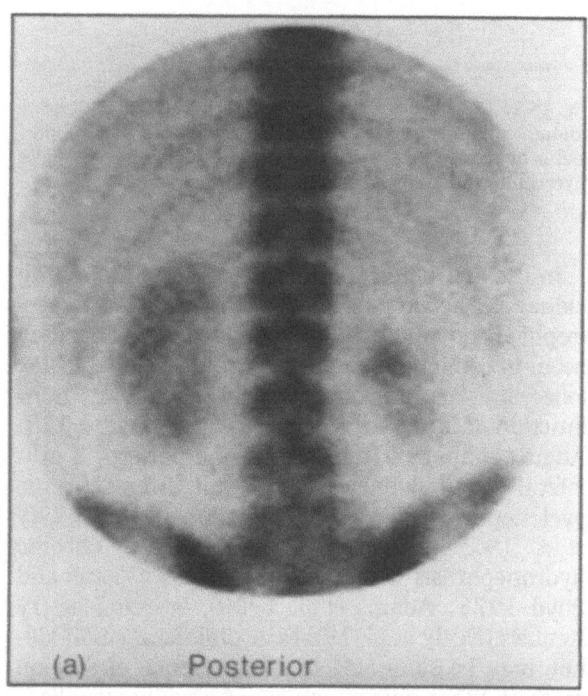

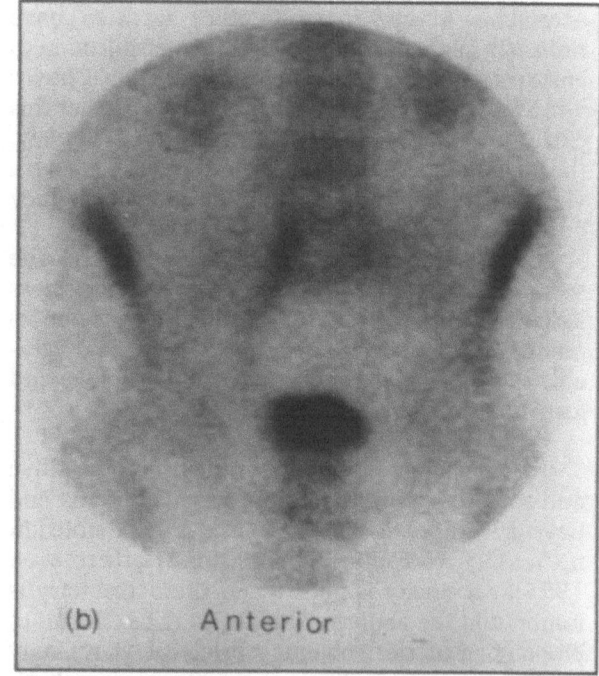

Fig. 15.3a,b. Small right kidney with ureteric dilatation secondary to chronic pyelonephritis.

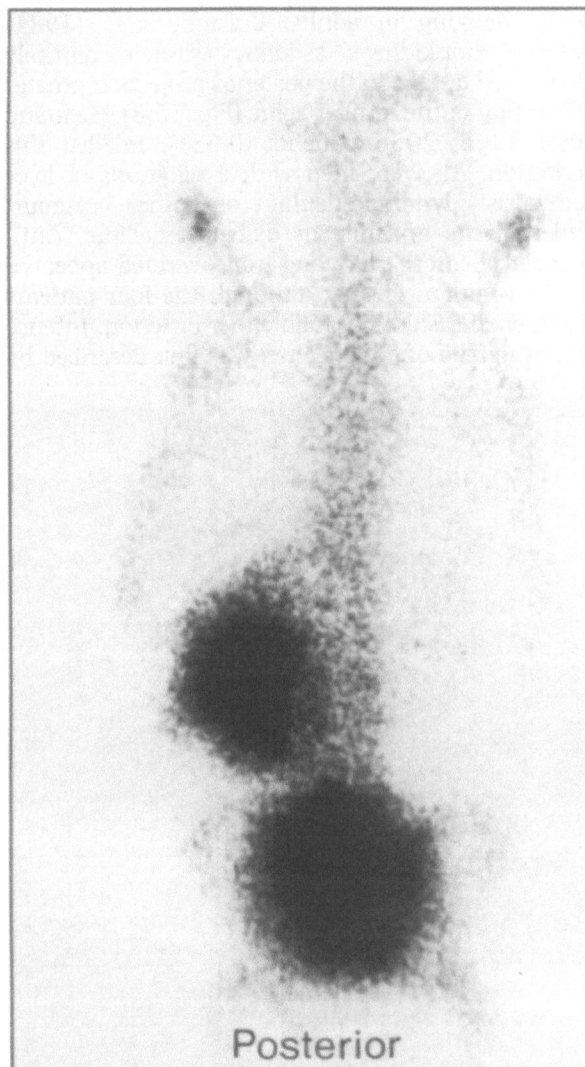

Fig. 15.4. An 8-year-old boy with uptake in a primary neuroblastoma mimicking an enlarged left kidney. (Courtesy of Dr. R. McKenzie)

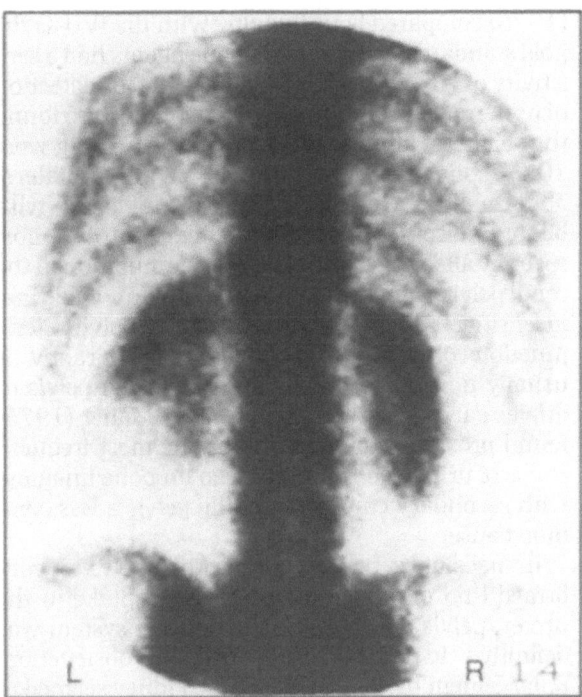

Fig. 15.5. Focal photon-deficient area in the lower pole of the left kidney caused by a renal cell carcinoma.

Biello et al. (1976) found that 10 of 20 mass lesions detected by intravenous urogram (IVU) were missed on bone imaging, providing a sensitivity of 50% and specificity of 100%. While some advocate renal flow studies during injection of bone agents to increase the sensitivity (Glass et al. 1980) and others propose an early blood pool image at 2 min after injection to increase the information density (Chaynes and Strashun 1980), there is no evidence at the present time that the increased workload is cost effective.

Obstructive Uropathy. The appearance of a dilated renal pelvis and ureter with increased tracer accumulation is the most common soft tissue abnormality on bone imaging (Fig. 15.7). Biello et al.

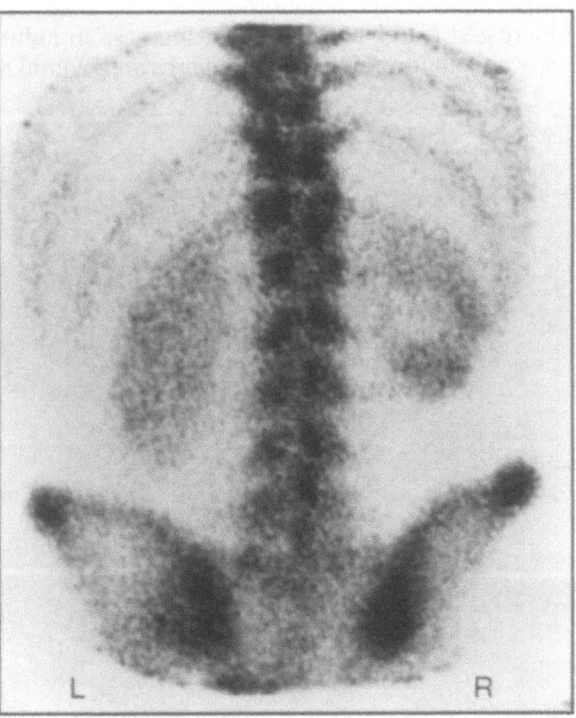

Fig. 15.6. Unsuspected secondary lesion of the right kidney in a patient with metastatic bronchogenic carcinoma.

(1976) compared bone imaging with the IVU as the gold standard and found that bone agents had a sensitivity of 73% with specificity of 100% for detection of ureteropyelocaliectasis. Those workers also found that bilateral abnormalities on bone scanning were 100% concordant with the IVU, while unilateral abnormalities were found in 50% of cases with bilateral disease, bone imaging detecting the most severely affected side. Increased accumulation in the renal pelvis alone was found to be an unreliable and insensitive (11%) indicator of true pelviureteric junction obstruction. Intravenous urography is usually normal or reveals an extra renal pelvis or duplex calyceal system in such cases. Maher (1975) found prostatic carcinoma to be the most frequent cause of urinary obstruction seen on bone imaging, with secondary carcinoma in the pelvis a less common cause.

In paediatric practice, Sty et al. (1979a) confirmed that dilatation and increased uptake in the ureter, pelvis and intrarenal collecting system was definitive in documenting urinary obstruction. Enlargement or contraction of the kidney seemed to depend upon the degree and duration of the obstruction, which was seen with congenital defects, calculi and blood clot, lymph node enlargement, pelvic and retroperitoneal masses and following surgery.

Abnormal Kidney Uptake, Size and Position. The miscellaneous renal abnormalities associated with increased tracer accumulation, increase in kidney size and abnormality of position are rarely found on

bone imaging in adults. Koizumi et al. (1981) defined "hot kidneys" as kidneys showing diffusely increased uptake in the posterior projection greater than that of the lumbar spine (Fig. 15.8). He found that 13 of 2056 patients (0.63%) fulfilled this criterion. All were men with a diagnosis of liver cirrhosis, lymphoreticular or other tumour, sideroblastic anaemia or diabetes mellitus. Anticancer chemotherapy and iron overload appeared to be common factors, although the four patients with cirrhosis did not fulfil either criterion. Intense renal uptake of bone agents was first described by

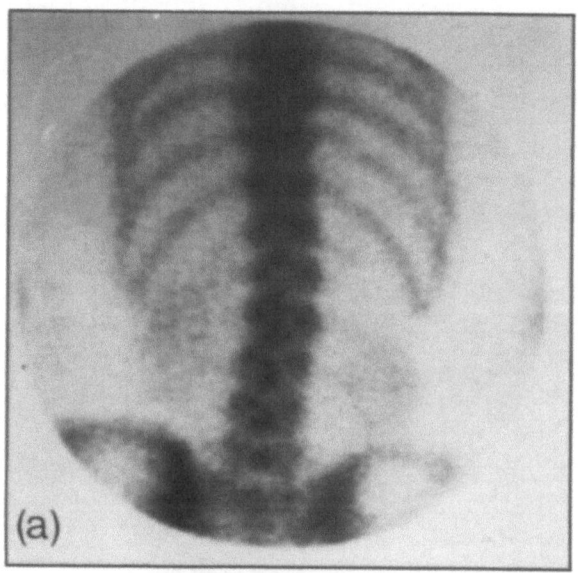

(a)

Posterior

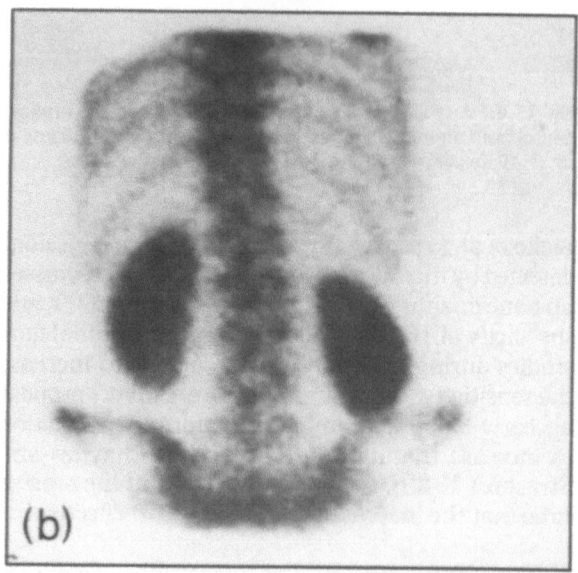

(b)

Fig. 15.8a,b. Renal uptake before (a) and 10 days after (b) receiving cyclophosphamide and doxorubicin. The diffuse increase in renal activity is thought to be related to drug nephrotoxicity.

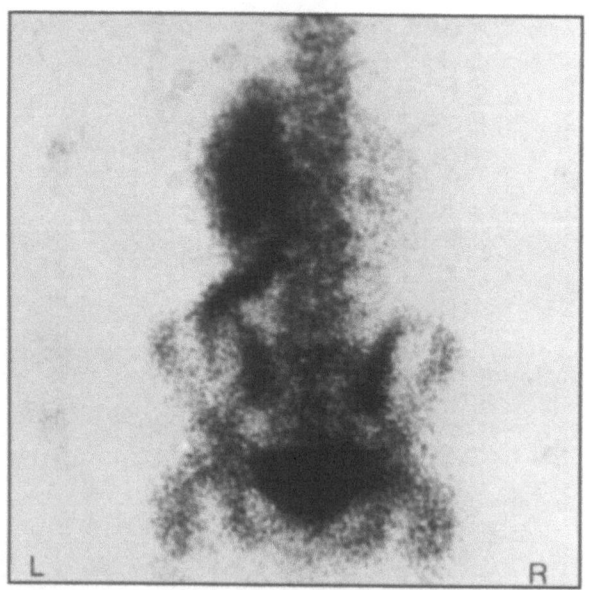

Fig. 15.7. Pelvic tumour in a 9-year-old girl resulting in a left obstructive uropathy. (Courtesy of Dr. R. McKenzie)

Lutrin et al. (1978) in children treated with cyclosporin, vincristine and doxorubicin within the previous 7 days. Trackler and Chinn (1982) reported similar findings after administration of amphotericin B and invoked tubular or interstitial damage with microcalcification as a likely mechanism. Iron overload following repeated blood transfusion or haemochromatosis has been noted to alter the biodistribution of bone agents with uptake at iron injection sites (Van Antwerp et al. 1975a; Byun et al. 1976) and intense concentration in kidney (Parker et al. 1976; Choy et al. 1981). Transchelation of ^{99m}Tc is thought to occur with synthesis of a renal rather than a bone-seeking agent (McRae et al. 1976).

Diffuse increase in kidney uptake has also been reported early after kidney irradiation (Lutrin and Goris 1979; Wistow et al. 1979), and in thalassaemia major (Valdez and Jacobstein 1980), nephrocalcinosis (Bossuyt et al. 1979), urinary obstruction at an early phase (Sty et al. 1979a), hypercalcaemia (Buxton-Thomas and Wraight 1983), myoglobinuria (Sty and Starshak 1982) and children with sickle cell disease (Sty et al. 1980).

Bilateral renal enlargement is uncommon in adults (Vieras and Boyd 1975; Adams et al. 1980) but is apparently the most common abnormality in children (Sty et al. 1979a). Sty recognised its association with many urological conditions in paediatrics and reported it in leukaemia, lymphoma, hyperuricaemic nephropathy and renal toxicity from chemotherapy. Bilateral enlargement in adults has been reported in thalassaemia major (Valdez and Jacobstein 1980) and myeloma (Adams et al. 1980).

A unilateral pelvic kidney (Fig. 15.9) is the congenital abnormality most likely to be encountered (Adams et al. 1980). Recognition is essential as it may mimic increased uptake in the lumbar spine. Polycystic (Fig. 15.10) and horseshoe kidneys (Fig. 15.11; Fink-Bennet and Dworkin 1977) are rare.

Renal displacement (Fig. 15.12) is a rarity (Vieras and Boyd 1975). Inferior displacement by a retroperitoneal mass (Neely et al. 1984) or neuroblastoma (Howman-Giles et al. 1979; Siddiqui et al. 1982) have been reported.

Abnormal tracer accumulation may be seen incidentally in the intraperitoneal (Neely et al. 1984) or retroperitoneal space (Dhawan et al. 1977; Lecklitner and Tauxe 1983) as a complication of renal surgery. The appearance is dramatic and unlikely to cause confusion.

Absent or Faint Renal Uptake. A low count density within kidneys during bone scanning is an unreli-

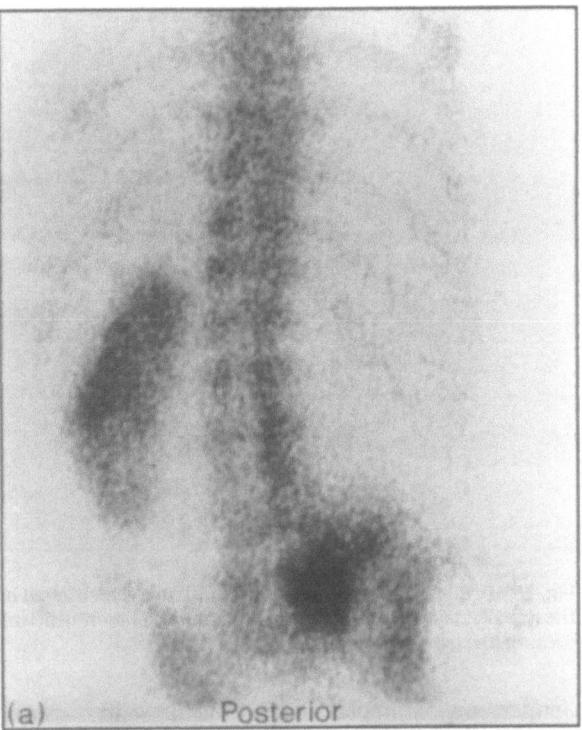

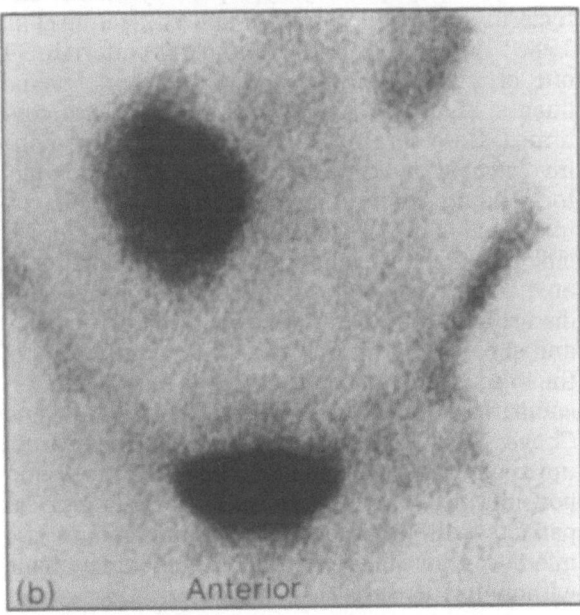

Fig. 15.9a,b. Pelvic kidney on the right. IVU confirmed stasis but no pelviureteric obstruction.

able sign of renal disease (Vieras and Boyd 1975). Sy et al. (1975) reported poor kidney visualisation secondary to rapid and enhanced uptake of radiopharmaceutical by abnormal bone, usually representing metastatic involvement (Fig. 15.13) but occasionally Paget's disease (Shirazi et al. 1974). It was later reported that similar

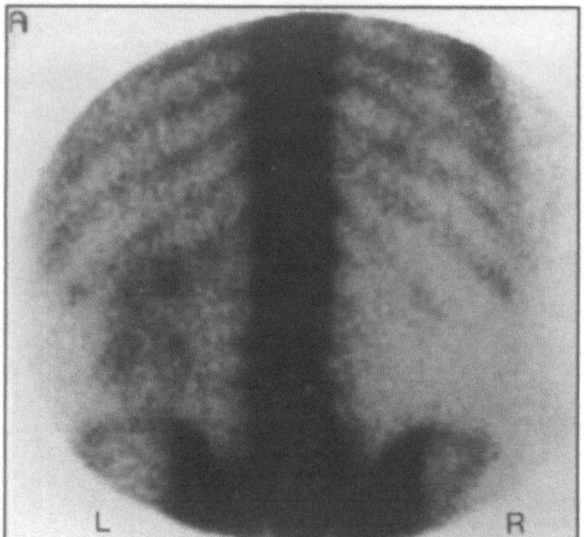

Fig. 15.10. Bilateral polycystic kidneys with non-visualisation of the right kidney and enlargement with multiple photon-deficient areas on the left.

"superscan" appearances occur in renal osteodystrophy, primary hyperparathyroidism and hyperthyroidism (Fogelman et al. 1977; Lunia et al. 1980). Adams et al. (1980) found this pattern in 34 out of 215 scans (16%) with abnormal renal images, and in no patient was renal disease confirmed. He commented that while extensive bone involvement by tumour was the most common factor in adults, intense epiphyseal concentration, cellulitis and neuroblastoma were the usual factors in children. Constable and Cranage (1981) differentiated "superscan" appearances caused by bone disease from the others with a bone/soft tissue index and showed that in the true "superscan", 10% of the injected dose of bone agent was excreted in 3 h compared with 60% in a normal patient. Kajubi and Chayes (1985) recognised a true superscan from unusually rapid vertebral uptake in a 3- to 8-min post-injection lumbar image. Accordingly, in patients with faint or absent renal images, no inference regarding kidney function should be made without further specific investigation.

Focal Uptake in Kidney. Focal areas of increased tracer accumulation in kidney (Fig. 15.14) are most often within the collecting system and provide an unreliable sign of renal disease (Vieras and Boyd 1975; Harbert et al. 1976) since they usually represent minor urinary stasis. Winter (1976a) cautioned against the adoption of supine imaging which favours postural pooling and reported that post-ambulatory or delayed views usually confirm the diagnosis.

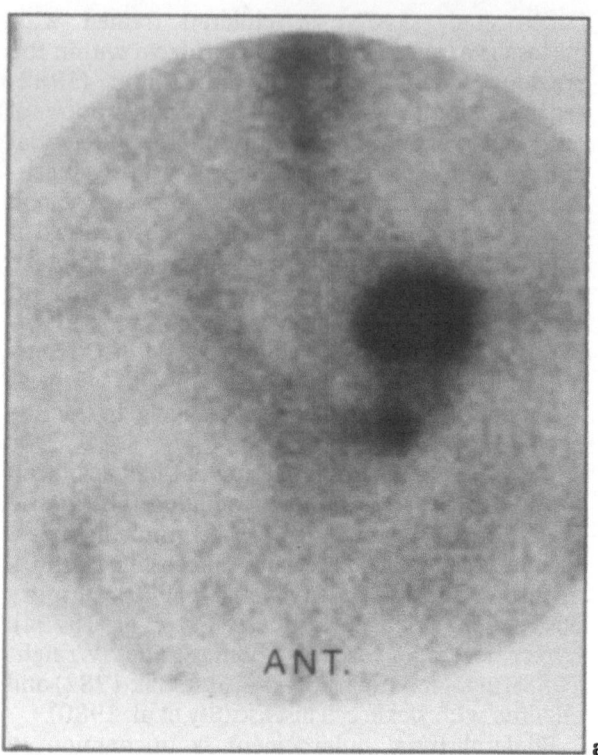

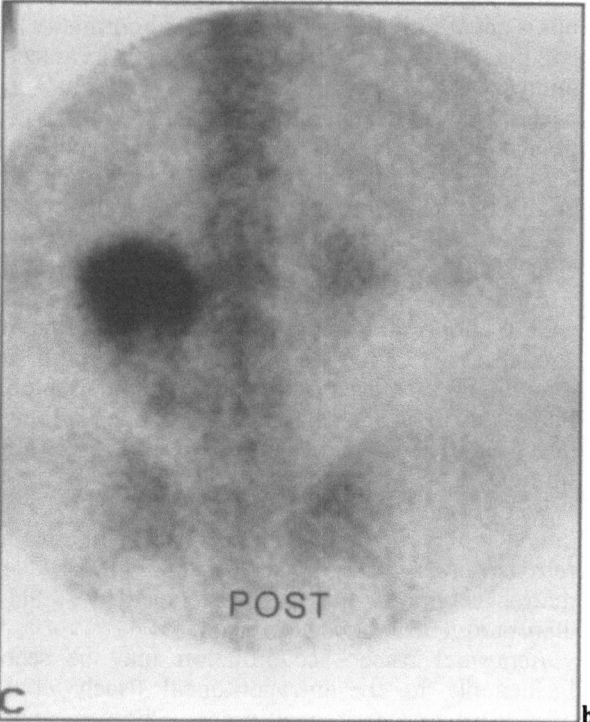

Fig. 15.11a,b. Horseshoe kidney.

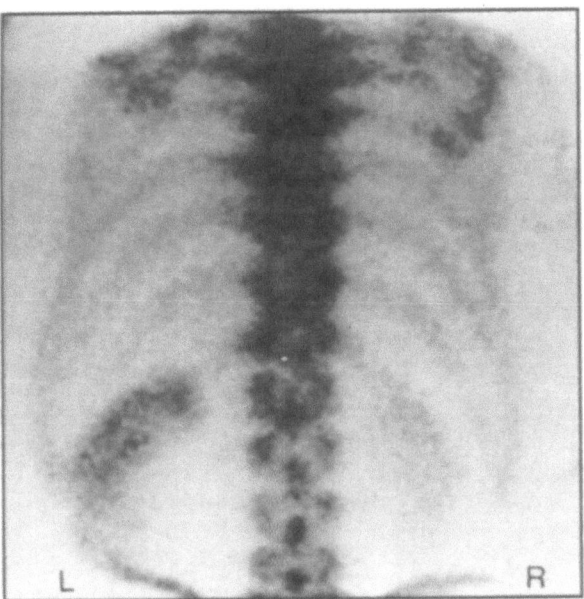

Fig. 15.12. Patient with large left hydronephrosis draining via a nephrostomy tube. Lateral displacement of the kidney has occurred.

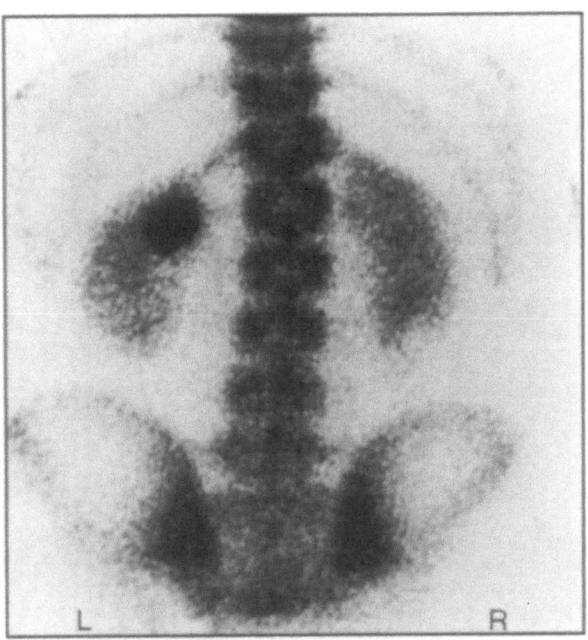

Fig. 15.14. Stasis at the left upper pole simulating a photon-rich lesion. IVU confirmed minor caliectasis.

Rarely, a lesion of the 12th rib may simulate a renal lesion (Neely et al. 1984), or stasis in an upper calyx may simulate a rib lesion (Fig. 15.15; Williamson 1979). There are also reports of focal uptake in primary renal tumours (Singh et al. 1977), in secondary renal tumours (Gerhold et al.

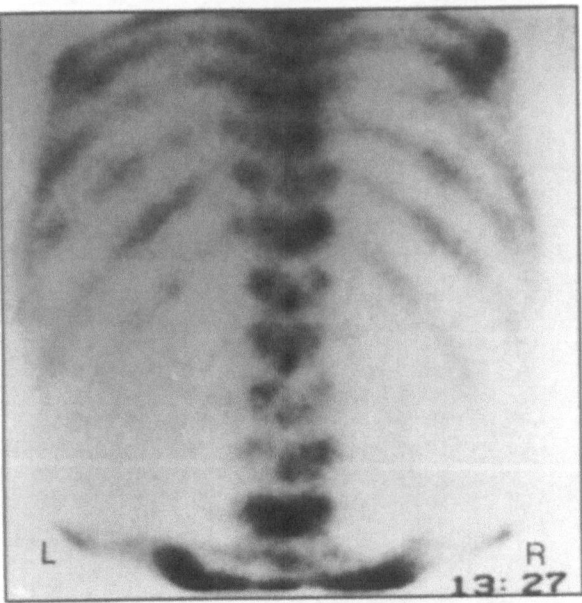

Fig. 15.13. Widespread bone involvement with metastatic prostatic carcinoma. There is markedly diminished renal uptake despite normal renal function.

1980), in renal metastasis from osteogenic sarcoma (Gilbert et al. 1983) and in a communicating cyst (Straub and Slasky 1982). Focal uptake in the renal bed has been noted in recurrent renal carcinoma simulating a normal kidney (Ozarda et al. 1983) and in neuroblastoma (Howman-Giles et al. 1979).

It is clear that valuable new information on kidney structure and function can be obtained by an alert analyst during bone scanning in at least 15% of patients. Renal asymmetry is the most common abnormality with mass lesions, and obstructive uropathy the most specific. Overall experience indicates that a renal abnormality on bone scan is unlikely to be a false-positive result and requires further investigation. However, normal renal images do not exclude renal abnormality.

Spleen

Unsuspected splenic visualisation during bone imaging usually results from homozygous or heterozygous sickle cell disease (Goy and Crowe 1976; Harwood 1978; Silberstein et al. 1984). Accumulation may be faint (Fig. 15.16) or striking (Fig. 15.17) and is related to the presence of splenic infarction, anoxia and/or a high local tissue concentration of iron.

Care should be taken to distinguish spleen from uptake in stomach (see Fig. 15.33), ribs, lung or a laterally displaced kidney (see Fig. 15.12). Adren-

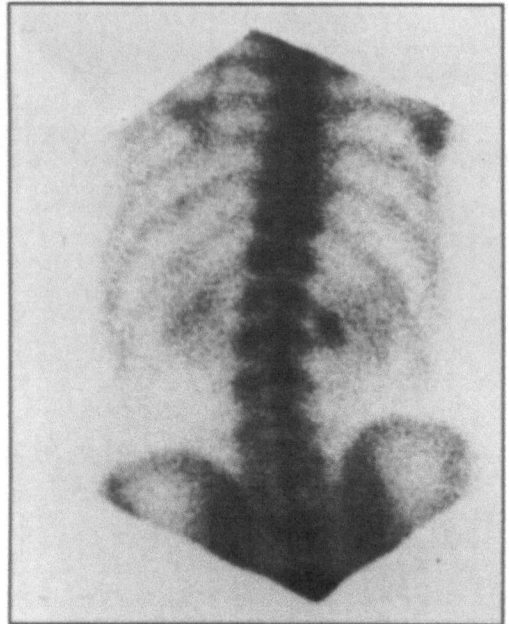

a

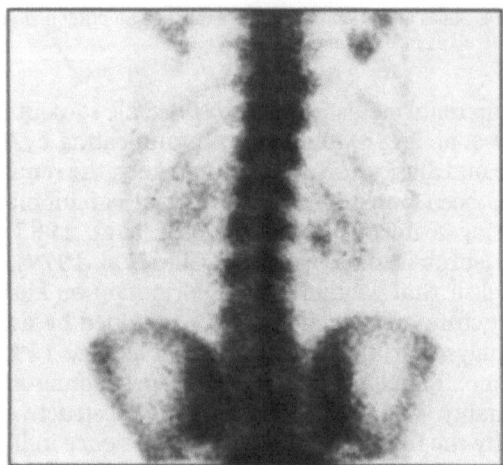

b

Fig. 15.15. **a** Lesion seen in region of right 12th rib posteriorly on supine scan. **b** On repeat scan erect it is apparent that activity is in renal pelvis.

al deposition may cause uncertainty but it is rare, with bilateral uptake and more medial position (Fig. 15.18). Other rare causes of splenic uptake include lymphoma or leukaemia (Winter 1976b; Nisbet and Maisey 1982), metastatic carcinoma (Costello et al. 1977) and trauma (Sty et al. 1982).

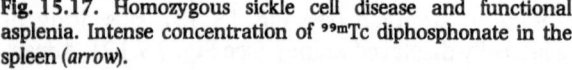

Fig. 15.17. Homozygous sickle cell disease and functional asplenia. Intense concentration of ^{99m}Tc diphosphonate in the spleen (*arrow*).

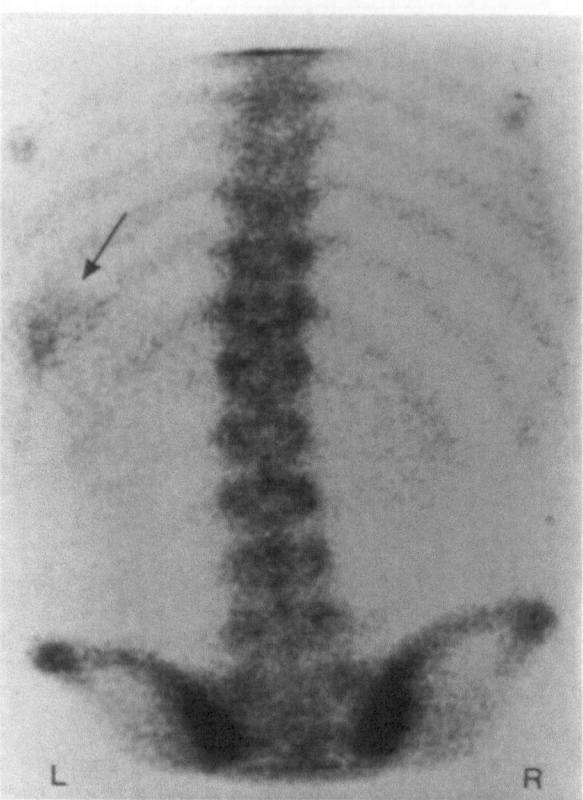

Fig. 15.16. Minor splenic uptake (*arrow*) in an asymptomatic patient with homozygous sickle cell disease.

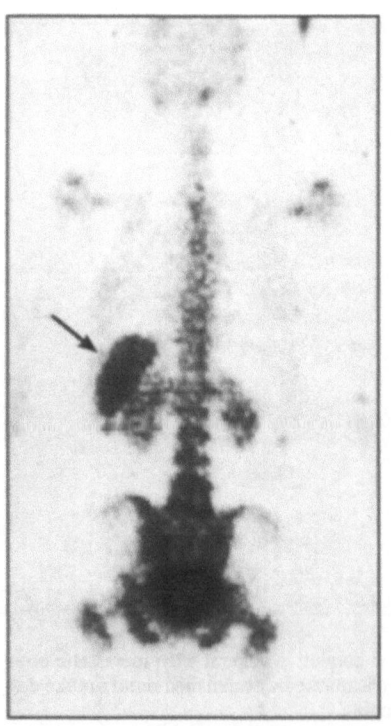

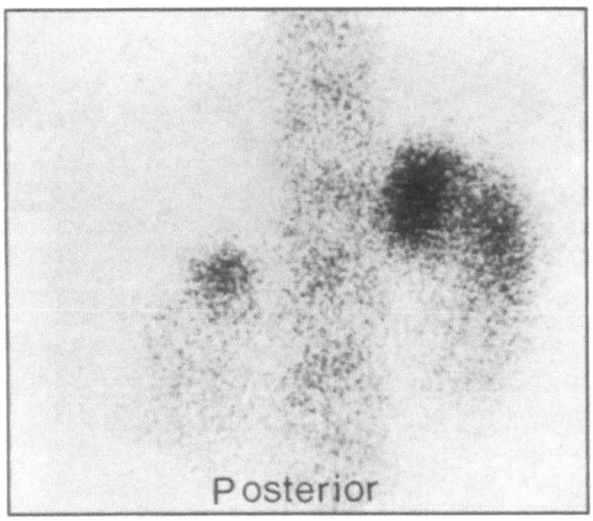

Fig. 15.18. Adrenal accumulation in a 25-year-old girl with nodular sclerosing Hodgkin's disease. No satisfactory explanation for the uptake. (Courtesy of Dr. M. V. Merrick)

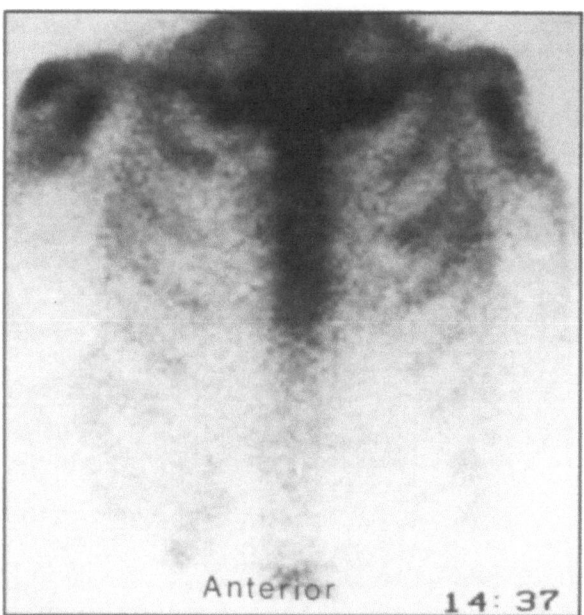

Fig. 15.19. Left-sided infiltrating breast carcinoma.

Breast

Breast uptake of bone agents is often seen incidentally (Fig. 15.19). The finding is quite non-specific and has been reported in the normal breast as well as in those harbouring benign or malignant disease (Berg et al. 1973; McDougall and Pistenma 1974; Serafini et al. 1974; Burnett et al. 1984). The mechanism of uptake is uncertain but may be related to high tissue calcium levels (Silberstein 1984) or to binding with receptor sites of acid phosphatase (Schmitt et al. 1974). In the largest series, Holmes et al. (1975) showed that 95% of benign lesions including fibroadenomas, mammary dysplasia and cystic mastitis had bilateral uptake, while 25% of malignant lesions showed a similar pattern. Those workers concluded that only unilateral breast uptake merited further investigation unless the uptake was seen in the contralateral breast following mastectomy. In this latter situation, malignancy was rarely found. As further caveats, Bledin et al. (1982) reported that non-mammary uptake in ribs on the mastectomy side was seen in 75% of patients and should not be confused with a pathological process, and Thrall et al. (1974) reported uptake in a pathological rib fracture simulating unilateral breast uptake.

Chest

Excluding uptake in breast, unilateral uptake over the chest during bone scanning is usually seen incidentally in malignant pleural effusion. Siegal et al. (1975) found bone radiopharmaceutical in the non-cellular fluid phase of the effusion, and other workers have confirmed the specificity for malignant rather than benign disease processes (Aprile et al. 1978; Lamki et al. 1982). The effusion can appear as diffuse uptake over the lower chest in erect views (Fig. 15.20a) or intense and well-circumscribed uptake when the effusion is loculated (Fig. 15.20b).

Less commonly, uptake in a hemithorax can result from a tumour of the chest wall (Fig. 15.21), lung and pleural uptake in bonchogenic carcinoma (Fig.15.22), radiotherapy to chest (Vieras 1977) and radiation pneumonitis (Sarreck et al. 1979). Metastatic disease in lung (Fig. 15.23) is readily identifiable by the more focal nature of the uptake (Hardy et al. 1976; Kim et al. 1980).

Brain

Localisation of ^{99m}Tc phosphates in brain is most commonly seen in cerebral infarction (Fig. 15.24). Less commonly, uptake may be noted in primary and metastatic carcinoma, chronic subdural haematoma, AV malformations and assorted inflammatory lesions (Matsui et al. 1973; Grames et al. 1975). Additional views may be necessary to exclude uptake in the calvaria.

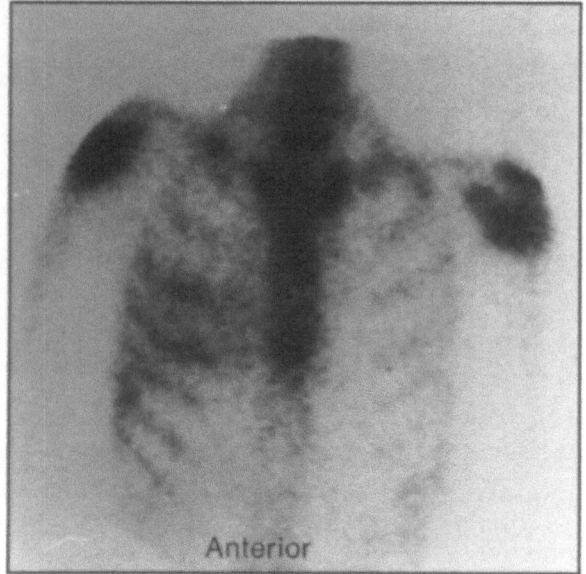

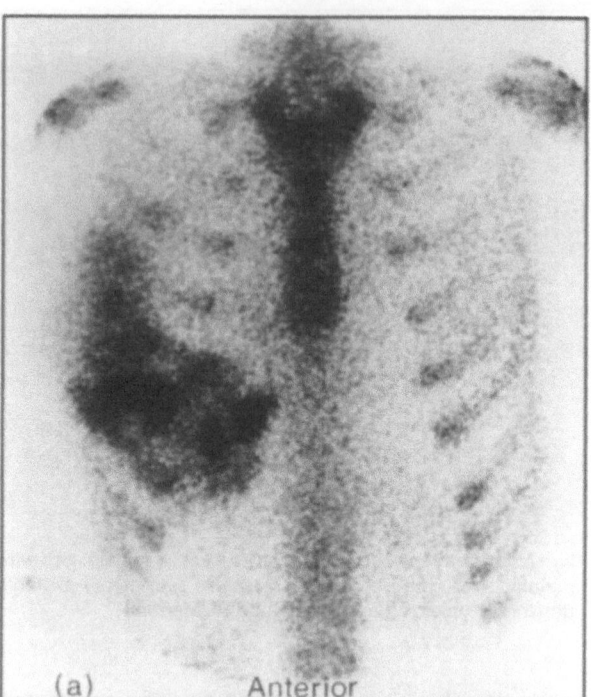

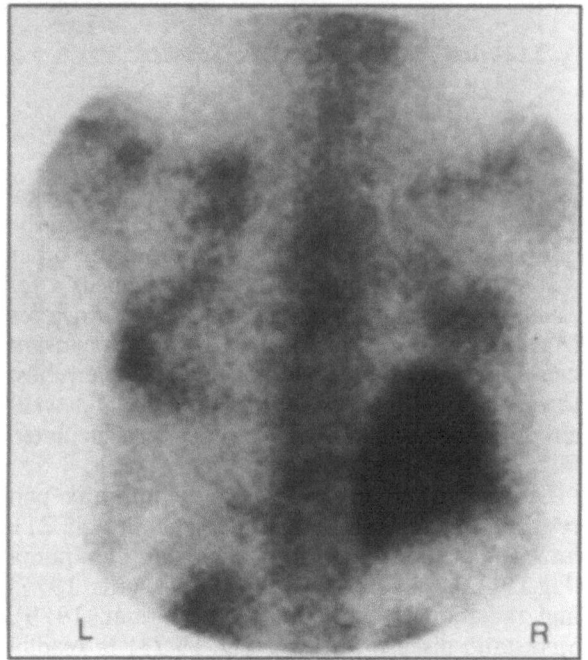

Fig. 15.20. a Malignant effusion secondary to disseminated mammary carcinoma. b Loculated malignant effusion secondary to a bronchogenic carcinoma.

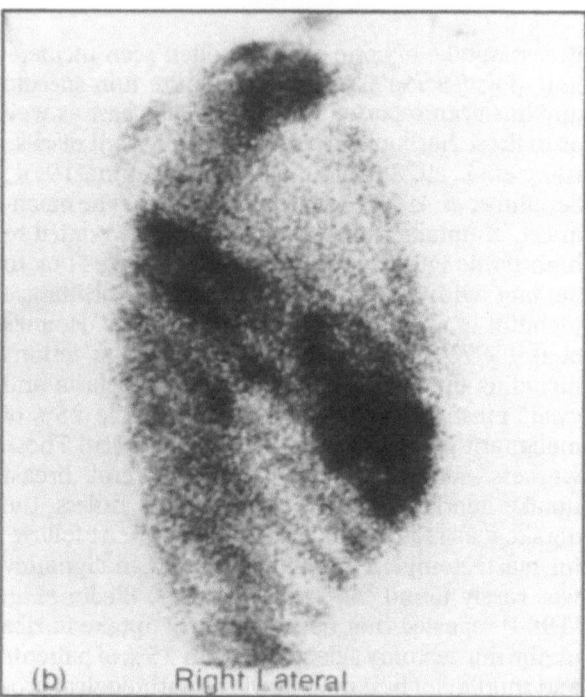

Fig. 15.21a,b. An 18-year-old girl who presented with a firm swelling of the anterior chest wall. Biopsy confirmed an anaplastic sarcoma with osteogenic features.

Uptake in brain occurs only when there is disorganisation of the blood–brain barrier. Since uptake of bone agents in cerebral infarction usually exceeds that of pertechnetate (Wenzel and Heasty 1974; Grames et al. 1975), the mechanism is likely to be related in part to the calcium content of the cerebral infarct. When computed tomography (CT)

is unavailable, greater intensity of ^{99m}Tc phosphate than ^{99m}Tc pertechnetate can be used to distiguish between infarct and tumour, if evaluation is made during the first month (Schauwecker et al. 1982).

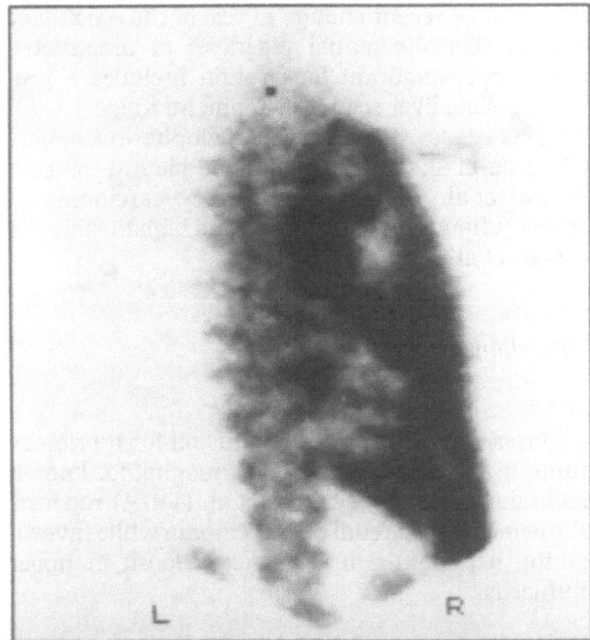

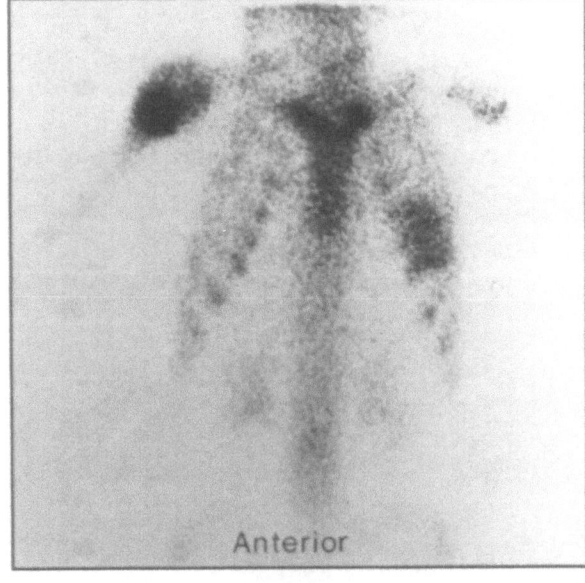

Fig. 15.23. A 10-year-old girl with a secondary deposit in the left lung from metastatic leiomyxoma. A further lesion is seen in the head of the right humerus. (Courtesy of Dr. R. McKenzie)

(Guiberteau et al. 1976; Garcia et al. 1977), lung (Oren and Uszler 1978; Que et al. 1980), oesophagus (Wilkinson and Gaede 1979), breast (Baumert et al. 1980) or prostate (Haseman 1983). The mechanism for uptake remains unclear. Wilson et al. (1983) found no association between localisation of bone agent and the presence of necrosis, cal-

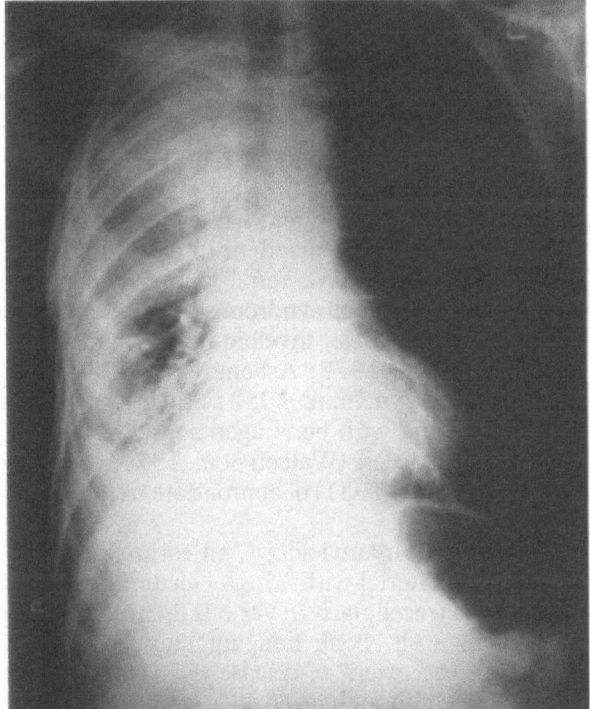

Fig. 15.22a.b. Lung and pleural uptake in a bronchogenic carcinoma. (Courtesy of Dr. M. V. Merrick)

Liver

Incidental detection of hepatic metastases on bone scanning (Fig. 15.25) is a relatively common occurrence. The primary tumour is usually found in colon

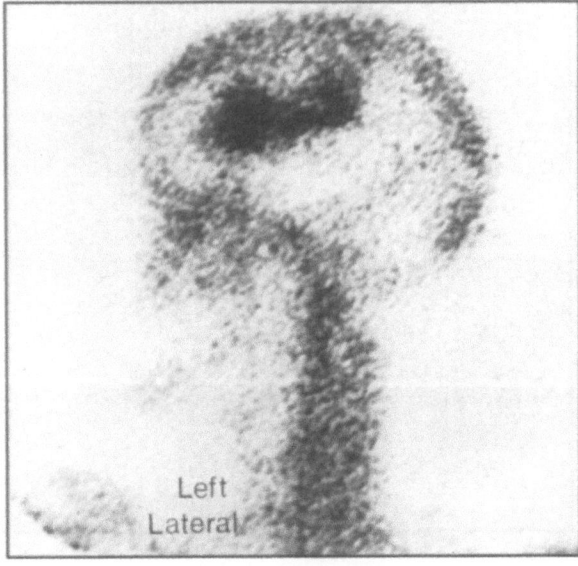

Fig. 15.24. Uptake in a large left cerebral infarct.

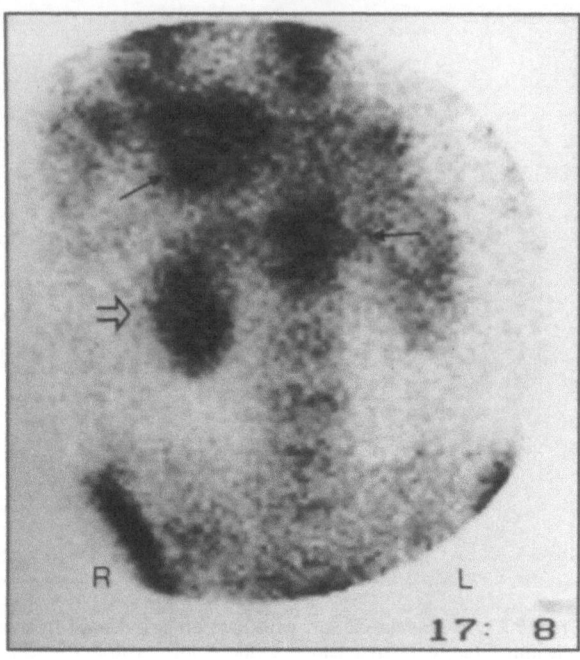

Fig. 15.25. Uptake in liver secondary deposits from breast adeno-carcinoma (*closed arrows*). The patient was normocalcaemic. Increased uptake in the right kidney (*open arrow*) relates to chemotherapy.

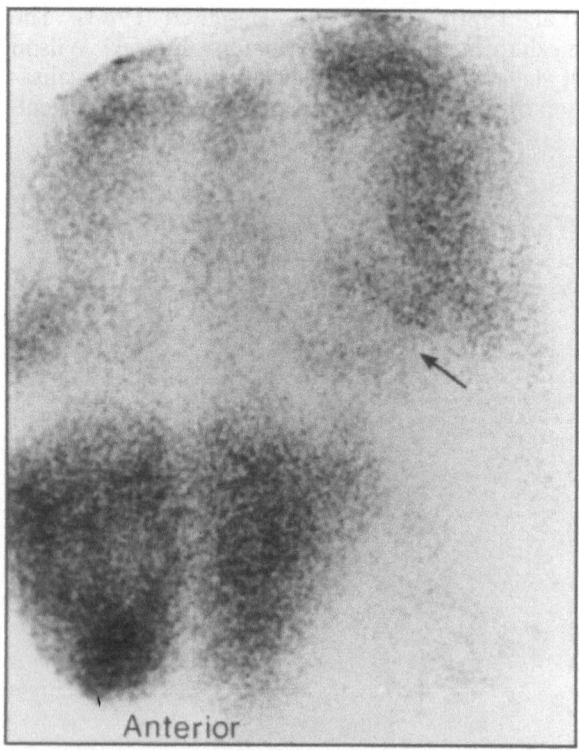

Fig. 15.26. Liver, lung and myocardial (*arrow*) uptake secondary to hypercalcaemia of malignancy.

cification or recent change in size of the secondary deposit. The differential diagnosis of unexpected right upper-quadrant localisation includes a previous colloid liver scan (Citrin and McKillop 1978), rib metastases, poor-quality radiopharmaceutical (Poulose et al. 1975), malignant pleural effusion (Seigal et al. 1975), inflammatory carcinoma of breast (Chaudhuri et al. 1974) and hepatic necrosis (Lyons et al. 1977).

Miscellaneous

Unsuspected Primary. It is unusual for a primary tumour to emerge during bone imaging for known secondary disease. Jackman et al. (1974) reported the detection of a renal cell carcinoma while investigating a photon-rich secondary deposit in upper humerus.

Metastatic Calcification. The diagnosis of metastatic calcification on clinical grounds is difficult; accordingly, the condition is often unrecognised (Holmes 1974; Chhabria et al. 1977). It is usually discovered incidentally (Richards 1975) when hypercalcaemic patients are screened for metastases by bone scanning (Fig. 15.26). Diffuse uptake of tracer is seen in lung but may also be noted in heart, liver, stomach and kidney and is a result of soft tissue microcalcification. In clinical practice it may occur in chronic renal failure, hyperparathyroidism, milk-alkali syndrome, hypervitaminosis D, bone metastases, myeloma and lymphoma (Rosenthal et al. 1977; Arbona et al. 1980; Seid et al. 1981; Wynchank 1982; Stone and Sisson 1985). Imaging with bone agents may be used to evaluate the success (Watson et al. 1977) or otherwise (Herry et al. 1981) of appropriate treatment.

Amyloidosis. In amyloidosis, an eosinophilic proteinaceous material with a high calcium content is deposited extracellularly in various tissues. After the biopsy diagnosis, bone imaging may be used to determine the extent of disease (Fig. 15.27; Yood et al. 1981); although insensitive, diffuse hepatic or cardiac uptake point to amyloid infiltration. Falk et al. (1983) selected patients with congestive cardiomyopathy and ventricular wall thickening on echocardiograph and found that uptake of bone agent was a sensitive and specific test for cardiac amyloid. Amyloid should be considered in any patient with diffuse hepatic and/or soft tissue uptake of bone-seeking agents with normal muscle enzymes (Van Antwerp et al. 1975b; Kula et al. 1977).

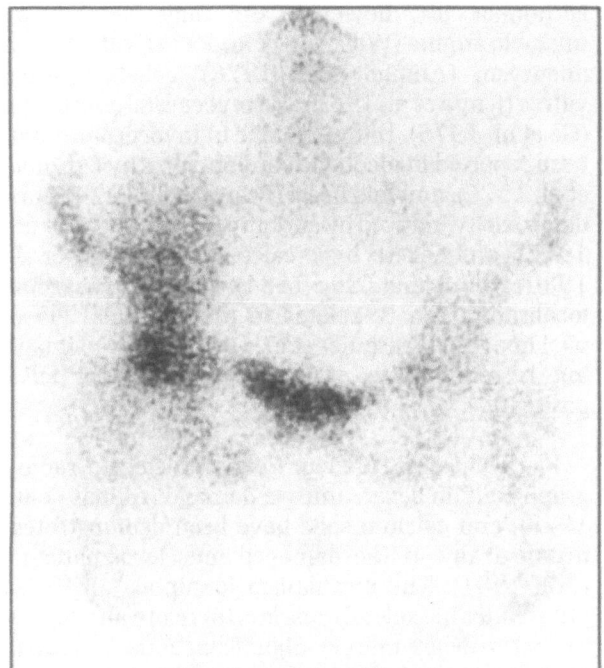

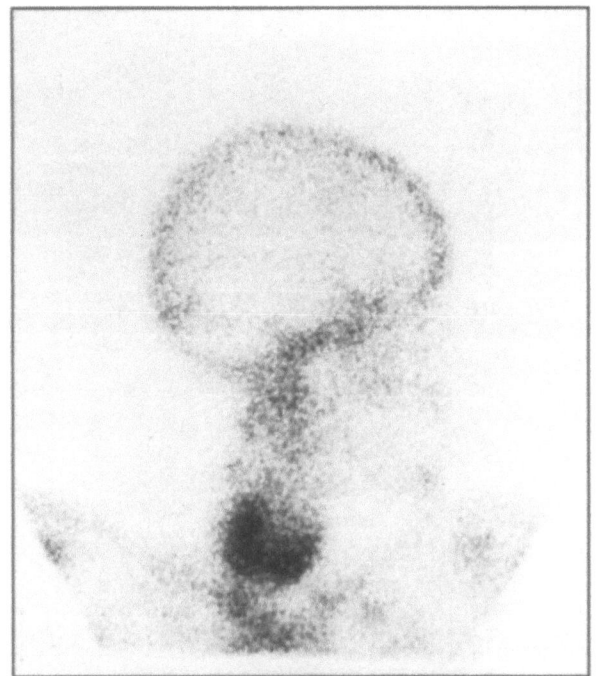

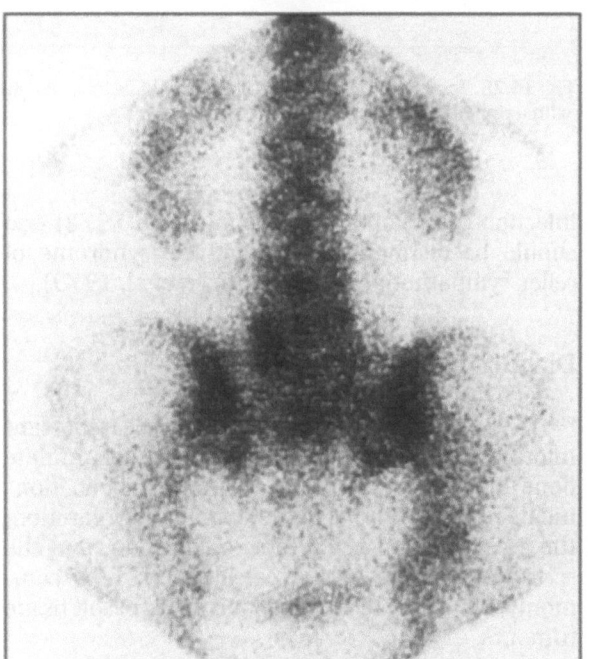

Fig. 15.27a–c. Amyloidosis. Functioning renal transplant seen (a). Tracer uptake, caused by amyloid, present in thyroid (b) and host kidneys (c).

Myopathy. Diffuse muscle uptake has been reported in a patient with carcinoma of the oropharynx (Lentle and Russell 1984). An incidental finding, the pattern of uptake pre-dated the onset of carcinomatous myopathy by several months; therefore, it may have an application in early diagnosis of this condition.

Lower Limb Uptake. An unusual increase in tracer accumulation is occasionally seen unilaterally in lower extremities during routine bone imaging (Fig. 15.28). The pattern may result from lymphoedema caused by lymphatic obstruction, circulation stasis caused by pelvic obstruction or deep vein thrombosis, or cellulitis caused by trauma,

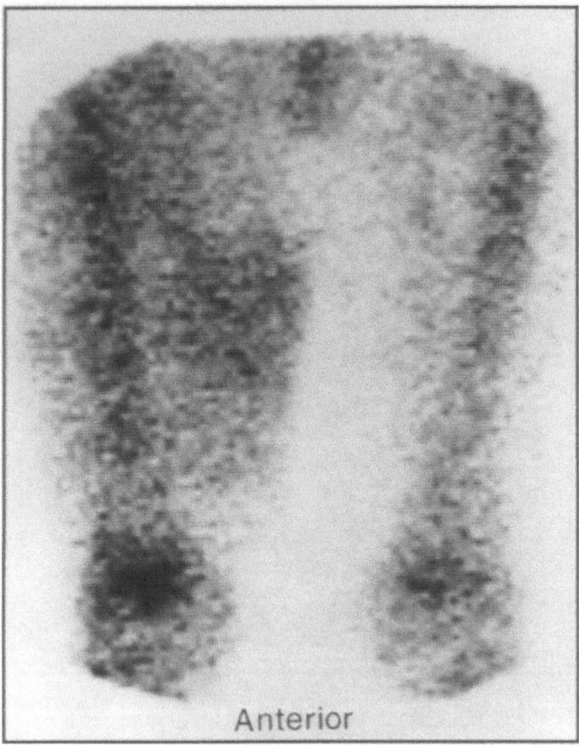

Anterior

Fig. 15.28. Increased uptake over the right thigh in a patient with a right ileofemoral venous thrombosis.

infection or radiation (Manoli and Soin 1978) and should be distinguishable from the syndrome of reflex sympathetic dystrophy (Kozin et al. 1979).

Diagnostic Applications

[99m]Tc phosphates may be used to provide important information on conditions known to accumulate bone agents in soft tissue. Common applications include the search for tissue damage or infarction, the assessment of heterotopic ossification, and the screening for soft tissue calcification. Less commonly, bone agents are used for staging of soft tissue tumours.

Tissue Damage or Infarction

Splenic infarction in sickle cell disease has already been discussed.

Myocardial Infarction. The technique of ^{99m}Tc pyrophosphate imaging for myocardial infarction (Bonte et al. 1974) has been widely applied (Bingham et al. 1983). Focal uptake in myocardium

is non-specific, however, and may be seen in unstable angina (Willerson et al. 1975), ventricular aneurysm (Ahmad et al. 1976), calcified heart valves (Jengo et al. 1977) and myocardial contusion (Go et al. 1975). Diffuse uptake in myocardium has been reported in alcoholic cardiomyopathy (Ahmad et al. 1976), amyloid heart (Braun et al. 1979), cardiac toxicity induced by adriamycin (Sty and Garrett 1977), and severe hypercalcaemia (Arbona et al. 1980; Atkins and Oster 1984). Diffuse myocardial localisation can be related to unintentional blood pool imaging (Prasquier et al. 1977). Delayed imaging is required to exclude this source of false positivity.

Rhabdomyolysis. Calcium can be detected radiographically in severe muscle damage (Akmal et al. 1978), and calcium salts have been demonstrated histologically in the damaged muscle of patients (Brill 1981). The mechanism for uptake of ^{99m}Tc phosphates in skeletal muscle is therefore analagous to that in heart muscle. Significant muscle uptake of bone agents has been reported in trauma (Silberstein 1984), ischaemia (Floyd and Prather 1977), idiopathic and alcohol-related rhabdomyolysis (Blair et al. 1975; Silberstein and Bove 1979), and after severe exercise (see Chap. 10; p 130), where it differentiates between joint or muscle injury, bone infarct or stress fracture (Matin et al. 1983). Cornelius (1982) found imaging with bone agents more sensitive than radiography, more specific than ultrasound for diagnosis of rhabdomyolysis and also useful in documenting muscle recovery. Diffuse muscle uptake may be found in inflammatory and collagen vascular diseases including polymyositis and scleroderma (Steinfeld et al. 1977) and carcinomatous myopathy (Lentle and Russell 1984). It is important to distinguish the curvilinear tracer uptake in femoral arteries from muscle uptake in thigh (Fig. 15.29). More common in older patients, vascular calcification is usually present on plain radiography or CT (Silberstein 1984).

Miscellaneous. Sfakianakis et al. (1978) have reported considerable success in detection of necrotising enterocolitis of the newborn with ^{99m}Tc diphosphonate. Barth et al. (1978) confirmed that good images of infarcted bowel can be obtained with bone agents in an experimental animal model.

Lyons et al. (1977) and Echeuarria et al. (1977) have independently reported intense concentration of bone tracer in severe centrilobular necrosis of liver. While as yet unreported, it is possible that the technique will be of value in the non-invasive detection of the Budd–Chiari syndrome.

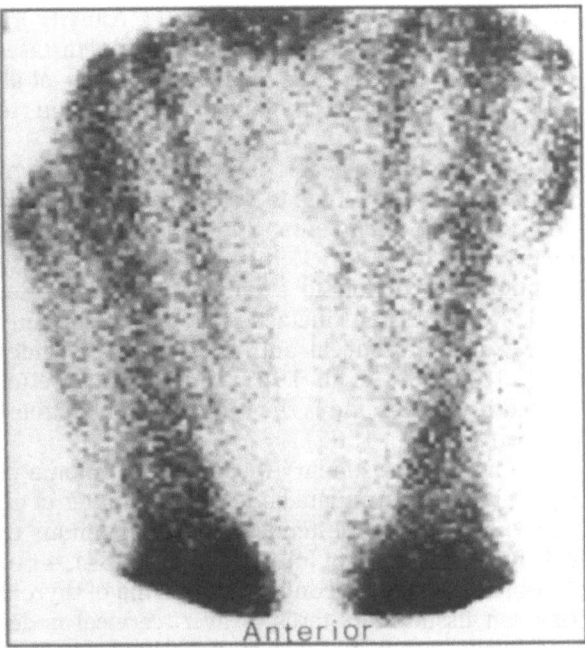

Fig. 15.29. Arteriosclerosis involving the femoral arteries in an elderly subject. Calcification was visible radiographically. Uptake of ^{99m}Tc-MDP is seen in the femoral arteries.

Heterotopic Bone Formation

The formation of bone outside the skeleton is unusual but readily detected on bone scanning. As myositis ossificans it occurs rarely as a congenital disorder, but most commonly after direct muscle trauma (Fig. 15.30; Suzuki et al. 1974), in patients with paraplegia (Tanaka et al. 1977) or following hip surgery (Russell and Kanis 1984). Uptake of

bone tracer is more sensitive than radiography in detecting ectopic bone formation and, if used serially, can indicate the optimum time for excision (Muheim et al. 1973). Ectopic bone formation around the hip in paraplegia can mimic deep vein thrombosis. Imaging is particularly valuable in identifying the nature of this complication (Prakash et al. 1978; Orzel et al. 1984).

Soft Tissue Calcification

Deposition of calcium phosphate in soft tissue (calcinosis) occurs in scleroderma and dermatomyositis. Sfakianakis et al. (1975) have shown that calcinosis universalis is common in the scleroderma and dermatomyositis of childhood and that bone tracers localise to the calcified lesion 18 months on average before they are seen on radiography. Uptake of bone agents occurs in calcinosis circumscripta, where small calcified deposits appear in the cutaneous and subcutaneous tissue over the extensor aspects of joints and fingertips (Fig. 15.31). Scintigraphy may also have a role in detecting calcinosis tumoralis, the localised but extensive calcification around joints and also in determining the effectiveness of dietary or steroid therapy (Leicht et al. 1979).

Staging of Soft Tissue Tumours

Most malignant and many benign tumours of soft tissue accumulate ^{99m}Tc phosphate (Chew et al. 1981). Preoperative staging with bone agents evaluates the relationship of the primary tumour to the adjacent bone. Increased tracer uptake in bone adjacent to a soft tissue sarcoma indicates bone

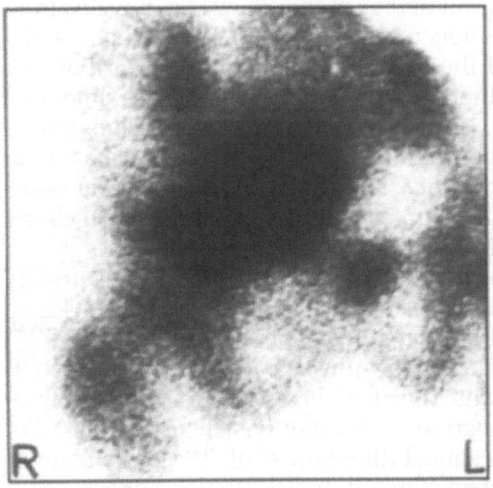
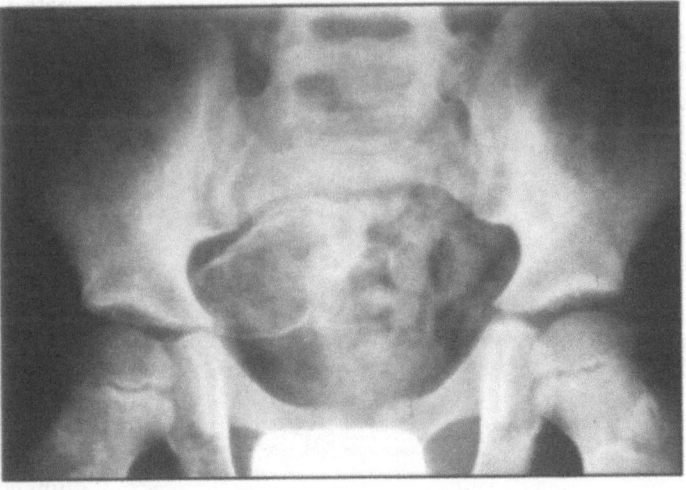

a   b

Fig. 15.30a,b. A 5-year-old boy with a 3-week history of a painful right hip. Radiography revealed the site of calcified muscle and biopsy confirmed myositis ossificans. Presumably, the history of trauma was concealed. (Courtesy of Dr. M. V. Merrick)

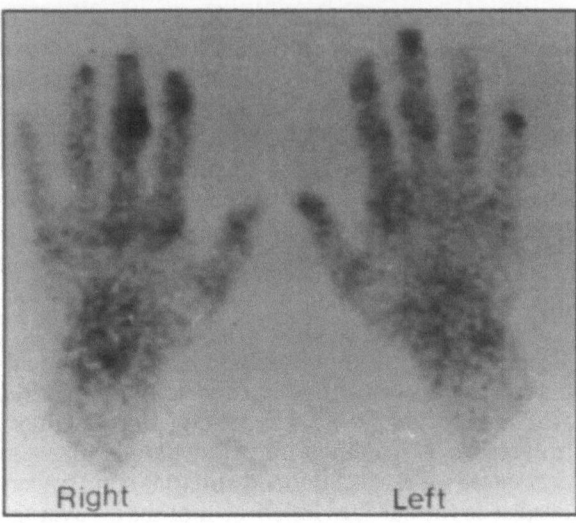

Fig. 15.31. A patient with calcinosis circumscripta without subcutaneous calcification on the radiograph. There are multiple photon-rich areas corresponding to the palpable subcutaneous nodules.

involvement by the tumour itself or by the reactive mesenchymal tissue around it. Such involvement may also be present when uptake in the soft tissue lesion is contiguous with the bone and cannot be separated even on appropriate multiple scan views.

Bone scintigraphy to determine the extent of an osteosarcoma and its bone metastases may be of value for detection of non-pulmonary soft tissue

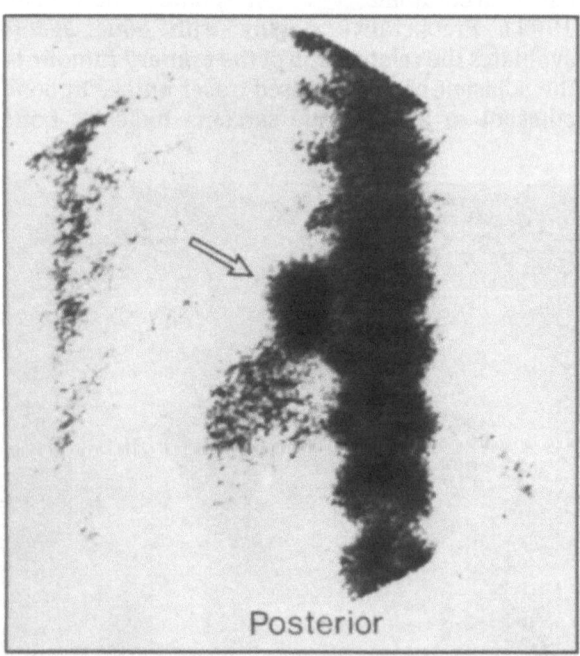

Fig. 15.32. Pulmonary deposit of osteogenic sarcoma (*open arrow*).

metastases (Teates et al. 1977). The sensitivity for scintigraphic detection of pulmonary metastases (Fig. 15.32) is only 21%, however (Vanel et al. 1984), CT providing the major contribution to diagnosis.

Bone imaging indicates the position and extent of a neuroblastoma in up to 90% of cases (Podrasky et al. 1983), documents the presence of bone metastases (Sty et al. 1979b) and picks up displacement or obstruction to a kidney (Howman-Giles et al. 1979). Distant metastases in soft tissue may be detected (Rosenfield and Treves 1974; Valdez et al. 1978; Sty et al. 1983), but CT has better spatial resolution and is the investigation of choice (Armstrong et al. 1982).

Primary and secondary medullary carcinoma of thyroid may accumulate bone agents (Reuter et al. 1983) because of the tendency for the tumour to calcify. In the series of Johnson et al. (1984), 4 out of 34 patients with medullary carcinoma of thyroid had soft tissue metastases in liver, cervical nodes and mediastinum detected by bone imaging. Two of these patients had soft tissue metastases without bone involvement. Further work is required to determine the role of bone imaging in the management of such patients, especially since ^{131}I-MIBG imaging may also be of value (Sone et al. 1985).

Artefacts

Sites of radiopharmaceutical injection or urine contamination on the lower pelvis, perineum and inner thighs are common mechanisms for soft tissue accumulation during bone scanning (Adams et al. 1980). Recording of the injection site by the technologist and use of lateral views should differentiate pathological uptake at the elbow (e.g. bursitis) from the injection artefact (Heck 1980), while caudal views of the pelvis may be required to distinguish contamination from a bladder diverticulum (see Fig. 15.1). Rare artefacts in the axilla include lymph node accumulation secondary to intradermal extravasation of injected bone agent (Penney and Styles 1982) and uptake secondary to hyperhydrosis (Ajmani et al. 1977).

Diffuse liver uptake on bone scanning is usually the result of a prior colloid scan (Citrin and McKillop 1978). Uptake in lung and bowel (Saha et al. 1977) or liver, gallbladder and bowel (Conway et al. 1979) may result from technical factors and is likely to cause diagnostic uncertainty. The pH of the radiopharmaceutical (Sherkow et al. 1984), its aluminium content (Chaudhuri 1976), the source of [99m]Tc (Conway et al. 1982), a prolonged time from make-up to injection (Van Duzee et al. 1982), and

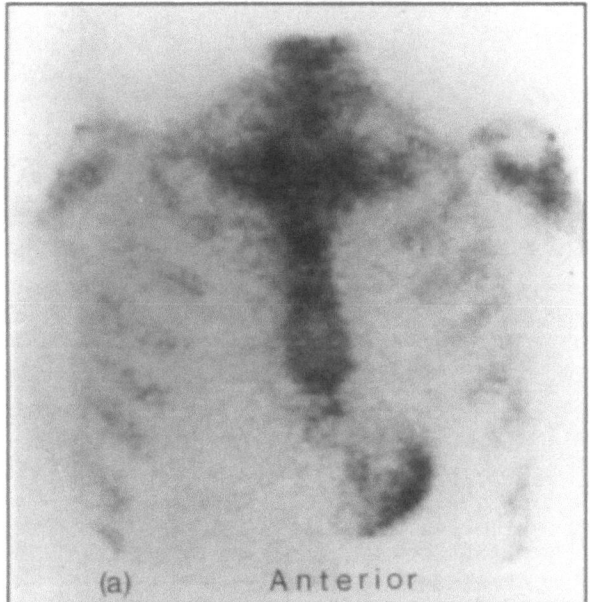

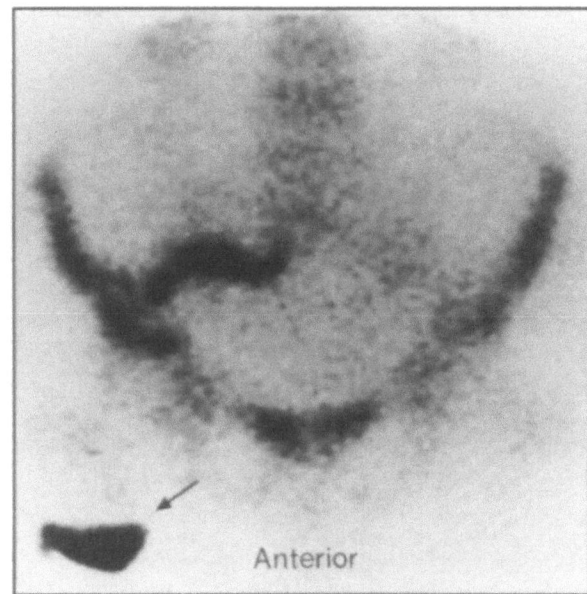

Fig. 15.34. Patient with an ileal conduit following total cystectomy for carcinoma of the bladder. The collecting bag is outlined (*arrow*).

choroid plexus. Stomach uptake (Wilson and Pollack 1981) can usually be recognised by the characteristic outline (Fig. 15.33) and must be distinguished from splenic or renal accumulation.

Fig. 15.33a,b. Stomach uptake of ^{99m}Tc during bone scanning. The anterior position (a) and curvilinear shape usually distinguishes stomach from kidney or spleen.

radiation-induced autodecomposition (Billinghurst et al. 1979) have all been reported to produce an unusual distribution of tracer which pointed to a failure in quality control. Drug interactions may have a similar effect (Crawford and Gumerman 1978).

The presence of unreduced pertechnetate will produce uptake in organs and tissues with an iodide trap such as thyroid, stomach, salivary glands and

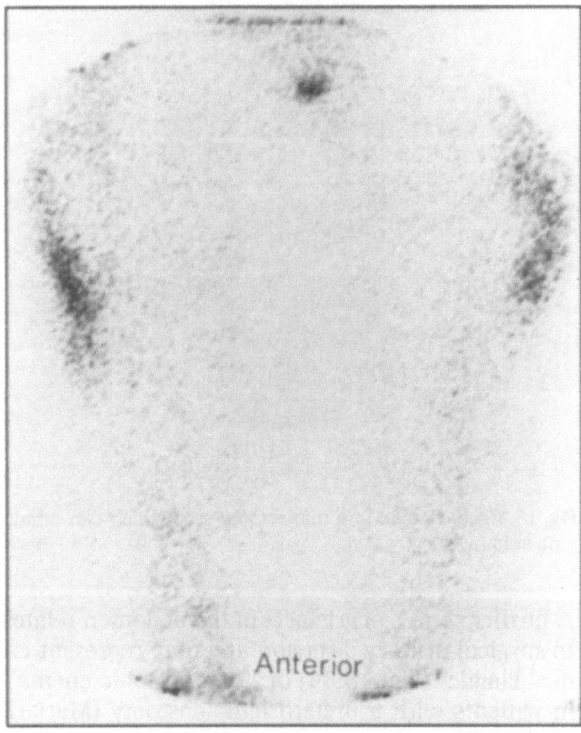

Fig. 15.35. Bilateral uptake in the soft tissue of the thighs following multiple injections of pethidine hydrochloride.

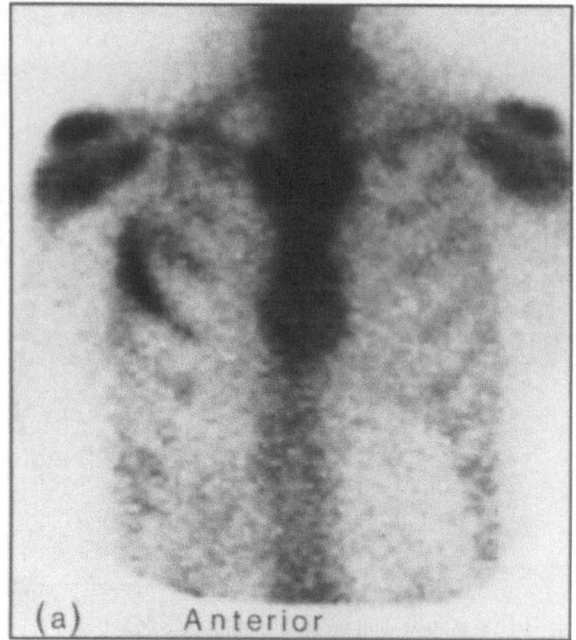

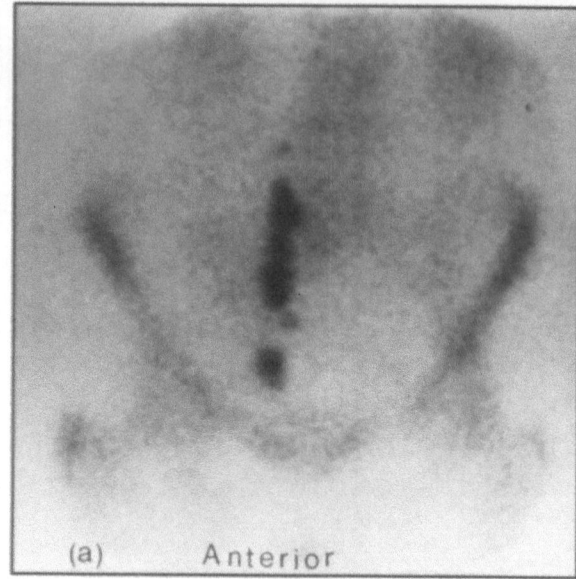

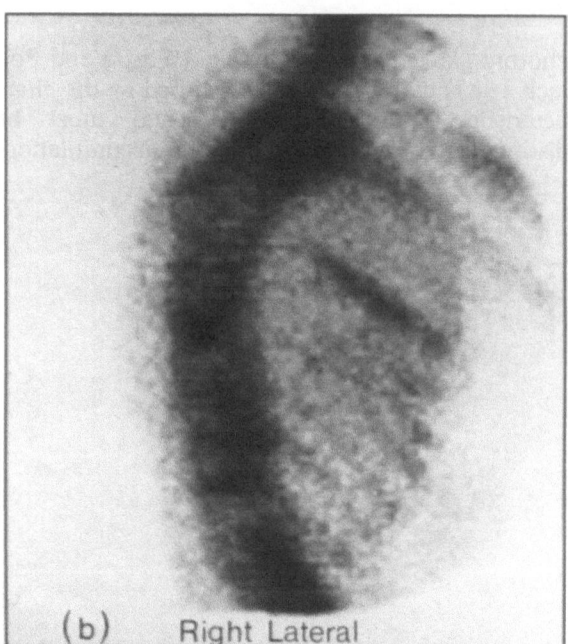

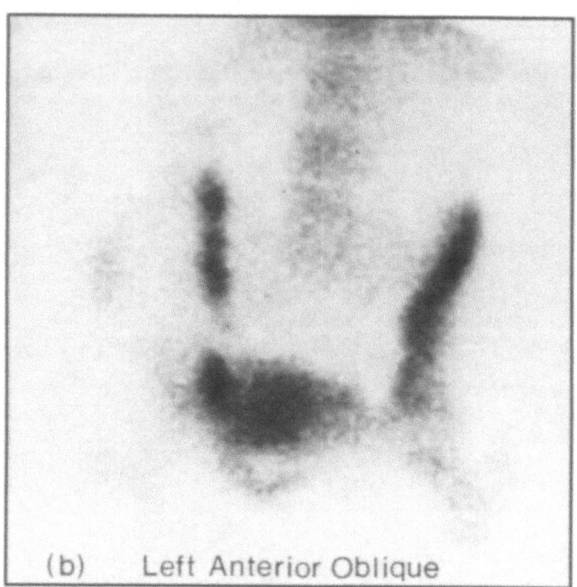

Fig. 15.37a,b. Uptake in a lower abdominal scar. Oblique views (b) are often required to rule out ureteric dilatation.

Fig. 15.36a,b. Uptake in a mastectomy scar which can mimic a rib lesion.

A further source of artefacts in the abdomen relates to surgical urinary diversion and may represent an ileal bladder (Fig. 15.34) or "scintigraphic enema" in patients with a ureterosigmoidostomy (Mariani et al. 1978).

Unusual uptake at injection sites has been reported with meperidine (Brill 1981), iron dextran (Van Antwerp et al. 1975a; Mazzola et al. 1976), and calcium heparinate (Planchon et al. 1983). The present author can record a similar pattern after multiple intramuscular injections of pethidine (Fig. 15.35).

Uptake in healing surgical scars (Poulose et al. 1975; Siddiqui and Stokka 1980) may simulate rib abnormality (Fig. 15.36) or dilatation of a ureter (Fig. 15.37). The artefactual nature of the uptake may not be recognised without oblique or lateral views.

References

Adams KJ, Shuler SE, Witherspoon LR, Neely HR (1980) A retrospective analysis of renal abnormalities detected in bone scans. Clin Nucl Med 5:1–7

Ahmad M, Dubiel JP, Verdon TA et al. (1976) Technetium-99m stannous pyrophosphate myocardial imaging in patients with and without left ventricular aneurysm. Circulation 58: 833–835

Ajmani SK, Lerner SR, Pirchen FJ (1977) Bone scan artifact caused by hyperhydrosis: case report. J Nucl Med 18:801–802

Akmal M, Goldstein DA, Telfer N, Wilkinson E, Massry SG (1978) Resolution of muscle calcification in rhabdomyolysis and acute renal failure. Ann Intern Med 89: 928–930

Alfrey AC, Solomons CC, Ciricillo J, Miller NL (1976) Extraosseous calcification: evidence for abnormal pyrophosphate metabolism in uraemia. J Clin Invest 57: 692–699

Aprile C, Bernardo G, Carena M et al. (1978) Accumulation of ^{99m}Tc-Sn-pyrophosphate in pleural effusions. Eur J Nucl Med 3: 219–222

Arbona GL, Antonmattei S, Tetalman MR, Scheu JD (1980) Tc-99m-diphosphonate distribution in a patient with hypercalcaemia and metastatic calcification. Clin Nucl Med 5: 422

Armstrong EA, Harwood-Nash DCF, Ritz CR, Chuang SH, Pettersson H, Martin DJ (1982) CT of neuroblastomas and ganglioneuromas in children. AJR 139: 571–576

Atkins HL, Oster ZH (1984) Myocardial uptake of a bone tracer associated with hypercalcaemia. Clin Nucl Med 9: 613–615

Barth KH, Alderson PO, Strandberg JD, Strauss HW, White RI (1978) ^{99m}Tc-pyrophosphate imaging in experimental mesenteric infarction: relationship of tracer uptake to the degree of ischaemic injury. Radiology 129: 491–495

Baumert JE, Lantieri RL, Horning S, McDougall IR (1980) Liver metastases of breast carcinoma detected on ^{99m}Tc-methylene diphosphonate bone scan. AJR 134: 389–391

Berg GR, Kalisher L, Osmond JD, Pendergrass HP, Potsaid MS (1973) ^{99m}Tc-diphosphonate concentration in primary breast carcinoma. Radiology 109: 393–394

Biello DR, Coleman RE, Stanley RJ (1976) Correlation of renal images on bone scan and intravenous pyelogram. Am J Roentgenol Radium Ther Nucl Med 127: 633–636

Billinghurst MW, Rempel S, Westendorf BA (1979) Radiation decomposition of technetium-99m radiopharmaceuticals. J Nucl Med 20: 138–143

Bingham JB, McKusick KA, Strauss HW (1983) Cardiovascular nuclear medicine In: Maisey MN, Britton KE, Gilday DL (eds) Clinical nuclear medicine. Chapman and Hall, London, pp 1–40

Blair RJ, Schroeder ET, McAfee JG, Duxbury CE (1975) Skeletal muscle uptake of bone seeking agents in both traumatic and non-traumatic rhabdomyolysis with acute renal failure. J Nucl Med 16: 515–516

Bledin AG, Kim EE, Haynie TP (1982) Bone scintigraphic findings related to unilateral mastectomy. Eur J Nucl Med 7: 500–501

Bonte FJ, Parkey RW, Graham KD, Moore J, Stokely EM (1974) A new method for radionuclide imaging of myocardial infarcts. Radiology 110: 473–474

Bossuyt A, Verbeelen D, Jonckheer MH, Six R (1979) Usefulness of ^{99m}Tc-methylene diphosphonate scintigraphy in nephrocalcinosis. Clin Nucl Med 4: 333–334

Braun SD, Lisbona R, Novales-Diaz JA, Sniderman A (1979) Myocardial uptake of ^{99m}Tc-phosphate tracer in amyloidosis. Clin Nucl Med 4: 244–245

Brill DR (1981) Radionuclide imaging of non-neoplastic soft tissue disorders. Semin Nucl Med 11: 277–288

Buja LM, Tofe AJ, Kulkarni PV et al. (1977) Sites and mechanisms of localisation of technetium-99m phosphorus radiopharmaceuticals in acute myocardial infarcts and other tissues. J Clin Invest 60: 724–740

Burnett KR, Lyons KP, Theron Brown W (1984) Uptake of osteotropic radionuclides in the breast. Semin Nucl Med 14: 48–49

Buxton-Thomas MS, Wraight EP (1983) High renal activity on bone scintigrams. A sign of hypercalcaemia. Br J Radiol 56: 911–914

Byun HH, Rodman, SG, Chung KE (1976) Soft tissue concentration of ^{99m}Tc-phosphates associated with injections of iron dextran complex. J Nucl Med 17: 374–375

Carlson DH, Simon H, Wegner W (1977) Bone scanning and diagnosis of reflex sympathetic dystrophy secondary to herniated lumbar discs. Neurology 27: 791–793

Charkes ND (1979) Mechanisms of skeletal tracer uptake. J Nucl Med 20: 794–795

Chaudhuri TK (1976) Liver uptake of ^{99m}Tc-diphosphonate. Radiology 119: 485–486

Chaudhuri TK, Chaudhuri TK, Gulesserian HP, Christie JH, Tonami N (1974) Extraosseous noncalcified soft tissue uptake of ^{99m}Tc-polyphosphate. J Nucl Med 15: 1054–1056

Chaynes ZW, Strashun AM (1980) Improved renal screening on bone scans. Clin Nucl Med 5: 94–97

Chew FS, Hudson TM, Enneking WF (1981) Radionuclide imaging of soft tissue neoplasms. Semin Nucl Med 11: 266–276

Chhabria PB, Stankey RM, Pinsky ST (1977) Extraskeletal uptake of ^{99m}Tc-Sn-pyrophosphate in hypercalcaemia associated with carcinoma of the urinary bladder. Clin Nucl Med 2: 87–88

Choy D, Murray IPC, Hoschi R (1981) The effect of iron on biodistribution of bone scanning agents in humans. Radiology 140: 197–202

Citrin DL, McKillop JH (1978) Atlas of technetium bone scans. Bohn, Scheltema and Holkema, Utrecht, pp 5–29

Citrin DL, Bessent RG, McGinley E, Gordon D (1975) Dynamic studies with ^{99m}Tc-HEDP in normal subjects and inpatients with bone tumours. J Nucl Med 16: 886–889

Conger JD, Alfrey AC (1976) Scanning for pulmonary calcification. Ann Intern Med 84: 224–225

Conger JD, Hammond WS, Alfrey AC, Contguglia SR, Stanford RE, Huffer WE (1975) Pulmonary calcification in chronic dialysis patients: clinical and pathologic studies. Ann Intern Med 83: 330–333

Constable AR, Cranage RW (1981) Pitfalls of absent or faint kidney sign on bone scan. J Nucl Med 22: 658

Conway JJ, Weiss SC, Khentigan A, Tofe AJ, Thane TT (1979) Gallbladder and bowl localisation of bone imaging radiopharmaceuticals. J Nucl Med 20: 622

Conway JJ, Weiss S, Van Duzee BF, Deprato DW (1982) A comparative study of the effects of instant and generator produced technetium-99m on the nonosseous localisation of skeletal imaging agents in children. J Nucl Med 23: P109

Cornelius EA (1982) Nuclear medicine imaging in rhabdomyolysis. Clin Nucl Med 7: 462–464

Costello P, Gramm HF, Steinberg D (1977) Simultaneous occurrence of functional asplenia and splenic accumulation of diphosphonate in metastatic breast carcinoma. J Nucl Med 18: 1237

Crawford SA, Gumerman LW (1978) Alteration of body distribution of ^{99m}Tc-pyrophosphate by radiographic contrast material. Clin Nucl Med 3: 305–307

Dewanjee MK, Kahn PC (1976) Mechanism of localisation of ^{99m}Tc-labelled pyrophosphate and tetracycline in infarcted myocardium. J Nucl Med 17: 639–646

Dhawan V, Sziklas JJ, Spencer RP, Gordon IJ (1977) Surgically related extravasation of urine detected on bone scan. Clin Nucl Med 2: 411

Echeuarria RA, Bonanno C, Davis DK (1977) Uptake of ^{99m}Tc pyrophosphate in liver necrosis. Clin Nucl Med 9: 322–323

Edeling CJ (1983) ^{99m}Tc-methylene diphosphonate uptake in a primary Wilms' tumour. Eur J Nucl Med 8: 30

Falk RH, Lee VW, Rubinow A, Hood WB, Cohen AS (1983) Sensitivity of technetium-99m pyrophosphate scintigraphy in diagnosing cardiac amyloidosis. Am J Cardiol 51: 826–830

Fink-Bennet D, Dworkin H (1977) Incidental detection of a horseshoe kidney on radionuclide bone images. Radiology 123: 392

Floyd JL, Prather JL (1977) ^{99m}Tc-EHDP uptake in ischemic muscle. Clin Nucl Med 2: 281–282

Fogelman I, McKillop JH, Boyle IT, Greig WR (1977) Absent kidney sign associated with symmetrical and uniformly increased uptake of radiopharmaceutical by the skeleton. Eur J Nucl Med 2: 257–259

Francis MD, Russell RGG, Fleisch H (1969) Diphosphonates inhibit formation of calcium phosphate crystals in vitro and pathological calcification in vivo. Science 165: 1264–1266

Garcia AC, Yeh SDJ, Benua SCD, Benua RS (1977) Accumulation of bone seeking radionuclides in liver metastases from colon carcinoma. Clin Nucl Med 2: 265–269

Gatter RA, McCartney DJ (1967) Pathological tissue calcifications in man. Arch Pathol 84: 346–353

Gerhold JP, Klingensmith WC, Loeffel SC (1980) Focal uptake of Tc-99m-MDP in renal metastases from squamous cell carcinoma of the lung. Clin Nucl Med 5: 522

Gilbert LA, Weiss MA, Gelfand MJ, Hawkins HH, Nishiyama H, Aron BJ (1983) Detection of renal metastasis of osteosarcoma by bone scan. Clin Nucl Med 7: 325–326

Glass EC, DeNardo GL, Hines HH (1980) Immediate renal imaging and renography with ^{99m}Tc-methylene diphosphonate to assess renal blood flow, excretory function and anatomy. Radiology 135: 187–190

Glimcher MJ, Krane SM (1968) The organisation and structure of bone and the mechanism of calcification. In: Ramachandron GN (ed) Treatise on collagen. Academic, New York, pp 137–153

Go RT, Doty DB, Chiu CL, Christie JH (1975) A new method of diagnosing myocardial contusion in man by radionuclide imaging. Radiology 116: 107–110

Goy W, Crowe WJ (1976) Splenic accumulation of ^{99m}Tc-diphosphonate in a patient with sickle cell disease: case report. J Nucl Med 17: 108–109

Grames GM, Jansen C, Carlsen EN, Davidson TR (1975) The abnormal bone scan in intracranial lesions. Radiology 115: 129–134

Guiberteau MJ, Potsaid MS, McKusick KA (1976) Accumulation of ^{99m}Tc diphosphonate in four patients with hepatic neoplasm: case reports. J Nucl Med 17: 1060–1061

Harbert JC, Vieras F, Boyd CM (1976) Focal renal activity on bone scans. J Nucl Med 17: 426–427

Hardy JG, Anderson GS, Newble GM (1976) Uptake of ^{99m}Tc-pyrophosphate by metastatic extragenital seminoma. J Nucl Med 17: 1105–1106

Harwood SJ (1978) Splenic visualisation using ^{99m}Tc-methylene diphosphonate in a patient with sickle cell disease. Clin Nucl Med 3: 308 309

Haseman MK (1983) Accumulation of a bone imaging agent in liver metastases from prostatic carcinoma. Clin Nucl Med 8: 488–489

Hattner RS, Miller SW, Schimmel D (1975) Significance of renal asymmetry in bone scans: experience of 795 cases. J Nucl Med 16: 161–163

Heck LL (1980) Extraosseous localisation of phosphate bone agents. Semin Nucl Med 10: 311–316

Herry JY, Chevet D, Moisan A, Le Pogamp P, Lejeune JJ, Kerdiles Y (1981) Pulmonary uptake of Tc-99m-labelled methylene diphosphonate in a patient with a parathyroid adenoma. J Nucl Med 22: 888–890

Holmes RA, (1974) Diffuse interstitial pulmonary calcification. JAMA 230: 1018–1019

Holmes RA, Manoli RS, Isitman AT (1975) Tc-99m labelled phosphates as an indicator of breast pathology. J Nucl Med 16: 536

Howman-Giles RB, Gilday DL, Ash JM (1979) Radionuclide skeletal survey in neuroblastoma. Radiology 131: 497–502

Jackman SJ, Maher FT, Hattery RR (1974) Detection of renal cell carcinoma with ^{99m}Tc polyphosphate imaging of bone. Mayo Clin Proc 49: 297–299

Jengo JA, Mena I, Joe SH, Criley JM (1977) The significance of calcific valvular heart disease in Tc-99m pyrophosphate myocardial infarction scanning: radiographic scintigraphic and pathological correlation,. J Nucl Med 18: 776–781

Johnson DG, Colman RE, McCook TA, Dale SK, Wells SA (1984) Bone and liver images in medullary carcinoma of the thyroid gland: concise communication. J Nucl Med 25: 419–422

Kajubi SK, Chayes ZW (1985) Superscan prediction—another benefit of early renal views in bone scans. J Nucl Med 26: 428–429

Kim EE, Domstad PA, Choy YC, DeLand FH (1980) Accumulation of Tc-99m phosphate complexes in metastatic lesions from colon and lung carcinoma. Eur J Nucl Med 5: 299–301

King WR, Francis MD, Michael WR (1971) Effect of disodium ethane-1-hydroxy-1, 1-diphosphonate on bone formation. Clin Orthop 78: 251–270

Koizumi K, Tonami N, Hisada K (1981) Diffusely increased Tc-99m MDP uptake in both kidneys. Clin Nucl Med 6: 362–365

Kozin F, Soin JS, Ryan LM, Carrera GF, Wortmann RL (1979) Bone scintigraphy in the reflex sympathetic dystrophy syndrome. Radiology 138: 437–443

Kula RW, Engel WK, Line BR (1977) Scanning for soft tissue amyloid. Lancet I: 92–93

Lamki LM, Wyatt JK (1983) Renal vein thrombosis as a cause of excess renal accumulation of bone seeking agents. Clin Nucl Med 8: 267–268

Lamki L, Cohen P, Driedger A (1982) Malignant pleural effusion and Tc-99m MDP accumulation. Clin Nucl Med 7: 331–333

Lantieri RL, Lin MS, Martin W, Goodwin DA (1980) Increased renal accumulation of Tc-99m MDP in renal artery stenosis. Clin Nucl Med 5: 305–309

Lecklitner ML, Tauxe WN (1983) Bone scintigraphy and postoperative ureteropelvic urine extravasation. Eur J Nucl Med 8: 346–347

Leicht E, Berberich R, Lauffenburger T, Haas HG (1979) Tumoral calcinosis: accumulation of bone seeking tracers in the calcium deposits. Eur J Nucl Med 4: 419–421

Lentle BC, Russell AS (1984) Uptake of Tc-99m MDP in muscle anticipating clinical evidence of a carcinomatous myopathy. J Nucl Med 25: 1320–1322

Lunia SL, Heravi M, Goel V, Tiv AS, Chodos RB (1980) Pitfalls of absent or faint kidney sign on bone scan. J Nucl Med 21: 894–895

Lutrin CL, McDougall IR, Goris ML (1978) Intense concentration of technetium 99m pyrophosphate in the kidneys of children treated with chemotherapeutic drugs for malignant disease. Radiology 128: 165–167

Lutrin CL, Goris ML (1979) Pyrophosphate retention by previously irradiated renal tissue. Radiology 133: 207–209

Lyons KP, Kuperus J, Green HW (1977) Localisation of Tc-99m pyrophosphate in the liver due to massive liver necrosis: case report. J Nucl Med 18: 550–552

Maher FT (1975) Evaluation of renal and urinary tract abnormalities noted on scintiscans. Mayo Clin Proc 50: 370–378

Manoli RS, Soin JS (1978) Unilateral increased radioactivity in the lower extremities of routine ^{99m}Tc pyrophosphate bone imaging. Clin Nucl Med 3: 374–378

Mariani G, Levorato D, Tuoni M, Giannotti P (1978) Incidental imaging of the large bowel in patients with uretero-sigmoidostomy during bone scintigraphy with ^{99m}Tc pyrophosphate. J Nucl Med Allied Sci 22: 153–157

Martin-Simmerman P, Cohen MD, Siddiqui A, Mirkin D, Provisor A (1984) Calcification and uptake of Tc-99m diphosphonates in neuroblastomas: concise communication. J Nucl Med 25: 656–660

Matin P, Lang G, Carretta R, Simon G (1983) Scintigraphic evaluation of muscle damage following extreme exercise: concise communication. J Nucl Med 24: 308–311

Matsui K, Yamada H, Chiba K, Iio M (1973) Visualisation of soft tissue malignancies by using ^{99m}Tc polyphosphate, pyrophosphate and diphosphonate (^{99m}Tc-P). J Nucl Med 14: 632–633

Mazzola AL, Barker MH, Belliveau RE (1976) Accumulation of ^{99m}Tc-diphosphonate at sites of intramuscular iron therapy: case report. J Nucl Med Tech 4: 133–135

McAfee JG, Silberstein EB (1984) Non-osseous uptake. In: Silberstein EB, McAfee JG (eds) Differential diagnosis in nuclear medicine. McGraw Hill, New York, pp 300–318

McCartney W, Nusynowitz ML, Reimann BEF, Prather J, Mazat B (1976) ^{99m}Tc-diphosphonate uptake in neuroblastoma. Am J Roentgenol Radium Ther Nucl Med 126: 1077–1081

McDougall IR, Pistenma DA (1974) Concentration of ^{99m}Tc diphosphonate in breast tissue. Radiology 112: 655–657

McLaughlin AF (1975) Uptake of ^{99m}Tc bone scanning agent by lungs with metastatic calcification. J Nucl Med 16: 322–323

McRae J, Hambright P, Valk P, Bearden AJ (1976) Chemistry of ^{99m}Tc tracers. (ii) In vitro conversion of tagged HEDP and pyrophosphate (bone seekers) into gluconate (renal agent). Effects of Ca and Fe (2) on in vivo distribution. J Nucl Med 17: 208–211

Muheim G, Donath A, Rossier AB (1973) Serial scintigrams in the course of ectopic bone formation in paraplegic patients. Am J Roentgenol Radium Ther Nucl Med 118: 865–869

Neely HR, Witherspoon LR, Shuler SE (1984) Genitourinary findings incidental to bone imaging. In: Silberstein EB (ed) Bone scintigraphy. Futura, Mount Kisko, NY, pp 371–397

Nisbet AP, Maisey MN (1982) Splenic accumulation of technetium 99m methylene diphosphonate. Br J Radiol 55: 454–455

Oren VO, Uszler JM (1978) Liver metastases of oat cell carcinoma of lung detected on ^{99m}Tc-diphosphonate bone scan. Clin Nucl Med 3: 355–358

Orzel JA, Rudd TG, Nelp WB (1984) Heterotopic bone formation (myositis ossificans) and lower extremity swelling mimicking deep venous disease. J Nucl Med 25: 1105–1107

Ozarda AT, Haynie TP, Gutierrez CR (1983) Recurrent renal cell carcinoma following nephrectomy mimicking a normal kidney on bone scan. Eur J Nucl Med 8: 148–149

Park CH, Glassman LM, Thompson NL, Mata JS (1973) Reliability of renal imaging obtained incidentally in ^{99m}Tc polyphosphate bone scanning. J Nucl Med 14: 534–536

Parker JA, Jones AG, Davis MA, McIlmoyle G, Tow DE (1976) Reduced uptake of bone seeking radiopharmaceuticals related to iron excess. Clin Nucl Med 1: 267–268

Penney HF, Styles CB (1982) Fortuitous lymph node visualisation after interstitial injection of Tc-99m MDP. Clin Nucl Med 7: 84

Planchon CA, Donadieu AM, Perez R, Cousins JL (1983) Calcium heparinate induced extraosseous uptake in bone scanning. Eur J Nucl Med 8: 113–117

Podrasky AE, Stark DD, Hattner RS, Godding CA, Moss AA (1983) Radionuclide bone scanning in neuroblastoma: skeletal metastases and primary tumour localisation with ^{99m}Tc-MDP. AJR 141: 469–472

Poulose KP, Reba RC, Eckelman WC, Goodyear M (1975) Extraosseous localisation of ^{99m}Tc pyrophosphate. Br J Radiol 48: 724–726

Prakash V, Lin MS, Perkash I (1978) Detection of heterotopic calcification with ^{99m}Tc pyrophosphate in spinal cord injury patients. Clin Nucl Med 3: 167–169

Prasquier R, Taradash MR, Botvinick EH, Shames DM, Parmley WW (1977) The specificity of the diffuse pattern of cardiac uptake in myocardial infarction imaging with technetium 99m stannous pyrophosphate. Circulation 55: 61–66

Que L, Wiseman J, Hales IB (1980) Small cell carcinoma of the lung: primary site and hepatic metastases both detected on Tc-99m pyrophosphate bone scan. Clin Nucl Med 6: 260–262

Ravin CE, Hoyt TS, De Blanc H (1977) Concentration of 99m-technetium polyphosphate in fibrothorax following pneumonectomy. Radiology 122: 405–408

Reuter E, Bethge N, Matthes M, Koppenhagen K (1983) ^{99m}Tc-phosphonates for imaging of amyloid in C-cell carcinoma. Eur J Nucl Med 8: 398–400

Richards AG (1975) Metastatic calcification and bone scanning. J Nucl Med 16: 1087

Richman LS, Gumerman LW, Levine G, Sartiano GP, Boggs SS (1975) Localisation of Tc-99m polyphosphates in soft tissue malignancies. Am J Roentgenol Radium Ther Nucl Med 124: 577–582

Rosenfield N, Treves S (1974) Osseous and extraosseous uptake of fluorine-18 and technetium-99m polyphosphates in children with neuroblastoma. Radiology 111: 127–133

Rosenthal DI, Chandler HL, Azizi F, Schneider PB (1977) Uptake of bone imaging agents by diffuse pulmonary metastatic calcification. Am J Roentgenol Radium Ther Nucl Med 129: 871–874

Rosenthall L (1984) Extraskeletal localisation of radiophosphate. In: Rosenthall L, Lisbona R (eds) Skeletal imaging. Prentice-Hall, London, pp 261–290

Rosenthall L, Kaye M (1975) Technetium 99m pyrophosphate kinetics and imaging in metabolic bone disease. J Nucl Med 16: 33–39

Rossier AB, Bussat PH, Infant F et al. (1973) Current facts on para-osteo-arthropathy (POA). Paraplegia 2: 35–45

Russell RGG, Kanis JA (1984) Ectopic calcification and ossification. In: Nordin BEC (ed) Metabolic bone and stone disease. Churchill Livingstone, Edinburgh, pp 344–365

Saha GB, Herzberg DL, Boyd CM (1977) Unusual in vivo distribution of ^{99m}Tc-diphosphonate. Clin Nucl Med 2: 303–305

Sarreck R, Sham R, Alexander LL, Cortez EP (1979) Increased ^{99m}Tc-pyrophosphate uptake with radiation pneumonitis. Clin Nucl Med 4: 403–404

Schauwecker DS, Burt RW, Richmond BD (1982) Imaging of brain tumours and other lesions utilising Tc-99m phosphates and Tc-99m pertechnetate. Clin Nucl Med 7: 493–496

Schmitt GH, Holmes RA, Isitman AI, Hensley Lewis JD (1974) A proposed mechanism for ^{99m}Tc-labelled polyphosphate and diphosphonate uptake by human breast tissue. Radiology 112: 733–735

Seid K, Lin D, Flowers WM (1981) Intense myocardial uptake of Tc-99m MDP in a case of hypercalcaemia. Clin Nucl Med 6: 565–567

Serafini AN, Raskin MM, Zard LC, Watson DD (1974) Radionuclide breast scanning in carcinoma of the breast. J Nucl Med 15: 1149–1152

Sfakianakis GN, Damoulaki-Sfakianaki E, Bass JC, Earl WC, Riccobond XJ (1975) Tc-99m polyphosphate scanning in calcinosis universalis of dermatomyositis. J Nucl Med 16: 568

Sfakianakis GN, Ortiz VN, Haase GM, Boles ET (1978) Tc-99m diphosphonate abdominal imaging in necrotising enterocolitis. J Nucl Med 19: 691–692

Shen AC, Jennings RB (1972a) Myocardial calcium and magnesium in acute ischaemic injury. Am J Pathol 67: 417–440

Shen AC, Jennings RB (1972b) Kinetics of calcium accumulation in acute myocardial ischaemic injury. Am J Pathol 67:

441–452

Sherkow L, Yunryo V, Fabich D, Patel GC, Pinsky S (1984) Visualisation of the liver, gallbladder and intestine on bone scintigraphy. Clin Nucl Med 9: 440–443

Shirazi PH, Ryan WG, Fordham EW (1974) Bone scanning in evaluation of Paget's disease of bone. CRC Crit Rev Clin Radiol Nucl Med 5: 523–558

Siddiqui AR, Stokka CL (1980) Uptake of Tc-99m methylene diphosphonate in a surgical scar. Clin Nucl Med 5: 274

Siddiqui AR, Cohen M, Moran DP (1982) Enhanced differential diagnosis of abdominal masses using inferior vena cava, renal and bone imaging with single foot injection of Tc-99m methylene diphosphonate (MDP) in children. J Nucl Med 23: P7

Siegel ME, Walker WJ, Campbell JL (1975) Accumulation of ^{99m}Tc-diphosphonate in malignant pleural effusions: Detection and verification. J Nucl Med 16: 883–885

Silberstein EB (1984) Nonosseous localisation of bone seeking radiopharmaceuticals. In: Silberstein EB (ed) Bone scintigraphy. Futura, Mount Kisco, NY, pp 347–370

Silberstein EB, Bove KE (1979) Visualisation of alcohol induced rhabdomyolysis: a correlative radiotracer, histochemical, and electron microscopic study. J Nucl Med 20: 127–129

Silberstein EB, Francis MD, Tofe AJ, Slough CL (1975) Distribution of ^{99m}Tc-Sn diphosphonate and free ^{99m}Tc-pertechnetate in selected hard and soft tissues. J Nucl Med 16: 58–61

Silberstein EB, Delong S, Cline J (1984) Tc-99m diphosphonate and sulphur colloid uptake by the spleen in sickle disease: interrelationship and clinical correlates: concise communication. J Nucl Med 25: 1300–1303

Singh BN, Ryerson TW, Kesala BA, Mehta SP (1977) ^{99m}Tc-diphosphonate uptake in renal cell carcinoma. Clin Nucl Med 2: 95–99

Sone T, Fukinaga M, Otsuka N et al. (1985) Metastatic medullary thyroid cancer: localisation with iodine-131 metaiodobenzylguanidine. J Nucl Med 26: 604–608

Steinfeld JR, Thorne NA, Kennedy TF (1977) Positive ^{99m}Tc-pyrophosphonate bone scan in polymyositis. Radiology 122: 168

Stone CK, Sisson JC (1985) What causes uptake of technetium 99m methylene diphosphonate by tumours? A case where the tumour appeared to secrete a hypercalcaemia-causing substance. J Nucl Med 26: 250–253

Straub WH, Slasky BS (1982) Accumulation of bone scanning agent in a communicating renal cortical cyst. Clin Nucl Med 7: 378

Sty JR Garrett R (1977) Abnormal myocardial image with ^{99m}Tc pyrophosphate in a child on chemotherapy. Clin Nucl Med 2: 65–66

Sty JR, Starshak RJ (1982) Abnormal Tc-99m MDP renal images associated with myoglobinuria. Clin Nucl Med 7: 476

Sty JR, Babbitt DP, Kun L (1979a) Atlas of ^{99m}Tc-methylene diphosphonate renal images in paediatric oncology. Clin Nucl Med 4: 122–127

Sty JR, Babbitt DP, Casper JT, Boedecker RA (1979b) ^{99m}Tc-methylene diphosphonate imaging in neural crest tumours. Clin Nucl Med 4: 12–17

Sty JR, Babbitt DP, Sheth K (1980) Abnormal Tc-99m methylene diphosphonate accumulation in the kidneys of children with sickle cell disease. Clin Nucl Med 5: 445–447

Sty JR, Starshak RJ, Hubbard A (1982) Accumulation of Tc-99m MDP in the spleen of a battered child. Clin Nucl Med 7: 292

Sty JR, Starshak RJ, Casper JT (1983) Extraosseous accumulation of Tc-99m MDP: metastatic intracranial neuroblastoma. Clin Nucl Med 8: 26–27

Suzuki Y, Hisada K, Takeda M (1974) Demonstration of myositis ossificans by ^{99m}Tc pyrophosphate bone scanning. Radiology 111: 663–664

Sy WM, Patel D, Faunce H (1975) Significance of absent or faint kidney sign on bone scan. J Nucl Med 16: 454–456

Tanaka T, Rossier AB, Hussey RW, Ahnberg DS, Treves S (1977) Quantitative assessment of para-osteo-arthropathy and its maturation on serial radionuclide bone images. Radiology 123: 217–221

Teates CD, Brower AC, Williamson BRJ (1977) Osteosarcoma extraosseous metastases demonstrated on bone scans and radiographs. Clin Nucl Med 2: 298–302

Thrall JH, Ghaed N, Geslien GE, Pinsky SM, Johnson MC (1974) Pitfalls in Tc-99m polyphosphate skeletal imaging. Am J Roentgenol Radium Ther Nucl Med 121: 739–747

Trackler RT, Chinn RYW (1982) Amphotericin B therapy. A cause of increased renal uptake of Tc-99m MDP. Clin Nucl Med 7: 293

Valdez VA, Jacobstein JG (1980) Visualisation of a malignant pericardial effusion with Tc-99m EHDP. Clin Nucl Med 5: 210–212

Valdez VA, Bonnin JM, Martini T, Herrera NE (1978) Abnormal liver and bone scans in a case of metastatic neuroblastoma. Clin Nucl Med 3: 337–338

Van Antwerp JD, Hall JN, O'Mara RE, Schuyler VH (1975a) Bone scan abnormality produced by interaction of Tc-99m diphosphonate with iron dextran (Imferon). J Nucl Med 16: 577

Van Antwerp JD, O'Mara RE, Pitt MJ, Walsh S (1975b) Technetium 99m diphosphonate accumulation in amyloid. J Nucl Med 16: 238–240

Van Duzee BF, Deprato DW, Cavanaugh DJ et al. (1982) A multi-site clinical study of factors influencing soft tissue localisation of skeletal imaging agents in children. J Nucl Med 23: 99

Vanel D, Henry-Amar M, Lumbroso J et al. (1984) Pulmonary evaluation of patients with osteosarcoma: roles of standard radiography, tomography, CT, scintigraphy and tomoscintigraphy. AJR 143: 519–523

Vieras F (1977) Radiation induced skeletal and soft tissue bone scan changes. Clin Nucl Med 2: 93–94

Vieras F, Boyd CM (1975) Diagnostic value of renal imaging incidental to bone scintigraphy with ^{99m}Tc-phosphate compounds. J Nucl Med 16: 1109–1114

Wahner HW, Dewanjee MK (1981) Drug induced modulation of Tc-99m pyrophosphate tissue distribution: What is involved? J Nucl Med 22: 555–559

Watson NW, Cowan RJ, Maynard CD, Richards F (1977) Resolution of metastatic calcification revealed by bone scanning: case report. J Nucl Med 18: 890–892

Wenzel WW, Heasty RG (1974) Uptake of ^{99m}Tc-stannous polyphosphate in an area of cerebral infarction. J Nucl Med 15: 207–209

Wilkinson RH, Gaede JT (1979) Concentration of Tc-99m methylene diphosphonate in hepatic metastases from squamous cell carcinoma. J Nucl Med 20: 303–305

Willerson JT, Parkey RW, Bonte FJ, Meyer SL, Atkins JM, Stokely EM (1975) Technetium stannous pyrophosphate myocardial scintigrams in patients with chest pain of varying aetiology. Circulation 51: 1046–1052

Williamson BRS, Teates CD, Bray ST, Lees RF, Croft BY (1979) Renal excretion simulating bone disease on bone scans—a technique for solving the problem. Clin Nucl Med 4: 200–201

Wilson MA, Pollack MJ (1981) Gastric visualisation and image quality in radionuclide bone scanning: concise communication. J Nucl Med 22: 518–521

Wilson MA, Liss LF, Studey C (1983) Calcification of hepatic metastases. J Nucl Med 24: P85

Winter PF (1976a) Focal renal activity in bone scans. J Nucl Med 17: 429

Winter PF (1976b) Splenic accumulation of ^{99m}Tc diphosphonate. J Nucl Med 17: 850

Wistow BW, McAfee JG, Sagerman RH, Thomas FD, Grossman

ZD (1979) Renal uptake of Tc-99m methylene diphosphonate after radiation therapy. J Nucl Med 20: 32–34

Wynchank S (1982) ^{99m}Tc methylene diphosphonate lung uptake in mixed small and large cell lymphoma. Eur J Nucl Med 7: 47–48

Yood RA, Skinner M, Cohen AS, Lee VW (1981) Soft tissue uptake of bone seeking radionuclide in amyloidosis. J Rheumatol 8: 760–766

Zimmer AM, Isitman AT, Holmes RA (1975) Enzyme inhibition of diphosphonate: a proposed mechanism of tissue uptake. J Nucl Med 16: 352–356

16 · Quantitative ^{99m}Tc Diphosphonate Uptake Measurements

M. L. Smith

Introduction

The isotope bone scan, using technetium-99m (^{99m}Tc) diphosphonate, is essentially a visual display of skeletal function. ^{99m}Tc diphosphonate is adsorbed onto any metabolically active bone with an intact blood supply. Uptake of ^{99m}Tc diphosphonate is believed to be primarily related to new bone formation; however, as bone formation and resorption are coupled, this uptake reflects skeletal metabolism. Any increase in bone turnover, whether focal or diffuse, will result in an increase in ^{99m}Tc diphosphonate uptake. Thus measurement of this uptake by bone provides a sensitive and objective means of quantifying skeletal metabolism (Holmes 1978).

Quantitative measurements of radiolabelled diphosphonate uptake have been widely applied to a variety of clinical problems. They have proved most valuable in the diagnosis and follow-up of patients with diffuse metabolic bone disease (MBD) where subtle changes in bone scan images may be difficult to appreciate (Fogelman et al. 1978, 1980; Caniggia and Vattimo 1980). Although of limited value in the initial diagnosis of focal bone disease where the abnormalities are usually easily identified, sequential diphosphonate uptake measurements may have a role to play in monitoring therapeutic response (Waxman et al. 1977; LaMont et al. 1981).

There are several different techniques currently in use for quantifying diphosphonate uptake by the skeleton. These can be considered in two main categories: local bone or whole-body uptake measurements. The choice of technique depends on the clinical problem being investigated and also on available equipment and expertise. The wide variety of approaches to diphosphonate quantitation ensures that these measurements can be obtained in almost any nuclear medicine department. This chapter discusses the general factors which may influence diphosphonate uptake measurements and outlines the techniques most relevant to current clinical practice.

Factors Influencing ^{99m}Tc Diphosphonate Uptake Measurements

There are many different factors which may influence skeletal uptake of diphosphonate and which must be taken into consideration when initiating and interpreting any such measurement.

Radiopharmaceutical

There are several different diphosphonates currently available for clinical use. Each diphosphonate has a different affinity for bone which results in a varying amount of diphosphonate being taken up by the skeleton (see Chap. 4, p. 36). It is therefore mandatory to use the same diphosphonate for all comparative uptake measurements.

The preparation of the radiopharmaceutical also requires consideration. There appears to be agreement in the literature that varying the amount of technetium in the radiopharmaceutical does not influence uptake measurements (Citrin 1977; Jarritt et al. 1984). It has also been reported with both hydroxyethylidene diphosphonate (HEDP; Citrin 1977) and methylene diphosphonate (MDP; Bull et al. 1977a) that varying the amount of diphosphonate does not affect uptake measurements. However, one report has suggested that large differences in the amount of diphosphonate may result in small changes in quantitative measurements (Jarritt et al. 1984). Small day-to-day variations in the preparation of commercial kits seem unlikely to result in significant changes in the amount of diphosphonate administered, provided eluate and injection volumes are kept constant.

The most important variable in the preparation of radiopharmaceutical seems to be the incubation time of the technetium/diphosphonate compound. Longer incubation times result in increased uptake measurements (Buell 1981; Buell et al. 1982). It has been suggested that 30 min is the optimal incubation period for MDP (Henkin et al. 1980). Whichever incubation time and diphosphonate are chosen, a standardised approach to the preparation of radiopharmaceutical for uptake measurements must be adopted.

Timing of Studies

Apart from the diphosphonate used, the single most important factor affecting uptake measurements is the time after administration of radiopharmaceutical that the measurement is made. The quantitative methods described in the literature vary from measurements made immediately after injection to those at 24 h. Most quantitative work based on routine bone scans has been performed at 1–6 h after administration of diphosphonate.

Makler and Charkes (1980) found that with MDP the contrast between bone and soft tissue plateaued at 6 h. Citrin et al. (1975) found that the net uptake of HEDP in normal bone stabilised at 2 h, but tumour uptake continued to increase even at 4 h. Fogelman et al. (1979) reported that lesion/bone and bone/soft tissue ratios using MDP also continued to rise up to 4 h.

As with preparation of radiopharmaceutical, the most important factor in the timing of uptake measurements is consistency. Measurements made at different times after injection cannot be reliably compared either sequentially in the same patient or on a cross-sectional basis in a large group of patients. The earlier the measurement, the more likely is a small variation in time to produce a significant difference in the result. As abnormal bone continues to concentrate diphosphonate even at 4 h, it

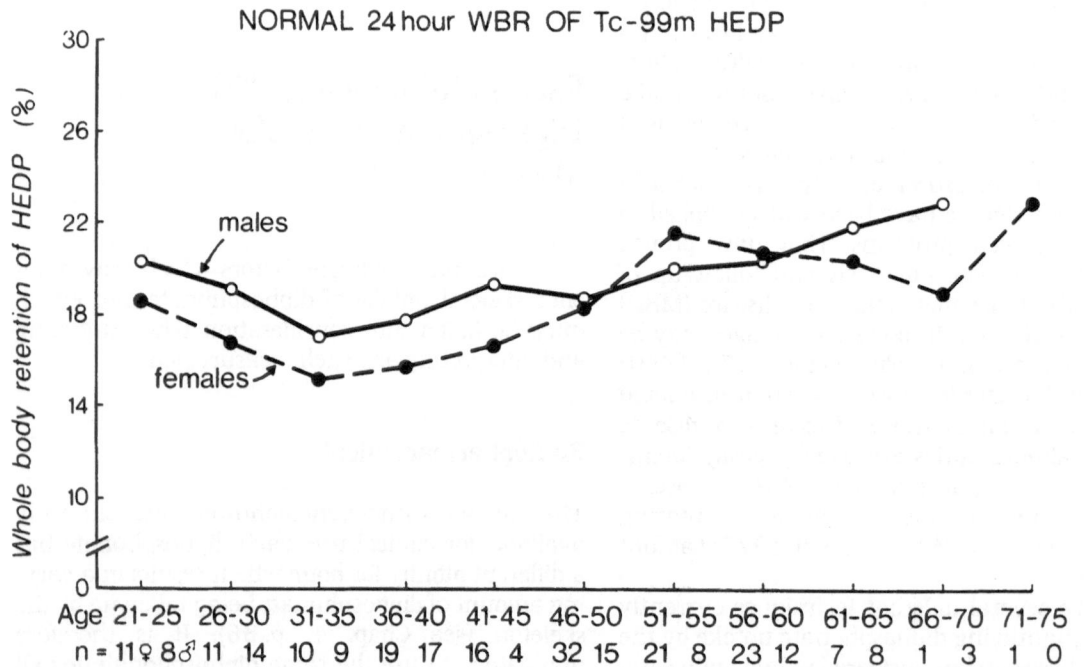

Fig. 16.1. Age- and sex-related changes in 24-h WBR of HEDP in 250 healthy volunteers. (Fogelman and Bessent 1982)

is probably best to perform uptake measurements at 4–6 h whenever this is possible.

Whole-body measurements of diphosphonate uptake are usually performed at 24 h after injection. This is an arbitrary choice, at a time when urinary excretion of diphosphonate is at a minimum and any variation in voiding pattern is unlikely to influence the results (Fogelman et al. 1978). It also ensures that the 24-h measurement can be obtained as part of the routine workload of the department. Once again standardisation of time is the most important factor.

Renal Function

As the diphosphonate not taken up by the skeleton is rapidly excreted in the urine (Citrin et al. 1975), it is clear that diphosphonate uptake measurements are influenced not only by skeletal metabolism but also by renal function. Patients with significant renal impairment will have increased uptake in soft tissue and perhaps bone, which often makes interpretation of quantitative measurements in patients with renal failure difficult. However, it has been shown that minor deterioration in renal function, as may occur in normal ageing, does not substantially affect quantitative measurements, provided the serum creatinine remains normal (Fogelman et al. 1982).

Age and Sex

It is now well established that alterations in skeletal metabolism resulting in loss of bone occur during normal ageing in both men and women. Bone loss in women is accelerated following the menopause (Eriksen et al. 1985). These normal alterations in bone turnover and the differences found between the sexes are reflected in quantitative diphosphonate uptake measurements, as shown by Fogelman and Bessent (1982) in a large study of 250 normal, healthy volunteers (Fig. 16.1). These differences in measurements with age and sex have obvious implications when establishing normal reference ranges.

Control Population

The choice of a control population depends to a large extent on the type of quantitative technique used. In some sequential studies individual patients may act as their own control and a true normal range

may not be required. However, in cross-sectional studies a normal reference range is essential.

The ideal control population would be healthy volunteers with no history of bone or renal disease. This is very difficult to achieve in practice, and normal ranges are frequently derived from patients referred for bone scan who have normal bone and renal biochemistry and who have no overt abnormality detected on the bone scan images. Care should be taken to exclude those patients being screened for secondary malignancy as there is increasing evidence that some of these patients have elevated diphosphonate uptake measurements (local and whole-body) even though their bone scans show no evidence of metastatic deposits (Bull et al. 1977a; Pfeifer et al. 1979; Buell et al. 1982; Jarritt et al. 1984). The cause and clinical relevance of this finding is as yet poorly understood; however, it does negate the use of such patients as normal controls.

When possible, control populations should be matched for age and sex to maximise both the sensitivity and specificity of diphosphonate uptake measurements in detecting altered skeletal metabolism. If this cannot be achieved, control ranges should span the whole spectrum of normal values. While this might theoretically result in slight loss of sensitivity, it would help to maintain the specificity of such measurements. It is absolutely mandatory for each department to establish their own normal ranges for each technique used to quantify skeletal uptake of diphosphonate.

Data Processing

Where several measurements are made during the course of a study and these are not acquired simultaneously, decay correction is necessary. Background correction may be required, particularly if low count rates are obtained (Fogelman et al. 1978). Correction for overlying soft tissue and attenuation is difficult and may even introduce further error into the measurement (Graham and Neil 1974). It is therefore usual to avoid any such corrections. Inter- and intra-observer variability in the processing of local uptake measurements should be established.

Methods of Quantitation

Local Measurements

Flow and Bone Clearance Measurements

Quantitation of diphosphonate uptake can commence at any time after injection of radiopharmaceutical. While most quantitative techniques measure "late" uptake of diphosphonate (i.e. more than 1 h after injection), some studies have looked at uptake during the early vascular phase (0–1 min) and early bone uptake phase (1–25 min) of the bone scan (Deutsch et al. 1981; Boudreau et al. 1983; Gandsman et al. 1983). Uptake curves over pathological bone can be obtained by dynamic data acquisition with a gamma camera interfaced to a computer. Such curves are generally compared with those obtained over a suitable control area imaged simultaneously on the same field of view.

An added dimension to quantitation of the early flow and uptake phase is the measurement of bone uptake of diphosphonate over the first 30 min after injection corrected for glomerular filtration rate measured using indium-113m (^{113m}In) diethylenetriamine pentaacetic acid (DTPA). Using this technique Schumichen et al. (1982) found increased bone clearance of diphosphonate in patients with renal osteodystrophy, but normal bone clearance rates in those patients with acute renal failure without bone disease.

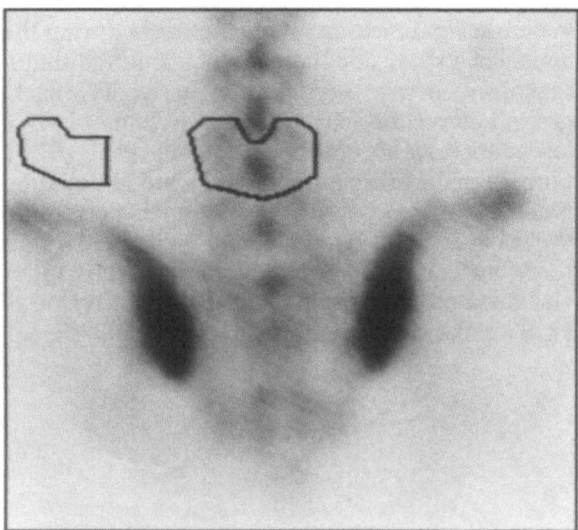

Fig. 16.2. Posterior image of lumbar spine showing ROI over bone (L–4) and soft tissue.

Another indirect method of quantifying bone clearance of diphosphonate is measurement of the plasma chromium-51(^{51}Cr)-EDTA/^{99m}Tc-MDP ratio (Nisbet et al. 1983, 1984). This relies on the assumption that ^{51}Cr-EDTA is cleared only by the kidneys, whereas ^{99m}Tc-MDP is removed from the plasma both by renal excretion and bone uptake. Thus by injecting ^{51}Cr-EDTA with MDP and measuring the ratio of the two radiopharmaceuticals in a single plasma sample an indirect measure of bone uptake can be obtained. As skeletal metabolism increases, MDP clearance from plasma increases and the ^{51}Cr-EDTA/^{99m}Tc-MDP ratio rises. This technique has the practical disadvantage of a 5-day delay before sample counting is complete. It also relies heavily on the assumption that renal handling of EDTA and MDP is identical in all circumstances; while this may be correct, it is as yet unproven and warrants further investigation.

Local Uptake Ratios

The simplest method of quantifying the uptake of diphosphonate in an area of diseased bone (the area of interest or lesion) is to express the count rate obtained in this area as a ratio of count rate in an area of comparable normal bone or soft tissue, acquired, when possible, on the same image. This use of an uptake ratio, rather than an absolute count rate, obviates any problems with differing amounts of injected activity, repositioning between different studies and changes in camera performance by using each patient as their own internal control.

Uptake ratios are now usually obtained from computerised bone scan images either by drawing a region of interest (ROI; Fig. 16.2; Rosenthall and Kaye 1975) around the area being studied or by obtaining a profile (Fig. 16.3) over it (Lentle et al. 1977). Count rates can then be obtained from the computer. Differences in area of ROI can be corrected for by expressing the count rate as mean counts per pixel.

The use of a profile rather than a ROI is probably a little more objective as the edge of the abnormal area can be more easily defined. This is of particular importance where the area of interest is small (e.g. in the hip) and may be difficult to draw (Lammer et al. 1982).

If a computer system is not readily available for all studies, similar uptake ratios can be obtained using a gamma camera/multichannel analyser system (Citrin et al. 1974), a probe counting system (Park et al. 1977) or by using a calibrated densitometer on routine scan films (Cranage 1984). While

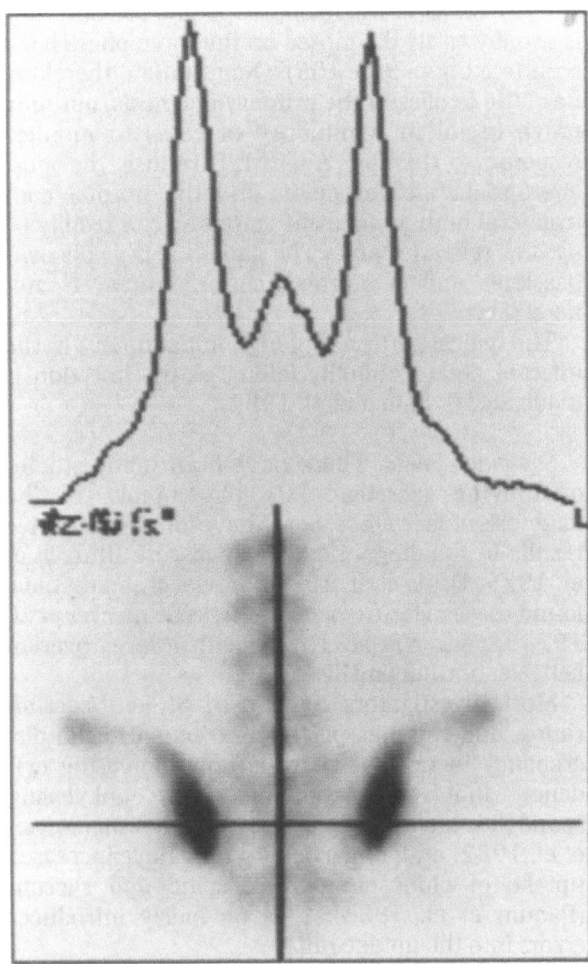

Fig. 16.3. Transverse profile through both SI joints and sacrum showing small central sacral peak flanked by higher uptake peaks of SI joints.

The ideal control region is a matched contralateral area of normal bone, or an adjacent normal vertebra if the abnormality is spinal. This technique does have two potential limitations, however. It is first of all necessary to define the abnormal area. This is easy if there are local symptoms (e.g. pain in one hip) or if the abnormality can be clearly seen on the scan, as in Paget's disease. However, in patients with metastatic disease very early lesions may not appear abnormal enough to quantify (Pitt and Sharp 1985). Measurement of L/B ratios also rely on the assumption that the "normal" bone is entirely unaffected by the disease process. This is a reasonable assumption in some instances, e.g. monostotic osteomyelitis, but is not valid in conditions such as rheumatoid arthritis or ankylosing spondylitis (Steven et al. 1982).

Bone/Soft Tissue Ratios. Several different areas in the skeleton have been used to determine bone/soft tissue (B/ST) ratios, e.g. high-uptake areas such as spine (Fogelman et al. 1981) and sacrum (Pfeifer et al. 1983) and low-uptake bone such as femur (Weigmann et al. 1977). These areas have been compared with a similar variety of soft tissues, e.g. thigh (Weigmann et al. 1977), kidney (Holmes 1978) and soft tissue below and lateral to the kidney (Fogelman et al. 1981).

B/ST ratios have been used to assess patients with MBD; however, the small area of bone chosen to represent the whole skeleton and the marked regional variations in soft tissue uptake caused by differences in bulk and vascularity both contribute to the marked overlap with normal seen in these patients (Fogelman et al. 1981). B/ST ratios are therefore of limited value in the investigation of MBD.

B/ST ratios have been used with rather more success in the detection of patients with specific malignancies. Pfeifer et al. (1983) found these measurements useful in detecting patients with haematological malignancies who had diffuse bone (or bone marrow) involvement. Constable and Cranage (1980) have also used B/ST ratios to confirm the presence of prostatic superscans.

Percentage Uptake Measurements

Local uptake ratios rely on an arbitrary choice of control area either in bone or soft tissue. As discussed already, this may be associated with potential errors, which can be avoided by referring uptake of diphosphonate in the area of interest to the administered dose (Hardy et al. 1980) or to the activity of a known external standard (Meindok et al. 1985).

the densitometer method is less reproducible than conventional ROI measurements, it has been suggested that it is adequate in most clinical situations.

Lesion Bone Ratios. In lesion/bone (L/B) ratios the term "lesion" denotes any focal area of bone which is considered to be potentially abnormal and "bone" denotes a suitable area of normal bone. L/B ratios have been extensively used to diagnose and, more commonly, monitor focal skeletal abnormality. They are easy to obtain and facilitate detection of small, but significant, changes in uptake (less than 20%) which may not be appreciated visually (Condon et al. 1981). Quantitation of rib lesions is difficult; however, the variability of L/B ratio measurements in other parts of the skeleton has been reported as less than 10% (Condon et al. 1981; Vellenga et al. 1984).

Lurye et al. (1977) determined uptake in multiple ROI as a percentage of administered activity and then displayed this visually as an Organ Uptake Image (OUI). Jarritt et al. (1984) have introduced a new technique using single photon emission computed tomography (SPECT) in which they measure uptake of MDP in the skull. They have found that this measurement is elevated in patients with MBD and patients with primary malignancy without skeletal secondaries. Although further studies would be required to establish the clinical value of this technique, it is likely that the specialised equipment necessary for this measurement will limit its application.

Where a gamma camera is not freely available to quantify diphosphonate uptake, a probe counter may be used to obtain percentage uptake measurements.

Clinical Use of Local Uptake Measurements

Avascular Necrosis. The three-phase bone scan is important in the early diagnosis of avascular necrosis in both children and adults (see Chap. 12, p. 157). Where the disease is unilateral or a well-defined "cold spot" is present in the affected femoral head the diagnosis can be made from scan images alone. However, in a small percentage of cases the disease may be bilateral, even though only one hip is symptomatic. In these cases the scan abnormality may be symmetrical and may be difficult to appreciate visually. In such cases quantitation of diphosphonate uptake in the femoral head on both flow and static phases may be valuable. At present the most suitable method of quantitation is L/B ratio. The difficulty lies in the choice of control area. Some workers have used the contralateral "normal" hip; however, in bilateral disease this may prove misleading. Others have chosen the femoral shaft (Dowsett et al. 1976; Conklin et al. 1983) or a vertebra (Cabarello-Carpena and Pardo-Montaner 1983). The best compromise is probably the ipsilateral femoral shaft as it can be easily included in the field of view and is unlikely to be significantly affected by alterations in weight bearing. Percentage uptake measurements may be useful in this condition and merit investigation.

If femoral head uptake measurements are being used for diagnostic purposes then an age-matched control population is necessary. However, when these measurements are used to monitor the progress of the disease the patient's baseline measurement will act as reference value, and a normal control range becomes less important.

Infection. After the neonatal period, osteomyelitis is usually easily diagnosed on the three-phase bone scan (see Chap. 9, p. 105). Quantitation, therefore, has little to offer in the primary diagnosis, but may prove useful in a minority of cases to monitor response to therapy. Again L/B ratio is the most appropriate measurement, and the normal contralateral limb or adjacent vertebrae can readily be used as reference area. The patient acts as his own baseline, and a normal control range is not necessary.

The typical pattern is of high initial uptake in the infected area, gradually falling as the infection is eradicated (Lammer et al. 1982).

Sacroiliac Joints. There have been many studies quantifying sacroiliac (SI) joint uptake in the diagnosis of sacroiliitis. Some have found favourable results in the diagnosis of early disease (Russell et al. 1975; Davis et al. 1984); however, many have found these measurements useless (Dequecker et al. 1978; Spencer et al. 1979), with a large overlap between normal and disease.

Most investigators have used SI joint/sacrum ratios, and this has partly contributed to the discrepancy in results. There is now increasing evidence that some patients with ankylosing spondylitis have altered skeletal metabolism (Steven et al. 1982) and, in particular, may have increased uptake of diphosphonate in spine and sacrum (Paquin et al. 1983). This obviously introduces errors into the uptake ratio.

Several workers have also found changes in SI joint/sacrum ratios with age (Agnew et al. 1982), with a difference between the sexes (Vyas et al. 1981). Thus differences in control populations in the various studies may also have contributed to the divergent results. The large overlap in SI joint/sacrum ratios between normal controls and patients with sacroiliitis has limited the clinical usefulness of such measurements. Percentage uptake measurements over the SI joints, with an age- and sex-matched control group might help to minimise the problems previously encountered.

Rheumatoid Arthritis. Joint uptake measurements have little place in the day-to-day management of patients with rheumatoid arthritis (RA) but have been used in research as an objective means of assessing joint inflammation. As diffuse changes in skeletal metabolism can also occur in RA, joint/bone ratios are inaccurate. Rosenspire et al. (1980) assessed four different methods of joint uptake quantitation and found that count rate per unit area in the joint normalised for dose of radiopharmaceutical and body weight was the measurement most likely to reflect disease activity. Fogelman and Bessent (1982) did not find any significant correlation between whole-body uptake measurements and weight. Thus correction for weight may not be necessary in joint uptake measurements; this requires further investigation.

Fracture and Graft Healing. There is some debate in the literature about the value of quantitative diphosphonate uptake measurements in evaluating fracture healing. Although O'Reilly et al. (1981) did not find these measurements useful in predicting delayed or non-union, Lund et al. (1978) and Jacobs et al. (1979) reported early detection of these complications by quantifying diphosphonate uptake.

Perhaps the most promising method of fracture quantitation is that described by Jacobs et al. (1979), who dissociated the vascular response to injury from bone healing by considering dynamic uptake in the 15 min following injection in two parts: 0–7.5 min and 7.5–15 min. Using the uptake ratio of fracture site to a control area in the same bone they found that normal healing resulted in an increase in bone uptake of 3% per month, delayed union 1.4% per month and non-union 0%.

Bone graft viability and healing can be assessed in a similar manner (Jacobs et al. 1979) or can be studied with a longitudinal profile through the graft. Where a large area of bone has been inserted, two peaks will be present on the profile at the graft–host junction which gradually coalesce as healing takes place (Stevenson et al. 1984).

Metastatic Disease. Quantitative diphosphonate uptake measurements have a limited place in the management of patients with malignant disease. B/ST ratios may improve the diagnostic accuracy of bone scans in patients suspected of having diffuse tumour infiltration in the skeleton (Constable and Cranage 1980; Pfeifer et al. 1983). However, in the majority of patients, metastatic deposits are multifocal and quantitation does not add to the diagnosis. The development of new lesions on sequential studies is the most important prognostic feature, and in such circumstances quantitation of pre-existing lesions is of little clinical relevance.

Diphosphonate uptake measurements have recently been used to try to differentiate between metastatic and degenerative spinal lesions in patients with malignancy. Israel et al. (1985) measured L/B uptake at 4 and 24 h and found that the 24/4-h ratio of these measurements was lower in patients with degenerative disease or treated metastases than in those patients with untreated secondary deposits. This interesting approach to quantitation merits further investigation.

Paget's Disease. Paget's disease is readily detected on routine bone scan images, and quantitative uptake measurements (flow and/or L/B ratios) have no diagnostic value. However, these measurements will provide a subjective index of disease activity and may be used on a sequential basis to assess response to therapy (Serafini et al. 1973; Espinasse et al. 1981; Vellenga et al. 1984).

Renal Osteodystrophy. Patients with chronic renal failure may have renal osteodystrophy, which results in increased bone turnover and increased skeletal uptake of diphosphonate. If the bone disease is severe, metabolic features are usually seen on routine bone scan images (see Chap. 7, p. 74). However, in the early stages, a mild increase in diphosphonate uptake may be difficult to appreciate visually, and a reliable method of quantifying this would be of value. Unfortunately, impaired renal excretion of diphosphonate results in high soft tissue retention in these patients, which makes interpretation of local bone uptake measurements difficult. Haemodialysis between administration of diphosphonate and scanning will help to reduce this, but may not normalise it completely. Thus B/ST ratios may be unreliable, and a percentage uptake measurement, either local (Hodson et al. 1981) or representative of total skeletal uptake (deGraaf et al. 1984), is more appropriate. An alternative method of quantifying bone uptake in these patients is measurement of early bone clearance of diphosphonate, corrected for glomerular filtration rate (Schumichen et al. 1982).

Clinical Comparison of ^{99m}Tc Diphosphonates. Many quantitative studies using both local (B/ST, L/B ratios) and whole-body uptake measurements have been performed to assess the relative merits of different diphosphonates in clinical practice. These have been discussed in Chapter 4.

Whole-body Measurements

Patients with MBD, in whom bone turnover is diffusely increased, often present a diagnostic problem on bone scanning. In severe disease skeletal uptake of diphosphonate is greatly increased and characteristic metabolic features may be seen on scan images. These may be associated with focal abnormalities, such as pseudofractures in osteomalacia, which also help to establish the correct diagnosis (see Chap. 7, p. 79). However, many patients with MBD have only mild to moderate increase in tracer uptake and this can be very difficult to appreciate visually. Quantitative diphosphonate uptake measurements thus have a potentially valuable role in the investigation of such patients.

Local uptake measurements have proved disappointing in reliably detecting patients with MBD (Fogelman et al. 1981). As skeletal abnormality in these patients is diffuse, a measurement of total skeletal uptake of diphosphonate is likely to be a more sensitive means of diagnosing MBD. As with local uptake measurements, there is more than one approach to quantitation of total skeletal uptake of diphosphonate.

Whole-body Bone Scan Quantitation

Computerised bone scan images can be analysed by drawing ROI around all the bones in the skeleton, summing the counts in these regions and presenting this sum as a percentage of the total counts obtained in the study. This is extremely time consuming and has no place in routine clinical practice. A slightly less time-consuming alternative is measurement of the Total Skeletal Activity Index (deGraaf et al. 1982) in which uptake of diphosphonate in a representative selection of ROI is measured and normalised for administered dose.

An easier method of evaluating total bone uptake of diphosphonate from a computerised bone scan is the contrast enhancement technique described by Smith et al. (1983). Each bone scan image is subjected to contrast enhancement until the bones (the "hot" areas) are above the upper display threshold (Fig. 16.4). The counts in these areas can then be obtained. Any areas of overlap or high soft tissue activity (such as kidneys and bladder) can be excluded using conventional ROI. By summing the bone counts and then the total counts for each view the percentage uptake in bone can be obtained.

Whole-body Retention of ^{99m}Tc Diphosphonate

The techniques described above are primarily of use as research tools. However, they are, too time consuming for routine clinical use. An alternative, more objective and much simpler method of quantifying total skeletal uptake of diphosphonate is measurement of the 24-h whole-body retention (WBR) of diphosphonate. This involves injecting a small amount of ^{99m}Tc diphosphonate (50 μCi; 1.85 MBq) and measuring 5-min and 24-h whole-body counts using a standard shadow-shield whole-body monitor (Fogelman et al. 1978). The percentage of diphosphonate retained in the body at 24 h can then readily be calculated after correcting for background activity and decay.

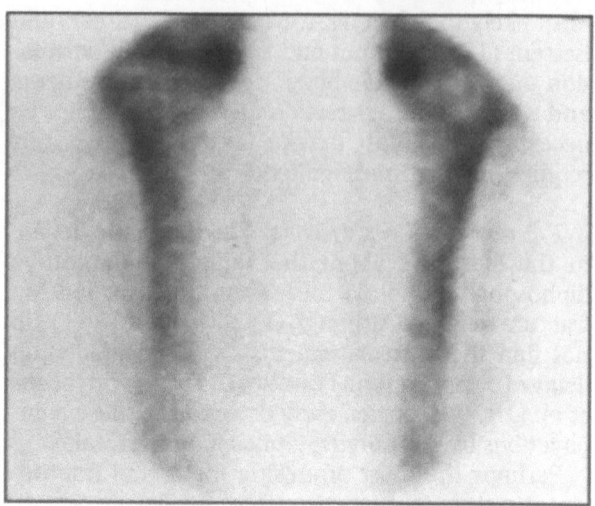

a

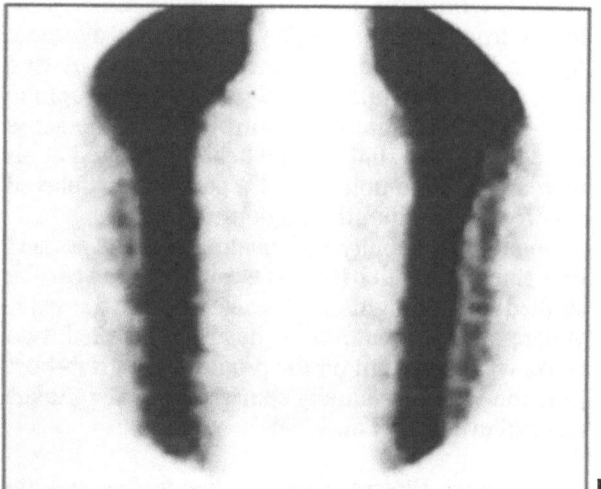

b

Fig. 16.4. a 4-h view of tibiae, before contrast enhancement; b 4-h view of tibiae, after contrast enhancement.

As the name implies, WBR measurements are a composite of both skeletal and soft tissue retention of diphosphonate. Although the soft tissue component is significant, it remains stable over a wide range of WBR measurements, and thus WBR does provide a reliable measure of osseous uptake of diphosphonate and can be used as a quantitative index of skeletal metabolism (Smith et al. 1983).

WBR measurements have been extensively investigated and have been found to be reproducible, with a standard deviation of only 1.2%. Results are unaffected by minor changes in positioning or small focal collections of diphosphonate (as found in fractures etc; Fogelman et al. 1982). However, WBR is only valid as an index of skeletal metabolism if the serum creatinine is normal (Fogelman and Bessent 1982) and therefore has no place in the investigation of patients in renal failure suspected of having renal osteodystrophy.

24 hr - WBR
99mTc - HEDP

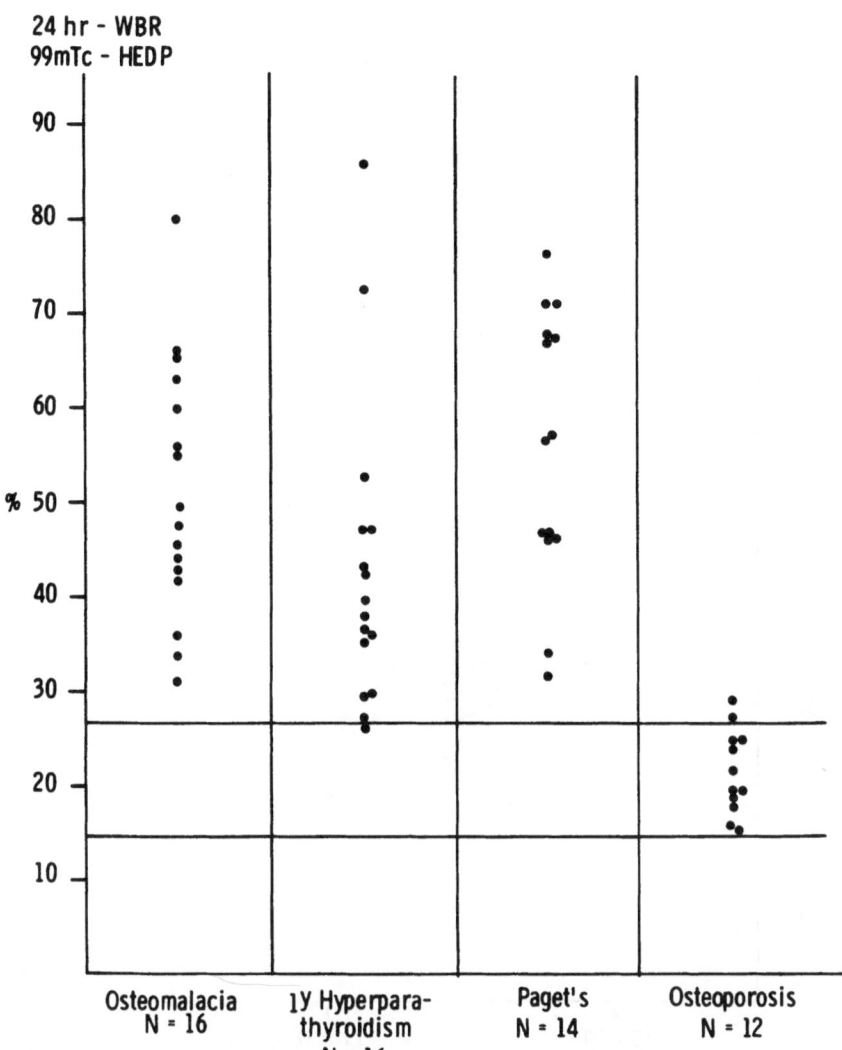

Fig. 16.5. 24-h WBR of HEDP in patients with MBD and Paget's disease. Normal range (Fogelman and Bessent 1982) indicated by horizontal lines.

An elevated WBR is diagnostic of accelerated bone turnover; however, it is non-specific and is found in osteomalacia, polyostotic Paget's disease and the majority of patients with primary hyperparathyroidism (Fogelman et al. 1977; Fogelman et al. 1978, Vattimo et al. 1981). Most osteoporotic patients will have a normal WBR, but a small percentage will have "high turnover" osteoporosis and this will be reflected by an elevated WBR (Fig. 16.5). It has been suggested that a normal WBR can be used to exclude a metabolic bone disorder such as osteomalacia (Fogelman 1980).

WBR can be used to assess the severity of skeletal involvement in patients with primary hyperparathyroidism (Fogelman et al. 1980). This may be important in patients undergoing parathyroidectomy, as those with severe bone disease often develop postoperative hypocalcaemia. WBR measurements may help to identify those patients at risk of this complication who would benefit from prophylactic preoperative vitamin D therapy. Sequential WBR measurements can be used following parathyroidectomy to monitor skeletal recovery (Fig. 16.6).

WBR has also been used to monitor response to therapy in patients with Paget's disease (Smith et al. 1984). In this situation sequential WBR measurements provide a simpler and more objective assessment of disease activity than local uptake measurements such as L/B ratio.

Much of the work done on WBR has used a shadow-shield whole-body monitor. This is a specialised piece of equipment which is not widely available. Because of this, other methods of quantifying WBR have been developed. As the diphosphonate that is not retained in the body is excreted in the urine, a 24-h urine collection following administration of ^{99m}Tc diphosphonate can be col-

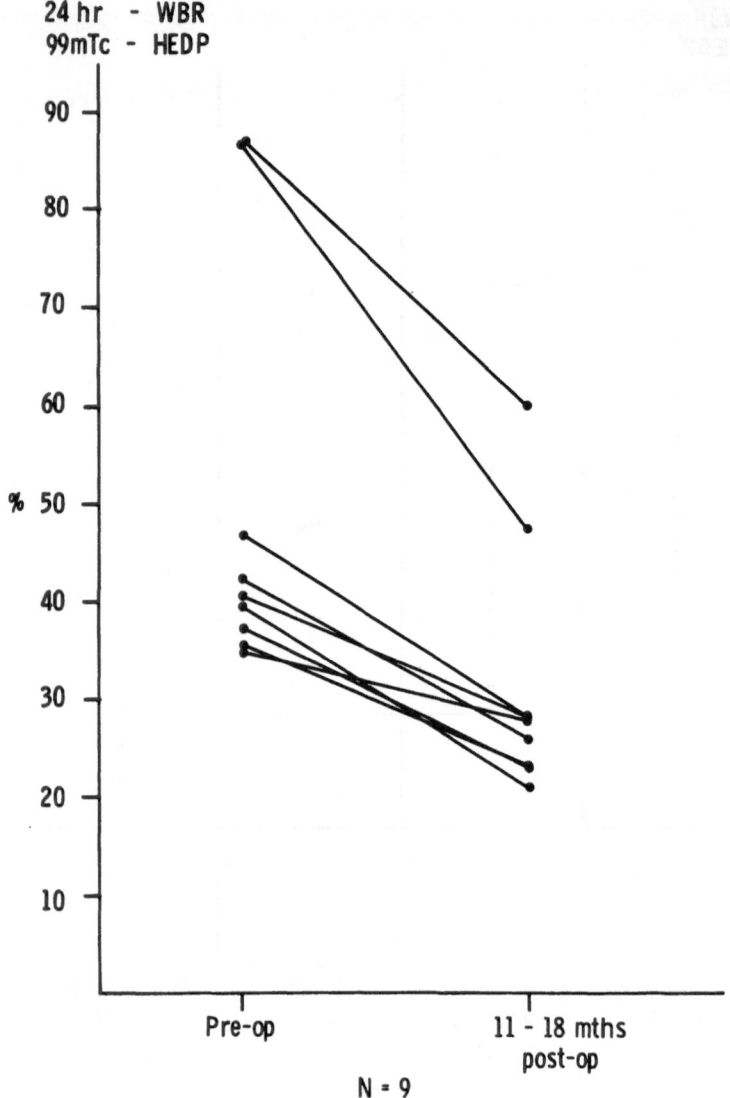

24 hr - WBR
99mTc - HEDP

Fig. 16.6. 24-h WBR of HEDP before and 11–18 months after parathyroidectomy in nine patients with primary hyperparathyroidism.

lected and counted against a standard to determine the percentage of administered dose excreted in the urine (Vattimo et al. 1981). An accurate WBR measurement thus relies on a complete urine collection which can sometimes be difficult to obtain, particularly in elderly or confused patients.

WBR can also be measured using either a gamma camera with a fishtail collimator (Martin et al. 1981) or an ordinary probe counter (Rosenthall and Arzoumanian 1983; Lang and Bull 1984). Both of these techniques require higher doses of technetium than is used with a whole-body monitor and can be effectively combined with a routine bone scan. As with any quantitative diphosphonate uptake measurement, normal control ranges must be established using the same equipment as for patient studies.

Summary

Quantitation of ^{99m}Tc diphosphonate uptake by bone provides a sensitive measurement of skeletal metabolism. Such measurements can be used to investigate and monitor both focal osseous abnormality and diffuse skeletal disease. Many different methods of quantitation are available, and the choice of technique depends to a large extent on the clinical problem being studied:

Local measurements. At present the most useful method of quantifying routine bone scans is measurement of L/B ratios using either a profile or ROI technique. This is of particular value in patients with avascular necrosis and is also useful in assessing fracture and bone graft healing. Current quantitative techniques have only a limited role in the diagnosis of sacroiliitis and in the routine management of patients with metastatic disease or rheumatoid arthritis.

Whole-body measurements. Measurement of 24-h WBR of diphosphonate is a sensitive index of overall bone turnover and is a useful means of detecting and monitoring patients with diffuse MBD.

Quantitation of diphosphonate uptake, whether local or whole body, provides a measure of skeletal metabolism which is often unobtainable by any other means. It adds a new dimension to conventional bone scanning and is within the scope of any nuclear medicine department.

References

Agnew JE, Pocock DG, Jewell DP (1982) Sacroiliac joint uptake ratios in inflammatory bowel disease: relationship to back pain and to activity of bowel disease. Br J Radiol 55: 821–826

Boudreau RJ, Lisbona R, Hadjipavlou A (1983) Observations on serial radionuclide blood-flow studies in Paget's disease: concise communication. J Nucl Med 24: 880–885

Buell U (1981) Tc99m methylene diphosphonate (MDP) bone imaging: optimum normal bone scan by optimum time delay? J Nucl Med 22: 95–96

Buell U, Zorn-Bopp E, Reuschel W, Muenzing W, Moser EA, Seiderer M (1982) A comparison of bone imaging with Tc-99m DPD and Tc-99m MDP: concise communication. J Nucl Med 23: 214–217

Bull U, Pfeifer JP, Niendorf HP, Togendorff J (1977a) A computer assisted comparison of ⁹⁹ᵐTc-methylene diphosphonate and ⁹⁹ᵐTc-pyrophosphate bone imaging. Br J Radiol 50: 629–636

Bull U, Schuster H, Pfeifer JP, Tongendorff J, Niendorf HP (1977b) Bone-to-bone, joint-to-bone and joint-to-joint ratios in normal and diseased skeletal states using region-of-interest technique and bone-seeking radiopharmaceuticals. Nuklearmedizin 16: 104–112

Cabarello-Carpena O, Pardo-Montaner J (1983) Contribution to the diagnosis of idiopathic femoral head necrosis by scintigraphy with ⁹⁹ᵐTc-MDP assessed quantitatively by computer. Nuklearmedizin 22: 232–236

Caniggia A, Vattimo A (1980) Kinetics of 99m technetium-tin-methylene diphosphonate in normal subjects and pathological conditions: a simple index of bone metabolism. Calcif Tissue Int 30: 5–13

Citrin DL (1977) An evaluation of the in vivo properties of ⁹⁹ᵐTc-HEDP. Radiology 122: 255–258

Citrin DL, Bessent RG, Tuohy JB, Greig WR, Blumgart LH (1974) Quantitative bone scanning: a method for assessing response of bone metastases to treatment. Lancet I: 1132–1133

Citrin DL, Bessent RG, McGinlay E, Gordon D (1975) Dynamic studies with ⁹⁹ᵐTc-HEDP in normal subjects and in patients with bone tumours. J Nucl Med 16: 886–890

Condon BR, Buchanan R, Garvie NW et al. (1981) Assessment of progression of secondary bone lesions following cancer of the breast or prostate using serial radionuclide imaging. Br J Radiol 54: 18–23

Conklin JJ, Alderson PO, Zizic TM et al. (1983) Comparison of bone scan and radiograph sensitivity in the detection of steroid-induced ischaemic necrosis of bone. Radiology 147: 221–226

Constable AR, Cranage RW (1980) Recognition of the superscan in prostatic bone scintigraphy. Br J Radiol 54: 122–125

Cranage RW (1984) A film densitometer method of bone scan quantitation. Br J Radiol 57: 831–832

Davis MC, Turner DA, Charters JR, Golden HE, Ali A, Fordham EW (1984) Quantitative sacroiliac scintigraphy. The effect of method of selection of region of interest. Clin Nucl Med 9: 334–340

deGraaf P, te Velde J, Pauwels EKJ, Schicht IM, Kleiverda K, deGraaf J (1982) Increased bone radiotracer uptake in renal osteodystrophy: clinical evidence of hyperparathyroidism as the major cause. Eur J Nucl Med 7: 152–154

deGraaf P, Pauwels EKJ, Vos PH, Schicht IM, te Velde J, deGraaf J (1984) Observations on computerized quantitative bone scintigraphy in renal osteodystrophy. Eur J Nucl Med 9: 419–425

Dequeker J, Goddeeris J, Walravens M, De Roo M (1978) Evaluation of sacroiliitis: comparison of radiological and radionuclide techniques. Radiology 128: 687–689

Deutsch SD, Gandsman EJ, Spraragen SC (1981) Quantitative regional blood flow analysis and its clinical application during routine bone-scanning. J Bone Joint Surg [Am] 63: 295–305

Dowsett DJ, Short MD, Morley TR (1976) A quantitative assessment of femoral head activity using Tc-99m-polyphosphate and a computer data collection system. Br J Radiol 49: 540–546

Eriksen EF, Mosekilde L, Melsen F (1985) Trabecular bone resorption depth decreases with age: differences between normal males and females. Bone 6: 141–146

Espinasse D, Mathieu L, Alexandre C, Chapuy MC, Meunier PJ, Berger M (1981) The kinetics of Tc99m labelled EHDP in Paget's disease before and after dichloromethylene-diphosphonate treatment. Metab Bone Dis Relat Res 2: 321–324

Fogelman I (1980) The value of 24 hour skeletal uptake of diphosphonate in the exclusion of metabolic bone disease. Nucl Med Comm 1: 351–356

Fogelman I, Bessent RG (1982) Age-related alterations in skeletal metabolism—24 hour whole-body retention of diphosphonate in 250 normal subjects: concise communication. J Nucl Med 23: 296–300

Fogelman I, Greig WR, Bessent RG, Boyle IT (1977) Skeletal uptake of Tc99m HEDP in primary hyperparathyroidism. J Nucl Med 18: 1040–1041

Fogelman I, Bessent RG, Turner JG, Citrin DL, Boyle IT, Greig WR (1978) The use of whole-body retention of Tc99m diphosphonate in the diagnosis of metabolic bone disease. J Nucl Med 19: 270–275

Fogelman I, Citrin DL, McKillop JH, Turner JG, Bessent RG, Greig WR (1979) A clinical comparison of Tc99m HEDP and Tc99m MDP in the detection of bone metastases: concise communication. J Nucl Med 20: 98–101

Fogelman I, Bessent RG, Beastall G, Boyle IT (1980) Estimation of skeletal involvement in primary hyperparathyroidism. Ann Intern Med 92: 65–67

Fogelman I, Bessent RG, Gordon D (1981) A critical assessment of bone scan quantitation (bone to soft tissue ratios) in the diagnosis of metabolic bone disease. Eur J Nucl Med 6: 93–97

Fogelman I, Bessent RG, Scullion JE, Cuthbert GF (1982) Accuracy of 24 hour whole-body (skeletal) retention of diphosphonate measurements. Eur J Nucl Med 7: 359–363

Gandsman EJ, Deutsch SD, Tyson IB (1983) Atlas of computerized blood flow analysis in bone disease. Clin Nucl Med 8: 558–563

Graham LS, Neil R (1974) In vivo quantitation of radioactivity using the Anger camera. Radiology 112: 441–442

Hardy JG, Kulatilake AE, Wastie ML (1980) An index for monitoring bone metastases from carcinoma of the prostate. Br J Radiol 53: 869–873

Henkin RE, Woodruff A, Chang W, Green AM (1980) The effect of radiopharmaceutical incubation time on bone scan quality. Radiology 135: 463–466

Hodson EM, Howman-Giles RB, Evans RA et al. (1981) The diagnosis of renal osteodystrophy: a comparison of technetium-99m-pyrophosphate bone scintigraphy with other techniques. Clin Nephrol 16: 24–28

Holmes RA (1978) Quantification of skeletal Tc-99m labelled phosphates to detect metabolic bone disease. J Nucl Med 19: 330–331

Israel O, Front D, Frenkel A, Kleinhaus U (1985) 24 hour/4 hour ratio of technetium-99m methylene diphosphonate uptake in patients with bone metastases and degenerative bone changes. J Nucl Med 26: 237–240

Jacobs RR, Jackson RP, Preston DF, Williamson JA, Gallagher J (1979) Dynamic bone scanning in fractures. Injury 12: 455–459

Jarritt PH, Cullum ID, Lui D, Ell PJ (1984) The measurement of absolute MDP concentration in the skull. The skull uptake test. In: Hofer R, Bergmann H (eds) Proceedings of international symposium: Radioaktive Isotope in Klinik und Forschung. Egermann, Vienna, pp 121–126

Lammer J, Nicoletti R, Fueger GF, Fink W (1982) Osteoscintimetry—a method of semiquantitative evaluation of skeletal scintigrams by use of profiles and macrofunction for computer processing. Eur J Nucl Med 7: 364–369

LaMont RL, Muz J, Heilbronner D, Bouwhuis JA (1981) Quantitative assessment of femoral head involvement in Legg–Calvé–Perthes disease. J Bone Joint Surg [Am] 63: 746–752

Lang P, Bull U (1984) Measurement of 24 hour whole body retention of Tc99m diphosphonate by a single thyroid probe. Nucl Med Comm 5: 627–632

Lentle BC, Russell AS, Percy JS, Jackson FI (1977) The scintigraphic investigation of sacro-iliac disease. J Nucl Med 18: 529–533

Lund B, Lund JO, Soerensen OH, Lund B (1978) Evaluation of fracture healing in man by serial ^{99m}Tc-Sn-pyrophosphate scintimetry. Acta Orthop Scand 49: 435–439

Lurye DR, Castronovo FP, Potsaid MS (1977) An improved method for quantitative bone scanning. J Nucl Med 18: 1069–1073

Makler PT, Charkes ND (1980) Studies of skeletal tracer kinetics IV. Optimum time delay for Tc-99m (Sn) methylene diphosphonate bone imaging. J Nucl Med 21: 641–645

Martin W, Fogelman I, Bessent RG (1981) Measurement of 24 hour whole-body retention of Tc-99m HEDP by a gamma camera. J Nucl Med 22: 542–545

Meindok H, Rapoport A, Oreopoulos DG, Rabinovich S, Meema HE, Meema S (1985) Quantitative radionuclide scanning in metabolic bone disease. Nucl Med Comm 6: 141–148

Nisbet AP, Mashiter G, Winn P, Hilson AJW, Maisey MN (1983) Quantitation of ^{99m}Tc MDP retention during routine bone scanning. Nucl Med Comm 4: 67–71

Nisbet AP, Edwards S, Lazarus CR et al. (1984) Chromium 51 EDTA/technetium 99m MDP plasma ratio to measure total skeletal function. Br J Radiol 57: 677–680

O'Reilly RJ, Cook DJ, Gaffney RD, Angel KR, Paterson DC (1981) Can serial scintigraphic studies detect delayed fracture union in man? Clin Orthop 160: 227–232

Paquin J, Rosenthall L, Esdaile J, Warshawski R, Damtew B (1983) Elevated uptake of 99m technetium methylene diphosphonate in the axial skeleton in ankylosing spondylitis and Reiter's disease: implications for quantitative sacroiliac scintigraphy. Arthritis Rheum 26: 217–226

Park HM, Terman SA, Ridolfo AS, Wellman HN (1977) A quantitative evaluation of rheumatoid arthritis activity with Tc-99m HEDP. J Nucl Med 18: 973–976

Pfeifer JP, Pfeifer H (1979) Quantitative assessment of ^{99m}Tc–MDP scans in the investigation of diffuse alterations in bone. Eur J Nucl Med 4: 407–412

Pfeifer JP, Hill W, Bull U, Burkhardt R, Kirsch CM (1983) Improvement of bone scintigraphy by quantitative evaluation compared with X-ray studies and iliac crest biopsy in malignant disease. Eur J Nucl Med 8: 342–345

Pitt WR, Sharp PF (1985) Comparison of quantitative and visual detection of new focal bone lesions. J Nucl Med 26: 230–236

Rosenspire KL, Kennedy AC, Russomanno L, Steinback J, Blau M, Green FA (1980) Comparison of four methods of analysis of ^{99m}Tc pyrophosphate uptake in rheumatoid arthritis joints. J Rheumatol 7: 461–468

Rosenthall L, Arzoumanian A (1983) Total body retention measurements of Tc-99m MDP using a simple detector. Clin Nucl Med 8: 210–213

Rosenthall L, Kaye M (1975) Technetium 99m pyrophosphate kinetics and imaging in metabolic bone disease. J Nucl Med 16: 33–39

Russell AS, Lentle BD, Percy JS (1975) Investigations of sacroiliac joint: comparative evaluation of radiological and radionuclide techniques. J Rheumatol 2: 45–51

Serafini A, Altman R, Sankey R, Coble C, Miale A (1973) Paget's disease: a method of evaluation of response to therapy using the Anger scintillation camera on-line to a computer. J Nucl Med 14: 449

Schumichen C, Fegert J, Gaede J, Straub E (1982) Improved diagnosis of renal osteodystrophy (ia) by the use of Tc99m MDP bone clearance. J Nucl Med 23: P50

Smith ML, Martin W, Fogelman I, Bessent RG (1983) Relative distribution of diphosphonate between bone and soft tissue at 4 and 24 hours: concise communication. J Nucl Med 24: 208–211

Smith ML, Fogelman I, Raston S, Boyce BF, Boyle IT (1984) Correlation of skeletal uptake of ^{99m}Tc-diphosphonate and alkaline phosphatase before and after oral diphosphonate therapy in Paget's disease. Metab Bone Dis Relat Res 5: 167–170

Spencer DG, Adams FG, Horton PW, Buchanan WW (1979) Scintiscanning in ankylosing spondylitis: a clinical, radiological and quantitative radioisotopic study. J Rheumatol 6: 426–431

Steven MM, Sturrock RD, Fogelman I, Smith ML (1982) Whole body retention of diphosphonate in rheumatoid arthritis. J Rheumatol 9: 873–877

Stevenson JS, Bright RW, Dunson GL, Nelson FR (1974) Technetium-99m phosphate bone imaging: a method of assessing bone graft healing. Radiology 110: 391–394

Vattimo A, Cantalupi D, Righi G, Martini G, Nuti R, Turchetti V (1981) Whole-body retention of Tc99m–MDP in Paget's disease. J Nucl Med Allied Sci 25: 5–10

Vellenga CJLR, Pauwels EKJ, Bijvoet OLM (1984) Comparison between visual assessment and quantitative measurement of radioactivity on the bone scintigram in Paget's disease of bone. Eur J Nucl Med 9: 533–537

Vyas K, Eklem M, Seto H et al. (1981) Quantitative scintigraphy of sacroiliac joints: effect of age, gender and laterality. AJR 136: 589–592

Waxman AD, Ducker S, McKee D, Siemsen JK, Singer FR (1977) Evaluation of Tc99m diphosphonate kinetics and bone scans in patients with Paget's disease before and after calcitonin treatment. Radiology 125: 761–764

Weigmann T, Rosenthall L, Kaye M (1977) Technetium-99m-pyrophosphate bone scans in hyperparathyroidism. J Nucl Med 18: 231–235

17 · Measurements of Bone Mineral by Photon Absorptiometry

H. W. Wahner

Introduction

The recognition of the socioeconomic impact of osteoporosis in our ageing population, with its associated morbidity and mortality from spinal, hip and radius fractures, has led to an increasing interest in bone mass and its measurement. As a result, several clinically tested methods are now available for diagnosing low bone mass, measuring the rate of bone loss and estimating the risk of fracture at specific skeletal sites.

Clinical Relevance of Bone Mass

In both sexes, maximal bone mass is reached sometime during the third decade, perhaps some years later in the cortical bone of the appendicular skeleton than in the trabecular bone of the axial skeleton. Because of physiological bone loss with age, the peak bone mass achieved is the single most important factor that determines how much bone can be lost before a critically low bone mass is reached and fracture occurs. The factors that determine peak bone mass result from genetic, mechanical, nutritional and hormonal forces. Heaney (1983) has stated that bone mass at any time after the age of 40 years is the result of the peak bone mass, the average remodelling balance of bone, the remodelling rate of bone, and the time

after peak bone mass has been achieved. The factors that modulate this bone loss with age are mechanical loading (as with exercise); nutritional status (particularly the intake of calcium); hormonal status (such as parathyroid hormone, somatotropin, calcitonin and oestrogen withdrawal at menopause); and, lastly, accumulated structural defects during remodelling.

The skeleton consists of about 80% cortical bone and 20% trabecular bone. From application of the different techniques to be discussed, the complex behaviour of bone mineral in the skeleton is gradually being understood. Not only cortical and trabecular bone respond differently to physical and abnormal stimuli; individual bones or parts of a bone may also vary in the degree of change. These differences explain why no single technique is applicable to all clinical questions regarding the mineral status of the skeleton and why the selection of the most appropriate site for a specific investigation is very important for obtaining meaningful results.

The morbidity and mortality associated with bone loss result from bone fractures. Measurements of bone mineral are ultimately used to assess the risk of fracture at specific sites. Although not identical, decreased strength of bone and increased susceptibility to fracture are related to the quantity of bone mineral in both the trabecular and the cortical bone. Geometrical changes in compact bone caused by ageing, predominant loss of either cortical or trabecular bone, the occurrence of microfractures in cortical bone, and bone size in relation to bone mass can all change the relationship between breaking strength and bone mineral. Muscle tone and skeletal instability leading to falls have additional influence on fracture occurrence. Despite these restrictions, measurements of bone mineral have been used successfully to predict the breaking strength of bone in the laboratory and to define the fracture risk in epidemiological studies.

Review of Different Techniques for Measuring Bone Mass

Several methods are available for the non-invasive measurement of bone mass. They all are based on the use of X-rays or gamma rays and range from the subjective interpretation of radiographs to sophisticated quantitative analysis such as neutron activation analysis (Table 17.1). The methods can be divided into those that measure the total skeletal mineral and those that sample the skeleton at a specific site. In the latter approach, conclusions about bone mineral in the entire skeleton or at other sites not measured are drawn from predictions based on documented experience. In the total skeleton approach, information is not obtained regarding specific sites. Both approaches have their indications and limitations (Wahner et al. 1984).

Some of these methods, such as neutron activation analysis, Compton scatter techniques, and radiographic photodensitometry, have been developed in research laboratories and may never become routine clinical tools. Other methods, such as photon absorptiometry, quantitative computed

Table 17.1. Summary of non-invasive methods used for estimations of bone mineral (adapted from Wahner et al. 1983)

1. *Estimation of total skeletal calcium:*
   Total body neutron activation analysis
   Total body bone mineral by dual photon absorptiometry
2. *Estimation of bone mineral at specific sites:*
   Radioscopy:
     biconcavity index
     Singh index
     Smith index
     fine-detailed radiographs
   Radiographic morphometry—cortical thickness
   Radiographic photodensitometry:
     visual interpretation
     reference wedge
   Absorptiometry:
     single photon
     dual photon
   Compton scattering
   Computed tomography:
     single energy
     dual energy

tomography, and perhaps radiographic morphometry, are more attractive as clinical tools for the routine management of patients with primary or secondary bone disease.

All methods are based on the assumption that qualitative changes in the composition of bone mineral are not associated with bone loss (with ageing or disease) and that the amount of bone mineral present represents the amount of bone. This assumption is not unchallenged. However, if qualitative changes in bone mineral composition caused by ageing and disease exist, they are very small and do not seem to influence the gamma-ray absorption characteristics of bone, as used in these techniques.

Requirements of a clinically useful method for longitudinal measurements include high precision or reproducibility; the coefficient of variation probably should not be more than 3%. This requirement allows the detection of bone loss of about 5%, with statistical significance. In comparison, standard radiographs of the spinal column show recognisable bone loss only when 30% or more is lost. There should be little chance for systematic error (such as with positioning), no contraindication for repeated measurements and good acceptability by the patient. For the detection of osteoporosis or bone loss, high accuracy is very important, and a statistically satisfactory normal population should be available for comparison. The method should also allow for the separate measurements of the cortical and the trabecular bone at sites of major fracture (hip, spine and radius). There are restrictions on the laboratory efforts and costs acceptable for a routine procedure. Because of their clinical relevancy, only photon absorptiometry and computed tomography will be reviewed. For a more detailed discussion of the different methods, the reader is referred to review articles on the subject (Dequeker and Johnston 1982; Mazess 1983; Wahner et al. 1984).

Single Photon Absorptiometry for the Evaluation of Cortical Bone in the Appendicular Skeleton

Single photon absorptiometry was first described by Cameron and Sorenson (1963), who were attempting to circumvent the problems inherent in methods based on film recording of density. The principle of using single photon absorptiometry is as follows: The thickness of bone mineral (T_b) in the path of

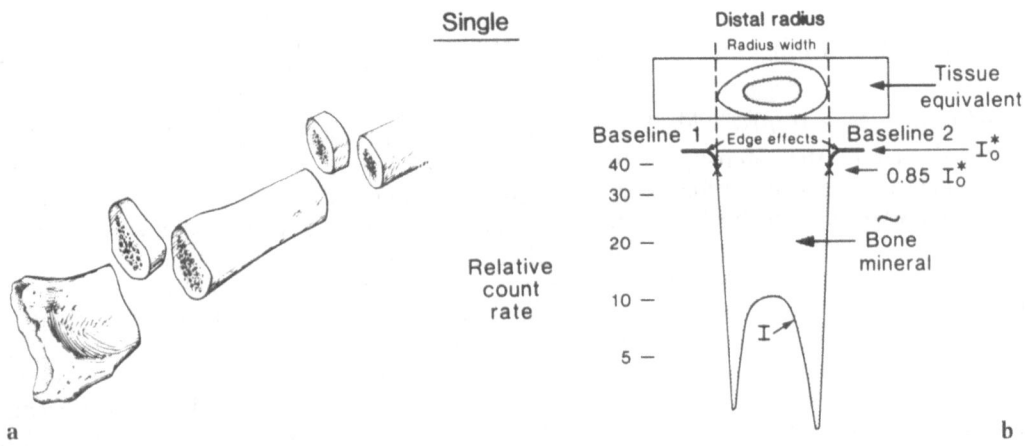

Fig. 17.1a,b. Single photon absorptiometry. **a** The units measured are grams of ashed bone in a cross-sectional piece of 1 cm of axial length. Commonly used measuring sites are the distal radius at 1/10 of forearm length and the mid-radius. **b** An absorption curve obtained from scanning across the distal radius. The area of the logarithmic plot is proportional to the bone mineral in the scanning path. Results are expressed in computer units and converted to bone mineral content (g/cm) using a standard curve obtained by scanning ashed bones or equivalent standards. (Wahner et al. 1984. By permission of the Society of Nuclear Medicine)

the photon beam is given by the following equation (Cameron and Sorenson 1963; Wahner et al. 1983):

$$T_b = [\ln(I_o^*/I)]/(\mu_b\,\rho_b - \mu_s\,\rho_s)$$

By convention, I_o is the beam intensity in air and I_o^* is the beam intensity after passage through tissue. I is the beam intensity after passage through bone and tissue. The mass absorption coefficients of bone mineral and tissue are μ_b and μ_s, and the density of bone mineral and tissue are ρ_b and ρ_s, respectively. These values are constants and are assumed not to change in bone disease and in different persons. Plotting I as a function of position across the bone gives a profile of the bone thickness of the radius (Fig. 17.1). The integration of this curve between the limits defined by I and corrected for edge effect, as shown in Fig. 17.1, yields a value proportional to the cross-sectional area of the radius and to the amount of bone mineral in the section of the radius scanned. The mineral content is determined from a calibration of the system with ashed human bones of different diameters and cortical thicknesses. Commercial instruments are available for single photon absorptiometry on the appendicular skeleton.

Dual Photon Absorptiometry for the Evaluation of Mineral in the Spinal Bone

Dual photon absorptiometry allows the evaluation of the axial skeleton, particularly the lumbar spine and hips. Because the axial skeleton is predominantly trabecular bone, this method allows a more specific evaluation of trabecular bone, in contrast to single photon absorptiometry, which evaluates cortical bone.

Dual photon absorptiometry was developed by Roos et al. (1970) and was adapted for the evaluation of whole-body calcium and the lumbar spine by Wilson and Madsen (1977) and Madsen and co-workers (1976) and for the evaluation of the hip by a group at the Mayo Clinic (Dunn et al. 1980; Riggs et al. 1982). The method is based on measurements of the radiation transmission of two separate photon energies through a medium consisting primarily of two different materials, bone and soft tissue. The gadolinium (^{153}Gd) energy spectrum has photoelectric peaks in NaI(T1) at approximately 44 and 100 keV (europium K X-rays at 42 and 48 keV; gamma rays at 97 and 103 keV).

Equations 1 and 2 describe the transmissions of each photon energy through a medium composed of bone and soft tissue.

$$I^{44}x,y =$$
$$I_0^{44}\exp[-(\mu/\rho)_{st}^{44} \cdot M_{st} - (\mu/\rho)_{bm}^{44} \cdot M_{bm}] \quad (1)$$

$$I^{100}x,y =$$
$$I_0^{100}\exp[-(\mu/\rho)_{st}^{100} \cdot M_{st} - (\mu/\rho)_{bm}^{100} \cdot M_{bm}] \quad (2)$$

$I^{44}x,y$ and $I^{100}x,y$ refer to the intensity of the transmitted radiation beam at a point x,y for 44-keV and 100-keV photon energies, respectively. I_0^{44} and I_0^{100} are the unattenuated photon intensities. The mass attenuation coefficients of soft tissue (st) and bone mineral (bm) at energy A are represented by $(\mu/\rho)_{st}$ and $(\mu/\rho)_{bm}$, respectively. The mass per unit area (g/cm²) of tissue and of bone mineral is indicated by M_{st} and M_{bm}. Solving these two equations simultaneously yields the following equation for bone mineral:

$$M_{bm} = \frac{RST(\ln I^{100}x,y/I_0^{100}) - (\ln I^{44}x,y/I_0^{44})}{(\mu/\rho)_{bm}^{44} - RST(\mu/\rho)_{bm}^{100}} \quad (3)$$

where $RST = (\mu/\rho)_{st}^{44}/(\mu/\rho)_{st}^{100}$.

In the measurement of bone mineral, the anatomical region of interest is scanned, and a point-by-point determination of bone mineral is made. The total bone mass is determined by summing the individual M_{bm} point values. The RST value (Wahner et al. 1983) is averaged over the extraosseous area scanned in some programmes or is determined on a line-by-line basis. The unit of measurement is either mass (g) for an exactly defined region such as L-2 to L-4, area density (g/cm²), or linear density, which is mass per axial length of spine scanned. Most frequently, area density is used (Fig. 17.2). Experiments with water, fat and ashed bone in phantoms have demonstrated that this procedure corrects for the presence of various amounts of fat and other changes in the tissue that surrounds the bone (Wahner et al. 1985). A commercial instrument and data output are illustrated in Fig. 17.3.

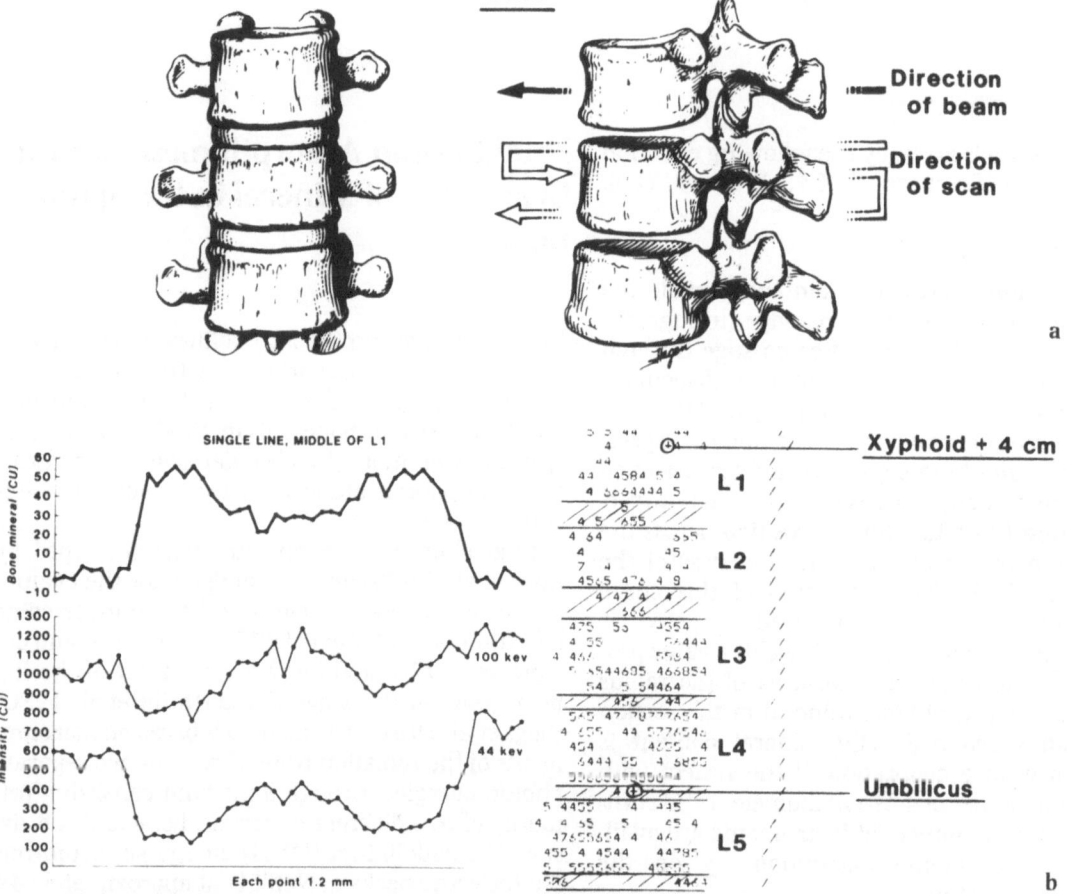

Fig. 17.2. Dual photon absorptiometry. a Measured units are grams of ashed bone in L-2 to L-4; intervertebral discs are included but transverse processes are omitted. The beam is passed in the anteroposterior direction. b Absorption curves for 44-keV and 100-keV gamma rays from ¹⁵³Gd and the calculated bone mineral, all for one pass across L-1. The character plot shows the final tracing of a scan from L-1 to L-5. A region of interest routine is used to select L-2 to L-4. (Wahner et al. 1984. By permission of the Society of Nuclear Medicine)

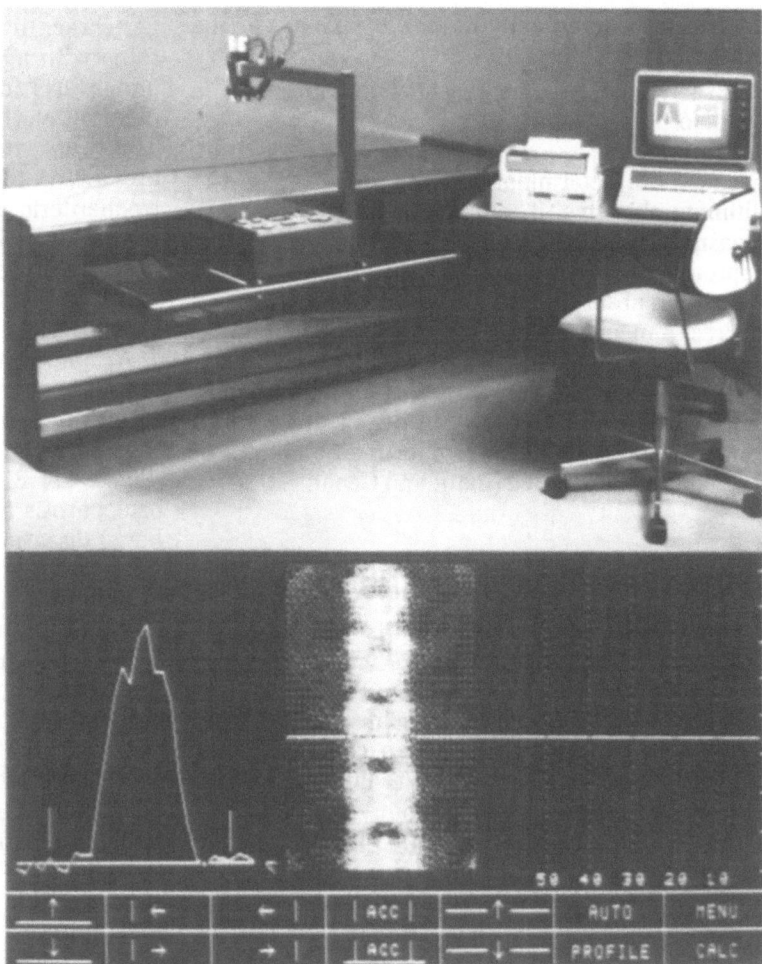

Fig. 17.3. *Top*: Illustration of the equipment and data output from a commercial bone mineral analyser. *Bottom*: Data analysis allows for display of bone mineral (in grams) in each scanning line (*left side*), a grey scale or colour scale of the bone mineral plot of the entire scan (*centre*) and a display of the baseline values outside the bone (*right side*).

Quantitative Computed Tomography

Computed tomography has been developed for the measurement of bone mineral along three different but closely related concepts. First, as a direct outgrowth of single photon absorptiometry, Rüegsegger et al. (1976) developed a forearm scanner that allows the separate measurement of cortical and trabecular bone mineral and displays the cross-sectional distribution of the bone mineral. Second, with the introduction of the commercial single-energy X-ray computed tomography (CT) scanners into radiological practice, Cann and Genant (1980) developed a technique to adapt these instruments, with minor modifications, for the measurements of bone mineral in the axial skeleton. Last, because of problems encountered with standard CT scanners,

dual-energy CT instruments are now being evaluated for bone mineral measurements (Genant and Boyd 1977). The clinical usefulness of such measurements with these rather expensive instruments awaits further evaluation.

These three techniques are based on a reconstruction of the cross-section of a bone slice a few millimeters thick and express the results in terms of the linear attenuation coefficient of the cortical and the trabecular bone. Source and detector assemblies are rotated around the bone to be scanned. The principle is the transmission of photons. The cost is in the image reconstruction, which requires extensive software and powerful computer support. However, there are three advantages:

1. A slice of the bone can be reconstructed and the bone mineral can be accurately determined per anatomical volume of bone, which is not possible with absorptiometry, in which approximations are made.

2. The trabecular and the cortical bone can be measured separately.

3. Exact relocation for repeated measurement is possible.

Because the determination of fracture risk is the ultimate objective, it remains to be seen whether measurement of trabecular bone alone is a superior approach over measurement of total bone mineral (as used in absorptiometry).

Precise measurements of vertebral bone mineral have been obtained by using conventional CT scanners with minor adaptations. A positioning capability within 1.5 mm has been demonstrated, and long-term precision in a human torso phantom of 2.8% has been reported (Cann and Genant 1980).

Clinical Applications of Photon Absorptiometry Methods

Bone loss in the axial skeleton (spine and hip) with age and in osteoporosis has been compared with bone loss in cortical bone of the radius (Riggs et al. 1981). In normal women, bone loss from the vertebrae begins at about age 30–35 years, and we have found the loss to be linear thereafter. In longitudinal studies, however, a slight increase in rate of loss, lasting from 5 to 8 years, was found at menopause. This loss has been obscured in our cross-sectional studies but has been documented by Krølner and Nielson (1982). Overall bone diminution throughout life is 47% for the lumbar

vertebrae. In normal men, bone diminution in the spine with ageing is less than in women, is linear and starts during the fourth decade. Similar observations have been made for the hip (Riggs et al. 1982). In women, the overall decreases during life are 58% in the femoral neck and 53% in the intertrochanteric region. For normal men, the age regression is linear but the decrease during life is only two-thirds that in women (Riggs et al. 1982). A summary of bone loss in normal women is given in Table 17.2.

A significantly better separation of patients with osteoporosis from normal subjects is achieved by using the bone mineral value of the lumbar spine than by using the bone mineral value of the radius (Fig. 17.4; Riggs et al. 1981). This suggests that osteoporosis is a predominantly spinal (trabecular bone) disease and it emphasises the importance of selecting the appropriate skeletal site.

Dual photon absorptiometry has been used successfully to study drug regimens for osteoporosis, bone loss after oophorectomy, metabolic bone disease (Seeman et al. 1982) and the effects of exercise (Krølner et al. 1983). The studies also allow definition of a fracture threshold for spinal compression fractures (Fig. 17.5). The 95th percentile for vertebral bone mineral of all patients studied who had non-traumatic compression fractures was 0.98 g/cm² (Riggs et al. 1981). More details are given in Table 17.2.

Used in the clinical environment, measurements of bone mineral give information on bone mineral mass at the time of the measurement, but these measurements give little information on the cause of bone loss and on when the loss has occurred. Low

Table 17.2. Bone data in normal women at different skeletal sites[a]

	Radius		Lumbar spine	Femur	
	Distal	Mid-shaft	(L-1 to L-4)	Neck	Intertrochanteric region
Trabecular bone content (%)	10–15	2–5	60–70	20–25	40–50
Bone loss at old age (% of maximal bone mass at age 30 years)	39	30	47	57	53
Average annual rate of bone loss (g/cm²)[b]	0.0067	0.0060	0.0082	0.0129	0.0018
Fracture threshold (g/cm²)	Not determined	Not determined	0.98	0.95	0.92
Fracture threshold compared with maximal bone mass[c]	Not determined	Not determined	2.3	2.4	2.2

[a] Data from Riggs et al. (1981).

[b] Bone loss calculated using cross-sectional data from age 20 to 90 years in a linear regression to the data. Actual bone loss is accelerated for 5–8 years at menopause.

[c] Standard deviations below mean bone mineral density at age 30 years; fracture threshold defined as 90th percentile of women with one or more non-traumatic compression fractures.

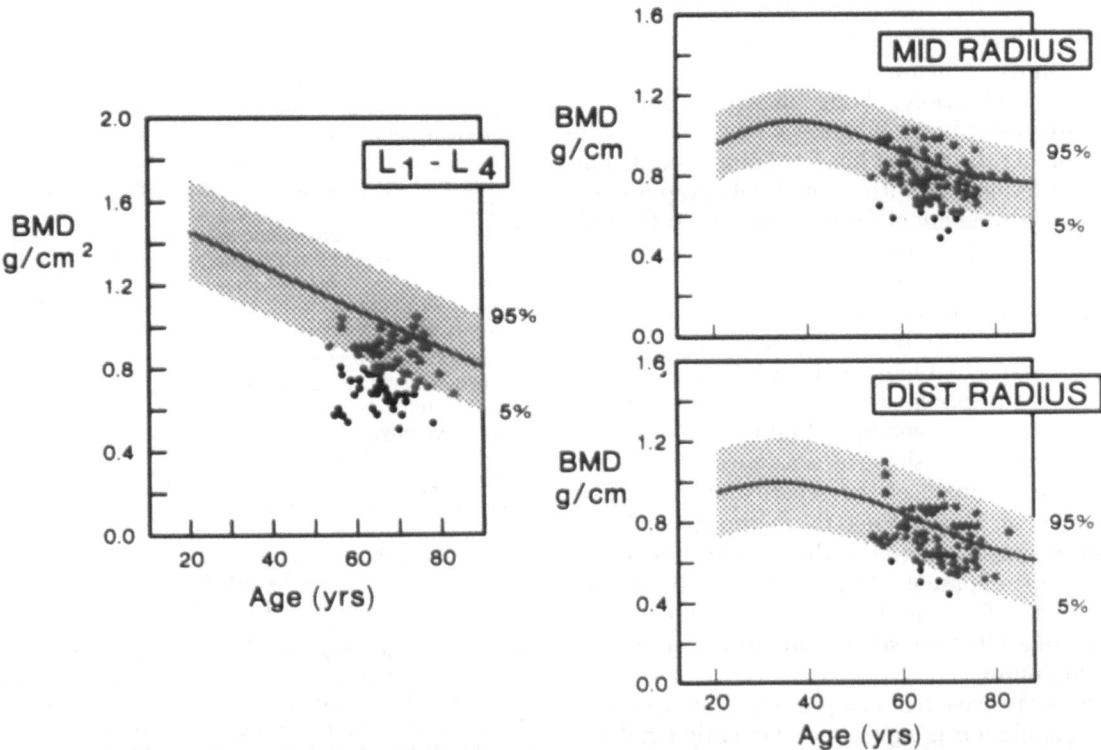

Fig. 17.4. Bone mineral in lumbar spine by dual photon absorptiometry and in radius by single photon absorptiometry in normal subjects (*shaded area*) and women with osteoporosis (*dots*). Note the better separation between the two populations with dual absorptiometry of the spine. *BDM,* bone mineral density. (Riggs et al. 1981. By permission of the American Society for Clinical Investigation)

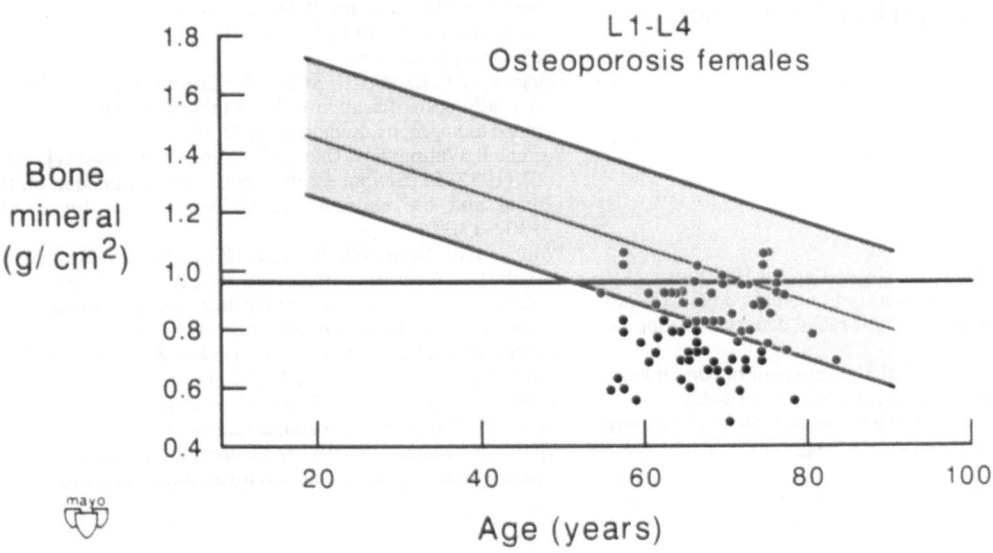

Fig. 17.5. Normal range (*shaded area*) with fracture threshold (*horizontal line*). The increasing number with age of normal subjects below the fracture threshold is illustrated. A young adult may be below the normal range but above or below the fracture threshold. The fracture threshold is 2.2 standard deviations below the mean maximal bone mass at young adult age. (Data from Riggs et al. 1981)

bone mineral does not distinguish between present ongoing abnormal bone loss and loss caused by a condition associated with a low peak bone mass in the past. Therefore, bone mineral should be measured early in the diagnostic work-up to establish whether the patient has low bone mineral. Particularly in patients with normal radiographs of the spine, measurement of the bone mineral is the only way to establish the presence of low bone mineral.

After low bone mineral has been confirmed, a specific history is taken and a clinical examination and relevant laboratory tests are performed. Occasionally, special radiographs and bone biopsy are needed for making a specific diagnosis or for defining the best therapeutic approach. Information on bone mineral can be translated into fracture risk, and this allows an estimate of the severity of the disease (Melton et al. 1985). When the method is used early in the diagnostic approach, the severity of bone loss is readily apparent. Diagnostic approach and therapeutic effort can then be selected and irreversible changes in bone such as fractures can be kept at a minimum.

An inexpensive and fast procedure for screening large population groups is not currently available. However, several studies (Awbrey et al. 1984) have suggested that measurements of bone mineral on the very distal radius by instruments that still have to be refined in order to give reproducible measurements may allow an estimation of spinal and hip-bone mineral from the distal radius with sufficient accuracy and sensitivity. Such methods should become available. Both computed tomography and absorptiometry are capable of these measurements.

References

Awbrey BJ, Jacobson PC, Grubb SA, McCartney WH, Vincent LM, Talmage RV (1984) Bone density in women: a modified procedure for measurement of distal radial density. J Orthop Res 2: 314–321

Cameron JR, Sorenson J (1963) Measurement of bone mineral in vivo: an improved method. Science 142: 230–232

Cann CE, Genant HK (1980) Precise measurement of vertebral mineral content using computed tomography. J Comput Assist Tomogr 4: 493–500

Dequeker J, Johnston CC Jr (eds) (1982) Non-invasive bone measurements: methodological problems. IRL Press, Oxford, p 250

Dunn WL, Wahner HW, Riggs BL (1980) Measurement of bone mineral content in human vertebrae and hip by dual photon absorptiometry. Radiology 136: 485–487

Genant HK, Boyd D (1977) Quantitative bone mineral analysis using dual energy computed tomography. Invest Radiol 12: 545–551

Heaney RP (1983) Prevention of age-related osteoporosis in women. In: Avioli LV (ed) The osteoporotic syndrome, detection, prevention, and treatment. Grune and Stratton, New York, pp 123–144

Krølner B, Nielsen SP (1982) Bone mineral content of the lumbar spine in normal and osteoporotic women: cross-sectional and longitudinal studies. Clin Sci 62: 329–336

Krølner B, Toft B, Nielson SP, Tondevold E (1983) Physical exercise as prophylaxis against involutional vertebral bone loss: a controlled trial. Clin Sci 64: 541–546

Madsen M, Peppler W, Mazess RB (1976) Vertebral and total body bone mineral content by dual photon absorptiometry. Calcif Tissue Res 21: 361–364

Mazess RB (1983) Noninvasive methods for quantitating trabecular bone. In: Avioli LV (ed) The osteoporotic syndrome, detection, prevention, and treatment. Grune and Stratton, New York, pp 85–114

Melton LJ, Wahner HW, Richelson LS, O'Fallon WM, Dunn WL, Riggs BL (1985) Bone density specific fracture risk: a population based study of the relationship between osteoporosis and vertebrae fractures. J Nucl Med 26: 24 (abstract)

Riggs BL, Wahner HW, Dunn WL, Mazess RB, Offord KP, Milton LJ III (1981) Differential changes in bone mineral density of the appendicular and axial skeleton with ageing. J Clin Invest 67: 328–335

Riggs BL, Wahner HW, Seeman E et al. (1982) Changes in bone mineral density of the proximal femur and spine with aging: differences between the postmenopausal and senile osteoporosis syndromes. J Clin Invest 70: 716–723

Roos B, Rosengren B, Sköldborn H (1970) Determination of bone mineral content in lumbar vertebrae by a double gamma-ray technique. In: Cameron JR (ed) Proceedings of bone measurement conference. United States Atomic Energy Commission, Chicago, pp 243–253

Rüegsegger P, Elsasser U, Anliker M, Gnehm H, Kind H, Prader A (1976) Quantification of bone mineralization using computed tomography. Radiology 121: 93–97

Seeman E, Wahner HW, Offord KP, Kumar R, Johnson WJ, Riggs BL (1982) Differential effects of endocrine dysfunction on the axial and the appendicular skeleton. J Clin Invest 69: 1302–1309

Wahner HW, Dunn WL, Thorsen HC, Griffin PA, Hockert NL (1983) Bone mineral measurements: review of various techniques. In: Wahner HW (ed) Nuclear medicine: quantitative procedures. Little, Brown, Boston, pp 107–132

Wahner HW, Dunn WL, Riggs BL (1984) Assessment of bone mineral: Part 2. J Nucl Med 25: 1241–1253

Wahner HW, Dunn WL, Mazess RB et al. (1985) Dual-photon Gd-153 absorptiometry of bone. Radiology 156: 203–206

Wilson CR, Madsen M (1977) Dichromatic absorptiometry of vertebral bone mineral content. Invest Radiol 12: 180–184

Subject Index